More information about this series at http://www.springer.com/series/13361

J. Michael Millis • Jeffrey B. Matthews
Editors

Difficult Decisions in Hepatobiliary and Pancreatic Surgery

An Evidence-Based Approach

Springer

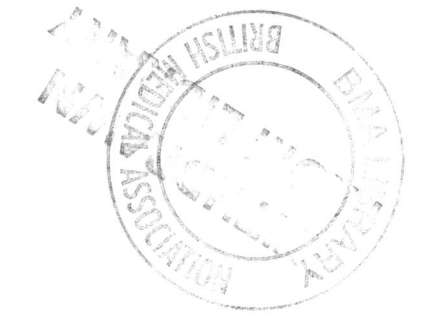

Editors
J. Michael Millis
The University of Chicago
Chicago, Illinois, USA

Jeffrey B. Matthews
The University of Chicago
Chicago, Illinois, USA

ISSN 2198-7750 ISSN 2198-7769 (electronic)
Difficult Decisions in Surgery: An Evidence-Based Approach
ISBN 978-3-319-27363-1 ISBN 978-3-319-27365-5 (eBook)
DOI 10.1007/978-3-319-27365-5

Library of Congress Control Number: 2016938792

Printed on acid-free paper

This Springer imprint is published by Springer Nature
The registered company is Springer International Publishing AG Switzerland

Preface

We are excited to present to the hepatobiliary and pancreatic multidisciplinary community a new format in assessing and making decisions for our patients. This volume expands on the successful editions of *Difficult Decisions in Thoracic Surgery*. The success of those editions has stimulated the University of Chicago surgical faculty to develop a series of *Difficult Decisions in XXX Surgery*. The *Difficult Decisions in Hepatobiliary and Pancreatic Surgery* volume is the first of several to be published over the next several years. Given that many difficult decisions in this field required multidisciplinary input, we have asked a number of leaders from interventional radiology, intervention endoscopy, gastroenterology/hepatology, and diagnostic radiology to provide and analyze the strength of the data regarding the underlying diseases, diagnostics, and the nonoperative therapy.

The format of this book follows its predecessor. The table of contents was developed that reflects the difficult decisions faced by busy, thoughtful surgeons specializing in the field of hepatobiliary and pancreatic surgery on controversial issues. We invited authors with national and international reputations on the specific topics to examine the evidence that hope to inform us on the correct path. When possible, we asked the authors to suggested best practice approaches to these challenging topics. We asked the authors to develop a PICO table (patient population, intervention, comparator group, and outcomes measured) to crystallize the question and data relevant to the decision.

As this concept is new to hepatobiliary and pancreatic surgery, all of the chapters presented are new and up to date with recent literature searches. The literature search terms are provided so that new information relevant to the topic can be easily identified as time progresses.

We are grateful to our busy colleagues who agreed to contribute to this volume and the publisher for supporting this volume as well as the entire planned series. As we know many of these difficult questions are initially asked by our trainees and students who stimulate us to think of different approaches and evaluate the evidence of our current decisions. Each of the authors in this volume epitomize the constant effort to evaluate all the current evidence to make the correct decisions and provide the best clinical care for our patients.

Chicago, IL, USA

J. Michael Millis
Jeffrey B. Matthews

Contents

Contributors

David B. Adams Department of Surgery, Medical University of South Carolina, Charleston, SC, USA

Syed A. Ahmad Pancreas Disease Center, University Cincinnati Cancer Institute, Cincinnati, OH, USA

Nobuhisa Akamatsu Hepato-Biliary-Pancreatic Surgery, and Artificial Organ and Transplantation Division, Department of Surgery, Graduate School of Medicine, University of Tokyo, Hongo, Bunkyo-ku, Tokyo, Japan

John Alverdy Department of Surgery, Pritzker School of Medicine, University of Chicago, Chicago, IL, USA

Andrew Aronsohn Center for Liver Diseases, University of Chicago Medical Center, Chicago, IL, USA

Marshall S. Baker Department of Surgery, Division of Surgical Oncology, University of Chicago, Pritzker School of Medicine, Chicago, IL, USA

NorthShore University Health System, Evanston, IL, USA

J. Camilo Barreto Section of General Surgery, University of Chicago Medicine, Chicago, IL, USA

Brian Bello Department of Surgery, Sinai Hospital of Baltimore, Baltimore, MD, USA

David J. Bentrem Department of Surgery, Northwestern University Feinberg School of Medicine, Chicago, IL, USA

Humberto Bohorquez Multi-Organ Transplant Institute, Department of Surgery, Ochsner Medical Center, New Orleans, LA, USA

Kimberly M. Brown Department of Surgery, University of Texas Medical Branch, Galveston, TX, USA

Darren S. Bryan Department of Surgery, Biological Sciences Division, The University of Chicago, Chicago, IL, USA

James R. Butler Department of Surgery, Indiana University School of Medicine, Indianapolis, IN, USA

Eugene A. Choi Department of Surgery, Baylor College of Medicine, Houston, TX, USA

Waldo Concepcion Department of Surgery, Stanford University, Stanford, CA, USA

Stanford University Medical Center, Palo Alto, CA, USA

Gregory A. Cote Division of Gastroenterology and Hepatology, Medical University of South Carolina, Charleston, SC, USA

Martin A. Croce Department of Surgery, University of Tennessee Health Science Center, Memphis, TN, USA

E. Patchen Dellinger Department of General Surgery, University of Washington, Seattle, WA, USA

Archita P. Desai University of Arizona, Tucson, AZ, USA

Daniel J. Deziel Department General Surgery, Rush University Medical Center, Chicago, IL, USA

Francesca M. Dimou Department of Surgery, University of Texas Medical Branch, Galveston, TX, USA

Department of Surgery, University of South Florida, Tampa, FL, USA

Shunda Du Department of Liver Surgery, Peking Union Medical College (PUMC) Hospital, Beijing, China

Cory Evans Department of Surgery, University of Tennessee Health Science Center, Memphis, TN, USA

Benjamin D. Ferguson Department of Surgery, University of Chicago Medical Center, Chicago, IL, USA

Zhi Ven Fong Department of Surgery, Massachusetts General Hospital, Harvard Medical School, Boston, MA, USA

Brian Funaki Department of Radiology, Section of Vascular and Interventional Radiology, University of Chicago Medical Center, Chicago, IL, USA

Shady F. Gad Division of Surgical Oncology and Department of Surgery, Moores Cancer Center, University of California San Diego, UC San Diego Health System, San Diego, CA, USA

John N. Gaetano Department of Gastroenterology, Section of Gastroenterology, Hepatology and Nutrition, The University of Chicago Medicine and Biological Sciences, Chicago, IL, USA

David A. Geller Department of Surgery, University of Pittsburgh, Pittsburgh, PA, USA

Andres Gelrud Center for Endoscopic Research and Therapeutics, Department of Medicine, University of Chicago, Chicago, IL, USA

Robert Gish Department of Medicine, Stanford University, Stanford, CA, USA

Ana Gleisner Department of Surgery, University of Pittsburgh, Pittsburgh, PA, USA

Mariano Gonzalez-Haba Center for Endoscopic Research and Therapeutics (CERT), Center for Care and Discovery, The University of Chicago Medicine and Biological Sciences, Chicago, IL, USA

Gabriella Grisotti Department of Surgery, Yale University School of Medicine, New Haven, CT, USA

Ashley N. Hardy Department of Surgical Oncology, Fox Chase Cancer Center, Philadelphia, PA, USA

Eric S. Hungness Northwestern University, Chicago, IL, USA

Mustafa Hussain Department of Surgery, Biological Sciences Division, The University of Chicago, Chicago, IL, USA

Alexander Itskovich Department of Surgery, The Brooklyn Hospital Center, Brooklyn, NY, USA

Sajid A. Khan Department of Surgery, Section of Surgical Oncology, Yale University School of Medicine, New Haven, CT, USA

Norihiro Kokudo Hepato-Biliary-Pancreatic Surgery, and Artificial Organ and Transplantation Division, Department of Surgery, Graduate School of Medicine, University of Tokyo, Hongo, Bunkyo-ku, Tokyo, Japan

Heather L. Lewis Department of Surgery, The University of Cincinnati Medical Center, Cincinnati, OH, USA

Keith D. Lillemoe Department of Surgery, Massachusetts General Hospital, Harvard Medical School, Boston, MA, USA

Jason B. Liu Department of Surgery, University of Chicago, Pritzker School of Medicine, Chicago, IL, USA

Jonathan M. Lorenz Department of Radiology, University of Chicago Medical Center, Chicago, IL, USA

Bill Ran Luo Department of Surgery, Northwestern Medicine, Chicago, IL, USA

Minh B. Luu Department General Surgery, Rush University Medical Center, Chicago, IL, USA

Deepa Magge Division of Surgical Oncology, University of Pittsburgh Medical Center, Pittsburgh, PA, USA

David M. Mahvi Department of Surgery, Northwestern University, Chicago, IL, USA

Grace Z. Mak Department of Surgery and Pediatrics, Pediatric Surgery Fellowship, The University of Chicago Pritzker School of Medicine, Chicago, IL, USA

Ajay V. Maker Department of Surgery, Division of Surgical Oncology, Department of Microbiology and Immunology, University of Illinois at Chicago, Chicago, IL, USA

Creticos Cancer Center, Advocate Illinois Masonic Medical Center, Chicago, IL, USA

Yilei Mao Department of Liver Surgery, Peking Union Medical College Hospital, Peking Union Medical College & Chinese Academy of Medical Sciences, Beijing, China

Jeffrey B. Matthews Department of Surgery, University of Chicago Medical Center, Chicago, IL, USA

Matthew T. McMillan Department of Surgery, University of Pennsylvania Perelman School of Medicine, Philadelphia, PA, USA

J. Michael Millis Department of Surgery, University of Chicago Hospitals, Chicago, IL, USA

David Caba Molina Department of Surgery, University of Chicago Hospitals, Chicago, IL, USA

Katherine A. Morgan Division of Gastrointestinal and Laparoscopic Surgery, Medical University of South Carolina, Charleston, SC, USA

Gareth Morris-Stiff Department of General Surgery, Division of Hepato-Pancreato-Biliary Surgery, Digestive Disease Institute, A100 Cleveland Clinic Foundation, Cleveland, OH, USA

Andreas Mykoniatis Department of Medicine, The University of Chicago Medicine, Chicago, IL, USA

Ankesh Nigam Department of Surgery, Albany Medical College, Albany, NY, USA

Aytekin Oto Department of Radiology, The University of Chicago Medicine, Chicago, IL, USA

Brodie Parent Department of General Surgery, University of Washington, Seattle, WA, USA

Mikin V. Patel Department of Radiology, University of Chicago Medical Center, Chicago, IL, USA

Thomas Pham Department of Surgery, Stanford University, Stanford, CA, USA

Mitchell C. Posner Section of General Surgery and Surgical Oncology, University of Chicago Medicine, Chicago, IL, USA

Vivek N. Prachand Department of Surgery, University of Chicago Medical Center, Chicago, IL, USA

Yudong Qiu Department of Hepatobiliary and Pancreas Surgery, Drum Tower Hospital, Medical School of Nanjing University, Nanjing, China

K. Gautham Reddy Department of Gastroenterology, Section of Gastroenterology, Hepatology and Nutrition, The University of Chicago Medicine and Biological Sciences, Chicago, IL, USA

Trevor W. Reichman Multi-Organ Transplant Institute, Department of Surgery, Ochsner Medical Center, New Orleans, LA, USA

KMarie Reid-Lombardo Division of Subspecialty General Surgery, Department of Surgery, Mayo Clinic, Rochester, MN, USA

John F. Renz University of Chicago Medicine, Chicago, IL, USA

Taylor S. Riall Department of Surgery, University of Arizona, Tucson, AZ, USA

Pierre F. Saldinger Department of Surgery, New York Presbyterian Queens, Weill Cornell Medical College, Flushing, NY, USA

B. Fernando Santos Geisel School of Medicine at Dartmouth, White River Junction Veterans Affairs Medical Center, Hartford, VT, USA

John Seal Multi-Organ Transplant Institute, Ochsner Medical Center, New Orleans, LA, USA

Baddr Shakhsheer Department of Surgery, Pritzker School of Medicine, University of Chicago, Chicago, IL, USA

Susan M. Sharpe Division of Surgical Oncology, Department of Surgery, University of Chicago Pritzker School of Medicine, Chicago, IL, USA

Jason K. Sicklick Division of Surgical Oncology and Department of Surgery, Moores Cancer Center, University of California San Diego, UC San Diego Health System, San Diego, CA, USA

Ajaypal Singh Center for Endoscopic Research and Therapeutics, Department of Medicine, University of Chicago, Chicago, IL, USA

Nathaniel J. Soper Department of Surgery, Northwestern Medicine, Chicago, IL, USA

Sadeesh K Srinathan Department of Surgery, University of Manitoba, Winnipeg, Manitoba, Canada

Steven C. Stain Department of Surgery, Albany Medical College, Albany, NY, USA

Yasuhiko Sugawara Hepato-Biliary-Pancreatic Surgery, and Artificial Organ and Transplantation Division, Department of Surgery, Graduate School of Medicine, University of Tokyo, Hongo, Bunkyo-ku, Tokyo, Japan

Malini D. Sur Department of Surgery, University of Chicago Medicine, Chicago, IL, USA

Shane Svoboda Department of Surgery, Sinai Hospital of Baltimore, Baltimore, MD, USA

Mark S. Talamonti Department of Surgery, North Shore University Health System, Evanston, IL, USA

Helen S. Te University of Chicago Medical Center, Chicago, IL, USA

May Chen Tee Department of Surgery, Mayo Clinic, Rochester, MN, USA

Ezra N. Teitelbaum Department of Surgery, Northwestern University, Chicago, IL, USA

Anouar Teriaky Center for Liver Diseases, University of Chicago Medical Center, Chicago, IL, USA

W. Grayson Terral Multi-Organ Transplant Institute, Department of Surgery, Ochsner Medical Center, New Orleans, LA, USA

Stephen Thomas Department of Radiology, The University of Chicago Medicine, Chicago, IL, USA

Tsuyoshi Todo Department of Medicine, Stanford University, Stanford, CA, USA

Darren van Beek Department of Radiology, Section of Vascular and Interventional Radiology, University of Chicago Medical Center, Chicago, IL, USA

Thuong G. Van Ha Section of Cardiovascular Interventional Radiology, Department of Radiology, University of Chicago, Chicago, IL, USA

Charles M. Vollmer Jr. Department of Surgery, University of Pennsylvania Perelman School of Medicine, Philadelphia, PA, USA

R. Mathew Walsh Department of General Surgery, Division of Hepato-Pancreato-Biliary Surgery, A100 Cleveland Clinic Foundation, Cleveland, OH, USA

Irving Waxman Center for Endoscopic Research and Therapeutics (CERT), Center for Care and Discovery, The University of Chicago Medicine and Biological Sciences, Chicago, IL, USA

Jeffrey D. Wayne Department of Surgery, Northwestern University Feinberg School of Medicine, Chicago, IL, USA

Stephan G. Wyers Section of General Surgery, University of Chicago Medicine, Chicago, IL, USA

Anthony D. Yang Department of Surgery, Northwestern University, Chicago, IL, USA

Amer H. Zureikat Division of Surgical Oncology, University of Pittsburgh Medical Center, Pittsburgh, PA, USA

Nicholas J. Zyromski Department of Surgery, Indiana University School of Medicine, Indianapolis, IN, USA

Chapter 1
Finding and Appraising the Evidence: EBM and GRADE

Sadeesh K. Srinathan

Abstract This chapter provides an overview of the principles of evidence based medicine (EBM) which will assist in making difficult decisions in the face of incomplete and inadequate evidence. The steps of searching for the evidence using the PICO format and an overview of the study design types which make up the body evidence will be discussed. A more detailed treatment of the GRADE system to make explicit the decisions on the quality of evidence and the nature of recommendations for interventions will be provided.

Keywords Evidence based medicine • EBM • GRADE • PICO

Introduction

Surgeons routinely make difficult decisions. In many cases, the difficulty lies in the need to make these decisions in the face of incomplete or unreliable information. An example of this in an individual patient is deciding to perform an exploratory laparotomy for an acute abdomen where the evidence from diagnostic studies may be incomplete or contradictory. Another example, in terms of policy, would be to decide on the appropriateness of screening for occult malignancies where the evidence for early detection may be closely matched by evidence for undesirable events such as overtreatment.

In this book, difficult scenarios commonly encountered by the hepatobiliary surgeon are presented. The authors lay out the available evidence and make a recommendation as to the appropriate responses in these scenarios. They have followed the principles of evidence based medicine in order to come to their recommendations

S.K. Srinathan (✉)
Department of Surgery, University of Manitoba,
GE 604 – 820 Sherbrook Street, Health Sciences Centre,
Winnipeg, Manitoba R3A 1R9, Canada
e-mail: ssrinathan@ex63change.hsc.mb.ca

J.M. Millis, J.B. Matthews (eds.), *Difficult Decisions in Hepatobiliary and Pancreatic Surgery*, Difficult Decisions in Surgery: An Evidence-Based Approach, DOI 10.1007/978-3-319-27365-5_1

and the purpose of this introductory chapter is to present an overview of the process which led their recommendations.

The phrase Evidence Based Medicine (EBM) came into widespread use after 1992 following a publication by Guyatt et al. [5], and is now commonly agreed to mean: '…the conscientious, explicit, and judicious use of current best evidence in making decisions about the care of individual patients. The practice of evidence based medicine means integrating individual clinical expertise with the best available external clinical evidence from systematic research" it also means that "… thoughtful identification and compassionate use of individual patients' predicaments, rights, and preferences in making clinical decision…" [13].

The practice of EBM can be carried out by using the following principles: (1) ask a clinical question, (2) locate the evidence, (3) appraise and synthesize the evidence, and (4) apply the evidence [12].

Ask the Clinical Question

On the face of it, asking the clinical question is straightforward. A patient problem is presented and a question arises. For example, Mrs. Smith is presenting with painless jaundice and a diagnosis of periampullary carcinoma. In considering the surgical options, you consider whether a pylorus preserving pancreaticoduodenectomy rather than a standard Whipple procedure should be performed.

Going directly to Google with the key words "pylorus preserving pancreaticoduodenectomy", we obtain 47,900 hits, while Wikipedia results in 2 hits. Clearly, neither of these extremes is satisfactory in determining a surgical approach. A useful step is to convert this specific clinical question about Mrs. Smith to a form that will allow us to search for the relevant evidence. The ***PICO*** format, which is used throughout this book, is a useful tool for this purpose.

The ***P*** stands for Patient or Population and specifies the patient group to which the question refers, in this case it may be: (a) all patients undergoing a pancreaticoduodenectomy, (b) women over the age of 50, (c) Caucasian women over 50, or (d) Caucasian women over 50 who have previously undergone a cholecystectomy. It is apparent that each iteration of the definition of the population is more and more specific. These details are important, but we may limit the information available to us if we define our population of interest too narrowly.

The ***I*** is for the Intervention or exposure of interest, and specifies what has happened to a group of patients such as an operation, or a diagnostic test. In our example the intervention we are considering is a pylorus preserving pancreaticoduodenectomy. However, there could also be specific issues that are considered important such as the specific method of reconstruction used or the use of drains.

The ***C*** refers to the comparator that we are interested in. In this case it is a standard Whipple procedure, but again we should be mindful of specific details of the standard procedure that may be important for our specific question.

O stands for the Outcome of interest. It is very important to be specific about the outcome of interest as it is likely that various studies may have used different outcomes in the study design than the one you are interested in. One study may have been focused on gastric emptying, whereas another may have been focused on blood loss during the procedure. It is worthwhile to identify each outcome of interest in the specific clinical scenario and to order them in order of importance to the patient and surgeon so that an overall assessment of the utility of an intervention can be made.

Taking these features of the clinical question into account, we can frame the scenario for Mrs. Smith in the following PICO question:

> In patients with periampullary carcinoma or carcinoma of the pancreatic head, does a pylorus preserving pancreaticoduodenectomy result in 1) less blood loss 2) lower incidence of delayed gastric emptying 3) lower operative mortality than a standard Whipple procedure?

P: Patients with a periampullary carcinoma or carcinoma of the pancreatic head
I: pylorus preserving pancreaticoduodenectomy with the use of drains
C: standard Whipple operation with the use of drains
O: (1) operative mortality, (2) delayed emptying, (3) blood loss

It is worth considering when reviewing the chapters in this book, whether the PICO questions chosen by the authors are sufficiently similar to your own formulation of the question for their findings and recommendations to apply to your specific case.

Find the Evidence

Often the first step in a literature search is to go to PubMed, the interface to access the Medline database of citations in the National Library of Medicine in the United States. However, a search of "pylorus preserving pancreaticoduodenectomy" produces 781 citations. This is more than we can reasonably go through for the purposes of answering a specific question for a patient. But, if we use the Clinical Queries page in PubMed which uses an algorithm to deliver focused studies relevant to clinical practice, [10] we obtain citations for 35 systematic reviews and 45 clinical studies, much better. Alternative search engines include TRIPdatabase (http://www.tripdatabase.com/) and SUMsearch (http://sumsearch.org/), which use multiple databases including Medline, EMBASE, and databases of guidelines and technology may also be used. Last, but certainly not least is the expertise available through your local medical librarian who will be well versed in the methods of constructing a PICO question and finding the relevant information from the medical literature.

Appraise the Studies

Once we have found the studies of interest, the next step is to identify the "best evidence". The concept of "best evidence" assumes a hierarchy of evidence. But in order to apply a hierarchy, it is important to understand the types of study designs and their use in answering specific types of clinical questions. Grimes et al. [7] provide a useful taxonomy of study designs (Fig. 1.1). In general, questions related to the superiority of one intervention over another (or no intervention) are best answered by experimental studies where one group of patients are assigned to the intervention by a bias free method, while another receive a comparison intervention. The gold standard for the experimental study is a well-designed randomized trial. Other types of clinical questions such as that of prognosis are appropriately answered using cohort studies, while questions of diagnosis rely on comparing the performance of a diagnostic test to a gold standard.

All study types have the potential for any number of biases which may lead to a finding which deviates from the "truth" [8]. The tools of critical appraisal are used

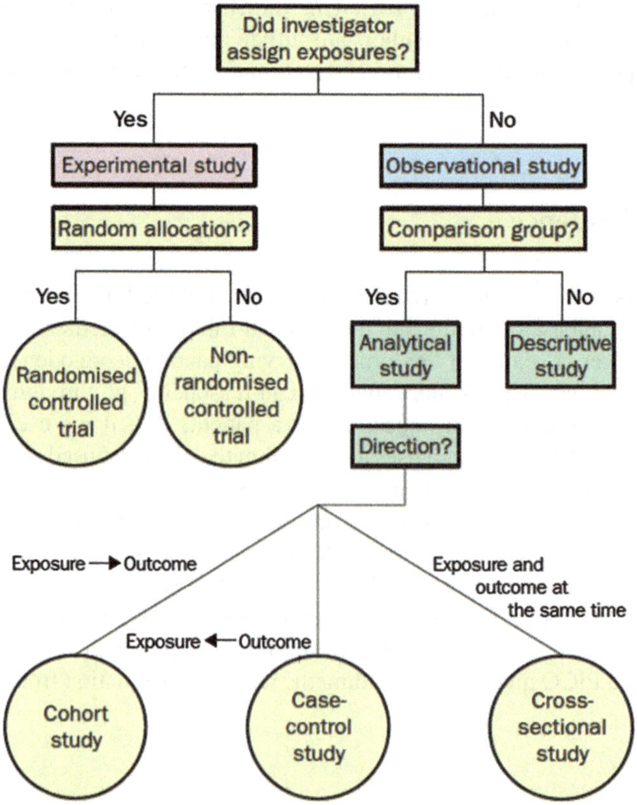

Fig. 1.1 Algorithm for classification of types of clinical research (Grimes and Schulz [7], Reprinted with permission from Elsevier)

determine the type and extent of these biases in the design and conduct of the study, and make a judgment of how it may have affected the findings of the study and the extent to which it undermines our confidence in the validity of the findings.

There are many excellent resources and tools to guide us in the specifics of appraising the medical literature and practicing EBM and these are listed in the recommended readings.

What happens when despite the best formulation of a question and literature search we are unable to find the high quality systematic review or randomized trial to guide us? Do we abandon the principles of EBM? Again from Sackett: "Evidence based medicine is not restricted to randomized trials and meta-analyses. It involves tracking down the best external evidence with which to answer our clinical questions.... However, some questions about therapy do not require randomized trials (successful interventions for otherwise fatal conditions) or cannot wait for the trials to be conducted. And if no randomized trial has been carried out for our patient's predicament, we must follow the trail to the next best external evidence and work from there" [13].

Although we can approach each problem we face by formulating a question and finding the best available evidence, individual clinicians are unlikely to have the time or resources to do this for all possible scenarios. To illustrate: our example PICO question generated 171 results using PubMed. There were 50 reviews, 74 relevant trials or studies, 3 guidelines and 44 other possibly relevant titles. This took an experienced medical librarian about 2.5 h to identify these studies, and does not include the time necessary to actually read these documents and appraise them.

The alternative to searching for each question has been standard textbooks, which seek to distill the evidence and guide clinical practice. The authors of these textbooks have always made decisions about which studies to consider and judgments about their confidence in making recommendation based on this evidence. However, these judgments and decisions have not been transparent. And although there are many schemes in use which grade the level of evidence and have been increasingly used in textbooks, it is not clear on what basis these decisions of grade were specifically arrived at [2]. A good systematic review makes transparent the question, the search strategy, and the rules for inclusion of studies and on what basis the quality of the study is determined. However, the final assessment of the overall quality of evidence and the subsequent recommendation arising from this evidence is often obscure.

In order to address this deficiency this book has adopted the GRADE system to make transparent the decision-making about the quality of evidence and the factors considered in making a recommendation and a statement about the strength of this recommendation. The reader may disagree with certain judgments made by the authors, but the reason for disagreement will hopefully be clear with the GRADE system and the reader can make up their own minds whether the conclusions drawn by the authors are on the whole reasonable or valid. The key component of GRADE is that it explicitly separates the process of evaluating the quality of the evidence for an intervention from the process of making a recommendation for its adoption (or not).

The GRADE System

The GRADE system defines quality in the following way: "In the context of a systematic review, the ratings of the quality of evidence reflect the extent of our confidence that the estimates of the effect are correct. In the context of making recommendations, the quality ratings reflect the extent of our confidence that the estimates of an effect are adequate to support a particular decision or recommendation" [3]. It is the latter definition that applies in this book, and the authors have included a discussion of their clinical experience that brings into play the necessity of balancing conflicting factors in making a recommendation. A more thorough discussion is provided by Andrews et al. and Brozek et al. [1, 4].

The GRADE table used in this book lays out the justification of why these decisions are made and it is instructive to describe in detail the components of the table. This example of a GRADE table is from Karanicalos et al.: (Tables 1.1 and 1.2) [9, 11]

Table 1.1 The GRADE system

Study design	Initial quality of the body of evidence		Lower if	Higher if	Quality of a body of evidence	
Randomized trials	High	→	Risk of bias	Large effect	High	⊕⊕⊕⊕
			−1 Serious	+1 Large		
			−2 Very serious	+2 Very large		
			Inconsistency	Dose response	Moderate	⊕⊕⊕
			−1 Serious	+1 Evidence of a gradient		
Observational studies	Low	→	−2 Very serious			
			Indirectness	All plausible residual confounding	Low	⊕⊕
			−1 Serious	+1 Would reduce a demonstrated effect		
			−2 Very serious	+2 Would suggest a spurious effect if no effect was observed		
			Imprecision		Very low	⊕
			−1 Serious			
			−2 Very serious			
			Publication bias			
			−1 Likely			
			−2 Very likely			

Derived from: Balshem et al. [3]

Table 1.2 GRADE profile for systematic review comparing pylorus preserving to standard Whipple procedure by Karanicolas et al.

	Quality assessment					Summary of findings			
# of studies (#of participants)	Study limitations[a]	Consistency	Directness	Precision	Publication bias	Relative effect (95 % CI)[d]	Best estimate of Whipple group risk	Absolute effect (95 %CI)	Quality
Five year mortality:									
3(229)	Serious limitations (−1)	No important inconsistency	Direct	No important imprecision	Unlikely	0.98 (0.87–1.11)	82.50 %	20 less/1,000;120 less to 80 more	+++, moderate
In-hospital mortality:									
6(490)	Serious limitations (−1)	No important inconsistency	Direct	Imprecision (−1)[c]	Unlikely	0.40 (0.14–1.13)	4.90 %	20 less/1,000; 50 less to 10 more	++, low
Blood transfusions (units):									
5(320)	Serious limitations (−1)	No important inconsistency	Direct	No important imprecision	Unlikely	–	2.45 units	−0.66 (−1.06 to −0.25); favours pylorus preservation)	+++, moderate
Biliary leaks:									
3(268)	Serious limitations (−1)	No important inconsistency	Direct	Imprecision (−1)[c]	Unlikely	4.77 (0.23–97.96)	0	20 more/1,000; 20 less to 50 more	++, low
Hospital stay (days):									
5(446)	Serious limitations (−1)	No important inconsistency	Direct	Imprecision (−1)[c]	Unlikely	–	19.17 days	−1.45 (−3.28 to 0.38); favours pylorus preservation	++, low

(continued)

Table 1.2 (continued)

	Quality assessment					Summary of findings			
# of studies (#of participants)	Study limitations[a]	Consistency	Directness	Precision	Publication bias	Relative effect (95 % CI)[d]	Best estimate of Whipple group risk	Absolute effect (95 %CI)	Quality
Delayed gastric emptying:									
5(442)	Serious limitations (−1)	Unexplained heterogeneity (−1)[b]	Direct	Imprecision (−1)[c]	Unlikely	1.52 (0.74–3.14)	25.50 %	110 more/1,000; 80 less to 290 more	+, very low

Derived from: Karanicolas et al. [11]

[a]Unclear allocation concealment in all studies, patients blinded in only one study, outcome assessors not blinded in any study, >20 % loss to follow-up in three studies, not analysed using intention to treat in one study

[b]$I^2=72.6$ %, $P=0.006$

[c]Confidence interval includes possible benefit from both surgical approaches

[d]Relative risks (95 % confidence intervals) are based on random effect models

The Header

The general title of the clinical question being considered.

Sub Heading

A question broken up into the PICO format of patient or population, the setting, the intervention and the comparison to which the intervention is being made. The question is that which is of interest to the author of the table and may or may not reflect the evidence which addresses this question.

Outcomes

The key component of the GRADE process is to focus on the outcomes to which the evidence applies. Individual studies may focus on differing outcomes that are of interest. It is often the case that many studies address common outcomes reflecting benefit, but do not reliably report on other outcomes, especially on harm. It is possible that with the same questions and same group of studies, the quality of evidence supporting an intervention is high for one outcome such but not others. This latter point is one of the reasons that during formulating the question it is useful to list in order of importance the outcomes of interest.

Justification for Quality Assessment

In the GRADE system, a judgment is made whether the overall quality of evidence for each outcome is High, Moderate, Low, or Very Low. Initially evidence from RCTs is considered to be High quality evidence while observational studies start off as Low quality. Whether the overall body of evidence moves up or down the ranking is determined by the extent to which the studies have features which move them up or down and (Table 1.1) [3], specifies the features which move a study up or down the list.

Study Limitation

The first judgment is related to the possible deficiency in the study designs themselves and these are determined during the critical appraisal process, features such as adequacy of randomization and blinding.

Inconsistency

Different studies may come to different conclusions either qualitatively e.g. the intervention works vs. it doesn't or the degree to which a treatment works, i.e. the effect size differs. A measure of this in systematic reviews is the degree of heterogeneity often reported as the I^2 value and this is illustrated in our example when examining delayed gastric emptying. This heterogeneity can be due to differences in the patient population studied, the nature of the intervention, means of measuring outcomes or other study design features.

Directness

This is the degree to which the studies actually address the question we are interested in. The results may be indirect because the study population is different from one we are interested in or the intervention is differs substantially from what we are interested in. This is slightly different from the above example the indirectness refers to the whole body of evidence in relation to our specific question.

Precision

Studies may report effects with wide confidence intervals where the values at the upper and lower bounds would suggest the different clinical actions. In our example, the mortality associated with PPP is expected to between 120 more deaths and 80 less deaths per 1000 patients. The wide confidence intervals are most often driven by too small a sample size in a study.

Publication Bias

We may suspect publication bias when the preponderance of the available evidence comes from a number of small studies, most of which have been commercially funded. This may suggest that studies which not showing an effect have not been published which biases the evidence.

Features Increasing Quality of Observational Studies

Large Magnitude of Effect

In well designed observation studies, if a large and plausible effect is observed (relative risk of greater than 5 or less than 0.2) there is reasonable confidence that the effect is not due to confounding. This is the reason why one doesn't really require a RCT to determine if parachutes are effective.

Dose Response Gradient

A finding in observational studies that increases our confidence in a cause effect relationship is the demonstration of a dose response effect. For example, an increased risk of bleeding with increasing INR.

All Plausible Confounding Would Reduce the Demonstrated Effect or Increase it if No Effect Was Observed

A confounder is a factor related to both a predictor and outcome, but is not in the causal link between the predictor and outcome. If a likely confounder acts opposite to the way one would expect, then it is possible that the true effect is underestimated. For example if high risk patients do at least as well with a surgical procedure as do those at low risk, it more strongly suggests that there is a true effect of the surgical intervention and would increase our confidence and thus the quality rating of the evidence.

Summary of Findings

The last column is a summary of findings where the estimate of relative effect, the baseline risk of the standard therapy and the absolute effects of the intervention are reported. A measure of the absolute effect is crucial for making a recommendation since one intervention may be more effective in comparison to another, the overall effect in terms of overall numbers may be small, in our example the absolute risk of bleeding is only decreased by 1 %. Another example is if the baseline risk of pneumonia is 1 % and with the addition of preoperative antibiotics drops down to .7 %. A change in absolute risk of .3 % is unlikely to be of clinical significance despite there being a 30 % relative risk reduction, which in many cases would be considered of considerable "clinical significance".

The final component of the GRADE system is to make a recommendation. In assessing the quality of the evidence necessary to make the recommendation, the ones making the recommendation should specify which of the various outcomes are crucial to making a recommendation, in our example it is reasonable to conclude that the evidence is low since that is the quality for the crucial outcome of perioperative mortality. It could be argued that the 5-year survival is more important in which case the quality of evidence is moderate (Tables 1.2).

From determining the quality of evidence, a recommendation is made. This is a separate process from determining quality of evidence. A recommendation is either strong or weak where "The strength of a recommendation is defined as the extent to which one can be confident that the desirable consequences of an intervention outweigh its undesirable consequences" [1]. A strong recommendation is one where from the clinicians' point of view; most patients should receive the intervention as

Table 1.3 Implications of the strength of recommendation for an intervention in the GRADE approach

Group	Strong recommendation	Weak recommendation
Patients	Most patients would want the course of action recommended, and only a small proportion would not	The majority of patients would want the recommended course of action, but many would not
Clinicians	Most patients should receive the recommended course of action	Different choices will be appropriate for different patients based on their values and preferences. Recognizing that you must make greater effort to help each patient to arrive a management decision
Policy makers	The recommendation can be adopted as policy in most situations	Policy making will require substantial debate and involve many stakeholders

the expected benefits comfortably outweigh the undesirable effects. In these situation there is usually little need for extensive discussions about the merits of the intervention. Weak recommendations on the other hand, may be appropriate in some patients, but requires more thorough discussions about the benefits and adverse effects of the treatment (Table 1.3) [4].

Ultimately, decisions about the care of individual patient falls to the surgeon and the patient which takes into account not just the external evidence for a particular course of action but crucially the patients own preferences and values and the practical ability for the surgeon to deliver on this decision in their own specific environment.

Acknowledgment I would like to acknowledge Tania Gottschalk and Gordon Guyatt for their advice and assistance.

Other Resources

JAMA Users Guide: Guyatt and Rennie

Author Gordon Guyatt, Drummond Rennie
Series Users' Guides to the Medical Literature
Publisher McGraw-Hill
Publication date: 2008
ISBN 978-0071590341
CEBM website: http://www.cebm.net/
GRADE website: http://www.gradeworkinggroup.org/index.htm
EPIQ: https://www.fmhs.auckland.ac.nz/en/soph/about/our-departments/epidemiology-and-biostatistics/research/epiq.html

References

1. Andrews J, Guyatt G, Oxman AD, Alderson P, Dahm P, Falck-Ytter Y, et al. GRADE guidelines: 14. Going from evidence to recommendations: the significance and presentation of recommendations. J Clin Epidemiol. 2013;66(7):719–25. doi:10.1016/j.jclinepi.2012.03.013.
2. Atkins D, Best D, Briss PA, Eccles M, Falck-Ytter Y, Flottorp S, et al. Grading quality of evidence and strength of recommendations. BMJ (Clin Res Ed). 2004;328(7454):1490. doi:10.1136/bmj.328.7454.1490.
3. Balshem H, Helfand M, Schünemann HJ, Oxman AD, Kunz R, Brozek J, et al. GRADE guidelines: 3. Rating the quality of evidence. J Clin Epidemiol. 2011;64(4):401–6. doi:10.1016/j.jclinepi.2010.07.015.
4. Brożek JL, Akl EA, Compalati E, Kreis J, Terracciano L, Fiocchi A, et al. Grading quality of evidence and strength of recommendations in clinical practice guidelines Part 3 of 3. The GRADE approach to developing recommendations. Allergy. 2011;66(5):588–95. doi:10.1111/j.1398-9995.2010.02530.x.
5. Evidence-Based Medicine Working Group. Evidence-based medicine. A new approach to teaching the practice of medicine. JAMA. 1992;268(17):2420–5. doi:10.1001/jama.1992.03490170092032.
6. GATE in ACP. 2013. GATE in ACP, 1–4.
7. Grimes DA, Schulz KF. An overview of clinical research: the lay of the land. Lancet. 2002;359(9300):57–61. doi:10.1016/S0140-6736(02)07283-5.
8. Grimes DA, Schulz KF. Bias and causal associations in observational research. Lancet. 2002;359(9302):248–52. doi:10.1016/S0140-6736(02)07451-2.
9. Guyatt GH, Oxman AD, Kunz R, Vist GE, Falck-Ytter Y, Schünemann HJ, GRADE Working Group. What is "quality of evidence" and why is it important to clinicians? BMJ (Clin Res Ed). 2008;336(7651):995–8. doi:10.1136/bmj.39490.551019.BE.
10. Haynes RB. Optimal search strategies for retrieving scientifically strong studies of treatment from Medline: analytical survey. BMJ (Clin Res Ed). 2005;330(7501):1179. doi:10.1136/bmj.38446.498542.8F.
11. Karanicolas PJ, Davies E, Kunz R, Briel M, Koka HP, Payne DM, et al. The pylorus: take it or leave it? Systematic review and meta-analysis of pylorus-preserving versus standard whipple pancreaticoduodenectomy for pancreatic or periampullary cancer. Ann Surg Oncol. 2007;14(6):1825–34. doi:10.1245/s10434-006-9330-3.
12. Sackett DL. Evidence-based medicine. Semin Perinatol. 1997;21(1):3–5.
13. Sackett DL, Rosenberg WMC, Gray JAM, Haynes RB, Richardson WS. Evidence based medicine: what it is and what it isn't. BMJ (Clin Res Ed). 1996;312(7023):71–2. doi:10.1136/bmj.312.7023.71.

References

Chapter 2
Is Surgery Indicated for Asymptomatic Giant Hepatic Hemangioma?

John Seal

Abstract Liver hemangiomas are the most common benign neoplasms of the liver and are often diagnosed incidentally on abdominal imaging. Most liver hemangiomas are small (<4 cm) indolent lesions that do not require further intervention or surveillance in the absence of symptoms. The management of giant liver hemangiomas (>4 cm), however, remains controversial. The natural progression of giant hemangiomas is not well defined and the risk of life-threatening complications, namely rupture and bleeding, is not clearly established. The development of symptoms such as abdominal pain, mass effects or life-threatening events such as rupture, bleeding or consumptive coagulopathy is an indication for surgical resection or intervention. Asymptomatic giant hemangiomas present a management dilemma as the risk of life-threatening complications is unknown. Several single centers studies have demonstrated the safety of expectant management of even very large asymptomatic hemangiomas. There is no evidence to support using size alone as an indication for resection. Although morbidity and mortality of liver resection for hemangioma has improved, the risks of surgical intervention need to be balanced against the rare risk of adverse events during expectant observation.

Keywords Hemangioma • Liver resection • Observation • Complications • Liver • Giant hemangioma • Cavernous hemangioma • Surgery • Resection

Introduction

Liver hemangiomas are the most common benign neoplasms of the liver and are often diagnosed incidentally on abdominal imaging. Most liver hemangiomas are small (<4 cm) indolent lesions that do not require resection or routine follow-up in the absence of symptoms or complications. The management of giant liver

J. Seal (✉)
Multi-Organ Transplant Institute, Ochsner Medical Center,
1514 Jefferson Highway, New Orleans, LA 70121, USA
e-mail: johnsealmd@gmail.com

J.M. Millis, J.B. Matthews (eds.), *Difficult Decisions in Hepatobiliary and Pancreatic Surgery*, Difficult Decisions in Surgery: An Evidence-Based Approach, DOI 10.1007/978-3-319-27365-5_2

hemangiomas (>4 cm), however, remains controversial [1–3]. In contrast to smaller lesions, giant hemangiomas can become quite large (>40 cm), symptomatic and even cause life-threatening complications. The most common symptoms of giant hemangiomas are abdominal pain and mass effects of the tumor such as biliary obstruction [4, 5], Budd Chiari syndrome [6], vena cava compression [7], and gastric outlet obstruction [8]. Although spontaneous rupture is very rare, traumatic rupture or intra-tumoral bleeding often necessitates emergency resection, trans-arterial embolization or both [9]. In some cases when hepatic resection is not anatomically feasible, both deceased and living donor liver transplantation have been reported for treatment of symptomatic giant hemangioma [10–12].

In the absence of significant symptoms, however, the rationale for surgical resection is less clear. The natural progression of hemangiomas and the risk of life-threatening complications, namely rupture and bleeding, is not well established. Several authors have advocated for preventive surgical resection or enucleation based on tumor size, rate of growth and perceived risk of rupture despite a lack of supporting evidence. Also, progress in surgical technique, anesthesia and peri-operative care has reduced the risk of death and major complications following liver resection, further lowering the risks associated with surgical intervention. An evidence-based approach to surgical management of asymptomatic giant hemangiomas must balance an estimate of the risk of expectant management in the absence of well-defined natural history of the disease with peri-operative morbidity and risks of surgical intervention.

Search Strategy

A literature search of English language publications from 1990 to 2014 was used to identity published data on management of liver hemangiomas using the PICO outline (Table 2.1). PubMed database was searched using the following terms [number of results]: "liver, hemangioma, surgery, observation" [36], "liver, giant, hemangioma, surgery, observation" [12], "surgical, approach, liver, hemangioima" [80], "giant, liver, hemangioma, surgery, technique" [17]. Articles that did not present new data with respect to observation versus surgical management were excluded. Retrospective studies of benign liver lesions were included if a separate analysis of hemangiomas was provided. In an effort to be more comprehensive in the analysis, studies that included smaller hemangiomas (<4 cm) were considered in the review.

Table 2.1 PICO table for management of giant liver hemangioma

P (Patients)	I (Intervention)	C (Comparator group)	O (Outcomes measured)
Patients with giant liver hemangioma (>4 cm) without symptoms	Surgical resection (anatomic resection, enucleation, liver transplantation)	Observation	Post operative complications, persistent or recurrent symptoms, life threatening adverse events

No prospective randomized studies comparing surgical resection and observation of asymptomatic giant hemangiomas were identified. The PubMed search yielded six single institution and one multicenter retrospective study comparing surgical resection and observation of hemangiomas and four single center retrospective reviews of benign liver lesions that included analysis of hemangiomas. An additional two retrospective single center reviews of resection for hemangioma were included to better assess the rate of complications following resection. The data were classified using the GRADE system.

Results

Resection Versus Observation for Giant Hemangiomas

Evidence comparing resection versus observation of asymptomatic giant hemangiomas is limited to retrospective single institution studies (Table 2.2) [13–20] and sub-analyses within single center retrospective studies of benign liver tumors (Table 2.3) [21–24]. The primary outcomes in most of these studies included perioperative morbidity and mortality, resolution of symptoms in the treatment group or development of new symptoms and adverse events in the observation cohorts. None of the studies describe deliberate changes in treatment algorithms during the study period and no explicit comparison of practices in different eras. Thus, the interpretation of the data is limited to center specific and often ill-defined practices in the management of giant hemangiomas. Nevertheless, the cumulative trends in outcomes offers insight into the risks and morbidity of resection compared with observation and the natural history of giant hemangiomas.

Table 2.2 Resection versus observation for liver hemangioma

	N	Resection		Observation	
Author (year)	(total)	N	% Complication	N	Finding
Yedibela (2013)	246	103	17 %	143	56 % new symptoms, 2 deaths from rupture
Giuliante (2010)	74	40	10 %	34	No significant increase in size of asymptomatic tumors during observation
Schnelldorfer (2010)	289	56	14 %	233	Size not associated with adverse events
Yoon (2003)	115	52	25 %	63	36 % resected patients to exclude presence of malignancy
Terkivatan (2002)	49	11	27.3 %	38	Symptoms resolved in 12 patients
Pietrabissa (1996)	78	16	NA	62	No rupture in observation group
Yamagata (1991)	33	13	23 %	20	Observation group tumors <5 cm diameter

Table 2.3 Studies of benign liver lesions: analysis of hemangiomas

Author (year)	N (total)	Resection N	Resection % Complication	Observation N	Observation Finding
Mezhir (2013)	151	60	NA	91	4.4 % of observed tumors were ultimately resected
Terkivatan (2001)	103	25	24 %	78	25 cm tumor followed without need for resection
Charny (2001)	97	39	21 %	58	63.3 % of pre-operative biopsies were indeterminate or incorrect
Weimann (1997)	238	103	18.8 %	135	No episodes of bleeding in observation group

The most recent report comparing resection and observation by Yedibela et al. [14] reviewed 307 hemangiomas referred for evaluation. Elective surgery was performed in 103 patients, 62 of which were symptomatic and 41 asymptomatic. Of the asymptomatic patients undergoing resection, 11 were for diagnostic uncertainty, 9 for tumor enlargement and 21 for patient fear of future complications. There was no mortality in the post-operative period and symptom resolution was achieved in 88 % of symptomatic patients. In contrast to other studies, they report a 9 % rate of major complications in the observation group with two fatalities from traumatic hemangioma rupture. In this study, the overall trend was toward lower rates of complications in the surgical treatment group.

Giuliante et al. [13] reviewed 74 consecutive referrals for hemangioma evaluation, with 34 undergoing observation and 40 treated surgically. As a regional hepatobiliary referral center, the authors discuss the bias that most giant hemangiomas were referred for symptoms, large size or diagnostic uncertainty and that the overall operative rate of 54 % is likely inflated with underrepresentation of asymptomatic lesions. The primary indications for resection were abdominal symptoms, diagnostic uncertainty and tumor growth. Tumor growth has been used by some centers as an indication for resection, but the trajectory of growth over long term follow-up and its implication for risk of tumor rupture is uncertain. In this study, only 7 of 14 tumors demonstrating growth underwent resection, 5 of which had additional indications for resection (abdominal pain and Kasabach-Merritt syndrome). Of the seven tumors demonstrating growth in the observation group, the tendency to enlarge decreased over time and among all tumors in the observation group, there was no significant increase in mean tumor size or development of new symptoms during the follow-up period.

Another single institution review by Terkivatan et al. [19] supported the safety of expectant management of asymptomatic giant hemangiomas. During the study period, 11 patients were treated with resection, all of whom had abdominal symptoms attributed to the hemangioma except for one asymptomatic lesion that exhibited 5 cm of growth over 36 months follow-up. Thirty-eight patients were managed with observation. Importantly, there was no significant difference in the mean diameter of tumors in the resection group compared with the observation group. Twelve of the observation patients had abdominal pain on initial assessment that was not attributed to the hemangioma and, in each case, the pain resolved during follow-up. None of the asymptomatic patients developed new symptoms during a mean follow-up period of 59 months.

Schnelldorfer et al. [16] report the only contemporary series to assess the impact of hemangioma management on quality of life. A quality of life survey was administered with responses from 289 of 492 patients treated for hemangioma at their center, including patients treated with surgical resection or observation. In the observation group, 20 % of patients developed new-onset symptoms with 2 % being life-threatening. Post-operative complications occurred in 14 % of resected patients with 7 % being life threatening. Interestingly, the size of the hemangioma was not associated with adverse events in either group, lending credence to the notion that risk of rupture is not necessarily related to tumor size or rate of growth. The subjective quality of life survey was similar for resected and observed patients leading the authors to conclude that observation is preferred in most patient and surgical resection should be reserved for patient with symptoms or hemangioma-related complications.

The consideration of tumor size and rate of growth have both been proposed as risk factors for tumor rupture and, thus, indications for resection in asymptomatic patients. Iwatsuki et al. [25] suggested benign hepatic lesions exceeding 10 cm should be resected based increased risk for internal bleeding, further growth or rupture, although this was not based on conclusive prospective observational data. In the more recent literature, an absolute size threshold as an indication for resection is not favored. The indication for resection of giant hemangioma was most often the development of symptoms. The rate of growth of the tumor remains a controversial indication for resection, although such recommendations are made without a clearly defined relationship between rate of growth and risk of rupture. Pietrabissa et al. [17] proposed resection for "rapidly growing" asymptomatic hemangiomas defined as a minimum 25 % increase in largest diameter over a period of 6 months. The rationale is based on the speculation that the risk for tumor rupture or diagnostic error is higher in patients with rapid growth. Although well reasoned, no clinical support is provided to substantial the claim of increased risk of rupture or diagnostic error with rapid growth, leaving the natural disease course of giant hemangiomas unresolved.

Diagnostic uncertainty has been used as an indication for resection of vascular lesions of the liver when a definitive diagnosis cannot be made from radiologic studies, particularly in the setting of known extra-hepatic malignancies or risk factors for the development of liver malignancy (cirrhosis, hepatitis, steatosis). With advances in imaging modalities and experience at high-volume centers, diagnostic uncertainty is much less common. In a subgroup analysis of a retrospective review of benign liver lesions at Memorial Sloan-Kettering Cancer Center, Mezhir et al. [22] report diagnostic uncertainty as the indication for surgical resection in 53.3 % of asymptomatic hemangiomas from 1992 to 2009. Importantly, though, only 12.5 % of patients resected for diagnostic uncertainty were seen in the last 10 years of the study, suggesting a significant impact of advances in medical imaging.

Treatment of Giant Hemangiomas: Operative Approaches and Non-surgical Therapies

The morbidity and mortality of hemangioma resection is an important consideration when determining appropriate treatment for giant hemangiomas, particularly asymptomatic lesions. Complications following surgical resection range from 10 % to 27.3 % in recent studies comparing resection and observation. In a recent multi-institutional review of surgical management of hepatic hemangiomas [26], the overall rate of Clavien grade 3 complication or higher was 5.7 % and included bile leaks and bleeding. The 30-day post-operative mortality was 0.8 % (N = 2). Although hepatic resections for hemangioma can be performed safely, post-operative complications can be significant with a nearly 1 % risk of death. The documented risks of surgery must be carefully weighted against the severity of symptoms and the very low risk of complications associated with observation.

Evolution in operative techniques and application of non-surgical therapies may lead to a less invasive and safer approach to management of hemangiomas in the future. Though technical aspects of resection may vary greatly between centers, a single center study by Lerner et al. [27] documented an intra-institutional evolution toward enucleation over resection for large hemangiomas over time with more liberal use of inflow occlusion, less intra-operative blood loss and less complications. Liver transplantation [10–12, 28] for life threatening symptoms attributed to giant hemangiomas has been reported, further expanding therapeutic options to include lesions anatomically unresectable by conventional approaches. Laparoscopic [29–32] and robotic [33] approaches have been reported by several centers, although the impact of a minimal access approach in reducing operative risk or complications is not defined.

The use of several non-surgical therapies for symptomatic giant hemangiomas has been reported. Transarterial embolization is widely used both in the setting of acute management of ruptured hemangiomas and as a pre-operative treatment to reduce vascular inflow and decrease size [34–38]. Radiofrequency ablation has also been reported for symptomatic control of giant hemangiomas with promising results. Gao et al. [39] report a single institution initial experience with RFA treatment in giant hemangiomas. In this series, use of RFA in lesions >10 cm diameter had a 100 % complication rate including life-threatening complications of lower esophageal fistula and acute respiratory distress syndrome. In smaller lesions (5–10 cm diameter), RFA was successful at controlling symptoms with only minor complications. Medical therapies such as the anti-angiogenic agent bevicizumab and the tyrosine kinase inhibitor sorafenib have also been reported to decrease the size of large hemangiomas, though published data is limited to case reports. Overall, even less invasive modes of treating giant hepatic hemangiomas will have some risk of complication that must be carefully considered in asymptomatic patients.

Recommendations

Surgical resection is a well established and accepted treatment of symptomatic giant hemangiomas. The relative risk of surgical intervention is balanced by a benefit to the patient with expected improvement or resolution of symptoms. Management of asymptomatic giant hemangiomas remains controversial as the natural progression of the disease in not well described. The hypothesis that tumor size contributes to the risk of rupture is not supported in the literature and should not be used alone as an indication for surgical resection. Retrospective studies from many centers demonstrate that expectant management of asymptomatic giant hemangiomas is safe. Surgical resection or an alternative treatment modality should be considered if symptoms develop. Though several centers consider rapid growth of tumors during observation periods as an indication for resection, there is no evidence to suggest that growth alone presents additional risk to the patient if a definitive radiographic diagnosis has been made.

A Personal View of the Data

Surgical resection of giant symptomatic hemangiomas is widely accepted as the risks of surgery are balanced by a direct benefit of symptom relief. Though resolution of symptoms after resection is not universal and varies in published reports, it is reasonable to expect a high rate of symptom resolution if the initial symptoms were appropriately attributed to the hemangioma. To that end, symptomatic patients with giant hemangiomas should be carefully assessed to ensure the symptoms, in particular non-specific abdominal pain, can be attributed to effects of the mass. The retrospective series highlighted in this chapter support the safety and prudence of deferring surgical resection in asymptomatic patients with giant hemangiomas. Yedibela et al. reported a higher rate of adverse events in patients under observation including two deaths from rupture, compared with other contemporary series that report no adverse events. Overall, the evidence indicates observation of even very large hemangiomas is safe. There is no evidence to support size alone as an indication for surgical resection in asymptomatic lesions. Impending complications such as vascular compression or gastrointestinal obstruction may be appropriate. Patient anxiety has been reported as an indication for surgical resection of asymptomatic lesions in some series. While anxiety can certainly be a significant symptom, it is the responsibility of the surgeon to reassure patients regarding the very low risk of adverse events associated with observation and to manage patient anxiety non-operatively. Finally, the risk of rupture related to tumor growth is unclear, but to date no series has demonstrated that rapid growth of hemangiomas presents an increased risk if a definitive radiologic diagnosis has been made. Rapid growth may prompt further investigation to confirm the diagnosis and exclude concern for malignancy, but there is insufficient evidence to support surgical resection on the basis of growth alone.

Recommendations

- Symptomatic liver hemangiomas should be surgically resected if symptoms are attributed to the hemangioma itself (evidence quality high, strong recommendation).
- Asymptomatic giant hemangiomas can be safely observed regardless of tumor size (evidence quality moderate, strong recommendation).
- The size of the hemangioma (greatest diameter) alone should not be used as an indication for resection. (evidence quality moderate, strong recommendation)
- Rate of growth alone should not be used as an indication for surgical resection (evidence quality low, weak recommendation).

References

1. Hoekstra LT, Bieze M, Erdogan D, Roelofs JJTH, Beuers UHW, van Gulik TM. Management of giant liver hemangiomas: an update. Expert Rev Gastroenterol Hepatol. 2013;7:263.
2. Belghiti J, Cauchy F, Paradis V, Vilgrain V. Diagnosis and management of solid benign liver lesions. Nat Rev Gastroenterol Hepatol. 2014;11:737–49.
3. Toro A, Mahfouz A-E, Ardiri A, et al. What is changing in indications and treatment of hepatic hemangiomas. A review. Ann Hepatol. 2014;13:327.
4. Losanoff JE, Millis JM. Liver hemangioma complicated by obstructive jaundice. Am J Surg. 2008;196:e3.
5. Tang L, Zhou W-P. Education and imaging. Hepatobiliary and pancreatic: large cavernous hemangioma with obstructive jaundice. J Gastroenterol Hepatol. 2009;24:930.
6. Kim DY, Pantelic MV, Yoshida A, Jerius J, Abouljoud MS. Cavernous hemangioma presenting as Budd-Chiari syndrome. J Am Coll Surg. 2005;200:470.
7. Akbulut S, Yilmaz M, Kahraman A, Yilmaz S. Bilateral lower limb edema caused by compression of the retrohepatic inferior vena cava by a giant hepatic hemangioma. Int Surg. 2013;98:229.
8. Aydin C, Akbulut S, Kutluturk K, Kahraman A, Kayaalp C, Yilmaz S. Giant hepatic hemangioma presenting as gastric outlet obstruction. Int Surg. 2013;98:19.
9. Donati M, Stavrou GA, Donati A, Oldhafer KJ. The risk of spontaneous rupture of liver hemangiomas: a critical review of the literature. J Hepatobiliary Pancreat Sci. 2011;18:797–805.
10. Meguro M, Soejima Y, Taketomi A, et al. Living donor liver transplantation in a patient with giant hepatic hemangioma complicated by Kasabach-Merritt syndrome: report of a case. Surg Today. 2008;38:463.
11. Ferraz AAB, Sette MJA, Maia M, et al. Liver transplant for the treatment of giant hepatic hemangioma. Liver Trans. 2004;10:1436.
12. Vagefi PA, Klein I, Gelb B, et al. Emergent orthotopic liver transplantation for hemorrhage from a giant cavernous hepatic hemangioma: case report and review. J Gastrointest Surg. 2011;15:209.
13. Giuliante F, Ardito F, Vellone M, et al. Reappraisal of surgical indications and approach for liver hemangioma: single-center experience on 74 patients. Am J Surg. 2011;201:741.
14. Yedibela S, Alibek S, Müller V, et al. Management of hemangioma of the liver: surgical therapy or observation? World J Surg. 2013;37:1303.

15. Yamagata M, Kanematsu T, Matsumata T, Utsunomiya T, Ikeda Y, Sugimachi K. Management of haemangioma of the liver: comparison of results between surgery and observation. Br J Surg. 1991;78:1223.
16. Schnelldorfer T, Ware AL, Smoot R, Schleck CD, Harmsen WS, Nagorney DM. Management of giant hemangioma of the liver: resection versus observation. J Am Coll Surg. 2010;211:724.
17. Pietrabissa A, Giulianotti P, Campatelli A, et al. Management and follow-up of 78 giant haemangiomas of the liver. Br J Surg. 1996;83:915.
18. Herman P, Costa MLV, Machado MAC, et al. Management of hepatic hemangiomas: a 14-year experience. J Gastrointest Surg. 2005;9:853.
19. Terkivatan T, Vrijland WW, Den Hoed PT, et al. Size of lesion is not a criterion for resection during management of giant liver haemangioma. Br J Surg. 2002;89:1240.
20. Yoon SS, Charny CK, Fong Y, et al. Diagnosis, management, and outcomes of 115 patients with hepatic hemangioma. J Am Coll Surg. 2003;197:392.
21. Charny CK, Jarnagin WR, Schwartz LH, et al. Management of 155 patients with benign liver tumours. Br J Surg. 2001;88:808.
22. Mezhir JJ, Fourman LT, Do RK, et al. Changes in the management of benign liver tumours: an analysis of 285 patients. HPB. 2013;15:156.
23. Weimann A, Ringe B, Klempnauer J, et al. Benign liver tumors: differential diagnosis and indications for surgery. World J Surg. 1997;21:983.
24. Terkivatan T, de Wilt JW, de Man RA, et al. Indications and long-term outcome of treatment for benign hepatic tumors: a critical appraisal. Arch Surg. 2001;136:1033.
25. Iwatsuki S, Todo S, Starzl TE. Excisional therapy for benign hepatic lesions. Surg Gynecol Obstet. 1990;171:240.
26. Miura JT, Amini A, Schmocker R, et al. Surgical management of hepatic hemangiomas: a multi-institutional experience. HPB. 2014;16:924.
27. Lerner SM, Hiatt JR, Salamandra J, et al. Giant cavernous liver hemangiomas: effect of operative approach on outcome. Arch Surg. 2004;139:818.
28. Longeville JH, de la Hall P, Dolan P, et al. Treatment of a giant haemangioma of the liver with Kasabach-Merritt syndrome by orthotopic liver transplant a case report. HPB Surg. 1997;10:159.
29. Acharya M, Panagiotopoulos N, Bhaskaran P, Kyriakides C, Pai M, Habib N. Laparoscopic resection of a giant exophytic liver haemangioma with the laparoscopic Habib 4× radiofrequency device. World J Gastrointest Surg. 2012;4:199.
30. Gadiyaram S, Shetty N. Laparoscopic resection of giant liver hemangioma using laparoscopic Habib probe for parenchymal transection. J Minim Access Surg. 2012;8:59.
31. Lanthaler M, Freund M, Nehoda H. Laparoscopic resection of a giant liver hemangioma. J Laparoendosc Adv Surg Tech A. 2005;15:624.
32. Patriti A, Graziosi L, Sanna A, Gullà N, Donini A. Laparoscopic treatment of liver hemangioma. Surg Laparosc Endosc Percutaneous Tech. 2005;15:359.
33. Giulianotti PC, Addeo P, Bianco FM. Robotic right hepatectomy for giant hemangioma in a Jehovah's witness. J Hepatobiliary Pancreat Sci. 2011;18:112.
34. Lupinacci RM, Szejnfeld D, Farah JFM. Spontaneous rupture of a giant hepatic hemangioma. Sequential treatment with preoperative transcatheter arterial embolization and conservative hepatectomy. G Chir. 2011;32:469.
35. Panis Y, Fagniez PL, Cherqui D, Roche A, Schaal JC, Jaeck D. Successful arterial embolisation of giant liver haemangioma. Report of a case with five-year computed tomography follow-up. HPB Surg. 1993;7:141.
36. Suzuki H, Nimura Y, Kamiya J, et al. Preoperative transcatheter arterial embolization for giant cavernous hemangioma of the liver with consumption coagulopathy. Am J Gastroenterol. 1997;92:688.

37. Vassiou K, Rountas H, Liakou P, Arvanitis D, Fezoulidis I, Tepetes K. Embolization of a giant hepatic hemangioma prior to urgent liver resection. Case report and review of the literature. Cardiovasc Interv Radiol. 2007;30:800.
38. Zhou J-X, Huang J-W, Wu H, Zeng Y. Successful liver resection in a giant hemangioma with intestinal obstruction after embolization. World J Gastroenterol. 2013;19:2974.
39. Gao J, Ke S, Ding X, Zhou Y, Qian X, Sun W. Radiofrequency ablation for large hepatic hemangiomas: initial experience and lessons. Surgery. 2013;153:78.

Chapter 3
What Is the Best Surgical Method of Addressing Hepatic Hemangiomas?

J. Michael Millis and David Caba Molina

Abstract Hepatic hemangiomas are the most common benign tumor of the liver and the second most common tumor following metastases. The diagnosis and management of hepatic hemangiomas has improved significantly for the past decade. The decision to treat this tumors surgically should be based mostly on symptomatology, inability to exclude malignancy, documented growth and less on feasibility for resection or patient anxiety. The decision for observation should be based on a thorough examination of asymptomatic tumors with benign characteristics on imaging. The surgical treatment of choice has evolved from formal hepatectomies to selected enucleation with improvement in outcomes regardless of the size of the lesion. Minimal invasive techniques have similar results as open surgery in appropriately selected patients with no difference in morbidity and mortality.

Keywords Hepatic hemangioma • Liver tumors • Enucleation

Introduction

Hepatic hemangiomas are the most frequent benign tumors of the liver with a frequency of 0.4–7.3 % in adults with a higher incidence in woman [1–3].

The accurate diagnosis of hemangiomas is a key component given the current high frequency of incidental findings on CT scans that lead to further workup to differentiate malignant neoplasms from benign tumors. The most sensitive studies are MRI (100 %), CT scan (98.3) and US (96.9 %) [4].

The most common indications for the treatment of hemangiomas are abdominal pain, diagnostic uncertainty, enlargement, occupations and hobbies that may entail abdominal trauma and the extremely rare Kasabach-Merrit syndrome. The definition of "giant hemangiomas" in the majority of the studies is a tumor with more than 4 cm in diameter [5, 6].

J.M. Millis (✉) • D.C. Molina
Department of Surgery, University of Chicago Hospitals, MC 5027, Chicago, IL 60637, USA
e-mail: mmillis@surgery.bsd.uchciago.edu

J.M. Millis, J.B. Matthews (eds.), *Difficult Decisions in Hepatobiliary and Pancreatic Surgery*, Difficult Decisions in Surgery: An Evidence-Based Approach, DOI 10.1007/978-3-319-27365-5_3

There are four classic surgical methods of treatment for hepatic hemangiomas: liver resection, enucleation, hepatic artery ligation and liver transplantation [7]. Enucleation refers to the creation of a plane between the normal liver parenchyma and the hemangioma without (or minimal) removal of normal hepatic parenchyma and it's though to decrease blood loss, bile leak and preservation of parenchyma [8].

Newer adjuvants in the surgical treatment had emerged in the past decade including laparoscopic ultrasonic resection and supraselective arterial embolization, those techniques are used to increase safety of surgery [9, 10]. Other non surgical treatments like radiotherapy, chemotherapy and transarterial embolization (TAE) had been proposed as successful alternatives when surgical resection is not indicated or feasible [11–13]. The resection can be achieved via an open or laparoscopic technique and new technology like RFA has been used as part of the surgical minimal invasive category.

Search Strategy

An online literature search on English Language of publications from 2000 to 2014 was used to identify and select published data on the surgical management of hepatic hemangiomas using the PICO outline (Table 3.1).

The Databases used for the search were PubMed, Cochrane Evidence Based Medicine, MEDLINE-MEDLINE plus/OVID, Science Citation Index Expanded (SCI-EXPANDED). The terms used for the search were: "liver/hepatic hemangioma treatment" "surgical treatment of liver/hepatic hemangioma" "management of liver/hepatic hemangioma" "resection of/for hepatic hemangioma", "treatment of liver/hepatic hemangioma". The search was expanded to use articles that included or addressed hepatic hemangiomas as part of benign tumors of the liver since hemangiomas tend to be clustered in that group as well, those terms include: "benign liver tumors" "treatment of benign liver tumors" and "management of benign liver tumors".

The studies showed were: Randomized controlled trials: 0, Retrospective cohort: 26.

Table 3.1 PICO table for surgical management of hepatic hemangiomas

P (Patients)	I (Intervention)	C (Comparator group)	Outcomes (Outcomes measured
Patients with diagnosed liver hemangioma (symptomatic or asymptomatic)	Surgical intervention (Open, Laparoscopic, mixed interventions with adjuvant treatment)	No surgical intervention (observation) vs Surgical intervention (enucleation vs hepatectomy, open vs Laparoscopic)	Perioperative complications

Results

Observation vs Surgical Treatment with Hepatectomy

The decision to treat hepatic hemangiomas surgically can be challenging when the indications are not well established and up to date guidelines are not encountered in the literature. Resection is indicated for symptoms and questionable diagnosis and the most widely methods studied are resection and enucleation [14–16].

A study from the University of Cincinnati from 2003 proposed an algorithm where the initial step is a triple phase CT, if there was any uncertainty of the diagnosis of hemangioma a tagged RBC/MRI scan was obtained, if the lesion was asymptomatic observation would be granted and surgery was indicated in symptomatic patients or increase in size along with large size hemangiomas. Ninety two percent of the entire series was properly diagnosed with this algorithm. Hemangiomas were 29 % of the cohort [17].

In 2001 Terkivatan et al. study aimed to prove that surgical treatment may not be justified during long term follow up of patient with benign tumors of the liver. This study involved other benign liver tumors and a total of 208 patients were analyzed of which 49.5 % (103) were hemagiomas and 24.2 % (25) of those patients underwent surgical resection. The main indication for resection in this subset of patients was abdominal pain (60 %) followed by suspected metastases. Non-anatomic resection (40 %) and segmental resections (28 %) were the most common procedures utilized. In terms of postoperative morbidity 24 % (6) had a reportable complication. The mean follow up for this group was 39 months. Of the conservative arm (non operative) a mean follow up of 45 months showed no mortality or coagulation, although there's no mention on growth or increased pain in the follow up [18].

In a retrospective cohort at the University of Miami including benign and solid tumors of the liver seen over 14 years a total of 130 cases where treated, 55 % were hemangiomas (71 patients). Surgical excision was performed in 49 %. The morbidity was 5 %. No rupture or progression of symptoms was observed in the asymptomatic group, although the follow up details are not specified in the study they concluded that resection in asymptomatic patients is not justified no matter the size [3].

In 2003 Yoon et al. at MSKCC published a large series where only hemangiomas where included. A total of 115 patients in the 8 year cohort were analyzed, 45.3 % (52 patients) presented with symptoms (abdominal pain) and underwent surgical resection, whereas 54.7 % (63) where observed. Inability to exclude malignancy was the indication in 29 %.

The median size of the resected group was 11 cm vs 4 cm unresected group, and of those more than half (58 %) had tumors larger than 10 cm. Enucleation was the treatment of choice in 60 %. Their complication rate was 25 %. In the observation arm only four patients had persistent symptoms without major complications [5].

In 2005 a paper from a group at the University of São Paolo presented a retrospective series of 249 patients over 14 years. In this series 31.7 % patient were symptomatic. The paper made emphasis in conservative treatment, only 3.2 % (n = 8) were treated with surgery, the main indication was pain. Giant hemangiomas (>4 cm) were present in 27.4 % of the cohort. The mean follow up was 78 months without any complications in the observation arm [19].

In the Amsterdam experience a cohort of 34 patients were identified and surgical resection was undertaken in 14 (41 %) after a mean follow up of 36.5 months due to progressive abdominal pain and suspected malignancy. Fifty eight percent of a group of tumors >5 cm underwent surgical treatment whereas in the group of smaller hemangiomas (<5 cm) only 20 %. The observation arm did not show any complications with a mean follow-up of 19.6 month [20].

A retrospective cohort from the Mayo Clinic in 2010 evaluated the rate of hemangioma-associated complications in patients with giant hemangiomas after clinical observation and after operative management to identify the optimal treatment algorithm. This series was based in a survey examination. A total of 233 patient (80.6 %) fell in the nonoperative group and 56 (19.4 %). Only 11 % of the nonoperative group had symptoms whereas 52 % on the operative group had abdominal pain. Nine percent of patient in the observation group developed symptoms or complications after diagnosis. Of the operative arm 34 patients had partial hepatectomy (60.7 %), 22 patients underwent enucleation (1 laparoscopic). The survey revealed that 93 % of patients undergoing surgery had good or better health status and there was no statistical significant difference in the overall rate of adverse events between the two groups. The long term risk of adverse events associated with non operative management is similar to the short term risk of operative intervention.

Based on this study, prophylactic intervention independent of the size without any clinical indication is not recommended due to the potential life-threatening event (2 % nonoperative vs 7 % operative) [6].

Yedibela et al. in 2013 published a large series of patients undergoing observation or surgical treatment of hemangiomas larger than >4 cm. A total of 103 patients underwent surgical resection mainly for abdominal pain (60 %). The indication for surgery in 51 % of asymptomatic patients was anxiety. There was resolution of symptoms in 88 % of patients. There was no statistical difference in the overall rate of adverse events between the surgical and observation group [21].

Enucleation vs Hepatectomy

In the year 2000 Özden published a study including 172 patients of which 42 underwent a surgical procedure for the treatment of hepatic hemangioma. Patients were evaluated to assess the effect of surgery (enucleation using Pringle maneuver). Abdominal pain was the major indication for elective surgery, 78.5 % underwent enucleation followed by formal hepatectomy Early morbidity occurred in 12 % (5 patients) bleeding being the most common. A total of 33 patients (78 %) were followed for a median interval of 53 months, of those patients 96 % (32) were symptomatic prior the intervention. Complete resolution of pain was achieved in

88 % (24) of patients and US revealed no recurrences. The evaluation method was not well standardized and enucleation was favored as a safer technique by the authors [22].

At the University of Chicago a cohort of benign tumors of the liver included 28 patients with benign tumors 35.7 % being hemangiomas (10 patients) the most common presenting symptom was pain and enucleation was performed in 64 % of patients. The complication rate was 10.7 % for the total cohort with no mention on hemangioma related complications [23].

A series from 2001 illustrated the changing indications for resection when patients are analyzed in a large cohort when indications changed (sixe, symptoms etc). This series included 57 patients undergoing resection for abdominal pain or size >4 cm, (criteria until 1996, cohort 1995–1999 after that only hemangiomas larger than 10 cm and pain were indications for surgery). Sixty six percent their cases were enucleation as it was favored over the course of the cohort. Their complication rate was 10.4 % without any mortality. A recurrence occurred in 5.2 % of their patients (3 patients) [24].

Another series of 2001 demonstrated the relationship between tumor size and presence of symptoms, this series included 155 patient with benign liver tumors, of which 63 % (97 patients) had been diagnosed with hemangiomas, 40 % of those patients underwent resection with the main indication being persistent symptoms (23 %). The majority (53 %) underwent enucleation, followed by segmentectomy (20 %). The median follow-up was 16 months and the series complication rate was 21 % [25].

A case series for giant cavernous hemangiomas including 52 patients was published to compare the outcomes on patients undergoing enucleation vs lobectomy. The series showed a higher complication rate with lobectomy (44 % vs 11 %), right lobe lesions more often treated with enucleation. Pringle flow occlusion was used far more frequently for enucleations (78 % vs 16 %). There was no statistical difference in operative times and transfusions, although there was a trend towards improvement with enucleation [26].

The second study to compare enucleation versus hepatic resection was published in 2005. A cohort of 22 symptomatic patients underwent enucleation (n = 10) or formal liver resection (n = 12). The operative time was longer in the resection group and blood loss along with need for transfusion was also greater in the resection group with no effect in length of stay. The complication rate was 14.2 %. In this study tumor localization and number of hemangiomas were the factors for the selection of surgery, being multiple and deep/central masses likely o have a formal resection [27].

A small cohort of 21 patients published in the 2007 showed that patients undergoing enucleation had less operative time (170 vs 230 min), blood loss (400 vs 1329 cc) and no morbidity with decreased length of hospital stay (5.6 vs 9.9 days) compared to liver resection. In this series the major indication were symptoms followed by uncertain diagnosis [28].

The approach for the surgical treatment with enucleation was addressed by the largest study available by Xiao-Hui regarding centrally of peripherally lesions and their respective outcomes, with the assumption that centrally located lesions (defined Couinaud's segments I, IV, V and VII) are more challenging to resect. A total of 172 patients underwent enucleation with Pringle maneuver for pain, lesions larger than 10 cm or enlarging tumors. A total of 76 (44.2 %) were centrally located and 96 (55.8 %) were peripherally located. Enucleation of centrally located hemangiomas required significantly longer vascular inflow occlusion time (45.3 vs 32.6 min)longer operating time (124.5 vs 89 min), higher volume of blood loss (800 vs 500 cc), greater blood transfusion (51 vs 42 pts, at least one unit of blood) and longer hospital stay (10.2 vs 9.1). The morbidity was 2.9 % for the entire series with no difference in the two groups, no mortality was registered. The median follow-up was 27 months and complete resolution of pain was achieved in 39.8 % and amelioration in 49.4 %.

This study is the only one to compare a crucial factor when deciding on resection of hemangiomas, the location of the hemangioma. As seen on previous papers, peripherally located lesions are more amenable for laparoscopic resection [8].

In 2011 a cohort of 74 patients was analyzed and were divided in two groups, for their management, operative (54.1 %) and nonoperative (45.9 %) with a median follow-up of 77.3 months. Abdominal pain was present in 37.8 % of the total cohort and in 62 % of the patients undergoing resection compared to 8.8 % in the nonoperative group. The mean size of the lesions was larger in the operative group (11.9 vs 6 cm). A total of 28 formal liver resections were made and 12 enucleations. This cohort includes a change after year 2000 when 50 % were resected by enucleations, size not being any different for enucleation vs formal resection. The decision was based on the location and the relationship with major vascular and biliary structures. The resection group had more pedicle clamping time than the enucleation subset, the rest of the intraoperative parameter did not show any statistical difference [29].

Minimal Invasive Approach

Minimal invasive techniques include laparoscopic and robotic resection with adjuvant technical instruments that facilitate the procedure [30].

One of the first laparoscopic liver resection series of benign tumors was published in 2003 to asses the feasibility, safety and outcomes in a multicenter setting in 18 centers in Europe. In this series of 87 patients only 13 patients (15 %) corresponded to hemangiomas. The main indication for resection was pain an undetermined nature of atypical features. In the overall series 95 % of the tumors were located in the left lobe or anterior segments. For the hemangiomas almost 60 % of the lesions where localized in segments II and II with a median size of 6 cm with a 10 % conversion to open procedures (bleeding being the major cause, 45 %). The main procedures were wedge resection followed by segmentectomy and major hepatectomy in three patients. Only one conversion was documented for a 13 cm hemangioma [31].

The first paper to describe a series a laparoscopic radiofrequency ablation of hepatic hemangiomas consisted of 27 patients with symptomatic and rapid-growth lesions. A total of 50 liver lesions were treated successfully. There was a median follow up of 21 months without any complications. An intraoperative laparoscopic ultrasound was used prior and at completion of the ablation. An abdominal US and CT were performed 7 days and a moth after RFA. Follow up CT scans were obtained 3–6 months achieving 100 % necrosis and relieve of symptoms in about 85 % of patients [32].

The use of other technology as adjuvant in surgical treatment has been addressed in paper utilizing ultrasonically activated device in 12 patients (8 formal resections, 4 enucleations) was published with no mortality or morbidity [33].

A most recent study from Ho et al. addressed factors determining surgical outcomes. The series includes 61 patients undergoing resection for giant hemangiomas (>4 cm), postoperative complications were associated with larger tumors, symptomatic presentation, increased blood loss and operative time and greater use of intraoperative inflow control. A Pringle maneuver was used in 50.8 %. The patients who had complications the majority had central tumors and required lobectomy. The complication rate was 4 % for enucleation and 19.4 % for resection [34].

A study by Yang et al. aimed to compare an important technical aspect of the surgical resection of hemangiomas, selective hepatic vascular exclusion (SHVE). A total of 273 patients had a hemangioma at least compressing one of the major hepatic veins from. Either SHVE (n = 120) or Pringle maneuver (n = 153) was used. No protocol was used for the selection. There was a significant difference favoring SHVE in the following intraoperative data: Blood loss (600 vs 1,000), blood transfusion units (2 vs 4). Major blood loss of 2000 L only happened in the Pringle group and 85 % in this group did not undergo a blood transfusion compared to 76 % in the Pringle group, also there was no air embolism and no conversion to total hepatic vascular exclusion (7.2 % in the Pringle group). The operative time was longer in the SHVE group (139.8 vs 124.2) The overall complication rate was higher in the Pringle group (30.7 % vs 20.8 %) [35].

More recently Miura et al. described a retrospective review from six major liver centers in the US. A total of 241 patients underwent open surgery (mainly hepatectomy or segmentectomy) but 17 % had a laparoscopic approach, showing the tendency to adopt this technique. A total of 63.2 % of the patient undergoing surgery for symptoms had improvement. Complication rate was 14 % with improvement of symptoms in 63.2 % [36].

A summary of the major published reports describing the various surgical options for hepatic hemangiomas is provided in Table 3.2.

Table 3.2 Hepatic hemangioma treatment

Author (year)	N	Age	Size (cm)	Operation	Complication rate	Other	Study type (QOE[a])
Özden et al. (2000) [22]	42	50	10	Enucleation	12 %		Retrospective cohort-low
Terkivatan et al. (2001) [18]	Total cohort: 208 103: Hemangiomas (25 operative, 78 observation)	48	9.0	Segmentectomy, Lobectomy, wedge resection	24 %	Includes other benign liver tumors	Retrospective cohort-low
Kammula et al. (2001) [23]	Total: 28 Hemangiomas: 10	35	7	Enucleation	10.7 %	Includes other benign liver tumors	Retrospective cohort-low
Reddy et al. (2001) [3]	Total: 130 Hemangiomas: 71 (35 operative, 36 observation)	49	6.9	Segmentectomy, Lobectomy trisegmentectomy	5 % 1.2 % mortality (pt with FNH)	Includes other benign liver tumors One unresectable hemangioma	Retrospective cohort-low
Charny et al. (2001) [25]	Total: 155 Hemangioma :97 (39 operative)	52	12.1	Enucleation. Segmentectomy, lobectomy	21 % (whole series)	Includes other benign liver tumors	Retrospective cohort-low
Popescu et al. (2001) [24]	57	44.2	9	Enucleation, segmentectomy and hepatectomy	10.3		Retrospective cohort-low
Yoon et al. (2003) [5]	115 (52 operative, 63 observation)	52	6	Enucleation, Segmentectomy	25 %	96 % symptom resolution Median ebl 400 cc	Retrospective cohort-low
Descottes et al. (2003) [31]	Total: 87 Hemangiomas: 13	41	6	Laparoscopic resection	5 % (whole series)	Includes other benign liver tumors. One conversion to open	Retrospective cohort-low
Tsai et al. (2003) [14]	43				Symptomatic vs suspicious diagnosis		Retrospective cohort. Low

Liu et al. (2004) [37]	Total : 107 Hemangiomas: 12	43	2.8 (whole series)	Lobectomy,Segmentectomy, wedge	16 %	Includes benign and malignant pathology	Retrospective cohort-low
Kim et al. (2004) [17]	Total: 71 Hemangioma: 21	41	NA	Lobectomy, wedge segementectomy	27 % (whole series)		Retrospective cohort-low
Lerner et al. (2004) [31]	52 (27 lobectomy, 25 enucleation)	48	10.9	Enucleation vs Lobectomy	27 %	Only giant hemangiomas, compared resection vs enucleation	Case series
Hamaloglu et al. (2005) [27]	22	46	9	Hepatectomy vs enucleation	14.2	Only giant hemangiomas compared enucleation vs resection	
Herman et al. (2005) [19]	249 (only 8 underwent surgery)	49	3.7	Lobectomy, segmentectomy	None	Surgical treatment granted to lesions >14 cm	Retrospective cohort-low
Fan (2005)	27	41	5.5	Laparoscopic RFA (50 lesions treated)	None	Complete necrosis achieved in 100 %	Retrospective cohort-low
Ibrahim et al. (2007) [38]	Total: 84 Hemangiomas: 46	43.6	8.2	Lobectomy, segmentectomy, wedge	8.3 (whole series)	Included patients with Hep-B	Retrospective cohort-low
Erdogan et al. et al. (2007) [20]	34 (14 operative)	48.5	12.9	Bisegmentectomy, lobectomy, segmentectomy	21 %		Retrospective cohort-low
Singh et al. (2007) [28]	21	42.5	9.5	Enucleation vs Hepatectomy	23 % (all in the resected group		
Belli et al. (2009) [33]	180 (12 surgical treatment	NA	NA	Enucleation		Enucleation using ultrasonically activated device in 4 cases	Retrospective cohort-low

(continued)

Table 3.2 (continued)

Author (year)	N	Age	Size (cm)	Operation	Complication rate	Other	Study type (QOE[a])
Fu Xiao-Hui et al. (2009) [8]	172 (96 peripheral, 76 central)	46/42	10/11	Enucleation	2.6	Centrally vs peripherally, impact of location	Retrospective cohort-low
Schnelldorfer et al. (2010) [6]	289 (233 non-operative, 56-operative)	51	8.4	Partial hepatectomy/enucleation/RFA	7.1 %		Retrospective cohort-low
Giuliante et al. (2011) [29]	74 (34 non-operative, 40 op	46.3	**6/11.9**	Partial hepatectomy/enucleation	10 %		Retrospective cohort-low
Ho et al (2012) [34]	61	47.3	10	Enucleation/lobectomy	13.1 %	Only giant hemangiomas	Retrospective cohort-low
Yedibela et al. (2013) [21]	246 (103 operative, 143 non operative)	52	9.1	hepatectomy, segmentectomy	17 %		
Yang Y et al. (2014) [35]	273	45/41	14.2/12.9	Lobectomy/Segmentectomy	26 %, 1.3 % mortality	Compares selective vascular exclusion vs Pringle maneuver	Retrospective cohort-low
Miura et al. (2014) [36]	241	46	8.5	Enucleation/hepatectomy/segmentectomy-	5.7 %, 0.8 % mortality		Retrospective cohort-low

[a]Quality of evidence

Recommendations

- The indication for the resection of hepatic hemangiomas has to be based on symptoms, suspicion of malignancy or growth, although no size increment or specific time interval is known (Evidence quality Moderate, strong recommendation)
- When feasible, enucleation is the method of choice to allow preservation of parenchyma, decreased blood loss and need for outflow control (Evidence quality Moderate, strong recommendation)
- Laparoscopic resection of hemangiomas is a safe procedure when patients are appropriately selected and the procedure is performed by an experienced surgeon. (Evidence quality low: weak recommendation)
- Alternative procedures like Radiation, Chemotherapy and TAE should be used as second line agents or for palliation purposes (Evidence quality low: weak recommendation)

References

1. Iwatzuki S, Starzl TE. Personal experience with 411 hepatic resections. Ann Surg. 1988;208:421–34.
2. Mortele KJ, Ros PR. Benign liver neoplasms. Clin Liver Dis. 2002;6:119–45.
3. Reddy KR, Kligerman S, Levi J, Livingstone A, Molina E, Franceschi D. Benign and solid tumors of the liver: relationship to sex, age, size of tumors and outcomes. Ann Surg. 2001;67:173–8.
4. Toro A, Mahfouz AE, Ardiri A, Malaguarnera M, Malaguarnera G, Loria F, Bertino G, Di Carlo I. What is changing in indications and treatment of hepatic hemangioma. A review. Ann Hepatol. 2014;13(4):327–39.
5. Yoon SS, Charny CK, Fong Y, Jarngin WR, Schwartz LH, Blumgart LH, DeMAtteo RP. Diagnosis, management, and outcomes of 115 patients with hepatic hemangioma. Am Coll Surg. 2003;3:392–402.
6. Schnelldorfer T, Ware AL, Smoot R, Schleck CD, Harmsen WS, Nagorney DM. Management of giant hemangioma of the liver: resection versus observation. Am Coll Surg. 2010;211(6):724–30.
7. Alper A, Ariogul O, Emre A, et al. Treatment of liver hemangiomas by enucleation. Arch Surg. 1988;123:660–1.
8. Fu xiao-Hui, Lai Eric Chun Hung, Yao Xiao-Ping, Chu Kai-Jian, Cheng Shu-Qun, Shen Feng, Meng Chao, Lau Wan Yee. Enucleation of liver hemangiomas: is there a difference in surgical outcomes for centrally or peripherally located lesions?. Am J Surg. 2009;198:184–87.
9. Suzuki H, Nimura Y, Kamiya J, Kondo S, Nagino M, Kanai M, Miyachi M. Preoperative transcatheter arterial embolization for giant cavernous hemangioma of the liver with consumption coagulopathy. Am J Gastroenterol. 1997;92:688–91.
10. Soyer P, Levesque M. Hemoperitoneum due to spontaneous rupture of hepatic hemangiomatosis: treatment by super selective arterial embolization and partial hepatectomy. Autralas Radiol. 1995;39:90–2.
11. Gaspar L, Mascarenhas F, da Costa MS, Dias JS, Alfonso JG, Silvestre ME. Radiation therapy in the unresectable cavernous hemangiomas of the liver. Radiother Oncol. 1993;29:45–50.

12. Giavroglou C, Economou H, Ioannidis. Arterial embolization of giant hepatic hemangiomas. Cardiovasc Interv Radiol. 2003;26:92–6.
13. Srivastava DN, Gandhi D, Seith A, Pande GK, Sahni P. Transcatheter arterial embolization in the treatment of symptomatic cavernous hemangiomas of the liver: a prospective study. Abdom Imaging. 2001;26:510–4.
14. Tsai HP, jeng LB, lee WC, Chen M. Clinical experience of hepatic hemangioma undergoing hepatic resection. Dig Dis Sci. 2003;48:916–20.
15. Borgonovo G, Razzeta F, Arezzo A, et al. Giant hemangiomas of the liver: surgical treatment by liver resection. Hepatogastroenterology. 1997;44:231–44.
16. Brouwers MA, Peeters PM, de Jong KP, et al. Surgical management of giant hemangioma of the liver. Br J Surg. 1997;84:314–6.
17. Kim J, Ahmad SA, Lowy AM, Buell JF, Pennington LJ, Moulton JS, et al. An algorithm for the accurate identification of benign liver lesions. Am J Surg. 2004;187:274–9.
18. Terkivaran T, de Wilt JH, de Man RA, van Rijin RR, Zondervan PE, Tilanus HW, et al. Indications and long term outcome of treatments for benign hepatic tumors: a critical appraisal. Arch Surg. 2001;136:1033–8.
19. Herman P, Costa MLV, Machado MA, Ougliese V, D'Albuquerque LA, Machado MC, Gama-Rodroguez JJ, Saad WA. Management of hepatic hemangiomas: a 14 year experience. J Gastrointest Surg. 2005;9:853–9.
20. Erdogan D, Busch OR, can Delden OM, Bennik RJ, ten Kate FJ, Gouma DJ, van Gulik TM. Management of liver hemangioma according to size and symptoms. J Gastroenterol Hepatol. 2007;11:1953–8.
21. Yedibela S, Alibek S, Muller V, Aydin U, Langheinrich M, Lohmuller C, Hohenberger W, Perrakis A. Management of hemangioma of the liver: surgical therapy or observation. World J Surg. 2013;37:1303–12.
22. Ozden I, Emre A, Alper A, et al. Long term results of surgery for liver hemangiomas. Arch Surg. 2000;135:978–81.
23. Kammula US, Buell JF, Labow DM, Rosen S, Millis JM, Posner MC. Surgical management of benign tumors of the liver. Int J Cancer. 2001;30(3):141–6.
24. Popescu I, Ciurea S, Brasoveaunu V, Hrehoret D, Boeti P, Georgecu S, Tulbure D. Liver hemangioma revisited: current surgical indications, technical aspects, results. Hepatogastroenterology. 2001;48(39):770–6.
25. Charny CK, Jarnagin WR, Schwartz LH, Fomeyer HS, De Matteo RP, Fong Y, et al. Management of 155 patients with benign liver tumors. Br J Surg. 2001;88:808–13.
26. Lerner SM, Hiatt Jr, Salamandra J, Chen PW, Farmer DG, Ghobrial RM, Busuttil RW. Giant cavernous liver hemangiomas: effect of operative approach on outcome. Arch Surg. 2004;139:818–21.
27. Hamaloglu E, Altun H, Ozdemir A, Ozenc A. Giant liver hemangioma: therapy by enucleation or liver resection. World J Surg. 2005;29:890–3.
28. Singh RK, Kapoor S, Sahni P, Chattapadhyay T. Giant haemangioma of the liver: is enucleation better than resection? Ann R Coll Surg Engl. 2007;89:490–3.
29. Giulainte F, Ardito F, Vellone M, Giordano M, Giuseppina R, Piccoli M, Giovannini I, Chiarla C, Nuzzo G. Am J Surg. 2011;201(6):741–8.
30. Giuliannotti PC, Adde P, Bianco FM. Robotic right hepatectomy for giant hemangioma in a Jehovah's Witness. J Hepato-Biliary-Pancreat Sci. 2011;18:112–8.
31. Descottes B, Glineur D, Lachachi F, Valleix D, Paineau J, et al. Laparoscopic liver resection of benign liver tumors. Surg Endosc. 2003;17:23–0.
32. Fan R-H, Chai F-L, He G-X, Wei L-X, Li R-Z, Wan W-X, Bai M-D, Zhu W-K, Cao M-L, Li H-M, Yan S-Z. Laparoscopic radiofrequency ablation of hepatic cavernous hemangioma-A preliminary experience with 27 patient. Surg Endosc. 2006;20:281–5.
33. Belli G, D'Agostino A, Fantini C, Cioffi L, Belli A, Limongelli P, Russo G. Surgical treatment of giant liver hemangiomas by enucleation using an ultrasonically activated device (USAD). Hepatogastroenterology. 2009;56(89):236–9.

34. Ho, Hui-Yu, Wu Tsung-Han, Yu Ming Chin, Lee Wei-Chen, Chao Tzu-Cjieh, Chen Miin-Fu. Surgical management of giant hepatic hemangiomas: complications and review of literature. Chang Gung Med J. 2012;35(1):70–78.
35. Yang Y, Zhao LH, Fu SY, Lau WY, Lai EC, Gu FM, Wang ZG, Zhou WP. Selective vascular exclusion versus pringle maneuver in partial hepatectomy for liver hemangioma compressing or involving the major hepatic veins. Am Surg. 2014;80(30):236–40.
36. Miura JT, Amini A, Schmocker R, Nichols S, Sukato D, Winslow ER, Spolverato G. Ejaz A, Squires MH, Kooby DA, Maithel SK, Li A, Wu M-C, Sarmiento JM, Bloomston M, Christians KK, Johnston FM, Tsai S, Turaga KK, Tsung A, Pawlik TM, Gamblin TC. Surgical managements of hepatic hemangiomas: a multi-institutional experience. HPB (Oxford). 2014 Oct;16(10):924–8.
37. Liu CL, Fan ST, Lo CM, Chan SC, Tso WK, Ng IO, et al. Hepatic resection for incidentaloma. J Gastrointest Surg. 2004;8:785–93.
38. Ibrahim S, Chen C-L, Shih-Ho W, Lin C-C, Yang C-H, Yong C-C, Jawan B, Cheng Y-F. Liver resection for benign liver tumors: indications and outcomes. Am J Surg. 2007;193:5–9.

Chapter 4
Which Diagnostic Modality is best to Assess Benign Hepatic Tumors?

Stephen Thomas and Aytekin Oto

Abstract Benign hepatic lesions are relatively common in the general population. The majority of these lesions are incidentally detected at imaging and don't pose any risk to the patient. Some of these lesions have characteristic imaging features while others can have atypical imaging features and can pose a diagnostic challenge. Utilizing the proper imaging modality and intravenous contrast agents can help better characterize them and minimize unnecessary workup of these lesions.

Benign hepatic lesions are classified according to their cell of origin. This article discusses common and uncommon benign hepatic tumors, their different imaging features, and the diagnostic modality that can best characterize them.

Keywords Hemangioma • Focal nodular hyperplasia • Hepatocellular adenoma • Biliary hamartoma • Medical imaging • Benign liver lesions

Introduction

There is high prevalence of benign hepatic lesions in the general population. While most of these lesions are usually asymptomatic and incidentally detected, they may pose a clinical dilemma in patients with systemic disease, chronic liver disease or in patients with a malignancy undergoing staging. These lesions may require additional imaging to prove benignity or in some cases may need resection due to their size or risk of hemorrhage. The benign hepatic neoplasms include hemangiomas, which are of mesenchymal origin; focal nodular hyperplasia (FNH), hepatocellular adenoma (HCA), and nodular regenerative hyperplasia (NRH) which are of hepatocellular origin; hepatic cysts, bile duct hamartoma which are of cholangiocellular origin.

S. Thomas (✉) • A. Oto
Department of Radiology, The University of Chicago Medicine,
5841 S. Maryland Avenue, MC 2026, Chicago, IL 60637, USA
e-mail: sthomas@hotmail.com

J.M. Millis, J.B. Matthews (eds.), *Difficult Decisions in Hepatobiliary and Pancreatic Surgery*, Difficult Decisions in Surgery: An Evidence-Based Approach, DOI 10.1007/978-3-319-27365-5_4

Imaging modalities commonly used for non-invasive liver lesion work-up and characterization includes ultrasonography (US), computed tomography (CT), magnetic resonance (MR) imaging. The tumor features being evaluated include their cystic or solid appearance; calcifications, fat and hemorrhage within the lesion; lesion border and capsule. The use of intravenous contrast agents allows evaluation of lesion vascularity, perfusion, hepatocyte function and biliary excretion.

There is a paucity of prospective studies comparing all modalities and their performance in detection and diagnosis of benign hepatic tumors in the literature. Imaging technologies were introduced at different decades with each modality undergoing significant technological advances over time leading to improved lesion conspicuity and characterization. In many cases, studies comparing the imaging findings of a particular modality with lesion histology have not been performed. Comparison with either another modality or following lesion stability over time would be considered the "gold-standard". Modalities such as US, CT and MR have improved lesion detection and characterization with the introduction of intravascular contrast agents, including selective hepatobiliary MR contrast agents, which have improved liver lesion characterization. Sonographic contrast agents have provided additional diagnostic capability to conventional ultrasonography. However, although these are widely available in Europe, their availability is limited in the US.

In this chapter, we will discuss the imaging features of cavernous hemangioma, focal nodular hyperplasia, hepatic adenoma, biliary hamartoma, and provide a preferred modality imaging in difficult cases.

Cavernous Hemangioma

Ultrasonography The 'typical' imaging features of a small hemangioma (<2 cm) on ultrasound is uniform hyperechogenicity (66 %), well defined margin and posterior acoustic enhancement [1]. Between 20 and 40 % (mostly larger lesions) can have an 'atypical' pattern with an echogenic border either as a thick rind or thin rim with a hypoechoic internal echo pattern or an anechoic/cystic pattern (Fig. 4.1) [2, 3]. Hemangiomas detected by ultrasound tend to be stable over time with 82 % having similar imaging characteristics. 18 % can show change in their sonographic appearance and they can also grow in size over the time [4]. The ultrasound appearance of hemangiomas can overlap with those of hepatocellular carcinoma (HCC) and some hypervascular hepatic metastases [5, 6]. As a result, patients with chronic liver disease or with a known or suspected extra-hepatic malignancy should undergo a confirmatory examination such as a contrast enhanced CT or MRI.

Computed Tomography Hemangiomas are well demarcated masses that are hypo-attenuating to liver parenchyma and are iso-attenuating to blood pool on non-contrast CT. Dystrophic calcifications can be present in approximately 10 % of lesions. With contrast administration, hemangiomas have a typical enhancement

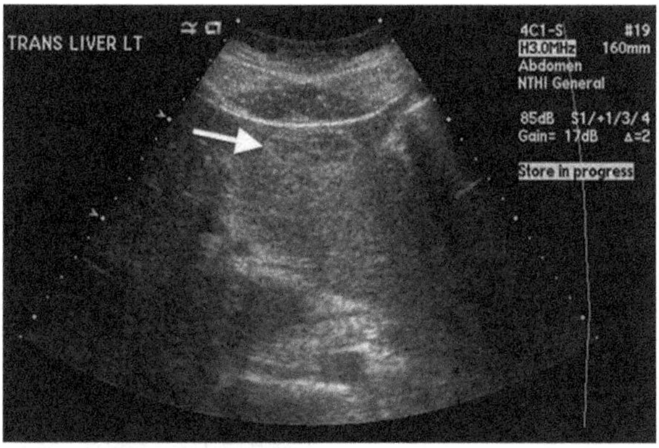

Fig. 4.1 Ultrasound of the liver shows a hypoechoic heterogeneous mass within the left lobe of the liver with a hyperechoic rim (*arrow*)

pattern with peripheral nodular discontinuous enhancement on the arterial and early portal venous phase with gradual centripetal filling on delayed phase images. This enhancement pattern is present in approximately 60 % of all hemangiomas, more commonly present in larger lesions and varies by size: >2 cm (85 %), 1–2 cm (55 %) and <1 cm (23 %) [7]. Smaller lesions can show diffuse hyper-enhancement, a pattern that can be seen in metastasis.

Magnetic Resonance Imaging A typical hemangioma is a well-demarcated homogenous mass that is hypointense on T1-weighted images and hyperintense on T2-weighted images (T2–WI) (Fig. 4.2). The very long T2 relaxation of hemangiomas is useful in distinguishing them from malignant hepatic neoplasms. Hemangiomas demonstrate a relative increase in signal intensity on heavily T2–WI sequences compared to moderately T2–WI sequences. In contradistinction, other solid hepatic masses show a relative decrease in signal intensity on more heavily T2–WI [8–11]. Using a 1.5 Tesla MR unit, MRI can characterize lesions as hemangiomas with an accuracy of 84–97 % based on T2 values, morphologic features and tissue homogeneity [8, 10, 11]. However, hypervascular metastasis from pheochromocytoma, carcinoid, and pancreatic islet-cell tumor can also be hyperintense on T2–WI and is a pitfall of this technique [12, 13]. Therefore, intravenous administered contrast agent is usually required to make a definitive diagnosis of hemangioma. Hemangiomas >4 cm can be heterogeneous in signal due to fibrosis, hemorrhage, thrombosis, hyalinization and cystic degeneration [14, 15].

Use of an intravenous gadolinium based contrast agent (GBCA) results in similar enhancement patterns as CT with arterial peripheral nodular or globular enhancement and progressive centripetal enhancement (Figs. 4.3 and 4.4). This pattern is seen in hemangiomas >2 cm; small lesions <2 cm may have a homogenous enhancement on early phase and may be indistinguishable from small hypervascular metastasis. Metastasis tends to have a continuous rim enhancement on later phases of imaging [12, 13, 16]. Contrast enhanced MRI is able to distinguish hemangioma from metastasis with an accuracy of 96 % [17].

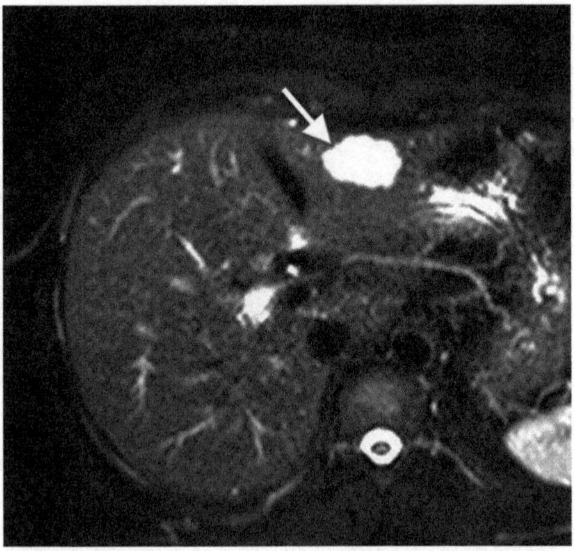

Fig. 4.2 Axial fat saturated T2-weighted MRI shows a well-demarcated T2 hyperintense mass in the left lobe of the liver (*arrow*)

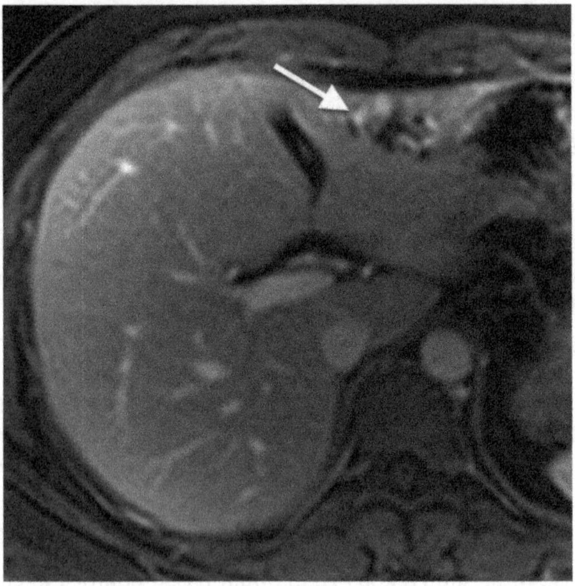

Fig. 4.3 Axial fat saturated T1-FSPGR post contrast MRI shows the classic peripheral nodular discontinuous enhancement on early arterial phase of imaging (*arrow*)

Strategy for Difficult Cases

MRI is the modality of choice in cases where the diagnosis is not certain. The use of heavily weighted T2–WI, multi-phasic contrast sequences with the ability to obtain multiple delayed phases without any ionizing radiation can help confirm the diagnosis of hemangioma. MRI can identify atypical features of hemangiomas,

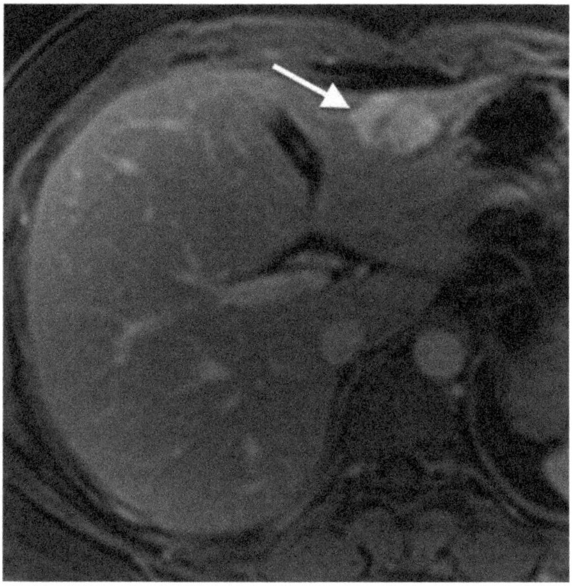

Fig. 4.4 Axial fat saturated T1-FSPGR post contrast MRI shows the progressive centripetal enhancement on portal phase of imaging with the mass filling in and remaining iso-intense to vasculature (*arrow*)

which include incomplete contrast filling, seen in hemangiomas larger than 3 cm due to central scarring. Lesions greater than 5 cm can have "flame shaped" discontinuous peripheral enhancement which may dominate or coexist with the typical nodular enhancement [18]. Hyalinized hemangiomas can be predominately fibrosed with obliterated vascular spaces and may not enhance. They may be only be slightly hyperintense on T2-WI, lack the early enhancement on dynamic contrast enhancement, with slight peripheral enhancement on late phase and may be confidently diagnosed on MR [19].

Focal Nodular Hyperplasia

Ultrasonography FNH are frequently first identified on US as the modality is commonly used to evaluate the liver and gallbladder. However, FNH echotexture can be quite variable. They can appear hyper, hypo, and isoechoic relative to hepatic parenchyma. Isoechoic lesions may only be detected if they deform the hepatic contour. Frequently, FNH are located in the subcapsular area of the liver and may deform the liver contour or rarely may be exophytic. The central scar, which is an important imaging feature, is only present in about 20 % of cases. Gray scale sonography is unable to reliably distinguish FNH from other neoplastic lesions [20].

Computed Tomography Detection and characterization of FNH is done using a tri-phasic contrast enhanced CT. On unenhanced CT, FNH is usually a homogenous isoattenuating or hypoattenuating mass. On arterial phase, FNH has marked arterial

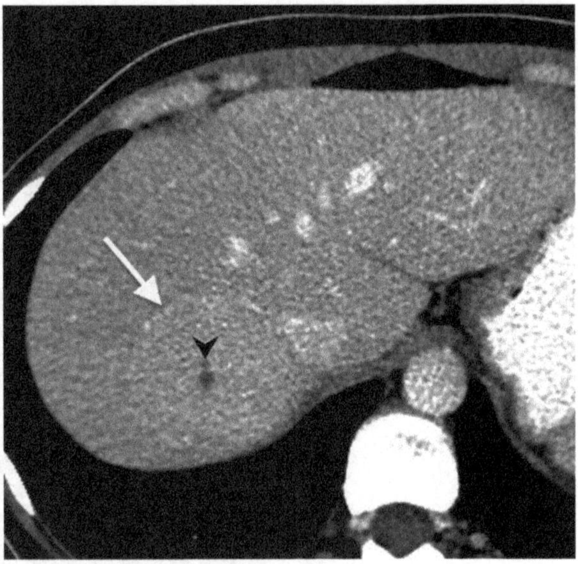

Fig. 4.5 Contrast enhanced CT shows a right hepatic lobe mass that is nearly iso-attenuating to the hepatic parenchyma (*arrow*). The lesion has a small hypo-attenuating central scar (*arrow head*)

enhancement that is homogeneous [20–22]. In about 30 % of cases a visible central scar is present which does not enhance on early phases of imaging and can be very small [20, 23]. In larger lesions, feeding hepatic arteries, small central and septal arteries, and early draining veins can be present [22, 24]. On portal venous and delayed phases, FNHs are iso-attenuating to hepatic parenchyma (Fig. 4.5). Enhancement of the central scar can be seen on delayed phases of imaging when it contains myxomatous stroma [23, 25]. While no prospective studies exist regarding the accuracy of CT to detect and characterize FNH, a small retrospective series (n = 20) showed that CT had a sensitivity of 70 % and specificity of 92 % and led to the correct characterization in 78 % of cases [26]. In a larger series of 86 patients with 99 foci of FNH, CT was able to correctly diagnose FNH in 60.3 % of cases [27].

Magnetic Resonance Imaging On unenhanced MR, FNH has similar characteristics to hepatic parenchyma on T1- and T2-weighted sequences [28]. Atypical features include hyperintense appearance on T1-WI due to steatosis, sinusoidal dilatation, or hemorrhage [28]. The central scar can be present in 25–43 % of lesions and is T1 hypointense and T2 hyperintense (Fig. 4.6) due to presence of vascular channels and bile ductules [29–32].

Using IV GBCA, typically FNH has homogenous arterial enhancement and is isointense to liver on portal venous phase. The central scar can be present in 79 % of FHN and is hyperintense due to enhancement on delayed phase of imaging (Figs. 4.7 and 4.8) [32].

Hepatobiliary contrast agents are unique MR contrast agents in that are taken up by functioning hepatocytes and excreted with bile. Hepatobiliary GBCAs such as

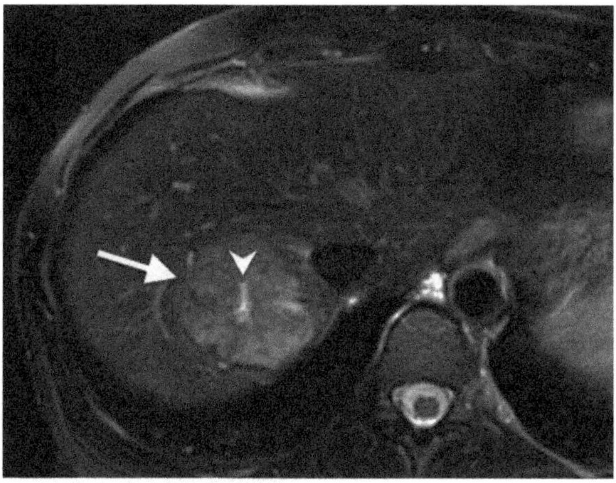

Fig. 4.6 Axial fat suppressed T2 weighted MRI shows a mildly hyperintense mass (*arrow*) with a hyperintense central scar (*arrow head*)

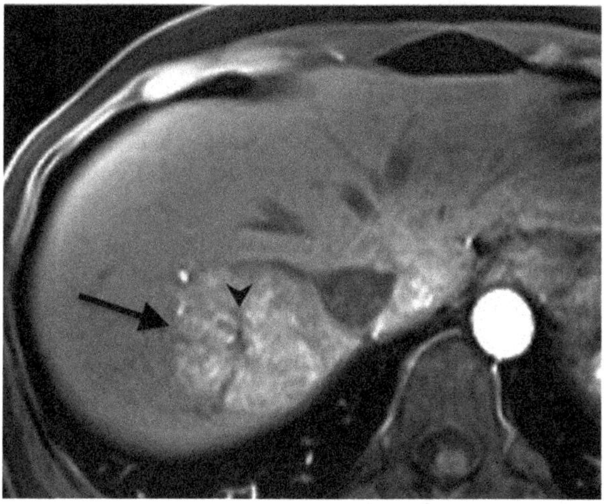

Fig. 4.7 Axial fat saturated T1-FSPGR post contrast MRI shows hyper-enhancement of the mass on arterial phase (*black arrow*). The central scar does not enhance (*arrow head*)

Gd-BOPTA and Gd-EOB-DTPA have properties of an extracellular contrast agent providing dynamic contrast enhancement information and biliary excretion for delayed hepatobiliary imaging performed 20 min after contrast bolus injection. Lesions that contain functioning hepatocytes show contrast uptake. Since FNH contain functioning hepatocytes, on delayed phase of imaging, they are typically hyperintense to isointense to hepatic parenchyma [31, 33].

The sensitivity and specificity of MRI in differentiating FHN from hepatocellular adenoma (HCA) is 96.9 %, and 100 %, and is primarily based on the contrast washout on hepatobiliary phase in hepatic adenomas when using Gd-BOPTA in a prospective study [34]. Using Gd-EOB-DTPA and the hepatobiliary phase the sensitivity to detect FNH was 96 % with a positive predictive value of 96 % when compared to HCA [35].

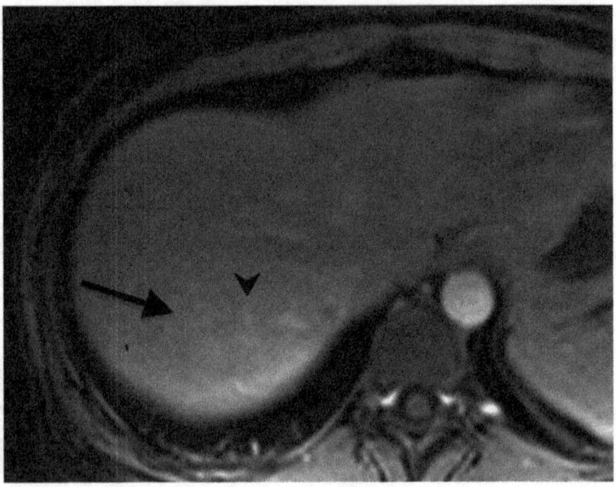

Fig. 4.8 Axial fat saturated T1-FSPGR post contrast MRI shows the mass to be iso-attenuating to the liver on portal venous phase (*black arrow*). The central scar now enhances, characteristic of focal nodular hyperplasia (*arrow head*)

Strategy for Difficult Cases

MRI using a hepatobiliary specific contrast agent may characterize lesions that cannot be otherwise characterized by CT. Atypical FNH lesions may show only mild arterial enhancement, and may be hypointense to liver parenchyma on late dynamic phase. For these lesions adding a hepatobiliary phase and calculating a signal intensity (SI) ratio improves diagnostic yield. Using a cutoff value of 0.87 for the SI ratio during the hepatobiliary phase, the sensitivity and specificity for differentiating FNH from HCA was 92 % and 91 % respectively [36].

Hepatocellular Adenoma

Ultrasonography HCA have a heterogeneous variable echotexture with 80 % having a mixed echogenicity and 20 % purely hypoechoic [37]. In a small study of 27 cases of HCA, the lesions were hypoechoic to hepatic parenchyma in 41 %, 30 % are hyperechoic, 22 % are isoechoic, and 7 % are of mixed echogenicity [21]. The utility of gray scale ultrasound to characterize HCA is limited due the overlap of imaging features with other benign and malignant hepatic lesions.

Computed Tomography HCAs have a variable appearance on unenhanced CT images. They may be hypoattenuating due to the presence of intracellular lipid, old hemorrhage or necrosis, or it may be hyperattenuating from acute hemorrhage or large amounts of glycogen [37]. HCA are sharply marginated – 85 %, nonlobulated – 95 %, sometimes encapsulated – 30 %, and rarely can calcify 5–10 %. Necrosis or hemorrhage can occur in 25 % of lesions [38, 39]. HCAs are almost uniformly (80–100 %) hyperattenuating on hepatic arterial phase and have variable appearance on portal venous phase with 31 % remaining hyperattenuating, 44 %

isoattenuating, and 25 % hypoattenuating [39, 40]. On delayed phase CT, HCAs characteristically are hypoattenuating to liver parenchyma with few (6 %) that are hyperattenuating [39]. The enhancement pattern helps differentiate FNH from HCA, which is important for patient management. HCA however have similar contrast enhancement characteristics as hepatocellular carcinoma (HCC) and differentiation between the lesions can be problematic especially in lesions that have undergone hemorrhage [41].

Magnetic Resonance Imaging HCAs have a variable appearance on MRI as there are sub-types including inflammatory, steatotic or those with β-catenin activation.

The inflammatory subtype accounts for 30–50 % of adenomas. These lesions are mildly hyperintense on T2–WI especially in the periphery of the lesion (Fig. 4.9), and iso to hypointense on T1–WI with heterogeneous signal intensity. There is characteristic T2 hyperintense rim like band termed the atoll sign in the periphery of the lesion that is isointense to surrounding liver toward the center of the lesion can be seen in 43 % of inflammatory HCAs [42].

Inflammatory HCAs are diffusely hyperintense on arterial enhancement persisting into the portal venous and delayed phases (Figs. 4.10 and 4.11). The T2 hyperintensity and persistent enhancement together are 85.2 % sensitive and 87.5 % specific for the diagnosis [43].

The steatotic subtype, shows diffuse signal loss on chemical shift sequence due to homogenous intratumoral fat. These lesions show moderate arterial enhancement not persisting into the portal venous phase [43]. The presence of intratumoral fat is not specific for HCAs as up to 40 % of hepatocellular carcinomas may contain fat [44].

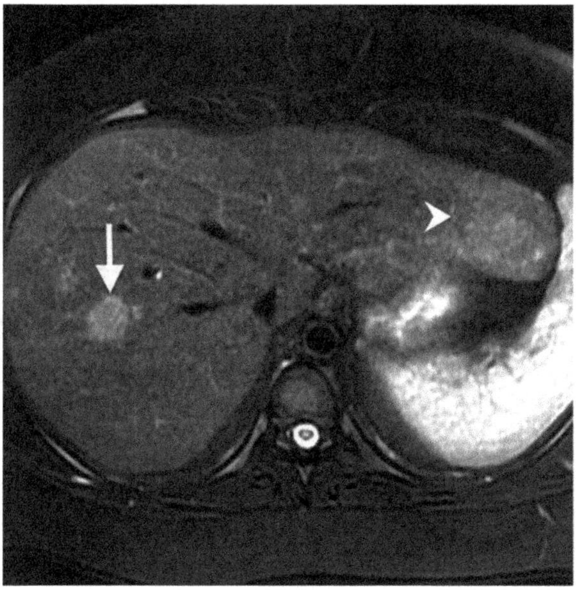

Fig. 4.9 Axial fat suppressed T2 weighted MRI shows a mildly hyperintense mass (*arrow*) in the right lobe of the liver and larger mass in the left lobe of the liver (*arrow head*)

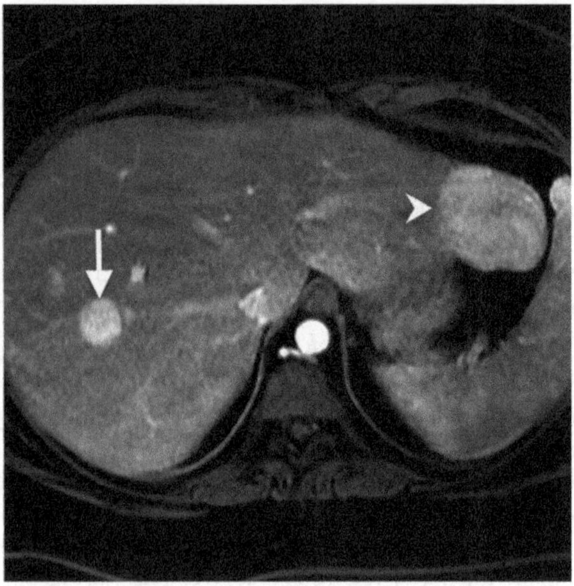

Fig. 4.10 Axial fat saturated T1-FSPGR post contrast MRI shows brisk homogenous enhancement of the right hepatic lobe mass (*arrow*) and the larger left hepatic lobe mass (*arrow head*) during arterial phase of imaging

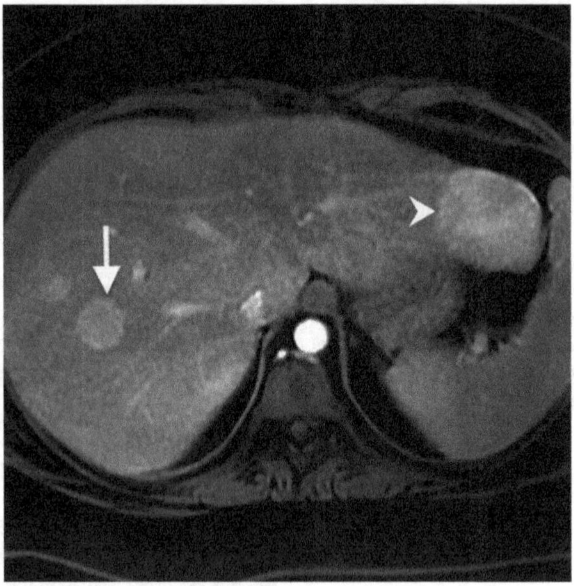

Fig. 4.11 Axial fat saturated T1-FSPGR post contrast MRI shows the right hepatic lobe mass (*arrow*) and the left hepatic lobe mass (*arrow head*) remain hyperintense to liver on portal venous phase

HCAs with β-catenin activation can have non-specific imaging features with strong arterial enhancement and portal venous washout. MRI may not be able to definitively characterize these lesions as the imaging features can overlap with HCC [43]. HCAs with activated β-catenin present a high risk of malignant transformation [45].

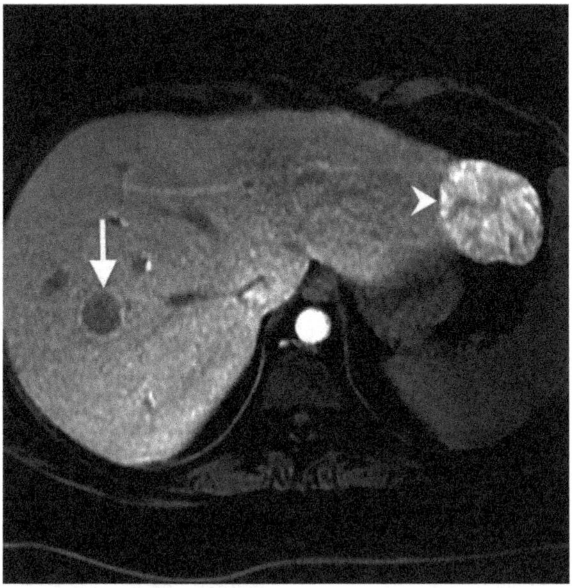

Fig. 4.12 Axial fat saturated T1-FSPGR post contrast MRI performed with a hepatobiliary contrast agent and imaged during the hepatobiliary phase (20 min after injection) shows no retention of contrast in the right hepatic lobe mass compatible with a hepatic adenoma (*arrow*). The left hepatic lobe mass retains contrast and is compatible with focal nodular hyperplasia (*arrow head*)

Strategy for Difficult Cases

Since HCAs can have several subtypes, undergo hemorrhage, and have variable imaging features on conventional MRI, they may not be easily discriminated from FNHs. Using hepatobiliary contrast agents on MR will improve the diagnostic performance of MRI. Delayed hepatobiliary phase images can be used to separate HCA from FNH with the former appearing hypointense to liver (Fig. 4.12) [34]. Follow-up studies have shown that up to 71 % of inflammatory HCAs can have areas of iso- or hyperintensity to the surrounding liver in the hepatocyte phase [46].

Biliary Hamartoma

Ultrasonography Biliary hamartomas have a variable appearance on ultrasound. They usually present as tiny hypoechoic or hyperechoic foci measuring less that 10 mm scattered through out the liver and may be associated with comet-tail artifacts (Fig. 4.13) [47, 48]. Their variable appearance on sonography may be mistaken for metastasis.

Computed Tomography At unenhanced CT, biliary hamartomas appear as well-marginated hypo or iso-attenuating lesions of nearly uniform size that do not enhance on contrast administration (Fig. 4.14) [48]. Their imaging features are important to recognize as they may simulate metastases or microabscesses [49, 50].

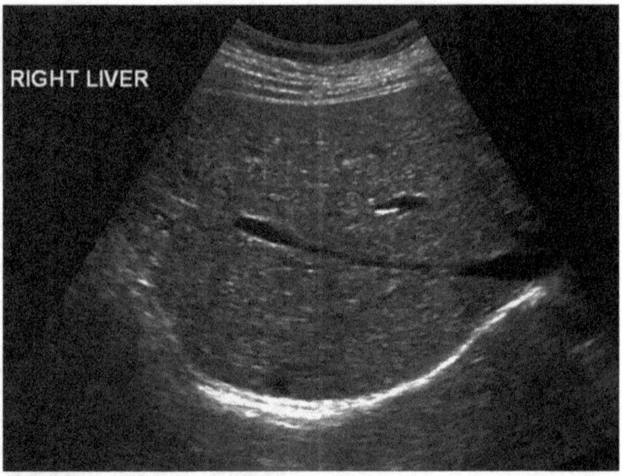

Fig. 4.13 Ultrasound of the liver shows increased parenchymal echogenicity of the right lobe with multiple small echogenic interfaces

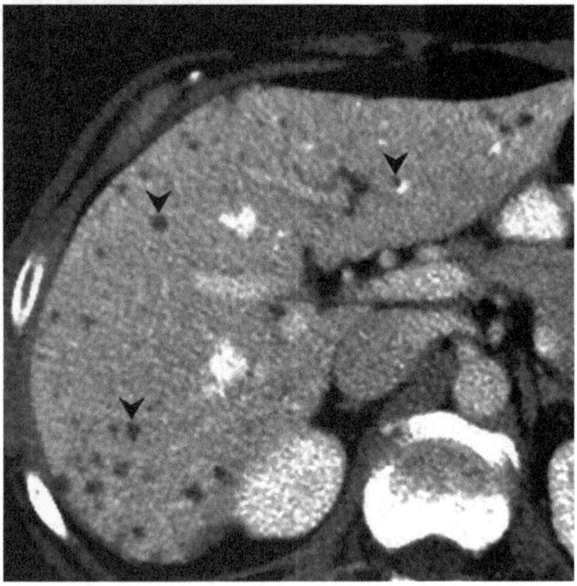

Fig. 4.14 Contrast enhanced CT shows multiple small nearly uniformly hypo-attenuating lesions in the liver (*arrow heads*). No clear enhancing wall is seen

Magnetic Resonance Imaging Biliary hamartomas have a characteristic appearance at MRI. They are hypointense on T1–WI, well defined and hyper-intense on T2–WI (Fig. 4.15). With GBCA they do not have central enhancement but may have a thin rim of peripheral enhancement, which may be from compressed hepatic parenchyma (Fig. 4.16) [51].

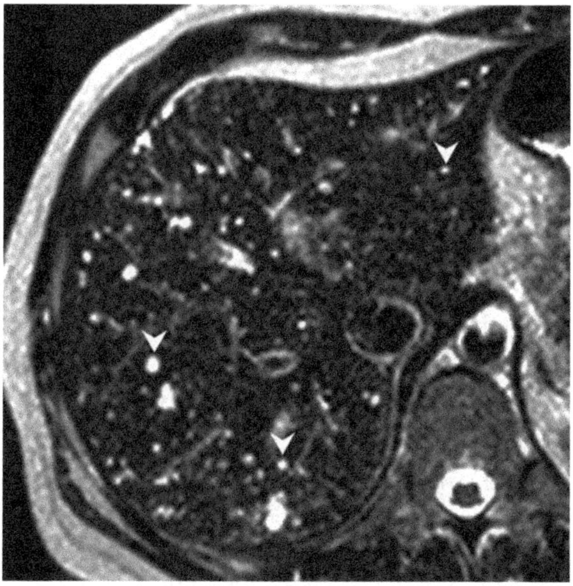

Fig. 4.15 Axial T2 weighted MRI shows multiple small nearly uniformly sized T2 hyperintense lesions (*arrow heads*)

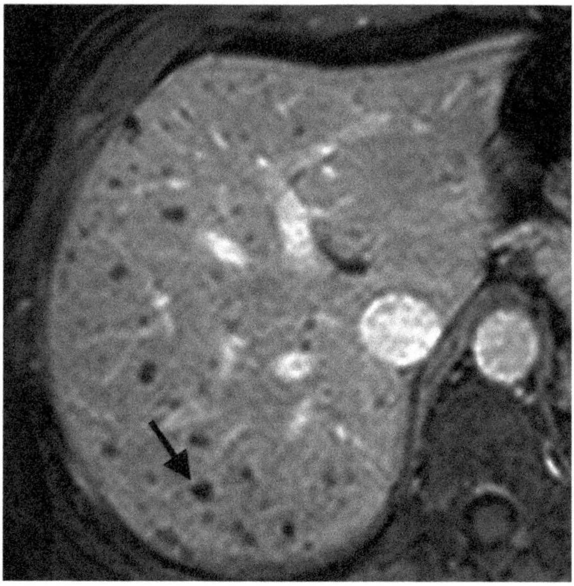

Fig. 4.16 Axial fat saturated T1-FSPGR post contrast MRI shows multiple small nearly uniformly sized hypo-intense lesions in the liver. Some have a subtle perceivable wall (*arrow*), which represents compressed hepatic parenchyma

Conclusion

Focal liver lesions are commonly encountered during routine imaging. While US and CT are able to detect and characterize many lesions, MR imaging with hepatocyte specific contrast agents can be used for difficult lesions an may be able to definitively characterize liver lesions so as to avoid biopsy or surgery. However, for lesions that do not have typical imaging features or those that are complicated by hemorrhage may have to undergo biopsy for accurate diagnosis.

References

1. Mirk P, Rubaltelli L, Bazzocchi M, et al. Ultrasonographic patterns in hepatic hemangiomas. J Clin Ultrasound. 1982;10:373–8.
2. Moody AR, Wilson SR. Atypical hepatic hemangioma: a suggestive sonographic morphology. Radiology. 1993;188:413–7.
3. Ricci OE, Fanfani S, Calabro A, et al. Diagnostic approach to hepatic hemangiomas detected by ultrasound. Hepatogastroenterology. 1985;32:53–6.
4. Gibney RG, Hendin AP, Cooperberg PL. Sonographically detected hepatic hemangiomas: absence of change over time. AJR Am J Roentgenol. 1987;149:953–7.
5. Leifer DM, Middleton WD, Teefey SA, Menias CO, Leahy JR. Follow-up of patients at low risk for hepatic malignancy with a characteristic hemangioma at US. Radiology. 2000;214:167–72.
6. Rapaccini GL, Pompili M, Caturelli E, et al. Hepatocellular carcinomas <2 cm in diameter complicating cirrhosis: ultrasound and clinical features in 153 consecutive patients. Liver Int. 2004;24:124–30.
7. Yun EJ, Choi BI, Han JK, et al. Hepatic hemangioma: contrast-enhancement pattern during the arterial and portal venous phases of spiral CT. Abdom Imaging. 1999;24:262–6.
8. McFarland EG, Mayo-Smith WW, Saini S, Hahn PF, Goldberg MA, Lee MJ. Hepatic hemangiomas and malignant tumors: improved differentiation with heavily T2-weighted conventional spin-echo MR imaging. Radiology. 1994;193:43–7.
9. Ohtomo K, Itai Y, Furui S, Yashiro N, Yoshikawa K, Iio M. Hepatic tumors: differentiation by transverse relaxation time (T2) of magnetic resonance imaging. Radiology. 1985;155:421–3.
10. Ohtomo K, Itai Y, Yoshikawa K, Kokubo T, Iio M. Hepatocellular carcinoma and cavernous hemangioma: differentiation with MR imaging. Efficacy of T2 values at 0.35 and 1.5 T. Radiology. 1988;168:621–3.
11. Stark DD, Felder RC, Wittenberg J, et al. Magnetic resonance imaging of cavernous hemangioma of the liver: tissue-specific characterization. AJR Am J Roentgenol. 1985;145:213–22.
12. Berger JF, Laissy JP, Limot O, et al. Differentiation between multiple liver hemangiomas and liver metastases of gastrinomas: value of enhanced MRI. J Comput Assist Tomogr. 1996;20:349–55.
13. Soyer P, Gueye C, Somveille E, Laissy JP, Scherrer A. MR diagnosis of hepatic metastases from neuroendocrine tumors versus hemangiomas: relative merits of dynamic gadolinium chelate-enhanced gradient-recalled echo and unenhanced spin-echo images. AJR Am J Roentgenol. 1995;165:1407–13.
14. Choi BI, Han MC, Park JH, Kim SH, Han MH, Kim CW. Giant cavernous hemangioma of the liver: CT and MR imaging in 10 cases. AJR Am J Roentgenol. 1989;152:1221–6.
15. Ros PR, Lubbers PR, Olmsted WW, Morillo G. Hemangioma of the liver: heterogeneous appearance on T2-weighted images. AJR Am J Roentgenol. 1987;149:1167–70.
16. Whitney WS, Herfkens RJ, Jeffrey RB, et al. Dynamic breath-hold multiplanar spoiled gradient-recalled MR imaging with gadolinium enhancement for differentiating hepatic hemangiomas from malignancies at 1.5 T. Radiology. 1993;189:863–70.
17. Mitchell DG, Saini S, Weinreb J, et al. Hepatic metastases and cavernous hemangiomas: distinction with standard- and triple-dose gadoteridol-enhanced MR imaging. Radiology. 1994;193:49–57.

18. Danet IM, Semelka RC, Braga L, Armao D, Woosley JT. Giant hemangioma of the liver: MR imaging characteristics in 24 patients. Magn Reson Imaging. 2003;21:95–101.
19. Cheng HC, Tsai SH, Chiang JH, Chang CY. Hyalinized liver hemangioma mimicking malignant tumor at MR imaging. AJR Am J Roentgenol. 1995;165:1016–7.
20. Shamsi K, De Schepper A, Degryse H, Deckers F. Focal nodular hyperplasia of the liver: radiologic findings. Abdom Imaging. 1993;18:32–8.
21. Mathieu D, Bruneton JN, Drouillard J, Pointreau CC, Vasile N. Hepatic adenomas and focal nodular hyperplasia: dynamic CT study. Radiology. 1986;160:53–8.
22. Choi CS, Freeny PC. Triphasic helical CT of hepatic focal nodular hyperplasia: incidence of atypical findings. AJR Am J Roentgenol. 1998;170:391–5.
23. Carlson SK, Johnson CD, Bender CE, Welch TJ. CT of focal nodular hyperplasia of the liver. AJR Am J Roentgenol. 2000;174:705–12.
24. Brancatelli G, Federle MP, Katyal S, Kapoor V. Hemodynamic characterization of focal nodular hyperplasia using three-dimensional volume-rendered multidetector CT angiography. AJR Am J Roentgenol. 2002;179:81–5.
25. Mortele KJ, Praet M, Van Vlierberghe H, Kunnen M, Ros PR. CT and MR imaging findings in focal nodular hyperplasia of the liver: radiologic-pathologic correlation. AJR Am J Roentgenol. 2000;175:687–92.
26. Procacci C, Fugazzola C, Cinquino M, et al. Contribution of CT to characterization of focal nodular hyperplasia of the liver. Gastrointest Radiol. 1992;17:63–73.
27. Shen YH, Fan J, Wu ZQ, et al. Focal nodular hyperplasia of the liver in 86 patients. Hepatobiliary Pancreat Dis Int. 2007;6:52–7.
28. Ferlicot S, Kobeiter H, Tran Van Nhieu J, et al. MRI of atypical focal nodular hyperplasia of the liver: radiology-pathology correlation. AJR Am J Roentgenol. 2004;182:1227–31.
29. Vilgrain V, Flejou JF, Arrive L, et al. Focal nodular hyperplasia of the liver: MR imaging and pathologic correlation in 37 patients. Radiology. 1992;184:699–703.
30. Rummeny E, Weissleder R, Sironi S, et al. Central scars in primary liver tumors: MR features, specificity, and pathologic correlation. Radiology. 1989;171:323–6.
31. Grazioli L, Morana G, Federle MP, et al. Focal nodular hyperplasia: morphologic and functional information from MR imaging with gadobenate dimeglumine. Radiology. 2001;221:731–9.
32. Mahfouz AE, Hamm B, Taupitz M, Wolf KJ. Hypervascular liver lesions: differentiation of focal nodular hyperplasia from malignant tumors with dynamic gadolinium-enhanced MR imaging. Radiology. 1993;186:133–8.
33. Huppertz A, Haraida S, Kraus A, et al. Enhancement of focal liver lesions at gadoxetic acid-enhanced MR imaging: correlation with histopathologic findings and spiral CT – initial observations. Radiology. 2005;234:468–78.
34. Grazioli L, Morana G, Kirchin MA, Schneider G. Accurate differentiation of focal nodular hyperplasia from hepatic adenoma at gadobenate dimeglumine-enhanced MR imaging: prospective study. Radiology. 2005;236:166–77.
35. Bieze M, van den Esschert JW, Nio CY, et al. Diagnostic accuracy of MRI in differentiating hepatocellular adenoma from focal nodular hyperplasia: prospective study of the additional value of gadoxetate disodium. AJR Am J Roentgenol. 2012;199:26–34.
36. Grazioli L, Bondioni MP, Haradome H, et al. Hepatocellular adenoma and focal nodular hyperplasia: value of gadoxetic acid-enhanced MR imaging in differential diagnosis. Radiology. 2012;262:520–9.
37. Welch TJ, Sheedy 2nd PF, Johnson CM, et al. Focal nodular hyperplasia and hepatic adenoma: comparison of angiography, CT, US, and scintigraphy. Radiology. 1985;156:593–5.
38. Grazioli L, Federle MP, Ichikawa T, Balzano E, Nalesnik M, Madariaga J. Liver adenomatosis: clinical, histopathologic, and imaging findings in 15 patients. Radiology. 2000;216:395–402.
39. Ichikawa T, Federle MP, Grazioli L, Nalesnik M. Hepatocellular adenoma: multiphasic CT and histopathologic findings in 25 patients. Radiology. 2000;214:861–8.

40. Grazioli L, Federle MP, Brancatelli G, Ichikawa T, Olivetti L, Blachar A. Hepatic adenomas: imaging and pathologic findings. Radiographics. 2001;21:877–92; discussion 892–874.
41. Hussain SM, van den Bos IC, Dwarkasing RS, Kuiper JW, den Hollander J. Hepatocellular adenoma: findings at state-of-the-art magnetic resonance imaging, ultrasound, computed tomography and pathologic analysis. Eur Radiol. 2006;16:1873–86.
42. van Aalten SM, Thomeer MG, Terkivatan T, et al. Hepatocellular adenomas: correlation of MR imaging findings with pathologic subtype classification. Radiology. 2011;261:172–81.
43. Laumonier H, Bioulac-Sage P, Laurent C, Zucman-Rossi J, Balabaud C, Trillaud H. Hepatocellular adenomas: magnetic resonance imaging features as a function of molecular pathological classification. Hepatology. 2008;48:808–18.
44. Paulson EK, McClellan JS, Washington K, Spritzer CE, Meyers WC, Baker ME. Hepatic adenoma: MR characteristics and correlation with pathologic findings. AJR Am J Roentgenol. 1994;163:113–6.
45. Bioulac-Sage P, Rebouissou S, Thomas C, et al. Hepatocellular adenoma subtype classification using molecular markers and immunohistochemistry. Hepatology. 2007;46:740–8.
46. Thomeer MG, Willemssen FE, Biermann KK, et al. MRI features of inflammatory hepatocellular adenomas on hepatocyte phase imaging with liver-specific contrast agents. J Magn Reson Imaging. 2014;39:1259–64.
47. Zheng RQ, Zhang B, Kudo M, Onda H, Inoue T. Imaging findings of biliary hamartomas. World J Gastroenterol. 2005;11:6354–9.
48. Lev-Toaff AS, Bach AM, Wechsler RJ, Hilpert PL, Gatalica Z, Rubin R. The radiologic and pathologic spectrum of biliary hamartomas. AJR Am J Roentgenol. 1995;165:309–13.
49. Sada PN, Ramakrishna B. Computed tomography of von Meyenburg complex simulating micro-abscesses. Australas Radiol. 1994;38:225–6.
50. Eisenberg D, Hurwitz L, Yu AC. CT and sonography of multiple bile-duct hamartomas simulating malignant liver disease (case report). AJR Am J Roentgenol. 1986;147:279–80.
51. Semelka RC, Hussain SM, Marcos HB, Woosley JT. Biliary hamartomas: solitary and multiple lesions shown on current MR techniques including gadolinium enhancement. J Magn Reson Imaging. 1999;10:196–201.

Chapter 5
Cystic Diseases of the Liver

John F. Renz

Abstract This manuscript provides a concise surgical review of cystic diseases of the liver. Attention is paid to diagnosis, pre-surgical evaluation, surgical techniques, including laparoscopy, and post-surgical care of the patient with cystic disease of the liver.

Keywords Liver cyst • Liver surgery • Hepatobiliary surgery • Cystic disease of the liver • Cystadenoma

Introduction

Cystic disease of the liver is a frequent indication for surgical consultation as modern cross-sectional imaging identifies some form of hepatic cystic disease in as high as 18 % of studies [1]. A myriad of conditions manifest cystic disease of the liver with an equally broad spectrum of prognoses; however, the overall management of cystic diseases within the liver is straightforward provided one adheres to several guiding principles. Furthermore, the widespread application of laparoscopy and intra-operative ultrasound has significantly improved therapeutic options for patients and surgeons.

Surgical Considerations

The approach to cystic diseases of the liver begins with recognition of four broad classifications based upon etiology. These categories are: congenital, neoplastic, traumatic, and infectious. Congenital cysts are, by far, the most prevalent and arise from a defect in production of bile duct basement membrane resulting in cystic

J.F. Renz (✉)
University of Chicago Medicine, 5841 S. Maryland,
Room J517 MC5027, Chicago, IL 60637, USA
e-mail: jrenz@surgery.bsd.uchicago.edu

J.M. Millis, J.B. Matthews (eds.), *Difficult Decisions in Hepatobiliary and Pancreatic Surgery*, Difficult Decisions in Surgery: An Evidence-Based Approach, DOI 10.1007/978-3-319-27365-5_5

malformation of intrahepatic bile ducts [2, 3]. These include simple cysts and adult polycystic liver disease (APLD) [3]. Neoplastic cysts may be primary or metastatic. Cystadenoma and cystadenocarcinoma may originate within the liver while cystadenocarcinomas from the ovary and pancreas often metastasize to the liver. Traumatic cysts form secondary to liver injury such as disruption of an intrahepatic bile duct or subcapsular hematoma. Infectious cysts include pyogenic liver abscess, hydatid disease, and amoebic abscesses as well as extra-hepatic cysts secondary to retained gallstones from a previous cholecystectomy [2]. Formulating a robust working hypothesis as to the origin of the cyst is essential to anticipating the optimal surgical therapy.

A second principle in approaching cystic liver disease is meticulous analysis of radiologic imaging. Often, patients presenting for surgical consultation have had diagnostic or potentially therapeutic procedures previously performed. These not only include interventional radiologic procedures such as biopsy, needle aspiration, and sclerotherapy but previous surgical fenestration. Complications such as bleeding or infection from these procedures can significantly alter subsequent imaging and the occurrence of a complication may not have been clinically recognized. In situations where any previous procedure has been performed upon a cyst, every effort should be made to obtain as much possible imaging, particularly cross-sectional imaging, that was performed prior to the intervention. If surgery is being entertained, recent cross sectional imaging (computed tomography or magnetic resonance imaging) will facilitate accurate cyst classification and symptom correlation while reducing the chance of an unanticipated change in surgical plan during surgery.

Cross sectional imaging analysis focuses upon four specific areas: number of cysts, cyst content, cyst wall architecture, and cyst location. Cysts may be single or multiple with a homogenous or heterogenous cyst content. The cyst wall architecture may be uniform in thickness or irregular in thickness with projections of the cyst wall into the lumen or septations. Lastly, does the cyst location support the patient's symptoms? Appreciation of multiple closely approximated cysts, heterogeneous cyst content without prior intervention, or any cyst wall architecture that is not completely uniform are indications for further investigation utilizing intra-operative ultrasound and a surgical approach that requires more than simple fenestration.

Correlation of cyst location to the patient's symptoms is particularly important in the management of congenital cysts. Common presenting symptoms include abdominal pain, epigastric bloating, early satiety, and dyspepsia [2]. Large size (>6 cm), pericapsular or ventral location, and heterogenous content suggesting previous hemorrhage are typically associated with abdominal pain while epigastric bloating, early satiety, and dyspepsia are associated with predominantly left lobe, dorsally located lesions may be symptomatic at a smaller size. Biliary disease, gastro-esophageal reflux disease, and other common indications of abdominal pain should be excluded prior to offering surgery for abdominal pain secondary to congenital cysts [2].

Congenital Cysts

Congenital cysts include simple cysts and APLD. Simple cysts are single or multiply scattered, uniform, thin-walled masses with a homogenous, low-viscosity cyst content. Histologically, the cyst lining is simple cuboidal or columnar epithelium that produces a serous fluid. Large cysts are more frequent in women with a female to male ratio of 4:1 and are uncommon under the age of 40 years. The average reported size of simple cysts is 3 cm and most are asymptomatic. Simple cysts on occasion may rupture into the abdominal cavity causing transient peritoneal discomfort but hemorrhagic rupture is exceedingly rare [2, 3].

Simple cysts are ideally approached laparoscopically. The cyst should be carefully examined utilizing intra-operative ultrasound to confirm a uniform thin lining with no papillary projections into the cyst lumen or hepatic parenchyma. The cyst wall typically demonstrates sharp sonographic echo demarcation secondary to the luminal fluid interface and compressed hepatic parenchyma [4]. Simple cyst fluid is clear and serous; however, a previous hemorrhage may produce a heterogeneous mix. In either case, the cyst should be aspirated and a generous excisional biopsy obtained for histologic evaluation. If a cystadenoma is excluded, the fenestration may proceed to wide excision of the cyst wall. Intra-operative ultrasound can be intermittently utilized to maximize wall excision without encountering major vascular structures. Argon beam coagulation of the remnant epithelial surface can be employed to destroy remaining biliary epithelia and recruit an inflammatory response but is not mandatory. When operating for a presumed simple cyst, if a cystadenoma cannot be excluded or the cyst content is overtly bilious, fenestration should be abandoned for hepatic resection. If there is a potential cystadenoma, the resection should include at least a 0.5 cm margin with pathologic confirmation. In the scenario of overtly bilious cyst fluid, the resection is indicated to completely remove the cyst lining so as to expose biliary radicle(s) for repair.

Percutaneous therapies for the management of simple cysts including aspiration and sclerotherapy are available. Aspiration as a diagnostic maneuver to assess symptom alleviation is potentially valuable but should not be considered definitive therapy due to a high recurrence rate [5]. Notably, aspiration will change the radiologic appearance of the cyst. Sclerotherapy may be applied in patients who are poor surgical candidates but its efficacy is lower than surgical fenestration [6].

APLD is most often identified in the presence of polycystic kidney disease and results from a mutation in the PKD-1 or PKD-2 gene. A rare mutant of the protein kinase C gene, 80 K-H, can manifest as isolated APLD. Cysts appear similar to simple cysts except they are far more numerous, generally smaller in size, bilobar in distribution, and are associated with numerous microcysts in their vicinity. A female predominance is observed with pregnancy and hormonal therapy implicated in APLD progression. Renal failure also correlates with APLD progression. APLD is associated with cerebral artery aneurysm, valvular heart disease, inguinal hernia, and diverticulosis [2, 3].

Symptoms may result from infection, traumatic rupture, intracystic hemorrhage, Budd-Chiari syndrome, dyspnea, or extrinsic compression of the biliary or digestive tracts [3]. Excluding infection, the occurrence of symptoms should be interpreted as the result of excessive abdominal volume and therapeutic options designed to significantly reduce volume rather than attention to an isolated cyst(s). Currently, there are no medical therapies to reduce disease burden or prevent progression [2].

Surgical therapy designed to substantially reduce abdominal volume offers the greatest promise for durable benefit. To this end, substantial knowledge in heptobiliary surgery is required to tailor procedures according to symptoms, cyst distribution, parenchymal preservation, biliary and vascular anatomy. Fenestration or dominant cyst wall excision is unlikely to yield long-term benefit. Instead, surgical resection, preferably laparoscopically, should be optimized to remove the highest concentration of cysts at the initial operation [7]. This yields the greatest chance of durable relief while preserving hepatic function as subsequent attempts at extensive resections following previous surgical procedures become significantly more difficult and risk parenchymal ischemia. For extensive disease, APLD progression mandates consideration of liver transplantation [7].

While not a true cystic disease, Caroli's disease does deserve mention as it may enter the differential diagnosis of a patient presenting with presumed intra-hepatic cysts. Caroli's disease is an autosomal recessive congenital malformation with a female predominance that results from incomplete gestational biliary duct formation. The biliary dilations are not true cysts as each communicates with the biliary system. Hence, a magnetic resonance cholangiopancreatography will demonstrate segmental dilatations in one or both hepatic lobes that often contain choledocholiths [2]. The most common presentation of Caroli's disease is cholangitis secondary to impaired biliary excretion. Caroli's disease may coexist with congenital hepatic fibrosis and predisposes to cholangiocarcinoma. When unilobar, more commonly the left hepatic lobe, surgical resection to include the extra-hepatic biliary tree with a Roux-en-Y hepaticojejunostomy is preferred. Extensive bilobar disease is a much more difficult condition that mandates ursodeoxycholic acid, surveillance imaging for cholangiocarcinoma, judicious instrumentation of the biliary tree when absolutely necessary and potential consideration of liver transplantation [2].

Neoplastic Cysts

Neoplastic cysts may be primary or metastatic. Primary cystadenocarcinoma of the liver is uncommon as is its precursor lesion a cystadenoma. Together, they comprise <1 % of intra-hepatic cystic lesions observed on cross-sectional imaging [2, 8]. Metastatic cystic lesions, most commonly from the pancreas or ovary are equally uncommon; however, both primary and metastatic cystic lesions carry a poor prognosis mandating precise surgical management from the onset to optimize outcome. Essential to properly managing these lesions is maintaining a high index of suspicion. This is best achieved from the very first examination of cross sectional imaging. As previously stated, every effort should be made to observe imaging that does not reflect interventions performed upon the cyst. The observation of heterogeneous or mucinous cyst content, septations, papillary projections, irregular wall thickness or the presence of a mass associated with the cyst is not consistent with congenital cystic disease. If any of the above are observed, serologic studies to exclude hydatid should be performed before proceeding to the operating room for excision of a presumed neoplastic cyst. While carbohydrate antigen 19-9 and carcinoembryonic antigen levels may be elevated in neoplastic cystic fluid, these findings are not diagnostic and attempts to obtain diagnostic cyst fluid sampling pre-operatively are not encouraged [9].

Surgical planning for a presumed neoplastic cyst involves formal hepatic resection to obtain an appropriate surgical margin. If a neoplastic cyst is entertained after initiating a fenestration procedure, conversion from a laparoscopic to an open procedure may afford improved source control and limit potential tumor distribution within the abdomen. Whenever one is contemplating reoperation for a recurrent cyst, particularly if the patient derived their initial care from another provider, caution in reviewing the surgical procedure and pathology is prudent as is the performance of a formal hepatic resection.

Traumatic Cysts

The incidence of traumatic cysts within the liver is increasing secondary to the widespread applicability of percutaneous diagnostic and therapeutic interventions. Traumatic cysts are a misnomer as they are technically pseudocyst cavities created secondary to hepatic injury without an epithelial lining. These cavities can be the result of a subcapsular hematoma, an intra-parenchymal hematoma, or coagulative necrosis following a parenchymal ablative procedure. Clinically, these patients present with constitutional signs of sepsis following bacterial superinfection of the pseudocyst. Initial treatment with broad-spectrum antibiotics and percutaneous drainage is often successful with surgical debridement and drainage (laparoscopic or open) reserved for unique circumstances [2, 10].

Infectious Cysts

Infectious cysts include pyogenic liver abscess, hydatid disease, fungal, and amoebic abscesses as well as extra-hepatic cysts secondary to retained gallstones from a previous cholecystectomy [10]. Irrespective of the etiologic agent, the approach to infectious cysts uniformly involves diagnosis, systemic treatment, cyst evacuation, and prevention of re-infection. Appropriate history and physical examination, in addition to serologic assay, are central to the early diagnosis of hydatid disease and amebiasis. An infectious etiology should also be appropriately excluded in the pre-operative evaluation of a neoplastic cyst. Following diagnosis, systemic treatment is initiated prior to evacuation of the cyst. Traditional operative therapy for infectious cysts is rapidly being replaced by percutaneous drainage with surgery reserved for larger cysts (>5 cm in diameter) or percutaneous treatment failures [11]. Following drainage, treatment is continued to prevent superinfection while the liver remodels.

Pyogenic liver abscess (PLA) has historically resulted from portal venous seeding of bacteria from appendicitis or diverticulitis. In immunocompromised patients, *Candida* should be a consideration; however, improved medical therapy has significantly lowered the incidence of PLA from these etiologies. Instead, PLA is now the most commonly the result of biliary tract disease or hepatic parenchymal ablation [2]. Hepatic parenchymal ablation with superinfection has been previously described but biliary tract manipulation, either instrumentation (ERCP) or stenting, along with obstruction from a benign or malignant stricture can incite a PLA [2, 10].

Attention to the patient's medical history in approaching a PLA guides therapy. In the setting of a PLA secondary to bacterial/fungal seeding, the routine algorithm advocated above with percutaneous aspiration/drainage is recommended. The decision to leave a drain should be tailored to the situation as repetitive aspiration has been demonstrated to be equivalent to drainage in smaller (<5 cm diameter) PLA [12]. When a PLA from a biliary source is suspected, the treatment should be surgical, typically a hepatic resection, and directed at the underlying biliary etiology.

Hydatid disease is caused by *Echinococcus granulosus* or *Echinococcus multilocularis* where humans are an intermediate host. Endemic areas include South America, Middle East, Far East, East Africa, Australia and the Mediterranean countries where sheep are plentiful. The most common presentation is persistent right upper quadrant pain secondary to cyst expansion and hepatic parenchymal compression; however, other serious complications from erosion of hydatid cysts into biliary and vascular structures have been reported. Cross-sectional imaging and an eosinophilia can be highly sensitive in conjunction with an appropriate history but the diagnosis is confirmed serologically. Surgical management has dramatically changed from traditional open hepatic resection to percutaneous drainage with laparoscopy as indicated according to the above infectious cyst protocol [2, 13, 14].

Amebic hepatic abscess secondary to *Entamoeba histolytica* should be considered in toxic patients a recent history of visiting tropical climates. The patients classically present with acute abdominal pain and fever. Cross sectional imaging demonstrates a single large loculated abscess with a heterogeneous content. The widespread parenchymal necrosis from the protozoan produces the "anchovy sauce" appearance of the cystic fluid. Diagnosis is by serology but, unlike hydatid disease, these patients do not exhibit eosinophilia. Treatment is as outlines for infectious cysts utilizing metronidazole, emetine hydrochloride, chloroquine phosphate, or diloxanide furoate. One unique consideration in amebic abscess is their proclivity to rupture. When located near the hepatic capsule, early aspiration and drainage is indicated [2].

Summary

Cystic diseases of the liver are common and multifactorial in origin. A standardized approach to an hepatic cyst, as outlined above, begins with a meticulous history and physical examination to broadly hypothesize the cyst etiology as congenital, neoplastic, traumatic, or infectious. Detailed radiologic analysis can then be incorporated evaluating the number, location, cyst content, cyst content heterogeneity, and wall characteristics to refine the hypothesis. Serologic studies add further data for differentiating complex infectious from neoplastic cysts. For infectious cysts, percutaneous drainage is becoming the standard while laparoscopy is the preferred method for all other cysts requiring surgery.

References

1. Carrim Z, Murchison J. The prevalence of simple renal and hepatic cysts detected by spiral computed tomography. Clin Radiol. 2003;58:626–9.
2. Reid-Lombardo K, Khan S, Sclabas G. Hepatic cysts and liver abscess. Surg Clin N Am. 2010;90:679–97.
3. Abu-Wasel B, Walsh C, Keough V, Molinari M. Athophysiology, epidemiology, classification, and treatment options for polycystic liver diseases. World J Gastroenterol. 2013;19:5775–86.
4. Charlesworth P, Ade-Ajayi N, Davenport M. Natural history and long-term follow-up of antenatally detected liver cysts. J Pediatr Surg. 2007;42:494–9.
5. Saini S, Mueller P, Ferrucci Jr J, Simeone J, Wittenberg J, Butch R. Percutaneous aspiration of hepatic cysts does not provide definitive therapy. Am J Roentgenol. 1983;141:559–60.
6. Erdogan D, van Delden O, Rauws E, et al. Results of percutaneous sclerotherapy and surgical treatment in patients with symptomatic simple liver cysts and polycystic liver disease. World J Gastroenterol. 2007;13:3095–100.
7. Schnelldorfer T, Torres V, Zakaria S, Rosen C, Nagorney D. Polycystic liver disease: a critical appraisal of hepatic resection, fenestration, and liver transplantation. Ann Surg. 2009;250:112–8.
8. Williams D, Vitellas K, Sheafor D. Biliary cystadenocarcinoma: seven year follow-up and the role of MRI and MRCP. Magn Reson Imaging. 2001;19:1203–8.
9. Koffron A, Rao S, Ferrario M, Abecassis M. Intrahepatic biliary cystadenoma: role of cyst fluid analysis and surgical management in the laparoscopic era. Surgery. 2004;136:926–36.
10. Lardiere-Deguelte S, Ragot E, Amroun K, et al. Hepatic abscess: diagnosis and management. J Visc Surg. 2015;466:1–13.
11. Pearce N, Knight R, Irving H, et al. Non-operative management of pyogenic liver abscess. HPB. 2003;5:91–5.
12. Yu S, Ho S, Lau W, et al. Treatment of pyogenic liver abscess: prospective randomized comparison of catheter drainage and needle aspiration. Hepatology. 2004;39:932–8.
13. Li H, Shao Y, Aji T, et al. Laparoscopic approach for total cystectomy in treating hepatic cystic echinococcus. Parasite. 2014;21:160–5.
14. Tuxun Y, Zhang J-H, Zhao J-M, Tai Q-W, Abudurexti M. World review of laparoscopic treatment of liver cystic echinococcus – 914 patients. Int J Inf Dis. 2014;24:43–50.

Chapter 6
When Should You Operate on Major Hepatic Trauma?

Cory Evans and Martin A. Croce

Abstract Hepatic trauma causes a significant amount of morbidity and mortality. The decision to on whether or not to operate is a key step in managing this problem. Operative management carries with it a higher rate of morbidity and mortality than non-operative management. However, clear indications do exist when an operation is needed. These include hemodynamic instability, continued bleeding, peritonitis, and other abdominal injuries requiring operation. Operative management involves a graded response to the injury. Selected angioembolization can be a useful adjunct to both operative and non-operative approach to hepatic trauma.

Keywords Hepatic trauma • Operative management • Non-operative management • Angioembolization

Introduction

Hepatic trauma is associated with a significant amount of morbidity and mortality. It is a complex and challenging problem to manage. Hemodynamically unstable patients with a blunt mechanism of injury to the liver should undergo operative management [1]. Similarly, patients with penetrating hepatic injuries mostly need operative management to search for associated intra-abdominal injury [2]. Non-operative management (NOM) of hemodynamically stable patients with blunt liver trauma has become the standard of care. This is a change in philosophy of management of these injuries began to evolve in the early 1990s. Spurred by case reports and results from the pediatric literature, several studies in this period showed a high rate of success of NOM for all American Association for the Surgery of Trauma (AAST) grades of blunt hepatic trauma [3–5]. More recently, several centers have

C. Evans • M.A. Croce (✉)
Department of Surgery, University of Tennessee Health Science Center, 910 Madison Ave, 2nd floor, Memphis, TN 38163, USA
e-mail: coryevans@gmail.com; mcroce@uthsc.edu

J.M. Millis, J.B. Matthews (eds.), *Difficult Decisions in Hepatobiliary and Pancreatic Surgery*, Difficult Decisions in Surgery: An Evidence-Based Approach, DOI 10.1007/978-3-319-27365-5_6

Table 6.1 PICO table for perioperative arrhythmia prophylaxis for lung resection

P (Patients)	I (Intervention)	C (Comparator group)	O (Outcomes measured)
Patients with traumatic liver injury	Operative management or angioembolization	Non-operative management	Failure of non-operative management, morbidity and mortality, liver related morbidity and mortality

been evaluating patients for non-operative management of penetrating hepatic trauma. These patients must be hemodynamically stable and carefully selected [6–8].

Patients who are managed with early operative management have higher Injury Severity Scores (ISS), higher rates of hypotension upon presentation, and higher mortality. Failure of NOM is also associated with higher overall mortality [4]. For this reason, the attempt will be made to manage most patients with blunt liver injury non-operatively. Angiography can be used as an adjunct to NOM or operative management of liver injury [1]. The failure of non-operative management can be due to the development of hemodynamic instability, failure to respond appropriately to transfusion or drop in hematocrit, suspicion of injury to other organs requiring operation, or clinical peritonitis [3]. Failures may be due to the liver injury itself or due to injuries to other intra-abdominal organs. Not surprisingly, higher grade injuries have a higher rate of failure. Grade IV and V injuries may have as high as two-third failure rate [2, 3]. Risk factors for failure are older age, lower admission mean SBP, worse base deficit, higher mean lactate, higher mean ISS, and hemoperitoneum extending into the pericolic gutter [3].

Operative management strategies can range from simple electrocautery and topical hemostasis to liver transplantation at the other extreme end of the spectrum. Most authors advocate a graded approach to the operative management of liver trauma. This begins with topical hemostasis for lower grade injuries, to suture ligation of bleeding vessels, to anatomic and non-anatomic liver resections. In the 1990s the concept of damage control laparotomy was reintroduced. Injuries to the liver are usually to the veins, which are a low pressure system. These can often be controlled simply with temporary gauze packing. This limits blood loss and allows for resuscitation of the patient. The patient can then return to the operating room in 24–72 h and definitive control if needed can be achieved.

Search Strategy

A literature search from the PubMed Database of English language publications from the last 10 years was used to identity published data on the operative management of liver trauma using the PICO outline (Table 6.1). Terms used in the search were "operative liver trauma", or "operative hepatic trauma". Articles were excluded if the full text was not available through the institution. Case reports were excluded.

Table 6.2 Failure of non-operative management and reasons for failure

Author (year)	N	op	NOM	Fail NOM	HD unstable	Hct. drop	Peritonitis	Other
Fang (2006)	278	64	214	30	0	24	0	6
Gaarder (2007)	114	41	73	11	ns	ns	ns	ns
Ghnnam (2013)	56	20	36	0	ns	ns	ns	ns
Kozar (2005)	337	107	230	12	0	1	0	11
Morales (2014)	117	19	98	7	0	2	2	3
Norrman (2009)	46	11	35	4	0	2	1	1
Parray (2011)	152	ns	152	8	8	0	0	0
Prichayudh (2013)	152	92	60	6	0	4	2	0
van der Wilden (2012)	393	131	262	23	0	7	10	6
Zago (2012)	120	55	65	6	2	0	4	0
Combined	1765	540	1225	107	10	40	19	27
%Combined	–	–	–	8.7	10.4	41.7	19.8	28.1

op operative management, *NOM* non-operative management, *ns* not studied

Twenty-six articles were selected to be used for the writing of this chapter. All studies used data from retrospective analysis, or data that was prospectively entered into a trauma database. Other cited articles were review articles or book chapters. The data was classified using the GRADE system.

Results

Non-operative Management

Hemodynamically stable patients with blunt liver injury can be managed non-operatively in up to 80 % of cases. All grades of liver injury except Grade VI can be managed non-operatively [2]. Cumulative results of reported NOM in the last 10 years shows a success rate of 91.3 %. This is including studies looking only at high grade liver injuries. Most common liver related reasons for the failure of NOM include continued drop in hematocrit or continued bleeding, hemodynamic instability, and biloma or bile leak (table). Non-liver related causes of failure of NOM are related to injury to other organs; mostly spleen, pancreas, or small bowel (Table 6.2).

Higher grades of liver injury according to AAST grading system are more likely to be managed operatively and tend to have a higher failure rate of NOM. The results of five studies were tabulated showing failure rates in Grade I of 0 %, Grade II of 0.8 %, Grade III of 3.0 %, Grade IV of 10.4 %, Grade V of 21.7 % [9–13]. Christmas et al. showed a similar trend of increasing operative management with higher grade injuries [14]. Cohn et al. also reported a poor sensitivity for predicting the need for operative management based on the AAST grading system for liver

Table 6.3 AAST grade of injury and failure of non-operative management based on grade

	Non-operative management total					Failure non-operative management				
Author (year)	Grade I	Grade II	Grade III	Grade IV	Grade V	Grade I	Grade II	Grade III	Grade IV	Grade V
Ghnnam (2013)	4	11	12	9	0	0	0	0	0	0
Kozar (2005)	na	na	130	92	8	na	na	0	7	4
Norman (2009)	24		11			3		1		
Parray (2011)	30	63	26	33	0	0	0	2	6	0
Saltzherr (2010)	20	43	30	10	1	0	1	4	2	0
van der Wilden (2012)	na	na	na	234	28	na	na	na	19	4
Zago (2012)	51				14	5				1
Combined	58	74	209	378	51	0	1	6	34	9

trauma. They did, however, report that the findings of lacerations involving more than two segments, lacerations extending into the hilum, and active extravasation correlate with a >90 % specificity for either angiographic or operative intervention. Furthermore they report a specificity of 85 % for intervention for >500 cc hemoperitoneum [15]. Interestingly, Fang et al. reported an operative rate of 100 % in 14 patients who had free extravasation of contrast into the peritoneal cavity [16] (Table 6.3).

Several factors are significantly associated with failure of NOM. These include hypotension on admission, worse base deficit, higher lactate, higher ISS, vascular blush on CT, and hemoperitoneum on CT scan extending into at least the paracolic gutters [3]. Polanco retrospectively analyzed the National Trauma Data Bank for isolated liver injuries. In over 3000 patients, increasing age, higher ISS, and hypotension on presentation were identified as risk factors in patients more likely to fail NOM [4]. In a smaller study, Norman et al. also found ISS and a lower presentation blood pressure in patients failing NOM [17]. One study identified only lower average blood pressure as a predictor of failure [20], while other studies failed to identify any variables as risk factors for failure of NOM [13, 18].

Penetrating trauma to the abdomen is generally managed with laparotomy, however case series do exist of the non-operative management of highly selective patients. Inaba et al. reported a series of eight patients with isolated liver injury and two patients with liver and kidney injury following gunshot wounds that were managed non-operatively. One patient with a isolated liver injury underwent non-therapeutic laparotomy and was discharged home after an 79 day recovery in the hospital [6]. MacGoey et al. presented a series of ten non-operatively managed patients with penetrating injuries with two failures of NOM due to hemodynamic instability [7]. Omoshoro-Jones et al. in a prospective study of 33 highly selected patients with gunshot wounds to the liver, had only two non-liver related failures of NOM [8]. These studies involved highly selected patients who were hemodynamically stable with right upper quadrant gunshot wounds and no clinical signs of peritonitis who had a reliable abdominal exam [6–8]. Based on the paucity of data, laparotomy is recommended for patients with penetrating hepatic trauma.

Angiography and Embolization

The EAST guidelines for management of liver trauma give a level 2 recommendation to the use of angiography and embolization as an adjunct to operative management of liver trauma or as a primary treatment modality for NOM in transient responders to resuscitation. They also give a level 2 recommendation to the use of angiography in patients who have an active blush on CT scan [1]. Sivrikoz et al. performed a retrospective analysis of over 6000 patients with isolated grade IV and V blunt hepatic injuries from the National Trauma Data Bank to investigate the role of angioembolization. Eleven percent of these patients underwent angiographic embolization. Angiographic embolization was shown to be an independent predictor of survival in both patients undergoing operation and patients managed non-operatively [19]. Saltzherr et al. showed a reduced mortality in high grade liver injuries and higher percentage of liver injuries successfully managed non-operatively after the introduction of angiographic embolization at their facility [11]. Christmas et al. showed embolization prevented failure of non-operative management in patients with persistent liver bleeding in 11 of 12 patients [14]. Van der Wilden et al. report successful non-operative management of grade IV and V while heavily relying on angiography and embolization. Embolization had a 93 % success rate for preventing FOM for persistent bleeding in 59 patients [20]. Dabbs et al. performed a retrospective analysis of 538 patients admitted with high grade liver injuries. One hundred sixteen of these underwent angiography and 71 had embolization. Forty-three of these patients had hepatic related complications including 100 % of patients with grade 5 injuries and thee were eight liver related deaths. The most common complication they observed was major hepatic necrosis which made up 42 % of the complications [21].

Outcomes

Published studies over the last 10 years were combined to determine the morbidity and mortality, liver related (LR) morbidity and mortality of operative, NOM and failure of NOM for blunt hepatic trauma. Not all studies consistently differentiated LR morbidity and mortality from all cause morbidity and mortality. Some only report LR morbidity and mortality or combined morbidity and mortality. Some studies focus only on high grade liver injuries. Not surprisingly, patients who were managed with an operation, either on presentation or after failure of NOM trended towards having higher morbidity and mortality. Morbidity of NOM was 18 % with mortality of 3.6 %. LR NOM morbidity was 2.2 % with no mortalities. Failure of NOM had a morbidity and mortality of 55 % and 14.4 %, respectively. LR failure NOM had morbidity of 44.8 % and mortality of 14.1 %. Operative morbidity and mortality were 79.9 % and 43.6 %. LR operative morbidity and mortality were 34.9 % and 21.3 % [9, 10, 13, 16–18, 20, 22–24] (Table 6.4). Christmas et al. showed a significantly higher mortality in grade III–V injuries managed operatively vs. non-operatively [14].

Surgical Strategies

Operative management of the liver first involves proper mobilization to allow for sufficient exposure to deal with the injury. This begins by dividing the ligamentum teres and mobilizing the falciform ligament off the abdominal wall. The right and left triangular and coronary ligaments should also be divided so that both lobes of the liver are freely mobile. The caveat is that the presence of a confined, nonexpanding retrohepatic hematoma should be a contraindication to mobilization of the liver in patients with blunt trauma. This often signifies an injury to the retrohepatic veins or inferior vena cava. Mobilizing the liver can lead to uncontrolled hemorrhage from these injuries [2].

Bleeding from minor lacerations to the liver can usually be controlled with manual compression, electrocautery, or topical hemostatic agents. The argon beam coagulator or Aquamantis may also be used to control hemorrhage, but should not be used for deep lacerations [25]. In damage control situations, packing the liver with gauze laparotomy pads and compression are the first line strategies to control bleeding [23, 25]. These will be removed at a planned second look laparotomy after the patient has been properly resuscitated, usually between 24 and 72 h after the initial operation. Often, the liver is packed in conjunction with other hemostatic procedures [3].

If persistent bleeding or bile leak is present despite packing, the injury will need further exploration. The Pringle maneuver is useful to control inflow while the wound is explored. In general, this should not be left in place for more than 30–45 min [2]. Intermittent clamping in a 15 min on 15 min off fashion is preferred [25]. If bleeding persists despite the Pringle maneuver, bleeding is most likely from a retrohepatic venous source. Visible bleeding vessels or bile ducts in the liver parenchyma should be suture ligated. Injuries to large veins can be repaired with 5–0 polypropylene suture. Often bleeding and bile leak is hidden deep within a laceration. To gain exposure, the finger fracture technique can be used to further open up the liver parenchyma, ligating and dividing vessels as they are exposed. However, this can be quite time consuming. Alternatively a laparoscopic stapler with vascular loads can be used to divide the liver more quickly [2, 25].

Every effort should be made to control bleeding from a retrohepatic venous injury by packing alone [23]. If forced to repair this type of injury, total vascular insolation needs to be achieved. This is accomplished by controlling the suprarenal

Table 6.4 Morbidity and mortality and liver related morbidity and mortality from liver trauma

Author (year)	N	op	NOM	Fail	NOM MB	LR NOM MB	NOM ML	NOM LR ML	Fail MB	LR fail MB	Fail ML	Fail LR ML	op MB	LR op MB	op ML	Op LR ML
Fang (2006)	278	64	214	30	3	3	ns	ns	7	3	8	8	ns	ns	ns	ns
Gaarder (2007)	114	41	73	11	ns	ns	ns	0	ns	ns	ns	0	ns	ns	ns	0
Ghnnam (2013)	56	20	36	0	ns	ns	0	0	na	na	na	na	ns	ns	2	2
Kozar (2005)	337	107	230	12	ns	2	ns	ns	ns	4	1	1	ns	ns	ns	ns
Morales (2014)	117	19	98	7	10	5	2	0	ns	ns	0	0	11	8	11	8
Norrman (2009)	46	11	35	4	9	ns	0	0	3	ns	1	1	7	ns	1	0
Parray (2011)	152	ns	152	8	ns	ns	0	0	4	4	0	0	ns	ns	ns	ns
Pricha-yudh (2013)	152	92	60	6	13	6	1	0	ns	ns	ns	ns	59	28	37	29
van der Wilden (2012)	393	131	262	23	91	ns	13	ns	23	ns	2	ns	112	ns	69	ns
Zago (2012)	120	55	65	6	7	0	0	0	2	2	1	1	57	22	23	ns
Combined	1765	540	1225	107	133	16	16	0	39	13	13	11	246	58	143	39

op operative management, *NOM* non-operative management, *fail* failure of NOM, *MB* morbidity, *ML* mortality, *LR* liver related

IVC, and suprahepatic IVC and the porta hepatis. The suprahepatic IVC is readily controlled within the pericardium either via a median sternotomy or by incising the tendinous portion of the diaphragm. The suprarenal IVC can be approached by performing a Kocher maneuver or by mobilizing the left lobe of the liver and entering the lesser sac along the lesser curvature of the stomach. Historically the Schrock atriocaval shunt has been advocated for addressing these injuries. However, survival is uniformly poor and this technique has all but been abandoned [2, 23].

Morales Uribe et al. discussed their operative management techniques for blunt liver trauma. Of 19 patients, three with grade I liver injuries required no intervention to the liver, one with a grade II injury was treated by suturing. Of the remaining high grade injuries, seven were treated with packing alone, two with packing plus suturing, two with packing plus non-anatomic resection, one with packing plus hepatic artery ligation. They had eight liver related mortalities including both patients undergoing resection and the patient undergoing hepatic artery ligation [18]. Polanco et al. reported a much lower mortality rate for operative management. In 144 patients with liver trauma, resection was performed in 56 patients, packing in 30 patients, hepatorrhaphy in 15, and no liver intervention in the remaining 16. They had an overall series mortality of 9 % including non-operatively managed patients and those who succumbed in the trauma bay. Patients managed by resection had an overall morbidity of 62.5 % and mortality of 17.8 %, but liver related morbidity and mortality were 30 % and 9 % respectively. Mortality for hepatic venous injury was only 25 %. The authors advocate resection for continued venous bleeding, devitalized tissue for which the injury has done a large portion of the resection, and major bile leaks [26].

Recommendations

Liver injuries should be operated on when a patient is hemodynamically unstable, develops peritonitis, continues to bleed, or has other abdominal injuries requiring an operation. Although some studies have shown successful NOM of penetrating liver injuries, this has been done in specialized centers with the resources to do so. Due to the high possibility of missing associated abdominal injuries, NOM of penetrating liver injuries is not recommended. NOM of blunt injuries should only be attempted in centers with units capable of continuous monitoring of patients with serial physical exams and laboratory studies. Angiographic embolization can be used as a modality to aid NOM or as an adjunct to operative management, but should not be used as a replacement for operative intervention in unstable patients. All hemodynamically stable patients with blunt liver injuries should undergo a CT scan. Although higher grade injuries are associated with higher failure of NOM, CT grading alone is not predictive of failure. Operative management of liver injuries should include a graded response to the injury using the simplest technique possible to manage the problem. Peri-hepatic packing should be used as a damage control strategy to allow time for appropriate resuscitation. Liver resection can be used for definitive management when required.

A Personal View of the Data

More recent studies confirm earlier data which resulted in a paradigm shift from operative to selective NOM of blunt liver injury. Characteristics of the liver injury which result in failure of NOM are not based on the radiographic severity of the injury, and the decision to operate should be based on the patients clinical status. While there is clearly a lower morbidity and mortality rate for patients in whom successful NOM can be achieved, one should not hesitate to operate when the situation calls for it.

Recommendations

- Trial of NOM for all patients who are hemodynamically stable with blunt liver injuries
- Operative management for penetrating liver injuries
- Operative management of blunt liver injuries who are or become hemodynamically stable, patients who develop peritonitis, patients with ongoing bleeding, or patients with associated injuries requiring an operation

References

1. Stassen NA, Bhullar I, Cheng JD, Crandall M, Friese R, Guillamondegui O, et al. Nonoperative management of blunt hepatic injury: an Eastern Association for the Surgery of Trauma practice management guideline. J Trauma Acute Care Surg. 2012;73(5 Suppl 4):S288–93.
2. Savage SA, Croce MA. The management of liver injuries. In: Cameron JL, editor. The management of liver injuries. Philadelphia: Elsevier Saunders; 2014.
3. Malhotra AK, Fabian TC, Croce MA, Gavin TJ, Kudsk KA, Minard G, et al. Blunt hepatic injury: a paradigm shift from operative to nonoperative management in the 1990s. Ann Surg. 2000;231(6):804–13.
4. Polanco PM, Brown JB, Puyana JC, Billiar TR, Peitzman AB, Sperry JL. The swinging pendulum: a national perspective of nonoperative management in severe blunt liver injury. J Trauma Acute Care Surg. 2013;75(4):590–5.
5. Croce MA, Fabian TC, Menke PG, Waddle-Smith L, Minard G, Kudsk KA, et al. Nonoperative management of blunt hepatic trauma is the treatment of choice for hemodynamically stable patients. Results of a prospective trial. Ann Surg. 1995;221(6):744–53; discussion 753–5.
6. DuBose J, Inaba K, Teixeira PG, Pepe A, Dunham MB, McKenney M. Selective non-operative management of solid organ injury following abdominal gunshot wounds. Injury. 2007;38(9):1084–90.
7. MacGoey P, Navarro A, Beckingham I, Cameron I, Brooks A. Selective non-operative management of penetrating liver injuries at a UK tertiary referral centre. Ann R Coll Surg Engl. 2014;96(6):423–6.
8. Omoshoro-Jones JA, Nicol AJ, Navsaria PH, Zellweger R, Krige JE, Kahn DH. Selective non-operative management of liver gunshot injuries. Br J Surg. 2005;92(7):890–5.

9. Ghnnam WM, Almasry HN, Ghanem MA. Non-operative management of blunt liver trauma in a level II trauma hospital in Saudi Arabia. Int J Crit Illn Inj Sci. 2013;3(2):118–23.
10. Parray FQ, Wani ML, Malik AA, Thakur N, Wani RA, Naqash SH, et al. Evaluating a conservative approach to managing liver injuries in Kashmir, India. J Emerg Trauma Shock. 2011;4(4):483–7.
11. Saltzherr TP, van der Vlies CH, van Lienden KP, Beenen LF, Ponsen KJ, van Gulik TM, et al. Improved outcomes in the non-operative management of liver injuries. HPB (Oxf). 2011;13(5):350–5.
12. Kozar RA, Moore JB, Niles SE, Holcomb JB, Moore EE, Cothren CC, et al. Complications of nonoperative management of high-grade blunt hepatic injuries. J Trauma. 2005;59(5):1066–71.
13. Zago TM, Pereira BM, Calderan TR, Hirano ES, Rizoli S, Fraga GP. Blunt hepatic trauma: comparison between surgical and nonoperative treatment. Rev Col Bras Cir. 2012;39(4):307–13.
14. Christmas AB, Wilson AK, Manning B, Franklin GA, Miller FB, Richardson JD, et al. Selective management of blunt hepatic injuries including nonoperative management is a safe and effective strategy. Surgery. 2005;138(4):606–10; discussion 610–1.
15. Cohn SM, Arango JI, Myers JG, Lopez PP, Jonas RB, Waite LL, et al. Computed tomography grading systems poorly predict the need for intervention after spleen and liver injuries. Am Surg. 2009;75(2):133–9.
16. Fang JF, Wong YC, Lin BC, Hsu YP, Chen MF. The CT risk factors for the need of operative treatment in initially hemodynamically stable patients after blunt hepatic trauma. J Trauma. 2006;61(3):547–53; discussion 553–4.
17. Norrman G, Tingstedt B, Ekelund M, Andersson R. Non-operative management of blunt liver trauma: feasible and safe also in centres with a low trauma incidence. HPB (Oxf). 2009;11(1):50–6.
18. Morales Uribe CH, Lopez CA, Cote JC, Franco ST, Saldarriaga MF, Mosquera J, et al. Surgical treatment of blunt liver trauma, indications for surgery and results. Cir Esp. 2014;92(1):23–9.
19. Sivrikoz E, Teixeira GP, Resnick S, Inaba K, Talving P, Demetriades D. Angiointervention: an independent predictor of survival in high-grade blunt liver injuries. Am J Surg. 2015;209(4):742–6.
20. van der Wilden GM, Velmahos GC, Emhoff T, Brancato S, Adams C, Georgakis G, et al. Successful nonoperative management of the most severe blunt liver injuries: a multicenter study of the research consortium of New England centers for trauma. Arch Surg. 2012;147(5):423–8.
21. Dabbs DN, Stein DM, Scalea TM. Major hepatic necrosis: a common complication after angioembolization for treatment of high-grade liver injuries. J Trauma. 2009;66(3):621–7; discussion 627–9.
22. Gaarder C, Naess PA, Eken T, Skaga NO, Pillgram-Larsen J, Klow NE, et al. Liver injuries – improved results with a formal protocol including angiography. Injury. 2007;38(9):1075–83.
23. Kozar RA, Feliciano DV, Moore EE, Moore FA, Cocanour CS, West MA, et al. Western Trauma Association/critical decisions in trauma: operative management of adult blunt hepatic trauma. J Trauma. 2011;71(1):1–5.
24. Prichayudh S, Sirinawin C, Sriussadaporn S, Pak-art R, Kritayakirana K, Samorn P, et al. Management of liver injuries: predictors for the need of operation and damage control surgery. Injury. 2014;45(9):1373–7.
25. Peitzman AB, Marsh JW. Advanced operative techniques in the management of complex liver injury. J Trauma Acute Care Surg. 2012;73(3):765–70.
26. Polanco P, Leon S, Pineda J, Puyana JC, Ochoa JB, Alarcon L, et al. Hepatic resection in the management of complex injury to the liver. J Trauma. 2008;65(6):1264–9; discussion 1269–70.

Chapter 7
Surgical Treatment of Hepatocellular Carcinoma: Resection Versus Transplantation

Thomas Pham, Tsuyoshi Todo, Robert Gish, and Waldo Concepcion

Abstract Hepatocellular carcinoma is the second most common cause of cancer mortality worldwide and its incidence is rising in North America, with an estimated 35,000 cases in the U.S. in 2014. The best chance for cure is surgical resection in the form of either segmental removal or whole organ transplantation although recent survival data on radiofrequency ablation approximates surgical resection and could be placed under the new moniker of "thermal resection". The debate between surgical resection and transplantation focuses on patients with "within Milan criteria" tumors, single tumors, and well compensated cirrhosis who can safely undergo either procedure. Although transplantation historically has had better survival outcomes, early diagnosis, reversal of liver disease, and innovations in patient selection and neo-adjuvant therapies have led to similar 5-year survival. Transplantation clearly has less risk of tumor recurrence but exposes recipients to long term immunosuppression and its side effects. Liver transplantation is also limited by the severe global limit on the supply of organ donors whereas resection is readily available. The current data does not favor one treatment over the other for patients with minimal or no portal hypertension and normal synthetic function. Instead, the decision to resect or transplant for HCC relies on multiple factors including tumor characteristics, biology, geography, co-morbidities, location, organ availability, social support and practice preference.

T. Pham
Department of Surgery, Stanford University, Stanford, CA, USA

T. Todo
Department of Medicine, Stanford University, Stanford, CA, USA

R. Gish
Stanford University Medical Center, 750 Welch Rd, Ste. 319 MC 5731, Palo Alto, CA 94304, USA

W. Concepcion (✉)
Department of Surgery, Stanford University, Stanford, CA, USA

Stanford University Medical Center, 750 Welch Rd, Ste. 319 MC 5731, Palo Alto, CA 94304, USA
e-mail: waldo1@stanford.edu

J.M. Millis, J.B. Matthews (eds.), *Difficult Decisions in Hepatobiliary and Pancreatic Surgery*, Difficult Decisions in Surgery: An Evidence-Based Approach, DOI 10.1007/978-3-319-27365-5_7

Keywords Hepatocellular carcinoma • Hepatic resection • Liver transplantation

Introduction

Liver transplantation and surgical resection have remained the key first-line therapies for hepatocellular carcinoma (HCC) as they hold the greatest chance for a cure. The Barcelona Clinic Liver Cancer (BCLC) staging and treatment guidelines best incorporate tumor, liver and patient characteristics to assess survival with all HCC-directed interventions [1]. According to this guideline, curative surgical resection and liver transplantation are reserved for patients with early stage disease whereas intermediate and advanced stage tumors are subject to palliative therapies [2] that may prolong life and occasionally be associated with a cure.

Patients with early stage tumors and advanced liver disease (Child-Pugh Class B and C), especially if multiple tumors, clearly benefit from liver transplantation as resection results in poor overall survival [3]. On the other hand, surgical resection is most beneficial for those patients with early stage tumors, single tumors and early cirrhosis or no underlying liver disease [4]. The debate lies within the small group of patients whose tumors are within Milan criteria, especially those with a single tumor, who have Child-Pugh Class A cirrhosis, who have no significant portal hypertension as determined by hepatic vein pressure gradient, and who are without liver dysfunction. Liver transplantation appears to be the obvious choice for cure as the entire tumor along with the field defect of cirrhosis is removed. However, transplantation is not available to everyone as fewer than 30 % of patients are eligible at the time of presentation and it is severely limited by the number of donor organs available [1]. For this reason, hepatic resection continues to play a significant role in the treatment of HCC even though it is applicable to only approximately 15 % of cases. It is readily available without the need for a waitlist and may be less restrictive than Milan criteria in regards to tumor size.

The aim of this discussion is to review the current data detailing outcomes such as overall survival, disease free survival, and recurrence following resection and/or transplantation for Milan criteria HCC. Numerous studies and meta-analyses have been performed addressing this topic but heterogeneous patient populations and retrospective observations have produced moderate to low quality data. Here we analyze current data, provide evidence-based recommendations for clinical practice and discuss future avenues of research.

Search Strategy

A literature search of peer-reviewed English language publications from 1996 to 2014 was used to identify data on liver resection and/or transplantation as the treatment for hepatocellular cancer. Databases searched were Pub Med and Cochrane Evidence Based Medicine. Terms used in the search were "hepatocellular carcinoma surgical treatment," "HCC resection versus transplantation," "HCC resection,"

"HCC transplantation," "HCC downstaging," "Milan Criteria expansion." "UCSF criteria," "salvage transplantation AND secondary transplantation." Articles were excluded if they included hepatocholangiocarcinoma, fibrolamellar HCC and non-cirrhosis HCC. Living donor liver transplantation for HCC was also excluded from this analysis. No randomized controlled trials were identified. Articles analyzed here include ten retrospective studies, two prospective cohort studies, three review articles, four meta-analyses and two clinical guidelines. The data was classified using the GRADE system.

Results

Resection of Hepatocellular Carcinoma

When considering patients for surgical resection, various factors such as tumor size, number, tumor biology, vascular invasion, underlying liver dysfunction, presence of portal hypertension, type of resection, and ability to treat the underlying liver disease help determine patient survival [5]. Reported 5-year overall survival and disease-free survival are 50–60 % and 25–35 %, respectively, in patients with HCC and preserved liver function [6, 7]. Preserved liver function refers to those with Child-Pugh Class A cirrhosis with or without portal hypertension (PHTN). According to the American Association for the Study of Liver Diseases (AASLD) and the European Association for the Study of the Liver (EASL), PHTN is a relative contraindication to resection because of increased morbidity and mortality following surgery [2]. Santambrogio et al. and others have challenged this dogma and have shown that patients undergoing resection who had clinically significant portal hypertension (splenomegaly >12 cm, platelet count <100 k/mm^3) and preserved liver function (INR, bilirubin, and albumin within normal limits) had 5-year survival equivalent to that of patients without PHTN who undergo resection, 65 % vs. 70 % [8]. Multivariate analysis identified albumin as an independent predictive factor for survival. Although not found to be significant in this study, bilirubin has been shown to be an independent predictor of survival in other studies [3, 7]. All patients included in the Santambrogio et al. study had transplantable tumors that were single lesions <5 cm, Child-Pugh Class A, BCLC stage Class A1 to A3. The study's findings helped establish a role for resection for HCC as patients with early tumors and well compensated cirrhosis can safely undergo resection.

Transplantation for Hepatocellular Carcinoma

Soon after liver transplantation was deemed successful, surgeons began using transplantation as a treatment for HCC. The benefits of transplantation over resection for cancer appeared obvious in that the entire organ-containing tumor was removed and in most cases the significant risk factor for malignancy (cirrhosis) was also removed.

Unfortunately, poor understanding of the biology of HCC resulted in high recurrence rates, as evidenced by studies showing recurrence as high as 74 % within 2 years [9, 10]. It was clear that simple removal of the tumor with transplantation was not sufficient to cure patients with HCC.

It was not until 1996 that Mazzaferro and colleagues published the results of a prospective cohort study that investigated 48 cirrhotic patients who underwent liver transplantation for HCC with single tumors ≤5 cm, or up to three tumors, the largest of which is ≤3 cm. Evident radiographical evidence of vessel and lymph node invasion were also excluded. Survival of these patients was comparable to that of patients who underwent transplantation for nonmalignant diagnoses (70 % at 5 years) [11]. In this cohort, 60 of 295 patients (20 %) were deemed candidates for liver transplantation. Forty-eight of these 60 patients were ultimately transplanted secondary to wait list drop off. This landmark article gave birth to the widely adopted Milan criteria which are used to guide decision making in most transplant centers today. Numerous retrospective studies have validated improved survival of patients transplanted within Milan criteria [12–14].

The difficulty in analyzing transplant outcomes is that patients are naturally selected when evaluated for transplant. This is seen in the landmark study by Mazzaferro et al. where 48 of 60 patients eventually underwent transplantation while the remaining 12 suffered from waitlist dropout. Although not specifically detailed in that study, the most commoh reasons for removal from the waitlist are tumor growth outside of Milan criteria, death and development of contraindications to transplant [15]. It is possible that patients who undergo transplant tend to have less aggressive tumors than those who exceed Milan criteria while on the wait list. To offset this selection bias seen in outcome studies where survival and tumor recurrence are measured at the time of transplant, intention to treat (ITT) analyses were performed where outcome is measured starting at the time of listing. Llovet et al. performed an ITT analysis in patients who underwent transplant (n=87) or resection (n=77) from the years 1989 to 1997 [7]. Upon analyzing patients with early HCC (single tumors ≤5 cm), survival between resection and transplant groups were similar at 74 % at 5 years when resection patients with clinically relevant portal hypertension were excluded. Interestingly, the most common causes of death in the transplant arm were wait list drop off (n=8) and post-transplant infections (n=8). The most common cause of death post- resection was tumor recurrence (n=26). This study sparked the debate on resection versus transplant for early stage tumors and several ITT analyses following it showed similar results [16, 17]. These studies included patients from the pre-Model for End Stage Liver Disease (MELD) era where HCC patients were allocated according to time on the waitlist which has been shown to be a poor predictor of death [18]. After MELD criteria were adopted by the United Network for Organ Sharing (UNOS) in 2002, special allocation was given to HCC patients which resulted in decreased wait time, with 87 % of patients being transplanted within 3 months [19]. To this date there have been no publications that compare resection to ITT survival in only MELD-era patients undergoing transplant for Milan criteria HCC.

Expanding the Milan Criteria

Since its induction in 1996, the Milan criteria have been the cornerstone for HCC transplant evaluation. Expansion of these criteria is underway so as to offer transplantation to a wider group of patients at initial presentation. Yao et al. have proposed the UCSF criteria which include solitary tumors ≤6.5 cm or no more than three tumors with the largest ≤4.5 cm not totaling more than 8 cm [20]. This finding was retrospectively determined by explant tumor characteristics and excluded tumors with gross vascular invasion. Survival at 5 years for 70 patients total was 75 % for those within UCSF criteria (n = 18) but only 50 % at 1 year for patients beyond their newly defined criteria. This 5-year survival was not significantly different from those transplanted within Milan criteria but not UCSF criteria. In a subsequent retrospective study by Duffy et al. encompassing 467 patients, 5-year survival again was not significantly different between those of UCSF criteria and Milan criteria [14]. More recently, a UNOS analysis by Patel et al. analyzed post-transplant survival of HCC patients who were within Milan criteria and those who were outside Milan but within UCSF [21]. Of the 3434 patients identified between 2002 and 2007 only 59 were within UCSF criteria and 1913 were within Milan criteria. Four year survival was 72 % for Milan and 51 % for UCSF with no statistical difference ($p = 0.21$). Opponents of criteria expansion suggest that the UCSF criterion applies to a small and clinically insignificant subset of patients and that they used explant pathology to stage the disease. This small number of patients that are within these criteria may contribute to the inability to detect significance in survival between UCSF and Milan criteria patients. Further evaluation with long term prospective studies are needed to elucidate this matter.

Salvage Transplantation

Salvage transplantation refers to transplantation after primary resection secondary to tumor recurrence or deterioration of liver function. The proposed benefit from this approach is that patients with resectable Milan tumors will be spared the morbidity and cost of organ transplantation and thus make more donor organs available for those who will clearly benefit from them (advanced liver disease, unresectable but transplantable tumors). One major drawback is that transplantation is only available to those who have recurrence within Milan criteria. Thus, patients who were transplantable at the time of presentation who undergo resection may then not be transplantable at the time of recurrence. Adam et al. retrospectively compared 17 patients undergoing salvage transplantation to that of 195 patients undergoing primary transplantation for HCC [22]. They found that secondary liver transplantation was associated with a significantly higher operative mortality, tumor recurrence and lower overall 5-year survival (41 % vs 61 % $p = 0.03$); 98 transplant eligible patients underwent resection and 69 (70 %) had recurrence. Only 17 (25 %) of the 69 patients had recurrence within Milan criteria. In an ITT analysis by Del Gaudio et al. comparing 10 patients undergoing salvage transplantation to 293 patients listed for transplantation, overall 5-year survival was 66 % following secondary transplant and 58 % following primary transplant with no significant difference observed [17]. One of the limiting factors in these retrospective ITT analyses is that patients listed for transplantation who forego resection have more advanced liver disease while those who undergo resection tend to have early liver disease but more advanced tumors (outside Milan criteria). This in part may explain the high recurrence rate seen after resection and the relatively few patients who have transplantable recurrence. It remains unclear whether the benefit of saving allografts by resecting first outweighs the number of patients who potentially would have been cured with primary transplantation but now have non-transplantable disease following resection.

Treatment Prior to Transplantation

The dropout rate while awaiting transplant has increased because of greater demand without significant increase in the supply of donor organs [7, 23]. Dropout rates are estimated to be between 12 and 20 % [15]. This has led most transplant centers to adopt the use of ablative therapies prior to transplant to halt tumor progression and thus prevent dropout although conclusive data showing decreased waitlist removal or improved post-liver-transplant survival has not been published. This bridge therapy includes radiofrequency ablation (RFA), transarterial chemoembolization (TACE), transarterial bead embolization (TABE), transarterial radioembolization (TARE) and percutaneous ethanol injection (PEI). Because PEI for the most part has been replaced by RFA, TACE, TABE, TARE, microwave and RFA are now the most common treatments used for pre-transplant ablative therapy [24]. Several studies have suggested that RFA, TACE and TABE are safe and efficacious treatments to prevent tumor progression and waitlist dropout [25, 26]. There are few studies that directly compare dropout rates in treated and untreated pre-transplant patients. Interpretation of these studies is difficult given their heterogeneous patient populations without clear criteria for treatment [27]. In one study that used a decision model based on a review of the current literature to simulate a randomized trial of treatment with TACE vs. no TACE in 600 virtual patients with HCC and cirrhosis, it was found that the benefit of neoadjuvant TACE may be limited to those patients transplanted from 4 to 9 months from first TACE [28]. In another study that used a Markov model to assess a hypothetical cohort of cirrhotic patients with early HCC, it was found that adjuvant therapies for HCC while waiting for liver transplantation provide moderate life expectancy gains and are cost effective for waiting lists of 1 year or more, but that only percutaneous treatment confers a relevant survival advantage for shorter waiting times [29].

Living Donor Liver Transplantation for HCC

Although living donor liver transplant (LDLT) for HCC has waned in frequency in the United States, it has gained popularity in Asian countries such as Japan, South Korea and China [30, 31]. This is because the paucity of deceased donors available in those countries makes LDLT a desirable option. LDLT has the potential advantage of decreased time to transplant as compared to those waiting for deceased donor livers. The major drawback is the risk to the donor who undergoes a major operation with a morbidity rate of 16 % and mortality estimated at one in 500 persons [32]. Studies comparing outcomes between LDLT and deceased donor liver transplant have shown that living donor recipients experience shorter wait times, are more likely to have tumors that exceed Milan criteria, have higher alpha fetoprotein levels and are less likely to have undergone pre-operative therapies such as embolic or thermal ablation [33]. This and other studies show little to no survival benefit of LDLT over deceased donor transplant [34, 35]. Although LDLT offers transplantation for those outside of Milan criteria who would not qualify for deceased donor transplant, the potential harm to the donor for similar outcomes results in its remaining controversial. This likely has contributed to the trend of performing less LDLT for HCC in the United States.

Comparative Outcomes Between Resection and Transplantation for HCC

The debate between resection and transplantation revolves around patients who have well compensated cirrhosis with Milan criteria resectable tumors. Patients within these criteria represent a very small proportion of those who initially present with HCC. This is especially true in western countries where hepatitis C is the most common cause of liver failure and HCC is a result of the progressive and in most cases advanced cirrhosis [15]. Given the need for a large number of patients to show statistical significance, it would be difficult to perform a high-quality prospective randomized controlled trial comparing resection and transplantation. In fact, our search of the literature revealed that no randomized controlled trials addressing this issue exist. Instead, outcomes of surgical treatment for HCC stem from retrospective analyses that have inherent detection, selection and attrition biases. Given the numerous articles available on this subject, several meta-analyses have been published to delineate the role of transplantation and resection for treatment of HCC [36–39]. However, there is reason to be wary of these meta-analyses because they pool data from heterogeneous populations with variable selection criteria and treatment protocols. One such meta-analysis by Dhir et al. focused their choice of articles to strict criteria which excluded studies with non-cirrhotic patients, fibrolamellar HCC and hepatocholangiocarcinomas but included those with HCC within Milan criteria and computation of 5-year survival; between 1990 and 2011 they identified ten articles that fit within these criteria, of which six were ITT analyses, six included only well-compensated cirrhotics (Child-Pugh Class A without liver dysfunction) and three were ITT analyses of well-compensated cirrhotics [37]. Analysis of the six ITT studies that included all cirrhotics (n=1118) (Child-Pugh Class A through C) showed no significant difference in survival at 5 years (OR=0.600, 95 % CI 0.291–1.237 l; p=0.166) but ITT analysis of only well-compensated cirrhotics (Child-Pugh Class A) revealed that patients undergoing transplant had a significantly higher 5-year survival as compared to those with resection (OR=0.521, 95 % CI 0.298–0.911; p=0.022). A more recent ITT retrospective analysis from Spain assessed long-term survival and tumor recurrence following resection or transplant for tumors <5 cm in 217 cir rhotics (Child-Pugh Class A, B and C) over the span of 16 years [40]. Recurrence at 5 years was significantly higher in the resection group (71.6 % vs. 16 % p<0.001) but survival at 4 years was similar (60 % vs. 62 %) which is likely explained by the evolving role of adjuvant therapies to treat post -resection recurrence.

Recommendations

When evaluating patients for surgical treatment of hepatocellular carcinoma several factors should be considered including age, size and location of tumor(s), presence of extrahepatic disease, presence of cirrhosis, comorbidities, organ waitlist time, blood type and degree of liver dysfunction. Patients with anatomically resectable single tumors and no cirrhosis or Child-Pugh Class A cirrhosis with normal bilirubin, HVPG (<10 mmHg), albumin and INR can be offered resection (evidence quality moderate; strong recommendation). Patients with Milan criteria tumors in the setting of Child- Pugh Class A with low platelets and either low albumin or high bilirubin or Child-Pugh Class B and C cirrhosis, especially those with more than one tumor, should be offered liver transplantation over resection (evidence quality moderate; strong recommendation). Those with Milan criteria tumors and Child-Pugh Class A cirrhosis without liver dysfunction should be considered for transplantation over resection (evidence quality low; weak recommendation). No recommendation can be made in regard to transplanting tumors beyond Milan criteria (evidence quality low) except to follow regional review board criteria. Pre-transplant therapies such as embolic or thermal ablation are safe and by expert opinion considered to be effective in decreasing transplant waitlist dropout and bridging patients to transplant (evidence quality low, weak recommendation). These interventions should be considered for those waiting longer than 6 months (evidence quality low, moderate recommendation). Living donor liver transplantation is a safe and effective option for treatment of HCC that are within and exceed Milan criteria (evidence quality moderate, weak recommendation).

A Personal View of the Data

The debate between resection and transplant for early stage tumors in patients with single tumors and well-compensated cirrhosis has persisted for decades without a clear winning strategy in sight. Fortunately, this accounts for only a small portion of the patients that present with HCC. A prospective randomized trial would require a large number of patients to find significance, something that would be further complicated by variable practice patterns between transplant centers. In addition, it would probably not pass IRB scrutiny due to the fact that thermal or embolic ablation is the standard of care at most institutions. As transplant experts at a high-volume center we prefer transplantation for patients with Milan criteria tumors and early cirrhosis because of superior disease-free survival as compared to resection. The significance of disease-free survival in the setting of chronic immunosuppression has yet to be determined. Survival after resection is steadily improving because of improvement in therapies such as TACE, RFA and possibly radioembolization to treat post-resection recurrence. In addition, the recent availability of highly effective therapy for hepatitis C (HCV) will lead to the elimination of chronic infection in many patients, reversing liver disease and improving liver function as well as decreasing portal hypertension [41] and will ultimately lead to reduced HCV-related HCC. Patients should have their underlying liver disease treated aggressively, including antiviral treatment for those with HBV or HCV infection, weight loss for patients with NASH and abstinence from alcohol for those with alcoholic liver disease. The treatment algorithm for HCC is ever changing with improvement not only in adjuvant therapies but with innovations in organ allocation, selection criteria and minimally invasive techniques which we have already observed in the past two decades. Prospective long term studies assessing outcomes of patients treated within the most recent era will help resolve this debate.

- Patients with single anatomically resectable tumors and no cirrhosis or Child-Pugh Class A cirrhosis with platelet counts over 100,000 and normal bilirubin, albumin and INR can be offered resection (evidence quality moderate, strong recommendation); patients with lower platelets need to have normal synthetic function to be considered for surgical resection
- Patients with Milan criteria tumors in the setting of Child-Pugh Class B and C cirrhosis should be offered liver transplantation over resection (evidence quality moderate, strong recommendation)
- Patients with Milan criteria tumors and Child-Pugh Class A cirrhosis without liver dysfunction should be considered for transplantation over resection (evidence quality low, weak recommendation).
- No recommendation can be made in regards to transplanting tumors beyond Milan criteria (evidence quality low).
- Pre-transplant therapy such as RFA and TACE are safe and effective and should be considered for those waiting longer than 6 months (evidence quality moderate, weak recommendation).

- Living donor liver transplantation is a safe and effective option for treatment of HCC that is within and exceeds Milan criteria (evidence quality moderate, weak recommendation).

References

1. Forner A, Reig ME, de Lope CR, Bruix J. Current strategy for staging and treatment: the BCLC update and future prospects. Semin Liver Dis. 2010;30(1):61–74.
2. Bruix J, Sherman M. American Association for the Study of Liver Diseases. Management of hepatocellular carcinoma: an update. Hepatology. 2011;53(3):1020–2.
3. Bruix J, Castells A, Bosch J, et al. Surgical resection of hepatocellular carcinoma in cirrhotic patients: prognostic value of preoperative portal pressure. Gastroenterology. 1996;111(4):1018–22.
4. Belghiti J, Kianmanesh R. Surgical treatment of hepatocellular carcinoma. HPB (Oxf). 2005;7(1):42–9.
5. Cauchy F, Fuks D, Belghiti J. HCC: current surgical treatment concepts. Langenbecks Arch Surg. 2012;397(5):681–95.
6. Cucchetti A, Qiao GL, Cescon M, et al. Anatomic versus nonanatomic resection in cirrhotic patients with early hepatocellular carcinoma. Surgery. 2014;155(3):512–21.
7. Llovet JM, Fuster J, Bruix J. Intention-to-treat analysis of surgical treatment for early hepatocellular carcinoma: resection versus transplantation. Hepatology. 1999;30(6):1434–40.
8. Santambrogio R, Kluger MD, Costa M, et al. Hepatic resection for hepatocellular carcinoma in patients with Child-Pugh's A cirrhosis: is clinical evidence of portal hypertension a contraindication? HPB (Oxf). 2013;15(1):78–84.
9. Iwatsuki S, Gordon RD, Shaw Jr BW, Starzl TE. Role of liver transplantation in cancer therapy. Ann Surg. 1985;202(4):401–7.
10. Olthoff KM, Millis JM, Rosove MH, Goldstein LI, Ramming KP, Busuttil RW. Is liver transplantation justified for the treatment of hepatic malignancies? Arch Surg. 1990;125(10):1261–6; discussion 1266–1268.
11. Mazzaferro V, Regalia E, Doci R, et al. Liver transplantation for the treatment of small hepatocellular carcinomas in patients with cirrhosis. N Engl J Med. 1996;334(11):693–9.
12. Shetty K, Timmins K, Brensinger C, et al. Liver transplantation for hepatocellular carcinoma validation of present selection criteria in predicting outcome. Liver Transpl. 2004;10(7):911–8.
13. Yoo HY, Patt CH, Geschwind JF, Thuluvath PJ. The outcome of liver transplantation in patients with hepatocellular carcinoma in the United States between 1988 and 2001: 5-year survival has improved significantly with time. J Clin Oncol. 2003;21(23):4329–35.
14. Duffy JP, Vardanian A, Benjamin E, et al. Liver transplantation criteria for hepatocellular carcinoma should be expanded: a 22-year experience with 467 patients at UCLA. Ann Surg. 2007;246(3):502–9; discussion 509–511.
15. Majno P, Lencioni R, Mornex F, Girard N, Poon RT, Cherqui D. Is the treatment of hepatocellular carcinoma on the waiting list necessary? Liver Transpl. 2011;17 Suppl 2:S98–108.
16. Facciuto ME, Rochon C, Pandey M, et al. Surgical dilemma: liver resection or liver transplantation for hepatocellular carcinoma and cirrhosis. Intention-to-treat analysis in patients within and outwith Milan criteria. HPB (Oxf). 2009;11(5):398–404.
17. Del Gaudio M, Ercolani G, Ravaioli M, et al. Liver transplantation for recurrent hepatocellular carcinoma on cirrhosis after liver resection: University of Bologna experience. Am J Transplant. 2008;8(6):1177–85.
18. Freeman Jr RB, Edwards EB. Liver transplant waiting time does not correlate with waiting list mortality: implications for liver allocation policy. Liver Transpl. 2000;6(5):543–52.

19. Sharma P, Balan V, Hernandez JL, et al. Liver transplantation for hepatocellular carcinoma: the MELD impact. Liver Transpl. 2004;10(1):36–41.
20. Yao FY, Ferrell L, Bass NM, et al. Liver transplantation for hepatocellular carcinoma: expansion of the tumor size limits does not adversely impact survival. Hepatology. 2001;33(6):1394–403.
21. Patel SS, Arrington AK, McKenzie S, et al. Milan Criteria and UCSF Criteria: a preliminary comparative study of liver transplantation outcomes in the United States. Int J Hepatol. 2012;2012:253517.
22. Adam R, Azoulay D, Castaing D, et al. Liver resection as a bridge to transplantation for hepatocellular carcinoma on cirrhosis: a reasonable strategy? Ann Surg. 2003;238(4):508–18; discussion 518–509.
23. Sarasin FP, Majno PE, Llovet JM, Bruix J, Mentha G, Hadengue A. Living donor liver transplantation for early hepatocellular carcinoma: a life-expectancy and cost-effectiveness perspective. Hepatology. 2001;33(5):1073–9.
24. Lesurtel M, Mullhaupt B, Pestalozzi BC, Pfammatter T, Clavien PA. Transarterial chemoembolization as a bridge to liver transplantation for hepatocellular carcinoma: an evidence-based analysis. Am J Transplant. 2006;6(11):2644–50.
25. Mazzaferro V, Battiston C, Perrone S, et al. Radiofrequency ablation of small hepatocellular carcinoma in cirrhotic patients awaiting liver transplantation: a prospective study. Ann Surg. 2004;240(5):900–9.
26. Chapman WC, Majella Doyle MB, Stuart JE, et al. Outcomes of neoadjuvant transarterial chemoembolization to downstage hepatocellular carcinoma before liver transplantation. Ann Surg. 2008;248(4):617–25.
27. Yao FY, Bass NM, Nikolai B, et al. A follow-up analysis of the pattern and predictors of dropout from the waiting list for liver transplantation in patients with hepatocellular carcinoma: implications for the current organ allocation policy. Liver Transpl. 2003;9(7):684–92.
28. Aloia TA, Adam R, Samuel D, Azoulay D, Castaing D. A decision analysis model identifies the interval of efficacy for transarterial chemoembolization (TACE) in cirrhotic patients with hepatocellular carcinoma awaiting liver transplantation. J Gastrointest Surg. 2007;11(10):1328–32.
29. Llovet JM, Mas X, Aponte JJ, et al. Cost effectiveness of adjuvant therapy for hepatocellular carcinoma during the waiting list for liver transplantation. Gut. 2002;50(1):123–8.
30. Clavien PA, Dutkowski P, Trotter JF. Requiem for a champion? Living donor liver transplantation. J Hepatol. 2009;51(4):635–7.
31. Kawasaki S, Makuuchi M, Matsunami H, et al. Living related liver transplantation in adults. Ann Surg. 1998;227(2):269–74.
32. Ishizaki Y, Kawasaki S. The evolution of liver transplantation for hepatocellular carcinoma (past, present, and future). J Gastroenterol. 2008;43(1):18–26.
33. Kulik LM, Fisher RA, Rodrigo DR, et al. Outcomes of living and deceased donor liver transplant recipients with hepatocellular carcinoma: results of the A2ALL cohort. Am J Transplant. 2012;12(11):2997–3007.
34. Grant RC, Sandhu L, Dixon PR, Greig PD, Grant DR, McGilvray ID. Living vs. deceased donor liver transplantation for hepatocellular carcinoma: a systematic review and meta-analysis. Clin Transplant. 2013;27(1):140–7.
35. Liang W, Wu L, Ling X, et al. Living donor liver transplantation versus deceased donor liver transplantation for hepatocellular carcinoma: a meta-analysis. Liver Transpl. 2012;18(10):1226–36.
36. Zheng Z, Liang W, Milgrom DP, et al. Liver transplantation versus liver resection in the treatment of hepatocellular carcinoma: a meta-analysis of observational studies. Transplantation. 2014;97(2):227–34.
37. Dhir M, Lyden ER, Smith LM, Are C. Comparison of outcomes of transplantation and resection in patients with early hepatocellular carcinoma: a meta-analysis. HPB (Oxf). 2012;14(9):635–45.

38. Rahman A, Assifi MM, Pedroso FE, et al. Is resection equivalent to transplantation for early cirrhotic patients with hepatocellular carcinoma? A meta-analysis. J Gastrointest Surg. 2012;16(10):1897–909.
39. Proneth A, Zeman F, Schlitt HJ, Schnitzbauer AA. Is resection or transplantation the ideal treatment in patients with hepatocellular carcinoma in cirrhosis if both are possible? A systematic review and metaanalysis. Ann Surg Oncol. 2014;21(9):3096–107.
40. Sapisochin G, Castells L, Dopazo C, et al. Single HCC in cirrhotic patients: liver resection or liver transplantation? Long-term outcome according to an intention-to-treat basis. Ann Surg Oncol. 2013;20(4):1194–202.
41. Afdhal N, Everson G, Calleja JL, et al. Sofosbuvir and ribavirin for the treatment of chronic HCV with cirrhosis and portal hypertension with and without decompensation: early virologic response and safety. J Hepatol. 2014;60(1 Suppl):S28.

Chapter 8
Hepatic Epithelioid Hemangioendothelioma

John F. Renz

Abstract This manuscript provides a concise surgical review of hepatic epitheliod hemangioendothelioma. A detailed review of diagnosis, pre-surgical radiologic evaluation, surgical techniques, including liver transplantation, and post-surgical care of the patient with hepatic epitheliod hemangioendothelioma is presented.

Keywords Hepatic epitheliod hemangioendothelioma • Liver surgery • Liver transplantation • Hepatobiliary surgery • Liver tumor

Introduction

Hepatic Epitheliod Hemangioendothelioma (HEHE) remains a diagnostic and therapeutic challenge to the practicing hepatobiliary surgeon. With less than 1000 reported cases since its initial description by Weiss and Enzinger in 1982 [1] and a widely variable clinical course, HEHE remains a diagnosis that affords the clinician a unique opportunity to tailor therapy to the patient. Infantile hemangioendothelioma, a rare neonatal vascular tumor associated with congestive heart failure, thrombocytopenia, and consumptive coagulopathy, is a unique clinical entity that will not be addressed in this manuscript [2].

Presentation

HEHE is a vascular tumor of endothelial cell origin with an incidence of approximately 1/1,000,000 population [3]. Since the initial series of 32 patients reported by Ishak in 1984 [4], our understanding of this rare disease has evolved through collective case reports, database surveys, and meta analyses. HEHE expresses a slight female

J.F. Renz (✉)
University of Chicago Medicine, 5841 S. Maryland, Room J517 MC5027,
Chicago, IL 60637, USA
e-mail: jrenz@surgery.bsd.uchicago.edu

J.M. Millis, J.B. Matthews (eds.), *Difficult Decisions in Hepatobiliary and Pancreatic Surgery*, Difficult Decisions in Surgery: An Evidence-Based Approach, DOI 10.1007/978-3-319-27365-5_8

preponderance (3:2) and is most often diagnosed in the fourth decade of life [5]. Presentation can vary widely from an incidental finding on routine imaging described in approximately 25 % of new cases to overt liver failure. Extra-hepatic involvement is present in over a third of patients at the time of diagnosis [5, 6]. The most frequent presentation includes a history of intermittent right upper quadrant pain, malaise, and weight loss. As the indolent tumor replaces more hepatic volume, late findings of hepatomegaly, jaundice, hepatic outflow obstruction (Budd-Chiari syndrome), Kasabach-Merritt syndrome, hemorrhage secondary to tumor rupture, and acute liver failure emerge [7–10]. The presence of symptoms at diagnosis has been validated as a poor prognostic indicator by MVA [11]. To date, no clear risk factors predisposing to HEHE have emerged; however, oral contraceptives, vinyl chloride, viral hepatitis, and trauma to the liver have been implicated in its development [5, 12]. Notably, HEHE is not associated with chronic liver disease [5]. This affords the physician typically normal hepatic parenchyma to accommodate medical, radiologic, or surgical therapy.

Diagnosis

As HEHE lies variably within the spectrum between hemangioma and angiosacroma, diagnosis requires integration of radiologic, histologic, and immunologic data. For the diagnosis of HEHE, magnetic resonance imaging (MRI) is emerging as the preferred therapy over ultrasound and computed tomography (CT) [13]. HEHE is described radiographically as two types: nodular and diffuse. The nodular type is an early manifestation of HEHE characterized by independent peripheral lesions, ranging from <1 cm to several centimeters in diameter, within the liver. Presentation typically involves both hepatic lobes with a preponderance of tumor in the right hepatic lobe. As the disease progresses, the multifocal tumors coalesce into bulky subcapsular disease throughout the liver defining the advanced diffuse form of HEHE. Capsular retraction develops secondary to scarring and fibrosis [14].

When evaluating a CT, the bulk of disease is best appreciated on unenhanced imaging where intra-tumoral calcification and capsular retraction can be appreciated. Contrast CT findings include arterial phase marginal enhancement that may appear target-like and is often described as a "halo." The concentric zonal or target-like appearance reflects the histology of an avascular, central stomal region with finger-like tumor projections extending peripherally along hepatic sinusoids. These areas become isodense to hepatic parenchyma on post-contrast imaging [14, 15]. On MRI, the central, hypocellular regions may demonstrate previous hemorrhage, thrombus, necrosis, or calcificiation with low signal T-1 weighting with T-2 hyperintesity. Gadolinium administration optimally demonstrates the peripheral halo with progressive centripetal filling on subsequent images. The key findings for any cross-sectional imaging modality are: multiple heterogeneous lesions, subcapsular location, capsular flattening or retraction, and peripheral delayed contrast enhancement with centripetal filling [16]. The utility of FDG-PET is variable.

FDG-PET has not proven sensitive in screening or diagnosis: however, when it is positive in approximately 40 % of cases, it can be useful in monitoring response to therapy [17].

Suggestive radiologic findings must be followed by histologic and immunologic analysis to secure the diagnosis of HEHE. Adequate tissue can be obtained by percutaneous, ultra-sound-guided liver biopsy or diagnostic laparoscopy. HEHE is an endothelial cell origin tumor with an appearance of spindle-shaped endothelial cells multiplying along vascular planes. The histology is variable within the spectrum of hemangioma to angiosarcoma but the tumor characteristically expresses Factor VIII-related antigen, CD34 (human hematopoietic progenitor cell antigen), and CD31 (platelet endothelial cell adhesion molecular 1). Immunoanalysis for at least two of these three antigens is necessary to secure the diagnosis. Therefore, precise pathologic interpretation is integral to identifying malignant features of HEHE and predicting clinical behavior [5].

Potential genetic translocations associated with HEHE have been postulated [18]; however, the rarity of the disease has impeded linkage analysis. Serum chemistries and standard tumor markers are non-diagnostic at presentation with one exception: an elevated CA19-9 is a negative prognostic factor for HEHE and should guide the clinician toward biliary origin malignancies [11].

Treatment

The wide clinical spectrum of disease at presentation and its variable biologic behavior afford the clinician the opportunity to utilize a variety of therapeutic modalities in "tailoring" therapy to the HEHE patient. The incidence of HEHE has prevented the establishment of guidelines and resulted in the application of a multitude of successful therapeutic endeavors ranging from chemotherapy to liver transplantation.

At the moment, the benchmark therapies remain surgical and, whenever possible, resection is preferred [5, 6]. Historically, the bulk of disease at diagnosis has favored liver transplantation; however, recent advances in surgical technique coupled with the fact that HEHE typically occurs in the setting of otherwise normal hepatic parenchyma have opened the possibility of good outcomes in the setting of repetitive surgical resection versus liver transplantation. Grotz et al. reported a retrospective series of 30 HEHE patients treated by surgical resection (SR), liver transplantation (LTX), medical therapy, or no therapy at the Mayo Clinic between 1984 and 2007 [6]. While patients were not randomized to SR or LTX, the group maintained a very aggressive protocol toward SR whenever possible. At a median follow-up of >41 months, the SR group, which contained approximately the same number of patients as the LTX group, demonstrated comparable disease-free survival and overall survival as LTX with a lower incidence of post-operative complications and period of hospitalization. The 1-, 3-, and 5-year overall survival for SR was 100 %, 86 %, and 86 % versus 91 %, 73 %, and 73 % for LTX, respectively. The 1-, 3-, and 5-year disease-free survival for the SR group was 78 %, 62 %, and 62 % versus 64 %, 46 %, and 46 % for LTX, respectively. Hospital stay and the occurrence of Clavien ≥ stage IV complications were lower in SR but did not achieve statistical significance.

Clinicopathologic predictors of prolonged disease-free survival have been proposed by Grotz et al. based upon their retrospective series data but have not been prospectively validated. These include: largest tumor size ≤10 cm, total tumor number ≤10, and hepatic involvement ≤4 segments [6]. This led the authors to advocate for SR as the surgically preferred option for patients with HEHE "regardless of bilobar distribution provided the hepatic disease can be resected [6]." The recent description of liver partition with portal vein ligation for staged hepatectomy described by Schlitt and others offers a new opportunity to dramatically extend the realm of hepatic resection and thereby avoid liver transplantation [19]. However, one must remember that HEHE is a widely variable disease entity and Grotz et al. concede the biologic behavior of each presentation factored largely into their decision to recommend curative surgical therapy [6]. An alternative strategy of hepatectomy followed by carbon-ion radiotherapy has also been advocated [20]. Intent to cure must remain the goal as palliative surgical debulking has been demonstrated to enhance progression [21].

Liver transplantation has proven a durable therapy for the treatment of HEHE. Initially described by Marino et al. in 1988 [22], the application of LTX to patients with extensive bilateral disease has yielded excellent results on three continents [11, 23, 24]. Mehrabi et al. performed a meta analysis from 1984 through 2005 identifying 402 cases [5]. Of this group, 45 % were treated by LTX, 25 % received no treatment, 21 % received chemotherapy and/or radiation therapy, and only 9 % SR. Within this group, the 1- and 5-year survival for LTX were 96 % and 55 % respectively. These results were bested only by the SR group that demonstrated 1- and 5-year survival of 100 % and 75 %, respectively. However, it is impossible to determine through meta analysis the extent of disease approached through SR. Notably, the authors identified extra-hepatic disease in 37 % of patients at the time of diagnosis but the presence of extra-hepatic disease did not portend a poor prognosis.

The unique finding of extra-hepatic disease not impacting long-term survival was confirmed by Lerut et al. who reported the results of the European Liver Transplant Registry in 2007 [23]. In their analysis of 59 patients followed for a median of greater than 6 years, the disease-free survival at 1-, 5-, and 10-years post-LTX were 90 %, 82 %, and 64 %, respectively. Overall recurrence in the cohort was 24 % with a median time to recurrence of 49 months. The extent of disease reported in referring to LTX included bilobar tumor 96 %, >15 tumor nodules 86 %, pre-LTX therapy 30 %, lymph node invasion 30 %, and extra-hepatic disease 17 %. In this context, the overall results obtained with LTX were excellent and led the authors to conclude pre-existing extrahepatic disease as well as lymph node localization are not contraindications to LTX. Vascular invasion upon histologic examination reduced overall patient survival but not disease-free survival. Thus, the pattern of continual treatment of a low grade malignant tumor with a slowly progressive phenotype re-emerged as the authors' inclusion of extra-hepatic disease was limited to that amenable to surgical resection with or without radiation therapy. The finding of carcinomatosis excluded LTX [23].

Data from the United Network for Sharing on 110 transplanted patients between 1987 and 2005 were reported by Rodriguez et al. in 2008 [24]. Their analysis was limited through inclusion of children transplanted for the infantile variant of HEHE and a relatively short median follow-up of only 24 months. The authors reported patient and allograft survival on a cohort including adults and children with an overall mortality related to HEHE recurrence of 16 %, presumably all in adults as the pediatric form is thought to be benign. Unfortunately, their study was not powered to determine the effect of extra-hepatic disease at LTX [24]. When considering LTX, it is imperative to exclude angiosarcoma as its biologic behavior is an absolute contraindication [25].

Disease recurrence has been widely reported as distant as 12 years following LTX and is best approached with surgery and radiation therapy where applicable [5, 26]. A role for adjuvant chemotherapy in the management of post-LTX recurrence is theoretically attractive but unproven.

Alternative Therapies

The epithelial-cell origin of HEHE and its consistent over-expression of vascular endothelial growth factor (VEGF) have made it a natural target for anti-angiogenic therapy [27]. To date, medical therapy alone has delivered inferior results to surgical therapy [5, 6]; however, a variety of chemotherapeutics have been reported to affect HEHE in individual cases. These include thalidomide, doxorubicin, 5-fluorouracil, vincristine, cyclophosphamide, interferon-alpha 2B, bevacizumab, sunitinib, and lenalidomide [28–33]. Chevreau reported results of a European multicenter, phase II trial of15 patients utilizing sorafenib [34]. Their early results were indeterminant, but as more information is elicited on the genetic composition of HEHE, the promise of medical therapy, particularly in highly aggressive disease prompting acute liver failure as well as very slowly progressing indolent disease is promising.

Summary

HEHE is a rare disease with a widely variable presentation and clinical course. Accurate diagnosis through a combination of radiology, histology, and immunochemistry is challenging but essential for anticipating the tumor's biologic behavior. Ultimately, the biologic behavior guides the practitioner to the most appropriate course of therapy with surgery, either resection or transplantation, the preferred avenue for cure. However, further scientific understanding of this unique biologic entity may yield superior outcomes through anti-angiogenic therapy.

References

1. Weiss S, Enzinger F. Epitheloid hemangioendothelioma: a vascular tumor often mistaken for a carcinoma. Cancer. 1982;50:970–81.
2. Dasgupta M, Das S, Patra C, Sarker S. Symptomatic infantile hepatic hemangioendothelioma succesfully treated with steroid. J Clin Neonatol. 2013;2:187–9.
3. Bioulac-Sage P, Laumonier H, Laurent C, Blanc J, Balabaud C. Benign and malignant vascular tumors of the liver in adults. Semin Liver Dis. 2008;28:302–14.
4. Ishak K, Sesterhenn I, Goodman M, Rabin L, Stromeyer F. Epithelioid hemangioendothelioma of the liver: a clinicopathologic and follow-up study of 32 cases. Hum Pathol. 1984;15:839–52.
5. Mehrabi A, Kashfi A, Fonouni H, et al. Primary malignant hepatic epithelioid hemangioendothelioma. Cancer. 2006;107:2108–21.
6. Grotz T, Nagorney D, Donohue J, et al. Hepatic epithelioid haemangioendothelioma: is transplantation the only treatment option? HPB. 2010;12:546–53.
7. Makhlouf H, Ishak K, Goodman Z. Epithelioid hemangioendothelioma of the liver. Cancer. 1999;85:562–82.
8. Frider B, Bruno A, Selser J, Vanessa R, Pascual P, Bistoletti R. Kasabach-Merritt syndrome and adult hepatic epithelioid hemangioendothelioma an unusual association. J Hepatol. 2005;42:282–3.
9. Hayashi Y, Inagaki K, Hirota S, Yoshikawa Y, Ikawa H. Epithelioid hemangioendothelioma with marked liver deformity and secondary Budd-Chiari syndrome: pathologic and radiologic correlation. Pathol Int. 1999;49:547–52.
10. Kim G, Kim Y, Kim H, et al. A case of primary hepatic hemangioendothelioma with spontaneous rupture. Korean J Hepatol. 2009;15:510–6.
11. Wang L, Zhou J, Zhou Y, et al. Clinical experience with primary hepatic epithelioid hemangioendothelioma: retrospective study of 33 patients. World J Surg. 2012;36:2677–83.
12. Dean P, Haggitt R, O'Hare C. Malignant epithelioid hemangioendothelioma of the liver in young women. Relationship to oral contraceptive use. Am J Surg. 1985;9:695–704.
13. Chen Y, Yu R-S, Qiu L-L, Jiang D-Y, Tan Y-B, Fu Y-B. Contrast-enhanced multiple-phase imaging features in hepatic epithelioid hemangioendothelioma. World J Gastroenterol. 2011;17:3544–53.
14. Amin S, Chung H, Jha R. Hepatic epithelioid hemangioendothelioma: MR imaging findings. Abdom Imaging. 2010;36:407–14.
15. Radin D, Craig J, Colletti P, Ralls P, Halls J. Hepatic epithelioid hemangioendothelioma. Radiology. 1988;169:145–8.
16. Roth C, Mitchell D. Hepatocellular carcinoma and other hepatic malignancies: MRI imaging. Radiol Clin N Am. 2014;52:683–707.
17. Dong A, Dong H, Wang Y, Gong J, Lu Z, Zou C. MRI and FDG PET/CT findings of hepatic epithelioid hemangioendothelioma. Clin Nucl Med. 2013;38:66–73.
18. Woelfel C, Liehr T, Weise A, et al. Molecular cytogenetic characterization of epithelioid hemangioendothelioma. Cancer Genet. 2011;204:671–6.
19. Schnitzbauer A, Lang S, Goessmann H, et al. Right portal vein ligation combined with in situ splitting induces rapid left lateral liver lobe hypertrophy enabling 2-staged extended right hepatic resection in small-for-size settings. Ann Surg. 2012;255:405–14.
20. Komatsu S, Iwasaki T, Demizu Y, et al. Two-stage treatment with hepatectomy and carbon-ion radiotherapy for multiple hepatic epithelioid hemangioendotheliomas. World J Gastroenterol. 2014;20:8729–35.
21. Ben-Haim M, Roayaie S, Ye M, et al. Hepatic epithelioid hemangioendothelioma: resection or transplantation, which and when? Liver Transplant Surg. 1999;5:526–31.
22. Marino I, Todo S, Tzakis A, et al. Treatment of hepatic epithelioid hemangioendothelioma with liver transplantation. Cancer. 1988;62:2079–84.

23. Lerut J, Orlando G, Adam R, et al. The place of liver transplantation in the treatment of hepatic epithelioid hemangioendothelioma: report of the European transplant registry. Ann Surg. 2007;246:949–57.
24. Rodriguez J, Becker N, O'Mahony C, Goss J, Aloia T. Long-term outcomes following liver transplantation for hepatic hemangioendothelioma: the UNOS experience from 1987 to 2005. J Gastrointest Surg. 2008;12:110–6.
25. Orlando G, Adam R, Mirza D, et al. Hepatic hemangiosarcoma: an absolute contraindication to liver transplantation-the European Liver Transplant Registry experience. Transplantation. 2013;95:872–7.
26. Rude M, Watson R, Crippin J. Recurrent hepatic epithelioid hemanioendothelioma after orthotopic liver transplantation. Hepatology. 2014;59:2050–2.
27. Emamaullee J, Edgar R, Toso C, et al. Vascular endothelial growth factor expression in hepatic epithelioid hemangioendothelioma: implications for treatment and surgical management. Liver Transpl. 2010;16:191–7.
28. Raphael C, Hudson E, Williams L, Lester J, Savage P. Successful treatment of metastatic hepatic epithelioid hemangioendothelioma with thalidomide: a case report. J Med Case Rep. 2010;22:1186–9.
29. Salech F, Valderrama S, Nervi B, et al. Thalidomide for the treatment of metastatic hepatic epithelioid hemangioendothelioma: a case report with a long term follow-up. Ann Hepatol. 2011;10:99–102.
30. Saada E, Saint Paul M-C, Gugenheim J, Follana P, Francois E. Metastatic hepatic epithelioid hemangioendothelioma: long-term response to sunitinib malate. Oncol Res Treat. 2014;37:124–6.
31. Pallotti M, Nannini M, Agostinelli C, et al. Long-term durable response to lenalidomide in a patient with hepatic epithelioid hemangioendothelioma. World J Gastroenterol. 2014;20:7049–54.
32. Lakkis Z, Kim S, Delabrousse E, et al. Metronomic cyclophosphamide: an alternative treatment for hepatic epithelioid hemangioendothelioma. J Hepatol. 2013;58(6):1254–7.
33. Sangro B, Inarrairaegui M, Fernandez-Ros N. Malignant epithelioid hemangioendothelioma of the liver successfully treated with Sorafenib. Rare Tumor. 2012;4:34–9.
34. Chevreau C, Cesne A, Ray-Coquard I, et al. Sorafenib in patients with progressive epithelioid hemangioendothelioma. Cancer. 2013;15:2639–44.

[illegible]

Chapter 9
What Is the Best Way to Screen Cirrhotic Patients for Hepatocellular Carcinoma in the United States?

Archita P. Desai and Helen S. Te

Abstract Hepatocellular carcinoma (HCC) continues to be a significant cause of mortality in the United States. However, HCC is curable if detected early in its course. Cirrhosis is a well-established risk factor for HCC, but direct evidence demonstrating the benefit of screening for HCC in this population remains under contention today. Ultrasound (US) every 6 months is currently the proposed screening methodology. Serum alpha-feto protein (AFP) has been dropped from screening guidelines, yet recent prospective data reported an added efficacy with the combination of serum AFP and US. Technological advances in cross-sectional imaging have dramatically impacted the field of hepatobiliary imaging, making them attractive alternatives for HCC screening in selected populations. While computed tomography (CT) does not appear to confer any significant advantage to US performed by trained personnel, magnetic resonance imaging (MRI) with hepatobiliary phase (HBP) and diffuse weighted imaging (DWI) offers the best sensitivity and specificity for HCC largely due to its superiority in detecting and characterizing lesions <2 cm. Its cost-effectiveness as a screening tool, however, remains to be seen.

Keywords Alpha-feto protein • Ultrasound • Computed tomography • Magnetic resonance imaging • Hepatocellular cancer • Screening • Surveillance • Liver transplantation

---

A.P. Desai
University of Arizona, 1501 N. Campbell Avenue, Rm 6309A, 245136, Tucson, AZ 85724, USA
e-mail: architadesai@deptofmed.arizona.edu

H.S. Te (✉)
University of Chicago Medical Center, 5841 S. Maryland Ave., MC 7120, Chicago, IL 60615, USA
e-mail: hte@medicine.bsd.uchicago.edu

J.M. Millis, J.B. Matthews (eds.), *Difficult Decisions in Hepatobiliary and Pancreatic Surgery*, Difficult Decisions in Surgery: An Evidence-Based Approach, DOI 10.1007/978-3-319-27365-5_9

Introduction

Despite the continuing medical advances in the management of chronic liver disease, the incidence of hepatocellular carcinoma (HCC) has steadily risen in the past two decades. Globally, HCC has become the fifth leading cause of cancer and the second leading cause of cancer-related death in adult men [1]. In the United States, the age-adjusted incidence rates have doubled since the mid 1980s [2], causing similar increases in HCC-related mortality and hospitalization rates [3, 4]. Although the incidence of HCC appears to have plateaued in the past decade, HCC-related deaths remain on the rise [5, 6].

Hepatocellular carcinoma is curable if detected early in its course. Liver transplantation for HCC cases that fall within the Milan criteria has demonstrated excellent results with 5-year survival rates exceeding 70 %. Hepatic resection in non-cirrhotic patients or in well-compensated cirrhotic patients with no portal hypertension and no significant liver functional impairment has led to 5-year survival rates exceeding 70 % as well [7]. However, to achieve a cure, the diagnosis must be made early, and early diagnosis is only possible if screening is performed.

Evidence demonstrating the benefit of screening for HCC remains under contention today. A meta-analysis found that evidence supporting the benefit of HCC screening in at-risk patients (cirrhotics and noncirrhotics) were of very low-strength [8]. While cirrhosis is a well-established risk factor for HCC, there has been no randomized controlled trial (RCT) performed in the US to validate the benefit of HCC screening in this population, partially due to ethical reasons and patient refusal [9]. Investigators have resorted to modeling techniques to demonstrate the cost-effectiveness of HCC surveillance in cirrhosis, and screening has been found to provide a survival benefit in targeted patients who are viable candidates for interventions at acceptable costs [10–15]. In fact, the American Association for the Study of Liver Diseases (AASLD) [7] and the European Association for the Study of the Liver (EASL) guidelines [16] recommend HCC surveillance with an ultrasound every 6 months for patients with cirrhosis of any cause, wherein the incidence of HCC is estimated to be 1.5 % per year or greater [7]. However, the question remains, does biannual ultrasound provide the best benefit in screening cirrhotic patients for HCC in the United States in 2014?

Search Strategy

A literature search of English language publications from 2000 to 2014 was used to identify published data on screening fot HCC in cirrhotic patients using the PICO outline (Table 9.1). Databases searched were PubMed, Medline and Cochrane Evidence Based Medicine. Terms used in the search were "hepatocellular carcinoma/screening/cirrhosis," "liver cancer/screening/cirrhosis." Manual searches of reference lists from applicable studies were performed to identify any studies that may have been missed by the computer-assisted search. As the quality of studies for each

Table 9.1 PICO table for screening for hepatocellular carcinoma in cirrhotic patients

P (Patients)	I (Intervention)	C (Comparator group)	O (Outcomes measured)
Patients with cirrhosis	Serum AFP assay	No screening	Diagnosis of hepatocellular carcinoma within Milan criteria, mortality
Patients with cirrhosis	Ultrasound examination	No screening or screening via another modality	Diagnosis of hepatocellular carcinoma, mortality
Patients with cirrhosis	CT examination	No screening or screening via another modality	Diagnosis of hepatocellular carcinoma, mortality
Patients with cirrhosis	MRI examination	No screening or screening via another modality	Diagnosis of hepatocellular carcinoma, mortality

screening modality varied, different inclusion criteria were used for the studies included in this review. For the performance of serum AFP, studies were excluded if they specifically addressed diagnosis of hepatocellular carcinoma after a lesion has been detected in the liver rather than screening, or if noncirrhotic patients were the only study subjects. For the performance of ultrasound as a screening test, only prospective studies of cirrhotic cohorts were included. For cross-sectional imaging, studies reviewed reflect the latest progress in the technology of computed tomography (CT) and magnetic resonance imaging (MRI). For CT, only studies assessing the performance of 16-slice or more multidectector CT (MDCT) with triple or quadruple phase imaging and explant pathology used as the reference standard were included. For MRI, studies using dynamic MRI with both hepatobiliary phase and diffusion weighted imaging MRI were included. The data was classified using the GRADE system.

Results

Clinical Relevance and Risk Factors of Hepatocellular Carcinoma

Screening is the administration of diagnostic tests to subjects who have a defined risk for developing HCC, but in whom there is no suspicion for HCC to be present prior to the screening. Surveillance is the repeated administration of screening tests. An intervention is considered effective if it provides an increase in longevity of about 100 days or 3 months [17], and interventions that can be achieved at a cost of <$50,000/year of life gained is considered to be cost-effective in 1992 [18], although this cost is likely higher in today's market rates.

Major advances in medicine have increased the ability to cure HCC when diagnosed early, although medical and locoregional interventions may still extend survival in later stages. Despite the absence of high quality data from RCT of HCC surveillance versus no HCC surveillance, the ability to change patient outcomes with appropriate interventions at acceptable costs is compelling reason to prompt the AASLD to recommend HCC surveillance in high-risk population. Cirrhosis is a well-established risk factor for HCC, wherein surveillance for an HCC incidence of 1.5 %/year is expected to increase survival by about 3 months [10]. Hepatitis B carriers who are Asian males aged over 40 years and Asian females aged over 50 years have an HCC incidence of 0.4–0.6 %/year, and those with a family history of HCC are known to have a higher HCC incidence than those without. African and North American Blacks with hepatitis B also are known to develop HCC at a younger age. Cirrhotic hepatitis B carriers have an HCC incidence of 3–8 %/year, while patients with hepatitis C cirrhosis and stage 4 primary biliary cirrhosis have an HCC incidence of 3–5 %/year. The HCC incidence in cirrhotics with genetic hemochromatosis, alpha 1- antitrypsin deficiency and other causes are not established but may approach >1.5 %/year for most cases [7]. Another growing group at risk for HCC is the population afflicted with non-alcoholic steatohepatitis, where the incidence is 2.6 %/year in one study [19, 20].

Screening Strategies

Serum Alpha-Feto Protein (AFP)

Serum AFP is the most widely tested biomarker in the diagnosis of HCC, but its performance as a surveillance tool has been suboptimal. The only RCT evaluating serum AFP alone as a screening tool for HCC was conducted in hepatitis B infected patients who were mostly non-cirrhotic; the findings included an earlier diagnosis of HCC [21]. Data in cirrhotic patients have been limited to case control studies, which have consistently shown a low sensitivity of a serum AFP cut-off of 20 ng/ml at about 60 % for detection of HCC (Table 9.2) [22–27]. Trevisani et al. reported the positive predictive value of a serum AFP cut-off value of >20 ng/ml to be dismal at 25.1 % in a population with an HCC prevalence of 5 % [25]. Currently, serum AFP is not part of the recommended screening process for HCC by both the AASLD [28] and the EASL guidelines [16, 28].

The potential value of measuring serial serum AFPs to survey for HCC has also been investigated in another case-control study involving hepatitis C-infected patients with advanced fibrosis or cirrhosis. Lee et al. found that both the standard deviation and the rate of increase of serum AFP were independently associated with HCC. Incorporation of these metrics along with patient-specific risk factors resulted in improved accuracy for HCC prediction to an area under the receiver-operating characteristic curve of 0.81 when compared with 0.76 when only the most recent serum AFP value was used [29]. However, these findings need to be validated further to determine its true value in HCC screening.

Table 9.2 Sensitivity and specificity of serum AFP in detecting early stage HCCs

Study	AFP cut-off (ng/ml)	Sensitivity (%)	Specificity (%)	Study type (quality of evidence)
Gamberin-Gelwan et al. [22]	≥20	58	91	Case-control (low)
Trevisani et al. [25][a]	>20	60	91	Case-control (low)
Nguyen et al. [24, 64]	>20	63	80	Case-control (low)
Snowberger et al. [27][b]	8.9	62	80	Case-control (low)
	50	31	96	
Marrero et al. [24]	>20	59	90	Case-control (low)
Lok et al. [23]	>20	61	81	Case-control (low)
Singal et al. [26]	>20	66	90	Prospective cohort (moderate)

[a]In a population with 50 % HCC prevalence
[b]Used explants as gold standard

Ultrasonography (US) with or Without Serum AFP

While US technology has been used for diagnostic purposes since the 1940s, its use for screening for liver masses was first reported in the early 1980s [30]. Since then, many studies evaluating the performance of US with or without serum AFP in surveillance programs aimed to detect early stages of HCC have been done [8, 31–33]. Despite a variety of study methodologies involved, a recent meta-analysis calculated the pooled odds of early detection as 2.08 (95 % CI 1.80–2.37). More importantly, screening increased the odds of receipt of curative therapy (OR 2.24, 95 % CI 1.99–2.52) and the odds of 3-year survival (OR 1.90, 95 % CI 1.90–2.17) [33]. It is important to note that this data has limited accuracy and applicability, as most of the studies included in the meta-analysis were observational studies susceptible to lead-time and selection bias, and these also included a wide variety of patient populations, utilized different screening programs and had largely different screening uptakes as well. Three randomized trials have been done in Europe and Asia to study the efficacy of screening with ultrasound with or without serum AFP [34–36], but cirrhotic patients were not included or defined [36] so these studies are not included in this discussion.

More recent data on HCC screening in patients with cirrhosis published after 2000 included prospective studies that assessed the performance of US with or without serum AFP in the real world. Overall, the sensitivity of US for detecting HCC has a wide range of 43–90 % and a specificity of 83–97 % (Table 9.3) [26, 34, 37–41]. While current guidelines do not recommend use of serum AFP, most studies included serum AFP testing in their surveillance program. In fact, one study attempted to assess the role of serum AFP by creating randomization arms that consisted of imaging surveillance without serum AFP, but discovered high usage rates of serum AFP assays in the imaging alone group, necessitating the final analysis to include imaging in combination with serum AFP [34]. The optimal interval

Table 9.3 Summary of prospective studies of hepatocellular carcinoma (HCC) screening in cirrhotics using ultrasonography (US) with or without serum alpha feto protein (AFP)

Study	Screening method	Cohort	Sensitivity	Specificity	Clinical effectiveness	Study type (quality of evidence)
Henrion et al. [37]	US and serum AFP assay every 6 months	Belgian cirrhotics	83 %	Insufficient data	Compliance to surveillance program overall was 66 % and was significantly higher in those with cirrhosis due to non-alcoholic causes	Prospective cohort (low)
Bolondi et al. [35]	US and serum AFP assay every 6 months	Italian Child-Pugh A or B cirrhotics	82 %	Insufficient data	Higher rate of unifocal and smaller HCC for screened vs control group (80 % vs. 53 %, $p<0.001$)	Prospective cohort (low)
					Longer 3-year survival for screened vs control group (45 % vs 31.7 %, $p=0.02$)	
					Similar rate of treatment for HCC in screened vs control group (58.6 % vs 68.8 %, p=NS)	
					Cost per year of life saved=$112,996	
Sangiovanni et al. [39]	Annual US and serum AFP assay[a]	Italian Child A and B cirrhotics, aged 36–72	Insufficient data	Insufficient data	Smaller nodules detected in latest study period with mean diameter of 2.2 cm (1997–2001) vs. 3.0 cm (1992–1996) vs. 3.7 cm (1987–1991)	Prospective cohort (low)
					Improved survival in those screened in the latest study period, linked to earlier diagnosis and improved linkage to treatment	

Trinchet et al. [32]	US every 3 or 6 months	French or Belgian Child-Pugh A or B cirrhotics	86.6 %	Insufficient data	No difference in diagnosis of early HCC or overall survival	Randomized control trial (high)
					Increased incidence of non-malignant focal lesions (especially those ≤10 mm) when US was completed every 3 months. If lesions were followed per EASL recommendations, the time of HCC diagnosis and treatment would not have changed	
Singal et al. [26]	US and serum AFP assay every 6–12 months[b]	American Child-Pugh A or B cirrhotics	US: 43.9 %	US: 91.5 %	38.7 % of study population received inconsistent or no surveillance	Prospective cohort (moderate)
			US + AFP: 90.2 %	US + AFP: 83.3 %	US sensitivity was lower in non-Caucasian race and lower MELD score	
					Majority of participants only had one positive surveillance study (AFP or US) prior to HCC diagnosis	
Di Martino et al. [36]	Doppler US followed by cross-sectional imaging	Italian OLT candidates over 3 year period who underwent all three imaging tests in 1 month[e]	71 %	62 %	US sensitivity decreased with decreasing nodule size, with only 22 % sensitivity for nodules under 10 mm	Prospective cohort (moderate)
					Lower specificity due to significant numbers of false positive examinations when state of the art US technology was used	

(continued)

Table 9.3 (continued)

Study	Screening method	Cohort	Sensitivity	Specificity	Clinical effectiveness	Study type (quality of evidence)
Pocha et al. [38]	US every 6 months vs. annual CT[c,d]	American Child A cirrhotics[f]	US: 71.4 %	US: 97.5 %	Significant number of participants went off-protocol	Randomized control trial (moderate)
			CT: 66.7 %	CT: 94.4 %	Ultrasound comparable to CT in detecting early stage HCC	
					AFP added little value to overall HCC detection	
					Cost of one HCC detected was significantly higher with CT ($35,383) vs US ($17,041)	

[a]If AFP >20 ng/dL, US and serum AFP assay frequency were increased to every 6 months
[b]Screening was obtained at the discretion of the treating hepatologist, no reminders were sent to patient or medical care providers
[c]computed tomography
[d]±AFP every 6 months in both arms
[e]Excluded three cholangiocarcinoma nodules (in two patients) and three hepatocholangiocarcinoma nodules (in one patient)
[f]Participants had to be potential candidates for treatment of HCC; advanced medical condition and those who were unable to receive IV contrast due to renal insufficiency or allergy were excluded

between screenings is not clear with most studies using 6 month or 12 month intervals. Shorter intervals appears to only increase detection of non-malignant focal lesions in the 3-month group, particularly those <10 mm in diameter, which did not impact clinical care or outcomes in most cases [34]. Although one study in a Veterans Administration hospital setting found no incremental benefit of the addition of serum AFP to imaging studies [40], one prospective cohort study involving 446 patients in real world practice reported substantial advantage of using serum AFP in conjunction with US than with US alone, with increased sensitivity to 90.2 % and specificity to 83.3 % [26].

Cross Sectional Imaging

The clinical effectiveness of US in screening for HCC is largely limited by low adherence rates, variability in operator experience, difficulty in visualization of the liver in patients with morbid obesity or very nodular livers, and poor sensitivity when identifying early HCC's (i.e., those <20 mm). These limitations have fueled the search for improved modalities in screening those at high risk for HCC. Both computed tomography (CT) and magnetic resonance imaging (MRI) of the abdomen have been used to further evaluate and diagnose liver lesions found during ultrasound examination. Therefore, both offer attractive alternatives for screening of those at risk for HCC.

Computed Tomography

Beginning in the 1990s, use of arterial-phase imaging during intravenous contrast medium-enhanced CT studies improved the sensitivity of small nodule detection [42]. In the 2000s, multidetector-row helical CT (MDCT) technology allowed for faster acquisition, thinner slices (0.5 mm for 64-slice MDCT vs. 5–10 mm for helical CT) in a single breath-hold and repetitive imaging during multiple perfusion phases after contrast material injection [42, 43]. In combination with four-phase CT protocols, which provide images during the pre-contrast, arterial, portal venous and delayed phases, 16-, 64- and even 128-slice MDCT has allowed for the detection of a significantly higher number of cases of HCC [42, 44]. Current UNOS policy outlines minimum criteria for the use of CT to accurately diagnose HCC radiographically [45]. Many of the studies assessing the sensitivity and specificity of triple phase 16- or 64-slice MDCT have been performed in individuals awaiting liver transplantation. Most are retrospective; however, many have used the explant pathology as the gold standard, thus increasing their validity with sensitivities of 77–89 % and specificities of 44–93 % (Table 9.4) [44, 46–48]. Due to the lack of prospective data, the screening interval for CT has yet to be established. Overall, even studies of the most advanced CT technology only show marginal superiority over US as a screening tool, largely due to better sensitivity for lesions <20 mm in size.

Table 9.4 Summary of studies using triple or four-phase protocols with 16- or greater slice multidetector-row helical computed tomography (MDCT) for the diagnosis of hepatocellular carcinoma (HCC) with explant pathology as gold standard

Study	Imaging method	Cohort	Sensitivity	Specificity	Clinical performance	Study type (quality of evidence)
Ronzoni et al. [48]	Triple-phase MDCT original reports vs. images reviewed retrospectively[a]	OLT recipients with CT within 6 months of OLT	Original report: 64 % by lesion, 77 % by patient	Original report: 75 % by patient[f]	32 % of false negative lesions were due to prior locoregional therapy and 70 % were <10 mm in size	Retrospective (low)
			Retrospective review: 73.3 % by lesion, 83.4 % by patient	Retrospective review: 77.5 % by patient[c]	14 % of the study population would have been denied or referred to OLT due to false-negative or false-positive results, respectively	
Denecke et al. [47]	Triple-phase MDCT images reviewed retrospectively by two radiologists	OLT recipients with HCC with CT within 100 days of OLT[c]	Observer 1: 78 %	Observer 1: 45 %	Sensitivity for both observers decreased with decreasing size of the nodule (43 % and 53 % observers 1 and 2 for nodules <10 mm, respectively, vs. 94 % for both observers for 11–20 mm nodules vs. 89 % and 95 %, respectively, for nodules >20 mm)	Retrospective (low)
			Observer 2: 83 %	Observer 2: 44 %	Poor specificity with high false positive rate for both observers noted	

Luca et al. [44]	Triple-phase MDCT images retrospectively reviewed by three blinded radiologists[b]	OLT recipients imaged with CT pre-transplant	Hypervascular lesion with washout on portal venous and/or delayed phase images: 43 %	Hypervascular lesion with washout: 93 %	Pattern of hypervascular nodule with washout has poor sensitivity but excellent specificity for the diagnosis of HCC	Retrospective (low)
			Overall: 89 %[e]		Limitation to hypervascular lesions with delayed phase washout only improved diagnostic accuracy	
					Pattern of hypervascular nodule with washout established an accurate staging of disease in 46 % of cases, underestimated in 52 % and overestimated in only 2 %	
					Hypervascular lesions >10 mm without washout and hypovascular lesions >20 mm have significant risk of HCC	
Addley et al. [46]	Triple-phase MDCT reviewed by three radiologist	OLT recipients with CT within 5 months of OLT[d]	Observer 1:78 %	Observer 1:47 %	Sensitivity for each radiologist was significantly lower if lesion <20 mm	Retrospective (low)
			Observer 2: 72 %	Observer 2: 69 %	Observer expertise and years of experience improved accuracy of HCC detection but decreased sensitivity	
			Observer 3: 65 %	Observer 3: 88 %		

[a]Diagnosis reached by consensus between two unblinded radiologists
[b]Diagnosis reached by consensus amongst three blinded radiologists
[c]Patients with incomplete histopathologic report and those who had intermittent tumor treatment were excluded
[d]Patients who had previously undergone treatment of HCC, those with malignancy other than HCC and those with multifocal HCC were excluded
[e]MDCT findings of hypervascular nodule with washout, hypervascular nodule without washout, and hypovascular nodules were included
[f]Specificity by lesion not reported

Magnetic Resonance Imaging

As with CT, MRI is evolving with new techniques allowing for improved diagnostic accuracy. With MR, however, there are a variety of techniques for imaging acquisition, image sequences and optimization, as well as image processing that can impact the ultimate performance of MR in liver lesion detection and accurate characterization. Current UNOS policy outlines specific minimum technical requirements for MRI in diagnosing HCC radiographically [49]. Of the recent advances in MR technology, dynamic imaging, hepatobiliary phase (HBP) imaging with hepatocyte-specific contrast agents, and use of diffusion weight image (DWI) characteristics have allowed MRI to evaluate tumor vascularity, increased tissue cellularity and absence of normal hepatocytes with greater detail and accuracy [50–54].

The reported sensitivity of dynamic contrast enhanced MR imaging (with an extracellular fluid contrast agent) is noted to be from 70 to 100 % in various studies with a pooled sensitivity of 81 % [31]. Even with dynamic, contrast-enhanced MRI, the detection of early HCC remains a challenge, particularly with the background of a cirrhotic liver where arterial enhancement of small <1 cm lesions is less diagnostically accurate for HCC. For these lesions, MRI offers several advantages over CT despite some inherent limitations [55–57].

Hepatobiliary phase (HPB) imaging may improve the ability to detect and diagnose early HCC. Use of gadoxetic acid (Eovist®) or gadobenate dimeglumine (MultiHance®) allows for both dynamic imaging during the extracellular phase and delayed imaging in the HBP phase, when the contrast is taken up by the hepatocytes [52, 53]. These agents can help differentiate arterial-enhancing pseudolesions. One study documented 95.5 % of HCC's displayed hypointensity during the HBP while 94.3 % of pseudolesions were isointense during the HBP. In this study, the sensitivity of MRI for diagnosing HCC was 93.9 % [58]. Another study showed lesions without arterial phase hyperenhancement, but with both venous phase hypoenhancement and HBP hypointensity, carry a higher probability of being well-differentiated HCC in cirrhotic livers [55]. A meta-analysis of gadoxetic acid-based MRI reported a pooled sensitivity of 91 % and specificity of 95 %. For studies focused on lesions <2 cm, performance continued to be excellent with a reported sensitivity range of 87–99 % and specificity range of 92–96 % [52].

Diffusion weighted imaging (DWI) in MRI is a functional MRI technique that offers its own advantages in the detection and diagnosis of HCC in those with cirrhosis. DWI capitalizes on the changes that accompany the development of HCC, such as changes in cellularity and extracellular space structure, to detect HCC lesions. A reported 70–80 % of HCC's, including those <1–2 cm in size, appear hyperintense on DWI [51]. The sensitivity and specificity of DWI were better at 91.2 % and 82.9 %, respectively, when compared to dynamic, gadolinium-based MRI at 67.6 % and 61 %, respectively [59]. A study also highlighted the utility of MRI enhanced with DWI as a screening tool for HCC for those in whom intravenous iodine contrast administration is contraindicated [54]. In another study, use of

DWI characteristics improved the sensitivity of conventional MRI from 83–85 % to 98 % in detecting HCC lesions <2 cm [60]. Furthermore, several studies that assessed the impact of combining HBP imaging with DWI to detect HCC concluded that DWI can incrementally improve the performance of MRI in the detection of HCC (Table 9.5) [61–63]. While these techniques are promising, the optimal interval of imaging and the cost of such a screening tool have not been examined. Therefore, evidence supporting the use of MRI for the screening and surveillance of cirrhotics for HCC is lacking, and their use has not been incorporated in the current practice guidelines.

Recommendations

While the clinical effectiveness of screening individuals with cirrhosis has yet to be determined, indirect evidence supports a survival benefit with screening of targeted individuals who are viable candidates for interventions. Biannual ultrasound with or without serum AFP is the most validated tool, offers good performance in the general population, and in experienced hands likely has similar performance to triple phase MDCT for the detection of tumors >2 cm. However, as locoregional therapy becomes more widely available, the detection of early HCC may offer a survival benefit. In this context, dynamic MRI with hepatobiliary phase and diffusion weighted imaging may be the best-performing screening test. Screening, regardless of modality, should be done in expert hands to optimize effectiveness of the test. The cost of such a surveillance program will have to be compared to its clinical effectiveness, which is largely dependent on uptake of screening and linkage to treatment.

A Personal View of the Data

Many advances have been made in the diagnosis of HCC over the past decade. Improvements in CT and MRI technology form the basis of this progress; however, translation into clinical practice and guidelines is limited by the quality of data supporting their use in screening and surveillance programs. Current data have created a strong platform for imaging-based screening of HCC, whereas the importance of tumor markers and invasive method such as biopsy has declined. In an era where the morbidity and mortality associated with HCC is rising, efforts to improve early diagnosis must be made in order to impact patient outcomes and reduce the healthcare burden associated with HCC. In this context, MRI-based imaging has the most promise for accuracy, although its cost is a major deterrence in its use as the first line tool.

Table 9.5 Summary of studies of the performance of gadoxetic acid-enhanced MRI with or without DWI in the detection of HCC

Study	Imaging method	Cohort	Sensitivity	Specificity	Clinical performance	Study type (Quality of evidence)
Park et al. [63]	Gadoxetic acid-enhanced MRI with or without DWI at 3.0-T as reviewed by three independent, blinded observers	HCC lesion <2 cm proven by surgical resection in those who had undergone MRI[a]	Gadoxetic acid alone: 81.4 %	Gadoxetic acid alone: 98.4 %	Adding DWI analysis to gadoxetic-acid enhanced MRI improved the sensitivity and specificity	Retrospective (very low)
			DWI alone: 78.8 %	DWI alone: 96.8 %		
			Combined: 92.4 %	Combined: 97.5 %	Sensitivity of combined image sets in the detection of lesions <1 cm is lower than for those lesions >1 cm (84.8 % vs. 95.7 %)	
					Specificity of combined image sets in the detection of lesions <1 cm is slightly lower than for those lesions >1 cm (94.5 % vs. 99.6 %)	
Park et al. [62]	Gadoxetic acid-enhanced MRI with or without DWI at 3.0-T as reviewed by two independent, blinded observers	Those with suspected lesion on MDCT or US with lesion <2.0 cm[b]	Combined: 98.5 %	Combined: 90.9 %	Arterial hyperintensity, hypointensity on HBP and hyperintensity on DWI was present in 65 % of <1 cm lesions	Retrospective (very low)
					The majority of lesions that did not have typical characteristics of HCC on MDCT were able to be characterized as HCC based on HBP and DWI characteristics	

Hwang et al. [61]	Gadoxetic acid-enhanced MRI with or without DWI at 3.0-T as reviewed by two independent, blinded observers	OLT recipients who underwent MRI within 90 days of OLT[c]	Gadoxetic acid alone: 72 %	Gadoxetic acid alone: 96 %	Adding DWI analysis to gadoxetic-acid enhanced MRI improved the sensitivity and specificity	Retrospective (low)
			Combined: 79 %	Combined: 93 %	Sensitivity of gadoxetic acid-enhanced MRI with and without DWI decreased with lesion size (for combined imaging, 93 % for lesions >2.0 cm vs. 61 % for lesions <1.0 cm)	
					Sensitivity of gadoxetic acid-enhanced MRI with and without DWI decreased with increasing severity of liver disease (for combined imaging, 97 % in Child-Pugh class A vs 56 % in Child-Pugh class C)	

[a]Control group included those with suspected HCC on initial imaging but with negative diagnostic work up
[b]Included individuals without cirrhosis. Individuals excluded if they had not had MDCT as well as MRI. Lesion deemed either HCC or benign hepatocellular nodule based on imaging criteria, biopsy, surgical resection or explant pathology
[c]Included 8/63 non-cirrhotics

Recommendations

1. MRI with HBP and DWI offers the best sensitivity and specificity of HCC largely due to its superiority in detecting and characterizing lesions <2 cm. While there are no data on screening interval for MRI, annual imaging in those with no worrisome lesions can be inferred based on tumor doubling time. The cost-effectiveness of this approach, however, remains to be studied.
2. In the general population, ultrasound with or without serum AFP every 6 months offers acceptable performance in the screening of HCC and should be used when cross-sectional imaging is not available or tolerated or is contraindicated. The combination of US with serum AFP has demonstrated increased accuracy in a larger prospective study than US alone. Furthermore, the interval change in serum AFP may offer more value in the detection of HCC than a single serum AFP assay alone.
3. In those awaiting liver transplantation, where accurate assessment of the burden of HCC can significantly alter management, MRI with HPB phase and DWI should be used, with the best performance noted in those with Child-Pugh class A and B cirrhosis.
4. Survival benefit of screening for HCC has yet to be established in randomized controlled trials, but it is unlikely for such trials to come to fruition due to difficulty with patient enrollment. Limiting screening to those individuals who are eligible for treatment will improve clinical effectiveness of surveillance program.

References

1. Jemal A, et al. Global cancer statistics. CA Cancer J Clin. 2011;61(2):69–90.
2. El-Serag HB, et al. The continuing increase in the incidence of hepatocellular carcinoma in the United States: an update. Ann Intern Med. 2003;139(10):817–23.
3. El-Serag HB. Hepatocellular carcinoma: recent trends in the United States. Gastroenterology. 2004;127(5 Suppl 1):S27–34.
4. Kim WR, et al. Mortality and hospital utilization for hepatocellular carcinoma in the United States. Gastroenterology. 2005;129(2):486–93.
5. Altekruse SF, et al. Changing hepatocellular carcinoma incidence and liver cancer mortality rates in the United States. Am J Gastroenterol. 2014;109(4):542–53.
6. Rahib L, et al. Projecting cancer incidence and deaths to 2030: the unexpected burden of thyroid, liver, and pancreas cancers in the United States. Cancer Res. 2014;74(11):2913–21.
7. Bruix J, Morris S. Management of hepatocellular carcinoma: an update. AASLD Practice Guidelines 2010 [cited 2014 9/17/14]; Available from: http://www.aasld.org/sites/default/files/guideline_documents/HCCUpdate2010.pdf.
8. Kansagara D, et al. Screening for hepatocellular carcinoma in chronic liver disease: a systematic review. Ann Intern Med. 2014;161(4):261–9.
9. Poustchi H, et al. Feasibility of conducting a randomized control trial for liver cancer screening: is a randomized controlled trial for liver cancer screening feasible or still needed? Hepatology. 2011;54(6):1998–2004.

10. Sarasin FP, Giostra E, Hadengue A. Cost-effectiveness of screening for detection of small hepatocellular carcinoma in western patients with Child-Pugh class A cirrhosis. Am J Med. 1996;101(4):422–34.
11. Andersson KL, et al. Cost effectiveness of alternative surveillance strategies for hepatocellular carcinoma in patients with cirrhosis. Clin Gastroenterol Hepatol. 2008;6(12):1418–24.
12. Arguedas MR, et al. Screening for hepatocellular carcinoma in patients with hepatitis C cirrhosis: a cost-utility analysis. Am J Gastroenterol. 2003;98(3):679–90.
13. Lin OS, et al. Cost-effectiveness of screening for hepatocellular carcinoma in patients with cirrhosis due to chronic hepatitis C. Aliment Pharmacol Ther. 2004;19(11):1159–72.
14. Mourad A, et al. Hepatocellular carcinoma screening in patients with compensated hepatitis C virus (HCV)-related cirrhosis aware of their HCV status improves survival: a modeling approach. Hepatology. 2014;59(4):1471–81.
15. Patel D, et al. Cost-effectiveness of hepatocellular carcinoma surveillance in patients with hepatitis C virus-related cirrhosis. Clin Gastroenterol Hepatol. 2005;3(1):75–84.
16. European Association For The Study Of The, L, R. European Organisation For, C. Treatment Of. EASL-EORTC clinical practice guidelines: management of hepatocellular carcinoma. J Hepatol. 2012;56(4):908–43.
17. Naimark D, Naglie G, Detsky AS. The meaning of life expectancy: what is a clinically significant gain? J Gen Intern Med. 1994;9(12):702–7.
18. Laupacis A, et al. How attractive does a new technology have to be to warrant adoption and utilization? Tentative guidelines for using clinical and economic evaluations. CMAJ. 1992;146(4):473–81.
19. Ascha MS, et al. The incidence and risk factors of hepatocellular carcinoma in patients with nonalcoholic steatohepatitis. Hepatology. 2010;51(6):1972–8.
20. Kim Y, et al. Temporal trends in population-based death rates associated with chronic liver disease and liver cancer in the United States over the last 30 years. Cancer. 2014;120(19):3058–65.
21. Chen JG, et al. Screening for liver cancer: results of a randomised controlled trial in Qidong, China. J Med Screen. 2003;10(4):204–9.
22. Gambarin-Gelwan M, et al. Sensitivity of commonly available screening tests in detecting hepatocellular carcinoma in cirrhotic patients undergoing liver transplantation. Am J Gastroenterol. 2000;95(6):1535–8.
23. Lok AS, et al. Des-gamma-carboxy prothrombin and alpha-fetoprotein as biomarkers for the early detection of hepatocellular carcinoma. Gastroenterology. 2010;138(2):493–502.
24. Marrero JA, et al. Alpha-fetoprotein, des-gamma carboxyprothrombin, and lectin-bound alpha-fetoprotein in early hepatocellular carcinoma. Gastroenterology. 2009;137(1):110–8.
25. Trevisani F, et al. Serum alpha-fetoprotein for diagnosis of hepatocellular carcinoma in patients with chronic liver disease: influence of HBsAg and anti-HCV status. J Hepatol. 2001;34(4):570–5.
26. Singal AG, et al. Effectiveness of hepatocellular carcinoma surveillance in patients with cirrhosis. Cancer Epidemiol Biomark Prev. 2012;21(5):793–9.
27. Snowberger N, et al. Alpha fetoprotein, ultrasound, computerized tomography and magnetic resonance imaging for detection of hepatocellular carcinoma in patients with advanced cirrhosis. Aliment Pharmacol Ther. 2007;26(9):1187–94.
28. Bruix J, Sherman M, D. American Association for the Study of Liver. Management of hepatocellular carcinoma: an update. Hepatology. 2011;53(3):1020–2.
29. Lee E, et al. Improving screening for hepatocellular carcinoma by incorporating data on levels of alpha-fetoprotein, over time. Clin Gastroenterol Hepatol. 2013;11(4):437–40.
30. Takashima T, et al. Diagnosis and screening of small hepatocellular carcinomas. Comparison of radionuclide imaging, ultrasound, computed tomography, hepatic angiography, and alpha 1-fetoprotein assay. Radiology. 1982;145(3):635–8.
31. Colli A, et al. Accuracy of ultrasonography, spiral CT, magnetic resonance, and alpha-fetoprotein in diagnosing hepatocellular carcinoma: a systematic review. Am J Gastroenterol. 2006;101(3):513–23.

32. Singal A, et al. Meta-analysis: surveillance with ultrasound for early-stage hepatocellular carcinoma in patients with cirrhosis. Aliment Pharmacol Ther. 2009;30(1):37–47.
33. Singal AG, Pillai A, Tiro J. Early detection, curative treatment, and survival rates for hepatocellular carcinoma surveillance in patients with cirrhosis: a meta-analysis. PLoS Med. 2014;11(4):e1001624–e1001624.
34. Trinchet J-C, et al. Ultrasonographic surveillance of hepatocellular carcinoma in cirrhosis: a randomized trial comparing 3- and 6-month periodicities. Hepatology. 2011;54(6):1987–97.
35. Wang J-H, et al. Hepatocellular carcinoma surveillance at 4- vs. 12-month intervals for patients with chronic viral hepatitis: a randomized study in community. Am J Gastroenterol. 2013;108(3):416–24.
36. Zhang B-H, Yang B-H, Tang Z-Y. Randomized controlled trial of screening for hepatocellular carcinoma. J Cancer Res Clin Oncol. 2004;130(7):417–22.
37. Bolondi L, et al. Surveillance programme of cirrhotic patients for early diagnosis and treatment of hepatocellular carcinoma: a cost effectiveness analysis. Gut. 2001;48(2):251–9.
38. Di Martino M, et al. Hepatocellular carcinoma in cirrhotic patients: prospective comparison of US, CT and MR imaging. Eur Radiol. 2013;23(4):887–96.
39. Henrion J, et al. Surveillance for hepatocellular carcinoma: compliance and results according to the aetiology of cirrhosis in a cohort of 141 patients. Acta Gastroenterol Belg. 2000;63(1):5–9.
40. Pocha C, et al. Surveillance for hepatocellular cancer with ultrasonography vs. computed tomography – a randomised study. Aliment Pharmacol Ther. 2013;38(3):303–12.
41. Sangiovanni A, et al. Increased survival of cirrhotic patients with a hepatocellular carcinoma detected during surveillance☆. Gastroenterology. 2004;126(4):1005–14.
42. Choi BI. The current status of imaging diagnosis of hepatocellular carcinoma. Liver Transpl. 2004;10(2 Suppl 1):S20–5.
43. Boone JM. Multidetector CT: opportunities, challenges, and concerns associated with scanners with 64 or more detector rows. Radiology. 2006;241(2):334–7.
44. Luca A, et al. Multidetector-row computed tomography (MDCT) for the diagnosis of hepatocellular carcinoma in cirrhotic candidates for liver transplantation: prevalence of radiological vascular patterns and histological correlation with liver explants. Eur Radiol. 2010;20(4):898–907.
45. United Network for Organ Sharing. HRSA/OPTN Policy 3.6 organ distribution: allocation of livers. Table 9–3: recommendations for dynamic contrast-enhanced CT of liver. Available at: http://optn.transplant.hrsa.gov/PoliciesandBylaws2/policies/pdfs/policy_8.pdf. Accessed on 10 Oct 2014.
46. Addley HC, et al. Accuracy of hepatocellular carcinoma detection on multidetector CT in a transplant liver population with explant liver correlation. Clin Radiol. 2011;66(4):349–56.
47. Denecke T, et al. Multislice computed tomography using a triple-phase contrast protocol for preoperative assessment of hepatic tumor load in patients with hepatocellular carcinoma before liver transplantation. Transplant Int. 2009;22(4):395–402.
48. Ronzoni A, et al. Role of MDCT in the diagnosis of hepatocellular carcinoma in patients with cirrhosis undergoing orthotopic liver transplantation. AJR Am J Roentgenol. 2007;189(4):792–8.
49. United Network for Organ Sharing. HRSA/OPTN Policy 3.6 organ distribution: allocation of livers. Table 1. Available at: http://optn.transplant.hrsa.gov/PoliciesandBylaws2/policies/pdfs/policy_8.pdf. Accessed 10 Oct 2014.
50. Barr DC, Hussain HK. MR imaging in cirrhosis and hepatocellular carcinoma. Magn Reson Imaging Clin N Am. 2014;22(3):315–35.
51. Lim KS. Diffusion-weighted MRI of hepatocellular carcinoma in cirrhosis. Clin Radiol. 2014;69(1):1–10.
52. Liu X, et al. Gadoxetic acid disodium-enhanced magnetic resonance imaging for the detection of hepatocellular carcinoma: a meta-analysis. PLoS ONE. 2013;8(8):e70896–e70896.
53. Seale MK, et al. Hepatobiliary-specific MR contrast agents: role in imaging the liver and biliary tree. Radiographics. 2009;29(6):1725–48.

54. Taouli B, Koh D-M. Diffusion-weighted MR imaging of the liver. Radiology. 2010;254(1):47–66.
55. Bartolozzi C, et al. Contrast-enhanced magnetic resonance imaging of 102 nodules in cirrhosis: correlation with histological findings on explanted livers. Abdom Imaging. 2013;38(2):290–6.
56. Bolondi L, et al. Characterization of small nodules in cirrhosis by assessment of vascularity: the problem of hypovascular hepatocellular carcinoma. Hepatology. 2005;42(1):27–34.
57. Hanna RF, et al. Cirrhosis-associated hepatocellular nodules: correlation of histopathologic and MR imaging features. Radiographics. 2008;28(3):747–69.
58. Sun HY, et al. Gadoxetic acid-enhanced magnetic resonance imaging for differentiating small hepatocellular carcinomas (< or =2 cm in diameter) from arterial enhancing pseudolesions: special emphasis on hepatobiliary phase imaging. Investig Radiol. 2010;45(2):96–103.
59. Vandecaveye V, et al. Diffusion-weighted MRI provides additional value to conventional dynamic contrast-enhanced MRI for detection of hepatocellular carcinoma. Eur Radiol. 2009;19(10):2456–66.
60. Xu P-J, et al. Added value of breath hold diffusion-weighted MRI in detection of small hepatocellular carcinoma lesions compared with dynamic contrast-enhanced MRI alone using receiver operating characteristic curve analysis. J Magn Reson Imaging. 2009;29(2):341–9.
61. Hwang J, et al. Pre-transplant diagnosis of hepatocellular carcinoma by gadoxetic acid-enhanced and diffusion-weighted magnetic resonance imaging. Liver Transpl. 2014;20(12):1436–46.
62. Park MJ, et al. Validation of diagnostic criteria using gadoxetic acid-enhanced and diffusion-weighted MR imaging for small hepatocellular carcinoma (<= 2.0 cm) in patients with hepatitis-induced liver cirrhosis. Acta Radiol. 2013;54(2):127–36.
63. Park MJ, et al. Small hepatocellular carcinomas: improved sensitivity by combining gadoxetic acid-enhanced and diffusion-weighted MR imaging patterns. Radiology. 2012;264(3):761–70.
64. Nguyen MH, et al. Racial differences in effectiveness of alpha-fetoprotein for diagnosis of hepatocellular carcinoma in hepatitis C virus cirrhosis. Hepatology. 2002;36(2):410–7.

Chapter 10
When Is Laparoscopic Liver Resection Preferred Over Open Resection?

Ana Gleisner and David A. Geller

Abstract Laparoscopic liver resection is being safely performed by surgeons worldwide for multiple indications. When compared to open liver resection, laparoscopic liver resection is associated with improvements in short-term outcomes such as decreased blood loss, transfusion rate, perioperative complications, length of stay, and overall cost. When laparoscopic is performed for malignancies such as hepatocellular carcinoma and metastatic colorectal cancer, oncological adequacy needs to be assured in order to avoid detrimental effects in long-term outcomes such as disease-free survival and overall survival. Current evidence suggests that in well-selected patients, the long-term oncologic outcomes achieved with laparoscopic liver resection are equivalent to those obtained with open liver resection. To date, there are no published randomized trials comparing laparoscopic to open liver resection, although two trials are ongoing.

Keywords Laparoscopic liver resection • Laparoscopic hepatectomy • Hepatocellular carcinoma • Metastatic colorectal cancer • Liver tumor

Introduction

Laparoscopic liver resections have been performed for several indications, including both benign lesions and malignancies, with low morbidity and mortality [1, 2]. When compared to open resections, laparoscopic liver resections are associated with decreased LOS, postoperative pain and complications [3–6]. Yet, when laparoscopic liver resections are used for the treatment of malignancies, concerns about the rates of positive margins and failure to recognize occult metastases have caused some to question the oncologic adequacy of the procedure [7]. Because oncologic

A. Gleisner • D.A. Geller (✉)
Department of Surgery, University of Pittsburgh,
3459 Fifth Avenue, Pittsburgh, PA 15213-2582, USA
e-mail: gellerda@upmc.edu

J.M. Millis, J.B. Matthews (eds.), *Difficult Decisions in Hepatobiliary and Pancreatic Surgery*, Difficult Decisions in Surgery: An Evidence-Based Approach, DOI 10.1007/978-3-319-27365-5_10

Table 10.1 PICO table for laparoscopic liver resection

P (Patients)	I (Intervention)	C (Comparator group)	O (Outcomes measured)
Patients with multiple indications for liver resection; patients with indication for liver resection for hepatocellular carcinoma and for metastatic colorectal cancer	Laparoscopic liver resection	Open liver resection	Short-term: EBL, transfusion rate, postoperative morbidity and mortality, LOS, surgical margins, cost
			Long-term: overall survival and disease-free survival for resection of malignancies

adequacy influences important long-term outcomes, such as recurrence and long-term survival, patient selection for laparoscopic liver resection is premised upon understanding which surgical indications are most likely to afford the improved short-term outcomes associated with the laparoscopic technique without compromising the oncologic adequacy of the procedure. This chapter addresses situations in which laparoscopic surgery is preferred over open liver resection, with discussion focused on the short-term outcomes of laparoscopic liver resection when compared to open liver resection for both benign and malignant liver disease as well as long-term outcomes for the most common primary liver malignancy and metastatic disease—hepatocellular carcinoma (HCC) and metastatic colorectal cancer to the liver (mCRC), respectively.

Search Strategy

A literature search of publications from 2001 to 2014 was performed to identify published data on laparoscopic liver resection using the PICO outline [8] (Table 10.1). Databases searched were PubMed, Embase, Science Citation Index and Cochrane Evidence Based Medicine, restricted for publications in English language. Terms used in the search were "laparoscopic liver resection," "laparoscopic hepatectomy," AND "open liver resection," "open hepatectomy," AND ("intraoperative complications" OR "perioperative complications" OR "postoperative complications" OR "overall survival" OR "disease-free survival" OR "long-term" OR "outcomes"). Articles were excluded if they were review articles or non-comparative. There were no randomized trials. We included 32 cohort studies and 3 meta-analyses that were classified using the GRADE system [9].

Results

Short-Term Outcomes of Laparoscopic Liver Resection

Several cohort studies have compared the perioperative outcomes of patients submitted to laparoscopic liver resection with those of patients who underwent open liver resection. In a study examining the comparative benefits of laparoscopic vs. open hepatectomy, Nguyen et al. analyzed 31 case-cohort matched comparative studies that compared laparoscopic liver resection in 1,146 patients to open liver resection in 1,327 patients [3]. The short-term benefits of laparoscopic liver resection were significantly less blood loss (14 studies), less pRBC transfusions (4 studies), less post-operative pain/narcotic use (8 studies), quicker resumption of diet (8 studies), less overall morbidity (7 studies), and shorter length of stay (24 studies). For HCC and mCRC, there was no difference in 3- or 5-year overall survival when compared with well-matched open hepatic resection cases. Thus, the short-term benefits of laparoscopic liver resection were realized without compromising long-term oncologic outcomes.

Several recent meta-analyses have addressed short-term benefits of laparoscopic liver resection compared to open liver resection by analyzing comparative series [4–6] (Table 10.2). These studies have included liver resections for multiple indications as well as those specifically performed for HCC and mCRC. Rao et al. [5] included 32 studies published between 1998 and 2009, including excision of malignant lesions, benign lesions or both, as well as one study in which the indication was live liver donation for transplantation. Most studies described different types of liver resections and matched the laparoscopic and open resection groups based on characteristics of the patients (i.e. age, gender, presence of cirrhosis and ASA classification), the lesions (i.e. size, location and etiology) and related to the operation (i.e. type of resection). A total of 2,466 patients were included, 1,161 (47.1 %) in the laparoscopic group and 1,305 (52.9 %) in the open group. Laparoscopic liver resection was associated with decreased postoperative morbidity (Odds Ratio [OR] 0.62; 95 % Confidence Interval [CI] 0.20–0.76), decreased length of stay (LOS) (Weighted mean difference [WMD] −2.96; 95 % CI −3.70 to −2.22 days) and decreased need for blood transfusion (OR 0.36; 95 % CI 0.23–0.74). The incidence of positive surgical margins for the resection of malignant lesions was also lower in the laparoscopic group (OR 0.30; 95 % CI 0.20–0.76), according to the data in 6 of the 32 studies. Mortality rate was reported in 18 of the 32 studies and was not significantly different between both groups ($p=0.80$).

Yin and colleagues [6] included 15 studies published between 2001 and 2011, where laparoscopic liver resection was compared to open resection exclusively for the treatment of HCC. Lesions were either solitary, restricted to the left lateral lobe or the peripheral subcapsular right segments of the liver and were treated by limited resection (three or fewer segments). Among patients treated with laparoscopic resection, there were significant decreases in EBL (WMD −225, 95 % CI −385 to −64 ml), need for blood transfusion (OR 0.36; 95 % CI 0.17–0.74), postoperative

Table 10.2 Short-term outcomes for patients submitted to laparoscopic liver resection

Author	Number of patients LLR/OLR	Indication	Number of studies (publication year)	pOR for postoperative morbidity (95 % CI)	EBL (95 % CI)	LOS (95 % CI)	pOR for Blood Transfusion	Study type (quality of evidence)
Rao (2012) [5]	1161/1305	Benign/malignant	32 (1998–2009)	0.35 (0.28–0.45)	−184[a] ml	−2.96 (−3.70 to −2.22)[a] days	0.36 (0.23–0.74)	Metaanalysis (moderate)
Yin (2013) [6]	485/753	HCC	15 (2001–2011)	0.37 (0.27–0.52)	−225 (−385 to −64)[a] ml	−4.81 (−6.66 to −2.96)[a] days	0.36 (0.17–0.74)	Metaanalysis (moderate)
Schiffman (2014) [4]	242/368	mCRC	8 (2009–2013)	0.70 (0.52–0.96)	−0.70 (0 to −1.41)[b]	−1.50 (−2.60 to −0.41)[b]	0.51 (0.32–0.81)	Metaanalysis (moderate)

LLR laparoscopic liver resection, *OLR* open liver resection, *HCC* hepatocellular carcinoma, *mCRC* metastatic colorectal cancer, *pOR* pooled odds ratio, *CI* confidence interval, *EBL* estimated blood loss, *LOS* length of stay

[a]Weighted mean difference

[b]Standard mean difference

complications (OR 0.37; 95 % CI 0.27–0.52) and LOS (WMD −4.81; 95 % CI −6.66 to −2.96 days). There was no significant difference in the rate of negative margins (OR 1.63; 95 % CI 0.82–3.22).

The most recent meta-analysis, by Schiffman and colleagues [4], summarized data published between 2009 and 2013 that compared laparoscopic surgery to open resection for the treatment of hepatic mCRC. Only matched cohorts were included, resulting in 8 studies with 242 patients submitted to laparoscopic surgery and 368 patients submitted to open resection. The findings also showed improvement in perioperative outcomes for patients who underwent laparoscopic surgery, including reduced EBL (standard mean difference [SMD] – 0.70; 95 % CI 0 to −1.41), need for blood transfusion (OR 0.51; 95 % CI 0.32–0.81), postoperative morbidity (OR 0.70; 95 % CI 0.52–0.96) and LOS (SMD −1.50; 95 % CI −2.60 to −0.41).

Although there is some redundancy in the articles included in the three meta-analyses, the effect of laparoscopic surgery in the perioperative outcomes is consistent and with large magnitude. It is possible, however, that important confounders have not been accounted for in these observational studies. For example, more accessible lesions may have been chosen for the laparoscopic approach, which could result in overestimation of its effect. Additionally, the determination of how accessible a tumor is can be hard to measure and varies considerably among surgeons. Further, inherent selection bias exists even in well-matched case cohort series.

In addition to the favorable perioperative outcomes associated with laparoscopic liver resection, there is evidence suggesting laparoscopic liver resections may be more cost-effective as well. In a retrospective cohort study, Vanounou and colleagues [10] found that laparoscopic left lateral sectionectomy was $1,527–2,939 more cost effective per patient compared to open left lateral sectionectomy. Bhojani and colleagues [11] reported results from 57 patients who underwent attempted laparoscopic resection matched to 2 open cases for multiple parameters including the number of segments removed. Eight (14 %) cases were converted to open and most perioperative outcomes were similar between the two groups. The median cost for laparoscopic surgery was lower when compared to open resections ($11,376 vs $12,523), but the difference did not achieve statistical significance ($p=0.077$). Another retrospective cohort by Cannon and colleagues [12] found an overall decrease in cost of liver resections performed laparoscopically (weighted average mean cost [WAMC] of $58,401 versus $69,728 for open resections). However, when only right hepatectomies were considered, the laparoscopic approach actually resulted in increased cost (WAMC $69,544 versus $68,266 for open resection), despite the fact that the patients in the laparoscopic group were more likely to have an "on course" hospitalization—suggesting that the cost effectiveness of laparoscopic surgery may vary according to the complexity of the procedure.

Long-Term Outcomes in Laparoscopic Liver Resection

Evaluation of the oncological adequacy of the laparoscopic approach to liver resection is crucial when this technique is applied to the treatment of malignancies. Concerns are mainly related to the rate of negative margins achieved and the ability to recognize occult metastasis, which would result in decreases in the disease-free and overall survival.

Hepatocellular Carcinoma

Several studies have reported long-term results on cohorts of patients who underwent laparoscopic resection of HCC. These studies included retrospective or prospective cohorts of patients submitted to laparoscopic surgery compared to retrospective cohorts of patients submitted to open resection (Table 10.3). With the exception of one study, which reported a significantly higher 3-year survival rate for those submitted to laparoscopic resection (89 % versus 55 % in the open resection group) [13], no significant differences in disease-free or overall survival were observed. The largest study, by Ker and colleagues, [14] included 116 patients submitted to laparoscopic resection and 208 patients submitted to open resection. Overall survival was comparable between both groups (3- and 5-year overall survival 70 % and 62 % for laparoscopic and 76 % and 72 % for open resection). The meta-analysis by Yin and colleagues [6] included 12 studies that reported long-term outcomes of patients operated for HCC. The pooled hazard ratio (HR) for 3- and 5-year overall survival for laparoscopic surgery was 0.98 (95 % CI 0.72–1.33) and 0.99 (95 % CI 0.74–1.33), respectively. Similarly, the pooled HR for 3- and 5-year recurrence free survival was not significantly different for those submitted to laparoscopic surgery when compared to open (HR 1.04; 95 % CI 0.81–1.34 and HR 1.01; 95 % CI 0.75–1.35, respectively). More importantly, no significant heterogeneity was found between the studies.

Metastatic Colorectal Cancer

Long-term results for patients submitted to laparoscopic and open liver resection for metastatic colorectal cancer are summarized in Table 10.4. Of the 11 cohort studies identified in the literature review, all but one matched with regard to clinical, tumor and/or procedure-related characteristics, and there were no difference in disease-free or overall survival between patients in the laparoscopic and open liver resection cohorts. The studies included a minimum of 13 and a maximum of 60 patients in the laparoscopic group. Disease-free survival was reported in seven studies, ranging between 14 % and 63 % in 3-years and 14 % and 42 % in 5-years for those who underwent laparoscopic resection, and between 18 % and 46 % in 3-years and 18 % and 38 % in 5-years for patients who underwent open resection.

Table 10.3 Long-term outcomes for patients submitted to laparoscopic liver resection for hepatocellular carcinoma

Author	Number of patients	Median follow-up (months)	Median DFS (months)	Median OS (months)	3-years DFS (%)	5-years DFS (%)	3-years OS (%)	5-years OS (%)	Study type (quality of evidence)
	LLR/OLR	LLR/OLR	LLR/OLR	LLR/OLR	LLR/OLR	LLR/OLR	LLR/OLR	LLR/OLR	
Kim (2014) [15]	29/29	48/60	NR	NR	62/61	54/40	100/92	92/88	Retrospective matched-cohort (low)
Cheung (2013) [16]	32/64	NR	79/29	92/71	73/50	55/44	88/73	77/57	Retrospective matched-cohort (low)
Kobayashi (2013) [17]	56/27	19/68	NR	NR	50/62	NR	100/100	NR	Retrospective matched-cohort (low)
Ker (2011) [14]	116/208	94/94	NR	NR	NR	NR	70/76	62/72	Retrospective cohort (low)
Truant (2011) [18]	35/53	36/36	NR	NR	NR	36/34	NR	70/46	Retrospective matched-cohort (low)
Lee (2011) [19]	33/50	35/29	NR	NR	51/56	45/56	82/81	76/76	Retrospective matched-cohort (low)
Hu (2011) [20]	30/30	NR	NR	NR	NR	NR	76/77	50/53	Retrospective cohort (low)
Kim (2011) [21]	26/29	22/25	NR	NR	NR	57/56	NR	NR	Retrospective matched-cohort (low)

(continued)

Table 10.3 (continued)

Author	Number of patients	Median follow-up (months)	Median DFS (months)	Median OS (months)	3-years DFS (%)	5-years DFS (%)	3-years OS (%)	5-years OS (%)	Study type (quality of evidence)
	LLR/OLR	LLR/OLR	LLR/OLR	LLR/OLR	LLR/OLR	LLR/OLR	LLR/OLR	LLR/OLR	
Tranchart (2010) [22]	42/42	30/35	NR	NR	61/54	46/37	74/73	60/47	Retrospective matched-cohort (low)
Aldrighetti (2010) [23]	16/16	32/32	23/31	40/48	NR	NR	NR	NR	Retrospective matched-cohort (low)
Belli (2009) [24]	54/125	24/24	38 /–	63 /–	52/55	NR	67/63	NR	Retrospective matched-cohort (low)
Sarpel (2009) [25]	20/56	24/18	NR	NR	NR	NR	NR	95/75	Retrospective matched-cohort (low)
Endo (2009) [26]	10/11	NR	NR	NR	NR	24/19	NR	57/48	Retrospective matched-cohort (low)
Lai (2009) [27]	25/33	29/29	NR	NR	52/56	NR	60/60	NR	Retrospective matched-cohort (low)
Cai (2008) [28]	31/31	NR	NR	70/61	NR	NR	67/74	56/54	Retrospective matched-cohort (low)
Kaneko (2005) [29]	30/28	NR	NR	NR	45/50	31/29	80/77	61/62	Retrospective and prospective matched-cohort (low)

Author	Number of patients	Median follow-up (months)	Median DFS (months)	Median OS (months)	3-years DFS (%)	5-years DFS (%)	3-years OS (%)	5-years OS (%)	Study type (quality of evidence)
	LLR/OLR	LLR/OLR	LLR/OLR	LLR/OLR	LLR/OLR	LLR/OLR	LLR/OLR	LLR/OLR	
Laurent (2003) [13]	13/13	NR	NR	NR	56/54	NR	89/55*	NR	Retrospective and prospective matched-cohort (low)
Shimada (2001) [30]	17/38	17/29	NR	NR	NR	72/72	NR	48/38	Retrospective and prospective matched-cohort (low)

DFS: Disease-free survival, *OS* Overall survival, *LLR* laparoscopic liver resection, *OLR* open liver resection, *NR* not reported

Table 10.4 Long-term outcomes for patients submitted to laparoscopic liver resection for metastatic colorectal cancer

Author	Number of patients	Median follow-up (mos)	Median DFS (mos)	Median OS (mos)	3-years DFS (%)	5-years DFS (%)	3-years OS (%)	5-years OS (%)	Study type (quality of evidence)
	LLR/OLR	LLR/OLR	LLR/OLR	LLR/OLR	LLR/OLR	LLR/OLR	LLR/OLR	LLR/OLR	
Montalti (2014) [31]	57/57	41/54	NR	NR	39/42	29/38	75/75	60/65	Retrospective matched-cohort (low)
Iwahashi (2014) [32]	21/21	NR	NR	NR	14/33	14/25	84/89	42/51	Retrospective matched-cohort (low)
Guerron (2013) [33]	40 /40	16/16	23/ 23	NR	NR	NR	89/81 (2-years)	NR	Retrospective matched-cohort (low)
Qiu (2013) [34]	30/30	NR	NR	NR	NR	NR	NR	NR	Retrospective matched-cohort (low)
Cannon (2012) [35]	35/140	NR	NR	NR	37/39	15/22	63/60	36/42	Retrospective matched-cohort (low)
Cheung (2013) [36]	20/40	NR	9.8/10.9	69/42	42/18	42/18	54/65	54/22	Retrospective matched-cohort (low)
Topal (2012) [37]	20/20	NR	NR	NR	NR	43/23	NR	48/46	Retrospective matched-cohort (low)
Hu (2012) [38]	13/13	NR	NR	NR	NR	NR	55/54	27/31	Retrospective matched-cohort (low)

Nguyen (2011) [3]	24/25	27/29	NR	NR	63/46	NR	75/79	NR	Retrospective matched-cohort (low)
Abu Hilal (2010) [39]	50/85	22/22	NR	NR	NR	NR	NR	NR	Retrospective cohort (low)
Castaing (2009) [40]	60/60	30/33	47/40	NR	47/40	35/27	82/70	64/56	Retrospective matched-cohort (low)

DFS Disease-free survival, *OS* Overall survival, *LLR* laparoscopic liver resection, *OLR* open liver resection, *NR* not reported

In the meta-analysis by Schiffman and colleagues [4], which included eight matched cohort studies comparing laparoscopic versus open resection of colorectal liver metastasis, long-term outcomes were reported in all studies. Again, there were no differences in disease-free and overall survival between laparoscopic and open resection cohorts. The 3- and 5-year mean disease-free survival was 47.1 % and 31.9 % in the laparoscopic group and 40.4 % and 25.5 % in the open resection group. The 3- and 5-year mean overall survival rate was 72.7 % and 51.4 % in the laparoscopic group and 67.2 % and 45.9 % in the open resection group. Importantly, the mean number of metastasis was 1.4 for the laparoscopic group and 1.5 for the open resection group ($p = 0.14$), implying that the data on long-term results of laparoscopic resection for mCRC cancer is only applicable to patients with limited disease (one or two tumors).

Of note, there have been no reports of peritoneal tumor seeding with laparoscopic liver resection of neither HCC nor mCRC.

The major limitation of the data on long-term outcomes comparing laparoscopic and open liver resections is the lack of randomized trials. Despite the fact that most cohorts were matched with regard to significant clinical, tumor and procedure-related factors, residual confounding and selection bias is certainly a possibility in these observational studies.

Recommendations

Laparoscopic liver resection is associated with decreased EBL, need for transfusion, perioperative morbidity, and LOS when compared to open liver resection. Although this data is entirely based on observational studies, the magnitude of the effects is high and there is consistency across several studies (evidence quality moderate). The rate of negative margins is at least equivalent between the two techniques (evidence quality low). Laparoscopic surgery seems to be cost-effective, especially for minor liver resections (evidence quality very low).

Long-term term outcomes, disease-free survival and overall survival, are equivalent in patients with either HCC or limited (one or ;two lesions) metastatic colorectal cancer submitted to laparoscopic liver resection when compared to open liver resection. Yet, the lack of randomized trials raises concerns regarding selection bias and residual confounding variables. It is plausible that surgeons selected patients with tumors with more favorable characteristics, such as tumor location, for laparoscopic procedures, which would overestimate the treatment effect of the laparoscopic procedure (evidence quality low).

We therefore make a weak recommendation for laparoscopic liver resection in patients with liver lesions, including hepatocellular carcinoma and limited metastatic colorectal cancer, for the potential benefits in perioperative outcomes and possibly cost, with no evidence showing compromise in long-term outcomes for patients with malignancy.

A Personal View of the Data

Laparoscopic liver resections have been performed safely in over 8,000 patients worldwide. Patient selection according to the surgeon's expertise is key to assure the short-term benefits of laparoscopic surgery. The current evidence also suggests long-term outcomes for laparoscopic liver resection are equivalent to those for open liver resections in well-selected patients, when the procedure can be performed without compromising the oncological adequacy. A more precise estimation of the treatment effect of laparoscopic liver resection in short- and long-term outcomes can only be determined by randomized trials, which may be difficult to perform when patients have a choice between laparoscopic and open resections.

Recommendations

- Laparoscopic liver resection should be considered for patients with benign liver lesions, as it is associated with decreased morbidity and LOS (evidence quality moderate; strong recommendation).
- Laparoscopic liver resection can be considered for patients with malignancies such as HCC or limited metastatic colorectal lesions (one or two tumors), as it is associated with improved short-term outcomes without detriment to long-term outcomes (evidence quality low; weak recommendation).

References

1. Nguyen KT, Gamblin TC, Geller DA. World review of laparoscopic liver resection-2,804 patients. Ann Surg. 2009;250(5):831–41.
2. Reddy SK, Tsung A, Geller DA. Laparoscopic liver resection. World J Surg. 2011;35(7):1478–86.
3. Nguyen KT, Marsh JW, Tsung A, Steel JJ, Gamblin TC, Geller DA. Comparative benefits of laparoscopic vs open hepatic resection: a critical appraisal. Arch Surg. 2011;146(3):348–56.
4. Schiffman SC, Kim KH, Tsung A, Marsh JW, Geller DA. Laparoscopic versus open liver resection for metastatic colorectal cancer: a metaanalysis of 610 patients. Surgery. 2015;157(2):211–22.
5. Rao A, Rao G, Ahmed I. Laparoscopic or open liver resection? Let systematic review decide it. Am J Surg. 2012;204(2):222–31.
6. Yin Z, Fan X, Ye H, Yin D, Wang J. Short- and long-term outcomes after laparoscopic and open hepatectomy for hepatocellular carcinoma: a global systematic review and meta-analysis. Ann Surg Oncol. 2013;20(4):1203–15.
7. Buell JF, Cherqui D, Geller DA, et al. The international position on laparoscopic liver surgery: the Louisville Statement, 2008. Ann Surg. 2009;250(5):825–30.
8. Haroon M, Phillips R. "There is nothing like looking, if you want to find something" – asking questions and searching for answers – the evidence based approach. Arch Dis Child Educ Pract Ed. 2010;95(2):34–9.

9. Brozek JL, Akl EA, Alonso-Coello P, et al. Grading quality of evidence and strength of recommendations in clinical practice guidelines. Part 1 of 3. An overview of the GRADE approach and grading quality of evidence about interventions. Allergy. 2009;64(5):669–77.
10. Vanounou T, Steel JL, Nguyen KT, et al. Comparing the clinical and economic impact of laparoscopic versus open liver resection. Ann Surg Oncol. 2010;17(4):998–1009.
11. Bhojani FD, Fox A, Pitzul K, et al. Clinical and economic comparison of laparoscopic to open liver resections using a 2-to-1 matched pair analysis: an institutional experience. J Am Coll Surg. 2012;214(2):184–95.
12. Cannon RM, Scoggins CR, Callender GG, Quillo A, McMasters KM, Martin 2nd RC. Financial comparison of laparoscopic versus open hepatic resection using deviation-based cost modeling. Ann Surg Oncol. 2013;20(9):2887–92.
13. Laurent A, Cherqui D, Lesurtel M, Brunetti F, Tayar C, Fagniez PL. Laparoscopic liver resection for subcapsular hepatocellular carcinoma complicating chronic liver disease. Arch Surg. 2003;138(7):763–9; discussion 9.
14. Ker CG, Chen JS, Kuo KK, et al. Liver surgery for hepatocellular carcinoma: laparoscopic versus open approach. Int J Hepatol. 2011;2011:596792.
15. Kim H, Suh KS, Lee KW, et al. Long-term outcome of laparoscopic versus open liver resection for hepatocellular carcinoma: a case-controlled study with propensity score matching. Surg Endosc. 2014;28(3):950–60.
16. Cheung TT, Poon RT, Yuen WK, et al. Long-term survival analysis of pure laparoscopic versus open hepatectomy for hepatocellular carcinoma in patients with cirrhosis: a single-center experience. Ann Surg. 2013;257(3):506–11.
17. Kobayashi T. Long-term survival analysis of pure laparoscopic versus open hepatectomy for hepatocellular carcinoma in patients with cirrhosis: a single-center experience. Ann Surg. 2013;257:506–11.
18. Truant S, Bouras AF, Hebbar M, et al. Laparoscopic resection vs. open liver resection for peripheral hepatocellular carcinoma in patients with chronic liver disease: a case-matched study. Surg Endosc. 2011;25(11):3668–77.
19. Lee KF, Chong CN, Wong J, Cheung YS, Wong J, Lai P. Long-term results of laparoscopic hepatectomy versus open hepatectomy for hepatocellular carcinoma: a case-matched analysis. World J Surg. 2011;35(10):2268–74.
20. Hu BS, Chen K, Tan HM, Ding XM, Tan JW. Comparison of laparoscopic vs open liver lobectomy (segmentectomy) for hepatocellular carcinoma. World J Gastroenterol. 2011;17(42):4725–8.
21. Kim HH, Park EK, Seoung JS, et al. Liver resection for hepatocellular carcinoma: case-matched analysis of laparoscopic versus open resection. J Kor Surg Soc. 2011;80(6):412–9.
22. Tranchart H, Di Giuro G, Lainas P, et al. Laparoscopic resection for hepatocellular carcinoma: a matched-pair comparative study. Surg Endosc. 2010;24(5):1170–6.
23. Aldrighetti L, Guzzetti E, Pulitano C, et al. Case-matched analysis of totally laparoscopic versus open liver resection for HCC: short and middle term results. J Surg Oncol. 2010;102(1):82–6.
24. Belli G, Limongelli P, Fantini C, et al. Laparoscopic and open treatment of hepatocellular carcinoma in patients with cirrhosis. Br J Surg. 2009;96(9):1041–8.
25. Sarpel U, Hefti MM, Wisnievsky JP, Roayaie S, Schwartz ME, Labow DM. Outcome for patients treated with laparoscopic versus open resection of hepatocellular carcinoma: case-matched analysis. Ann Surg Oncol. 2009;16(6):1572–7.
26. Endo Y, Ohta M, Sasaki A, et al. A comparative study of the long-term outcomes after laparoscopy-assisted and open left lateral hepatectomy for hepatocellular carcinoma. Surg Laparosc Endosc Percutan Tech. 2009;19(5):e171–4.
27. Lai EC, Tang CN, Ha JP, Li MK. Laparoscopic liver resection for hepatocellular carcinoma: ten-year experience in a single center. Arch Surg. 2009;144(2):143–7; discussion 8.
28. Cai XJ, Yang J, Yu H, et al. Clinical study of laparoscopic versus open hepatectomy for malignant liver tumors. Surg Endosc. 2008;22(11):2350–6.

29. Kaneko H, Takagi S, Otsuka Y, et al. Laparoscopic liver resection of hepatocellular carcinoma. Am J Surg. 2005;189(2):190–4.
30. Shimada M, Hashizume M, Maehara S, et al. Laparoscopic hepatectomy for hepatocellular carcinoma. Surg Endosc. 2001;15(6):541–4.
31. Montalti R, Berardi G, Laurent S, et al. Laparoscopic liver resection compared to open approach in patients with colorectal liver metastases improves further resectability: oncological outcomes of a case-control matched-pairs analysis. Eur J Surg Oncol. 2014;40(5):536–44.
32. Iwahashi S, Shimada M, Utsunomiya T, et al. Laparoscopic hepatic resection for metastatic liver tumor of colorectal cancer: comparative analysis of short- and long-term results. Surg Endosc. 2014;28(1):80–4.
33. Guerron AD, Aliyev S, Agcaoglu O, et al. Laparoscopic versus open resection of colorectal liver metastasis. Surg Endosc. 2013;27(4):1138–43.
34. Qiu J, Chen S, Pankaj P, Wu H. Laparoscopic hepatectomy for hepatic colorectal metastases – a retrospective comparative cohort analysis and literature review. PLoS One. 2013;8(3):e60153.
35. Cannon RM, Scoggins CR, Callender GG, McMasters KM, Martin 2nd RC. Laparoscopic versus open resection of hepatic colorectal metastases. Surgery. 2012;152(4):567–73; discussion 73–4.
36. Cheung TT, Poon RT, Yuen WK, et al. Outcome of laparoscopic versus open hepatectomy for colorectal liver metastases. ANZ J Surg. 2013;83(11):847–52.
37. Topal B, Tiek J, Fieuws S, et al. Minimally invasive liver surgery for metastases from colorectal cancer: oncologic outcome and prognostic factors. Surg Endosc. 2012;26(8):2288–98.
38. Hu MG, Ou-yang CG, Zhao GD, Xu DB, Liu R. Outcomes of open versus laparoscopic procedure for synchronous radical resection of liver metastatic colorectal cancer: a comparative study. Surg Laparosc Endosc Percutan Tech. 2012;22(4):364–9.
39. Abu Hilal M, Underwood T, Zuccaro M, Primrose J, Pearce N. Short- and medium-term results of totally laparoscopic resection for colorectal liver metastases. Br J Surg. 2010;97(6):927–33.
40. Castaing D, Vibert E, Ricca L, Azoulay D, Adam R, Gayet B. Oncologic results of laparoscopic versus open hepatectomy for colorectal liver metastases in two specialized centers. Ann Surg. 2009;250(5):849–55.

Chapter 11
Clinical Management of Pyogenic Liver Abscesses

Trevor W. Reichman and W. Grayson Terral

Abstract Pyogenic liver abscesses are rare but if handled inappropriately can be life-threatening. Early experiences with the management of these liver abscesses yielded high morbidity and mortality. However, over the last three decades, treatment has moved away from surgery as the front-line therapy and has evolved to include less invasive interventional radiologic procedures. This change in paradigm has been accompanied by shorter length of hospital stay and decreased morbidity and mortality. Despite these findings in the general population, patients that develop pyogenic liver abscesses following a liver transplant have a much higher morbidity and mortality, with some ultimately requiring retransplantation. When managed appropriately and in many cases with a multi-modality approach, patients with pyogenic liver abscesses can achieve excellent clinical outcomes.

Keywords Liver abscess • Pyogenic • Percutaneous aspiration • Percutaneous drainage • Hepatectomy of liver abscess

Introduction

Pyogenic liver abscesses are relatively uncommon occurrences, with an incidence ranging from 1.1 to 2.3 cases per 100,000 based on the most recent population-based studies [1, 2]. Although liver abscesses are uncommon, if left untreated, risk significant morbidity and mortality. Liver abscesses were first described by Ochsner and Debakey in 1938, and surgical drainage was the primary treatment recommendation [3]. Despite intervention, overall mortality was 77 %. Since then, therapy has evolved with the advent of improved diagnostic imaging, antibiotics, and percutaneous intervention and this has improved the mortality in more recent studies to between 6 % and 14 % [4–6]. In the past 30 years, the advent and wide spread acceptance of

T.W. Reichman (✉) • W.G. Terral
Multi-Organ Transplant Institute, Department of Surgery, Ochsner Medical Center,
1514 Jefferson Highway, New Orleans, LA 70121, USA
e-mail: treichman@ochsner.org

J.M. Millis, J.B. Matthews (eds.), *Difficult Decisions in Hepatobiliary and Pancreatic Surgery*, Difficult Decisions in Surgery: An Evidence-Based Approach, DOI 10.1007/978-3-319-27365-5_11

percutaneous aspiration and percutaneous drainage along with antibiotic regimens has supplanted surgical intervention as the primary treatment modality.

As the etiology of pyogenic liver abscess has evolved, the appropriate treatment modality has evolved as well. Appropriate patient selection based on etiology, nutritional status, abscess characteristics, and institutional interventional options should be considered. This chapter addresses the indications for surgical intervention, percutaneous aspiration or drainage, and antibiotics therapy alone.

Search Strategy

A literature search of English language publications from 1980 to 2014 was used to identity published data on pyogenic liver abscess using the PICO outline (Table 11.1). Databases searched were PubMed, Ovid MEDLINE, and Cochrane Reviews. Terms used in the search were "pyogenic liver abscess, etiology", "pyogenic liver abscess, treatment", "pyogenic liver abscess AND percutaneous drainage or percutaneous aspiration", "pyogenic abscess, antibiotics", "pyogenic liver abscess risk", "pyogenic liver abscess AND surgery versus drainage".

Etiology of Liver Abscesses

In review of the etiology by Johannsen et al. and Rahimian et al. abscesses can be classified by the presumed route: biliary, portal venous, hepatic artery, direct extension, and traumatic [7, 8]. Biliary causes include suppurative cholangitis, the most common identifiable cause, Caroli's disease, and *Ascaris lumbricoides* invasion in the developing world. According to Seeto and Rockey's review, 52 of 142 identifiable causes (37 %) were attributed to biliary disease [9]. Eleven of the 52 had malignant lesions, 31 had cholelithiasis or choledocholithiasis, 8 had strictures, and 2 with biliary cirrhosis. Appendicitis, historically the most common identifiable cause, along with diverticulits, pancreatitis, inflammatory bowel disease, and abdominal surgery all represent common portal venous causes of abscesses. Again, Seeto and Rockey's review identified 16 of 142 patients with a portal venous system etiology as the cause for their liver abscess: 5 from diverticulitis, 4 from appendicitis, 3 with perforation of the small bowel, 2 patients with IBD, and 2 with other intra-abdominal infections [9]. Any systemic bacterial infection can lead to liver abscess, but as found at autopsy, these abscesses are typically micro-abscesses and

Table 11.1 PICO table for assessment of treatment of pyogenic liver abscesses

P (Patients)	I (Intervention)	C (Comparator)	O (Outcomes)
Patients with pyogenic liver abscess	Surgical drainage	Percutaneous drainage or aspiration, antibiotics alone	Mortality, morbidity, resolution of abscess

are not identifiable by imaging. Direct extension includes cholecystitis, perinephric abscesses, and subdiaphragmatic abscesses. Traumatic causes include penetrating trauma but also include ingestion of foreign objects, blunt trauma with resultant infected hepatic hematoma, tumor necrosis, and sickle cell disease. Lastly, cryptogenic liver abscesses have become the most common finding and predominated in reviews from both Rahimian et al. and Rockey and Seeto with cryptogenic causes as 48 % and 40 % respectively [8, 9].

Predicting Prognosis

Several attempts have been made to try to stratify patients into risk categories in attempt to identify patients that might have a higher risk of mortality and/or a more complicated clinical course. Theoretically, stratifying patients should help to identify individuals that warrant more aggressive clinical management of their abscess up front rather then taking a more conservative approach. Chen et al. studied 298 patients with pyogenic liver abscesses with an overall mortality rate of 10 % [10]. The authors demonstrated by multivariate analysis that the Acute Physiology and Chronic Health Evaluation II (APACHE II score), SAPS II score, the presence of a gas-forming abscess, or an anaerobic infection was associated with higher mortality. These findings were further substantiated in a study by Hsieh et al. which found that a more aggressive approach in patients with APACHE II scores greater than 15 were associated with better clinical outcomes [11].

In addition to mortality, Alvarez Pérez et al. examined 133 patients in an attempt to identify risk factors associated with a complicated clinical course from a pyogenic abscess [12]. They found by multivariate analysis that patients that present with shock, a hemoglobin <10 g/dl, an elevated PT (>17) and/or polymicrobial infections were more likely to have a complicated clinical course. In this study, the overall rate of patients with a complicated clinical course was 36 %. In addition, the authors also identified factors that were associated with patient mortality. Pyogenic abscesses associated with a biliary origin, multiple abscesses, a low hemoglobin (<10 g/dl), or an elevated BUN (>28 mg/dL) were associated with death by multivariate analysis. In addition, the presence of shock was the highest predictor of mortality by multivariate analysis with an odds ratio of 22.66. An additional study by Ruiz-Hernández et al. also reported similar findings in that patients that develop sepsis and/or are in septic shock are at high risk of mortality [13].

Treatment Options

Interventions for pyogenic hepatic abscesses range in degree of invasiveness from antibiotic therapy alone to more aggressive therapies such as hepatic resection. Trials comparing methodologies to manage pyogenic liver abscesses are presented in Table 11.2.

Table 11.2 Trials comparing treatment modalities for pyogenic liver abscesses

First author, year	Study type	n	Comparison	Outcome
Yu, 2004	RCT	64	Percutaneous aspiration vs. qCD	Equivalent
Zerem, 2007	RCT	60	Percutaneous aspiration vs. CD	Improved with CD
Rajak, 1998	RCT	50 (11 with PLA)	Percutaneous aspiration vs. CD	Improved with CD
Tan, 2005	RR	80 (PLA >5 cm)	CD vs. surgery	Improved with Surgery
Hsieh, 2008	RR	81 (APACHE II ≥15)	CD vs. surgery	Improved with surgery
Chou, 1997	RR	483 (single vs. multiple PLA)	CD vs. surgery	Single = CD
				Multiple = surgery
Hope, 2008	RR	107	Abx vs. CD vs. surgery	≤3 cm = Abx
				>3 cm, UL = CD
				>3 cm, ML = surgery

RCT randomized controlled trial, *CD* catheter drainage, *PLA* pyogenic liver abscess, *RR* retrospective review, APACHE II, *Abx* antibiotics, *UL* uniloculated, *ML* multiloculated

Antibiotic Therapy

Antibiotic therapy is almost universally used in conjunction with other treatment modalities. However, in the absence of positive blood cultures, the disadvantage to treatment of liver abscesses without any intervention is a lack of the ability to identify the offending organism(s) in which antibiotic therapy can be tailored. Current recommendations for antibiotic treatment of pyogenic hepatic abscesses include empiric coverage of *Enterobacteriaceae*, enterococci, anaerobes, and in certain situations staphylococci and streptococci. Empiric regimens should include a beta-lactam/beta-lactamase inhibitor combination, carbapenem, or second-generation cephalosporin with anaerobic coverage. Metronidazole or clindamycin should be included in the antibiotic regimen to cover *Bacteroides fragilis* if not covered by the initial antibiotic(s). Systemic antifungal agents should also be initiated if a fungal abscess is suspected. Once cultures and sensitivities are available, the antibiotic regimen should be tailored appropriately. The recommended duration of antibiotic therapy should be 4–6 weeks. However, this may potentially be shortened in patients that have undergone drainage and an uncomplicated clinical course [14].

Earlier reports demonstrated inferior results in patients treated with antibiotics alone versus an intervention plus antibiotics [12]. However, in appropriately selected patients, antibiotic therapy alone can be effective in the treatment of certain pyogenic abscesses. In a series by Hope et al. the authors stratified 107 patients with pyogenic liver abscesses into 3 categories: (1) <3 cm, (2) Unilocular, >3 cm, and (3) Complex, multilocular, >3 cm [15]. Patients were also stratified into three treatment algorithms that included one of the following treatment arms: (1) Antibiotics alone, (2) Percutaneous drainage plus antibiotics, or (3) Surgery. In this series, antibiotic therapy alone was effective in 100 % of patients with hepatic abscesses <3 cm in size. Hsieh et al. also demonstrated successful treatment of <3 cm abscesses with antibiotics alone, even in patient with high APACHE II scores [11]. Similarly, Rahimian et al. reported successful treatment of approximately 17 % of their patients (14 of 70 patients) treated for pyogenic liver abscess with no treatment failures requiring additional interventions [8].

Radiologic Intervention

Percutaneous radiologic interventions (e.g. aspiration or placement of an indwelling catheter) are becoming more commonly the modality of choice for patients with pyogenic liver abscesses. Percutaneous interventions serve two purposes: (1) They drain the underlying infection and (2) They provide abscess contents for culture and sensitivity. There have been several studies that have demonstrated similar or decreased mortality rates in patients treated with percutaneous intervention versus open surgical drainage or resection [8, 9, 12, 16].

The optimal percutaneous approach to abscess drainage (intermittent needle aspiration versus continuous indwelling catheter and drainage) is still debated. Intermittent needle aspiration has the advantage in that it is easier and more cost effective to perform and is also less painful for the patient. The one disadvantage is that it typically requires multiple interventions. In a randomized-controlled trial by Yu et al. the authors compared intermittent needle aspiration to continuous catheter drainage in 64 consecutive patients with a pyogenic liver abscess. There was no statistically significant difference in outcomes from either treatment modality, however, there was a trend toward higher treatment success rate, shorter hospital stay, and lower mortality rate in patients treated with needle aspiration [6]. However, a similar randomized study by Rajak et al. demonstrated an improved outcome using percutaneous catheters versus needle aspiration. However, this report has been criticized due to the low sample size of confirmed pyogenic abscesses (n = 11) and the limitation on the number of aspirations allowed (≤2). A more recent study however appeared to confirm these findings and again demonstrated improved outcomes with catheter drainage versus intermittent needle aspiration in a randomized controlled trial with no treatment failures occurring in the percutaneous catheter group [17].

Previously, the effectiveness of catheter-based drainage has been questioned in patients with multiloculated abscesses. However, a recent publication by Liu et al. compared 109 patients with either uniloculated or multiloculated abscesses who were all treated with percutaneous catheter drainage [18]. Clinical success ranged between 87 and 92 % regardless of whether the patient had single or multiple abscesses or the abscess was uniloculated or multiloculated, indicating potentially all abscesses regardless of their characteristics should have a trial of percutaneous drainage. Overall mortality reported in this series was 3.5 %. However, no comparison to other modalities was made.

In a series from Memorial Sloan-Kettering, Mezhir et al. examined their series of hepatic abscesses (n = 51) of which 88 % occurred the setting of a history of cancer.

Twenty-two percent of the patient had previously underwent local-regional therapy (transarterial chemoembolization or radiofrequency ablation). Percutaneous drainage was successful in 66 % of patients; 9 % of patients required surgical intervention. The presence of yeast and/or communication with the biliary tree was associated with poorer outcomes. Overall mortality was 26 %, however many of these patients (60 %) died of progression of disease [19].

Surgical Therapy

Prior to the advent of percutaneous radiology-based interventions, surgery was the mainstay of treatment for patients with pyogenic liver abscesses. However, based on review of the current literature, the paradigm has clearly switched from surgical drainage to percutaneous procedures. However, in certain subsets of patients, surgical intervention might still be the most appropriate first line therapy. In patients with large abscesses (>5 cm), there may still be a role for open surgical drainage. Tan et al. compared PD to surgical drainage (SD, 36 patients versus 44 patients, respectively) in patients with pyogenic liver abscesses greater then 5 cm in size [20]. The authors examined time to defervescence of fever, treatment failure, secondary procedures, length of hospital stay, morbidity and mortality. Of these endpoints, patients that had SD had less treatment failures, less secondary procedures performed, and shorter length of stays. There was no statistical difference between morbidity and mortality. Hope et al. also noted a high treatment failure rate in patients with large, multiloculated abscesses (67 %). In comparison, patients treated with surgery up front had no recurrence of their abscess [15]. In contrast to this, a recent publication from 2009 noted a 87 % clinical success rate in patients treated percutaneous drainage with an average abscess size of 8.3 cm [18]. No comparison to other treatment modalities was made in this series.

Patients also who score high on a severity-of-disease classification system may also warrant a more aggressive approach. Hsieh et al. compared the outcomes of patients with an APACHE II score that underwent initial percutaneous drainage versus surgical drainage [11]. The authors found a higher treatment success rate and a lower mortality rate in patients treated initially treated with surgery. In addition, less antibiotic use and a shorter length of stay were also noted in the group in which surgery was performed upfront.

Additional clinical findings might also warrant a surgical approach. Chou et al. demonstrated a high failure rate in patients that underwent catheter-based therapy in the setting of multiple abscesses [21]. The presence of fungus in the abscess culture also appears to increase catheter-based treatment failure. On multivariate analysis, yeast in the abscess culture was identified as a risk factor for treatment failure via a percutaneous approach [19]. Strong et al. also reviewed there experience with patients treated for abscess and concluded that a non-surgical approach should be undertaken for patients with pyogenic liver abscesses. However, for patients that present with an initial intraperitoneal abscess rupture or in cases of hepatobiliary pathology causing multiple abscesses above an obstructed duct system, primary surgical treatment of pyogenic liver abscess is likely indicated [22].

Liver Abscess After Liver Transplantation

Although rare, pyogenic liver abscesses following liver transplantation can be challenging to manage, with many of these occur in the setting of vascular compromise to the liver graft. Hepatic artery thrombosis is almost always the cause and is often associated with biliary tree necrosis and/or biliary strictures [23]. Management of these abscesses can be challenging since with a compromised blood supply, the infection is very difficult to clear. In addition, clinicians are often faced managing these patients in the setting of chronic immunosuppression. Tachopoulou et al. reviewed their experience at the Cleveland Clinic from 1990 to 2000 in solid organ transplant patients and identified 12 patients, all liver transplant recipients, with hepatic abscesses [24]. Thirteen patients underwent aspiration of the abscess from which 30 microbial isolates were obtained. Of these, 15 were gram-positive aerobic bacteria, 9 were gram-negative aerobic bacteria, and 3 were anaerobic. All patients except one were initially treated with percutaneous intervention. The overall mortality of the infected patients in this series was 36 %, significantly higher then that reported for non-transplant patients. Five patients required retransplantation. Similarly, Nikeghbalian reviewed their experience and identified 5 patients out of 560 liver transplant recipients with a hepatic abscess. Overall mortality in their series was 40 % [25].

Personal Experience

As detailed by the authors of several of the quoted manuscripts in this chapter, although now rare in the United States, in our experience, pyogenic abscesses when diagnosed can be challenging to manage, often occurring in older, debilitated patients. A combination approach which includes broad-spectrum antibiotics and percutaneous intervention is typically performed. Although it is ideal to obtain cultures prior to the initiation of antibiotic therapy, it is rarely the case as many of these patients present in extremis and empiric antibiotics have already been started prior to any workup being initiated. Once antibiotic therapy has started, percutaneous aspiration plus or minus placement of a pigtail catheter depending on the size of the abscess is almost routinely performed. Patients are typically reimaged 5–7 days following catheter placement to assess for adequate drainage; sooner if the patients clinical course is not improving. Repeat interventions are performed including upsizing of catheters as needed to maximize drainage. Antibiotics are eventually tailored once cultures and sensitivities have been obtained. Surgery is rarely indicated, and is only reserved for patients that have failed multiple attempts at percutaneous interventions. In patients with a prior liver transplant, liver abscesses can be challenging. Hepatic arterial thrombosis should always be ruled out, either by CT angiogram or ultrasound. Interrogation of the biliary system either via MRCP or ERCP should also be performed to rule out biliary necrosis and/or biliary stricturing. In patients that fail intervention, many will require liver retransplantation especially if biliary or vascular complications are present.

Summary

Excellent outcomes can be obtained from patients with pyogenic liver abscesses when managed appropriately. First-line therapy should include a percutaneous aspiration or trans-catheter drainage of the abscess in order to control the infection and obtain a sample for culture and sensitivity. All patients should be treated with broad spectrum antibiotics which can be tailored to the organism once identified for a duration of 4–6 weeks. Surgery should be reserved for patients that fail first line therapy, but can also be warranted in patients with large (>5 cm) abscesses or patients who present with high APACHE II scores, depending on the experience and expertise of the interventional radiology department.

Recommendations

- Percutaneous drainage is first line therapy for the treatment of pyogenic liver abscesses and surgical drainage or resection should be considered in patients who fail initial therapy especially in patients with a large, multi-loculated (>5 cm) abscess (evidence quality good – strong recommendation)
- Surgery should be considered for patients with high APACHE II scores (evidence quality poor – weak recommendation).
- Antibiotics alone are suitable first line therapy for abscesses less then 3 cm, however, aspiration should be considered in order to tailor antibiotics if possible (evidence quality good – strong recommendation)

References

1. Hansen PS, Schonheyder HC. Pyogenic hepatic abscess. A 10-year population-based retrospective study. APMIS. 1998;106(3):396–402.
2. Kaplan GG, Gregson DB, Laupland KB. Population-based study of the epidemiology of and the risk factors for pyogenic liver abscess. Clin Gastroenterol Hepatol. 2004;2(11):1032–8.
3. Ochsner A, DeBakey M, Murray S. Pyogenic abscess of the liver. An analysis of 47 cases and review of the literature. Am J Surg. 1938;40:292–319.
4. Mohsen AH, Green ST, Read RC, McKendrick MW. Liver abscess in adults: ten years experience in a UK centre. QJM. 2002;95(12):797–802.

5. Pitt HA. Surgical management of hepatic abscesses. World J Surg. 1990;14(4):498–504.
6. Yu SC, Ho SS, Lau WY, Yeung DT, Yuen EH, Lee PS, et al. Treatment of pyogenic liver abscess: prospective randomized comparison of catheter drainage and needle aspiration. Hepatology. 2004;39(4):932–8.
7. Johannsen EC, Sifri CD, Madoff LC. Pyogenic liver abscesses. Infect Dis Clin North Am. 2000;14(3):547–63, vii.
8. Rahimian J, Wilson T, Oram V, Holzman RS. Pyogenic liver abscess: recent trends in etiology and mortality. Clin Infect Dis. 2004;39(11):1654–9.
9. Seeto RK, Rockey DC. Pyogenic liver abscess. Changes in etiology, management, and outcome. Medicine. 1996;75(2):99–113.
10. Chen SC, Huang CC, Tsai SJ, Yen CH, Lin DB, Wang PH, et al. Severity of disease as main predictor for mortality in patients with pyogenic liver abscess. Am J Surg. 2009;198(2):164–72.
11. Hsieh HF, Chen TW, Yu CY, Wang NC, Chu HC, Shih ML, et al. Aggressive hepatic resection for patients with pyogenic liver abscess and APACHE II score > or =15. Am J Surg. 2008;196(3):346–50.
12. Alvarez Perez JA, Gonzalez JJ, Baldonedo RF, Sanz L, Carreno G, Junco A, et al. Clinical course, treatment, and multivariate analysis of risk factors for pyogenic liver abscess. Am J Surg. 2001;181(2):177–86.
13. Ruiz-Hernandez JJ, Leon-Mazorra M, Conde-Martel A, Marchena-Gomez J, Hemmersbach-Miller M, Betancor-Leon P. Pyogenic liver abscesses: mortality-related factors. Eur J Gastroenterol Hepatol. 2007;19(10):853–8.
14. Carpenter CF, Gilpin DO. Hepatic abscess. In: Bartlett JG, Auwaerter PG, Pham PA, editors. John Hopkins ABX Guide 2012. 3rd ed. Johns Hopkins Medicine; 2011.
15. Hope WW, Vrochides DV, Newcomb WL, Mayo-Smith WW, Iannitti DA. Optimal treatment of hepatic abscess. Am Surg. 2008;74(2):178–82.
16. Yinnon AM, Hadas-Halpern I, Shapiro M, Hershko C. The changing clinical spectrum of liver abscess: the Jerusalem experience. Postgrad Med J. 1994;70(824):436–9.
17. Zerem E, Hadzic A. Sonographically guided percutaneous catheter drainage versus needle aspiration in the management of pyogenic liver abscess. AJR Am J Roentgenol. 2007;189(3):W138–42.
18. Liu CH, Gervais DA, Hahn PF, Arellano RS, Uppot RN, Mueller PR. Percutaneous hepatic abscess drainage: do multiple abscesses or multiloculated abscesses preclude drainage or affect outcome? J Vasc Interv Radiol. 2009;20(8):1059–65.
19. Mezhir JJ, Fong Y, Jacks LM, Getrajdman GI, Brody LA, Covey AM, et al. Current management of pyogenic liver abscess: surgery is now second-line treatment. J Am Coll Surg. 2010;210(6):975–83.
20. Tan YM, Chung AY, Chow PK, Cheow PC, Wong WK, Ooi LL, et al. An appraisal of surgical and percutaneous drainage for pyogenic liver abscesses larger than 5 cm. Ann Surg. 2005;241(3):485–90.
21. Chou FF, Sheen-Chen SM, Chen YS, Chen MC. Single and multiple pyogenic liver abscesses: clinical course, etiology, and results of treatment. World J Surg. 1997;21(4):384–8; discussion 8–9.
22. Strong RW, Fawcett J, Lynch SV, Wall DR. Hepatectomy for pyogenic liver abscess. HPB (OXf). 2003;5(2):86–90.
23. Rabkin JM, Orloff SL, Corless CL, Benner KG, Flora KD, Rosen HR, et al. Hepatic allograft abscess with hepatic arterial thrombosis. Am J Surg. 1998;175(5):354–9.
24. Tachopoulou OA, Vogt DP, Henderson JM, Baker M, Keys TF. Hepatic abscess after liver transplantation: 1990–2000. Transplantation. 2003;75(1):79–83.
25. Nikeghbalian S, Salahi R, Salahi H, Bahador A, Kakaie F, Kazemi K, et al. Hepatic abscesses after liver transplant: 1997–2008. Exp Clin Transpl. 2009;7(4):256–60.

Chapter 12
Which Is Better Local Therapy for HCC, RFA or TACE?

Thuong G. Van Ha

Abstract Loco-regional therapies such as radiofrequency ablation and transarterial chemoembolization have been used in the treatment of hepatocellular carcinoma not suitable for resection and have proven to increase survival. To improve outcomes, it is important to identify patient populations who can be appropriately treated with these modalities.

Keywords Hepatocellular carcinoma (HCC) • Radiofrequency ablation (RFA) • Transarterial chemoembolization (TACE)

Introduction

Worldwide, hepatocellular carcinoma (HCC) is the sixth most common cancer and third leading cause of cancer-related deaths [1]. Historically, the rates of HCC have been lower in the United States compared to other countries. However, the incidence in the US tripled between 1975 and 2005 [2]. Given current screening protocols of patients with known cirrhosis, HCC is now increasingly recognized at an early stage [3]. Still, most patients are diagnosed in late stages so that less than one-third of the patients are candidates for surgical treatments such as resection or liver transplantation [4–6]. For patients who do not qualify for resection or liver transplantation, loco-regional therapies such as transcatheter arterial chemoembolization (TACE) and thermal ablation are accepted treatments that prolong survival by eradicating or controlling tumor while preserving liver function [7]. Both techniques have limitations in treating HCC, with incomplete necrosis of tumor and subsequent tumor recurrence using TACE, and inadequate control of medium to large size HCC for both TACE and ablative therapy.

T.G. Van Ha (✉)
Section of Cardiovascular Interventional Radiology, Department of Radiology, University of Chicago, MC 2026 5841 South Maryland Ave, Chicago, IL 60615, USA
e-mail: tgvanha@radiology.bsd.uchicago.edu

J.M. Millis, J.B. Matthews (eds.), *Difficult Decisions in Hepatobiliary and Pancreatic Surgery*, Difficult Decisions in Surgery: An Evidence-Based Approach, DOI 10.1007/978-3-319-27365-5_12

The Barcelona-Clinic Liver Cancer classification groups patients into five stages and allocates treatment according to their status [8–10]. Briefly, very early stage refers to HCC with tumor <2 cm in diameter, and early stage refers to with single tumor =/>2 cm or up to three satellite nodules, each </= to 3 cm. Intermediate HCC refers to multinodular asymptomatic patients and advanced HCC with symptomatic tumor, macrovascular tumoral involvement, or extrahepatic disease. Advanced stage and terminal stage are the last two stages where surgery and loco-regional therapy do not have a role.

Surgery when possible is the mainstay of therapy for HCC. Resection is considered first line treatment option for patients with a single tumor and well preserved liver function. For patient within Milan criteria or with mild portal hypertension not suitable for liver transplantation, resection can be performed though there is no strong evidence for this strategy. Liver transplantation is considered first line for patients meeting Milan criteria who cannot undergo resection. Loco-regional therapy is considered if waiting list exceeds 6 months.

Local ablation is considered standard of care for patients with BCLC 0-A (very early-early stages) with tumors not suitable for surgery. This advocacy is based on studies showing good results with smaller tumors. Currently radiofrequency ablation (RFA) is considered the modality of choice due to evidence of better control than percutaneous ethanol injection (PEI) [11]. Evidence with other modalities such as microwave ablation (MWA) is lacking though their use is increasing [12]. RFA can be performed by open surgery, through laparoscopic approach, or more commonly using the percutaneous approach under radiologic guidance. RFA works by ionic agitation creating local rise in temperature and in the process causes cell death through coagulative necrosis [13]. However, RFA has limitations, including size threshold of the treated area and the "heat sink effect," where tumor adjacent to blood vessels is spared as the heat is carried away by the flowing blood.

TACE has been recommended for patients with BCLC stage B (intermediate). The use of TACE is recommended in part due to two radomized control trials (RCT) that showed survival benefit of TACE in unresectable HCC, though the numbers of subjects were small and the chemotherapeutic agents used in each trial was different [14, 15]. TACE is a transarterial technique, usually through a common femoral arterial approach, that delivers chemotherapeutic agent or agents through a catheter placed in the hepatic artery feeder vessels to the tumor, followed by embolization which blocks further flow to the tumor. The goal of this technique is to deliver a high dose of chemotherapeutic agent to the tumor while sparing the rest of the liver parenchyma (i.e., chemotherapy is injected directly into the tumor) and to decrease washout of the agent (i.e., by embolization) thereby prolonging drug effect while limiting systemic toxicity [13].

We seek to see whether there is any evidence comparing the use of ablative therapy to TACE in patients who are in BCLC 0-A and BCLC B stages.

Search Strategy

A literature search of English language publications was performed in the time period of 2000–2014. Publications were identified on the subject of chemoembolization and radiofrequency ablation for hepatocellular carcinoma.

Terms used: Transarterial chemoembolization, TACE, chemoembolization, RFA, radiofrequency ablation, thermal ablation, AND hepatocellular carcinoma OR HCC.

Databases used were PubMed and Embase.

Articles were excluded if they addressed surgical treatment of HCC or comparison between surgical resection TACE and/or RFA. In addition, studies involving sorafenib or adjuvant and neoadjuvant chemotherapy were also excluded.

Results

No randomized control trials were identified comparing RFA to TACE head to head. There were three retrospective studies comparing RFA to TACE (Table 12.1).

Hsu et al. [16] retrospectively analyzed data that were prospectively collected in an 8 year period, in two cohorts of patients who met the Milan criteria. Three hundred fifteen patients underwent RFA and 215 received TACE. From each arm, 101 matched patients were selected to create a propensity score model. Long term survival significantly favored the RFA group (P=0.048). However, in the propensity score model, there was no significant difference in long term survival between the two groups. The study also found that total tumor volume less than 11 cm^3 have significantly longer survival with RFA treatment (P=0.032).

Kim et al. [17] reported a retrospective study of RFA versus TACE in the treatment of single HCC smaller than 2 cm (BCLC very-early stage HCC). There were 165 patients treated initially with RFA and 122 patients who were initially treated with TACE. There were no significant differences in overall survival (P=0.079). However, there was a difference in response rates favoring the RFA group (100 % vs. 95.9 %). In addition, the RFA group had a more favorable time to progression (27 vs 18 months; P=0.013).

Liu et al. [18] in a retrospective analysis of 424 patients undergoing RFA and 282 patients receiving TACE, all within Milan criteria, evaluated for overall survival. Patients were stratified by ECOG performance status (PS) into two cohorts, one with ECOG PS 0 and the other with PS =/>1. Overall, the RFA patients had better survival than the TACE patients with the 3 year survival of 71 % and 59 % respectively (P=0.001). Of the initial patient population, 167 pairs of patients with PS of 0 and 68 pairs with PS of 1 or greater were entered into propensity score matching analysis. For the PS 0 group, RFA had significantly better survival then the TACE group. However, in the analysis of the PS 1 or greater propensity matched patients, there was no significant difference in survival.

Table 12.1 Studies comparing RFA to TACE directly

Studies	HCC size	RFA cohort (Number of patients)	TACE cohort (Number of patients)	Overall survival (%) RFA/TACE	Median TTP (months) RFA/TACE	Tumor regression % RFA/TACE
Hsu et al. [16]	Within Milan Criteria	315	215	3 years: 72/63	Not given	Not given
				5 years:		
				55/43 (p=0.048)		
	Propensity Score analysis	101	101	3 years: 60/55	Not given	Not given
				5 years: 41/36 (p=0.476)		
Kim et al. [17]	<=2 cm	165	122	3 years:	27/18	100/95.9
				86.7/75.4		
				5 years: 74.5/63.1 (p=0.079)		
Liu et al. [18]	Within Milan Criteria	424	282	3 years:		
				71/59 (p=0.001)		
	PS 0	319	197	77/63 (p=0.006)		
	PS >=1	105	85	38/47 (p=0.812)		

PS ECOG Propensity score, *TTP* Time to progression

One additional study [19], though not a comparative analysis, evaluated patients who were eligible for RFA but instead underwent TACE. The study retrospectively analyzed 114 patients, who would have qualified for RFA, with HCC, the largest less than 5 cm in diameter up to three nodules who have undergone TACE as initial treatment. Many of these patients were treated when RFA was not readily available. The 1-, 3-, 5-year survival rates were 80 %, 43 %, and 23 % respectively, which the authors concluded as being comparable to historical rates of survival for RFA treated patients.

Recommendations

RFA has been shown to be effective in the treatment of HCC with tumor size </= 3 cm with good complete response rate of 90 %. As tumor size increases, there is a decrease in the response rate to RFA. Though complete ablation can be achieved with medium size tumors, from 3 to 5 cm, tumors larger than 5 cm have poor response rate [13]. RFA is also not recommended in central locations where risk of bile duct or vascular injury is high. Tumors abutting large vessel can be less effective as the flow of blood can carry the heat away and therefore offer protection to the adjacent tumor margin [20]. Additionally, peripheral lesions adjacent to other organs such as bowel or pericardium, should not undergo ablation if protective measures such as hydro-dissection or CO_2 insufflation cannot be adequately provided [21, 22]. TACE, on the other hand, received validation through two RCT and numerous meta-analysis as having a survival benefit in the treatment of unresectable HCC [14, 15, 23].

The EASL-EORTC Clinical Practice Guidelines

The EASL-EORTC clinical practice guidelines recommend that the BCLC staging system, as described above be used for prognostic prediction and treatment allocation [7]. Surgical treatments include hepatic resection and liver transplantation. Resection is considered first line treatment for patients with solitary tumors and very well preserved function, defined as normal bilirubin level and either hepatic venous pressure gradient </= 10 mmHg or platelet count >/= 100,000 plt/mcL. For patients with multifocal tumors, within the Milan criteria but not suitable for transplantation, resection could be performed, but no definitive recommendation can be made at this point due to lack of prospective comparison with loco-regional therapies. Liver transplantation is considered first line treatment option for patients within Milan criteria but not candidates for surgical resection. Loco-regional treatments can be considered if the waiting list exceeds 6 months, even though long term outcomes are uncertain due to level of available evidence.

According to the guidelines, local ablation is considered first line treatment option for patients with early stage HCC who are not candidates for surgical resection. Percutaneous ethanol injection has been shown to be inferior to RFA in lesions larger than 2 cm and is associated with high recurrence rate in lesions larger than 3 cm. Therefore, RFA is preferred over PEI as an ablative technique [24], but PEI can be employed where use of RFA is not possible. Other ablative therapies including microwave ablation and cryoablation are being used but strong evidence is currently lacking. Though there are studies comparing RFA and surgical resection of small solitary HCC, the results are mixed and ablation could not be recommended as alternative therapy to hepatic resection. TACE is recommended as first line treatment for intermediate stage HCC, more specifically, those with multinodular HCC but without cancer related symptoms, vascular invasion, or extrahepatic spread. Although there is a lack of definitive evidence, chemotherapeutic agents recommended are doxorubicin and cisplatin and that TACE can be repeated 3–4 times per year. To minimize affecting non-tumoral hepatic tissue in an attempt to preserve liver function, it is also recommended that superselective chemoembolization, i.e. treatment limited to tumoral feeder vessels and sparing vessels to normal liver, be used.

Other Recommendations

Similar to EASL recommendations, CEPO, an oncologist group of specialists who provide evidence based guidelines for clinicians in the province of Quebec, Canada, recommends that TACE be considered standard of practice for palliative treatment of HCC in eligible patients [25]. CEPO also states that DEB-TACE be considered an alternative and equivalent treatment to TACE. Bland embolization and radioembolization are not considered standard treatments for HCC currently by either group. Sorafenib, an oral agent, inhibitor of multi-tyrosine kinase, is the only systemic drug that has shown survival benefit [26] and it is recommended for patients with well-preserved liver function (Child-Pugh A) and with advanced HCC, or tumors progressing on loco-regional therapies. No recommendation can be made with sorafenib in Child-Pugh B patients at this point.

Outside these recommendations, there are a few RCT favoring the use of TACE/RFA combination therapy over RFA alone. In a meta-analysis [27] consisting of 7 RCTs that included 571 patients who were treated with TACE and RFA or RFA alone, found that there was a significant differences in the 1- and 3-year survival rates favoring the combination group. Recurrence free survival at 1 and 3-year also favors the combination group.

In a more recent publication, a meta-analysis consisting of 12 studies and 1952 patients comparing clinical outcome of small HCC among the various treatment, divided the study group into two different cohorts [28]. One arm consisted of patients receiving surgical resection and the other arm patients undergoing non-surgical loco-regional treatment or treatments including RFA, PEI, TACE, and

TACE plus RFA combination. The results showed that there were no significant survival advantage at 1 and 3 year, but the 5 year survival rate favored the surgical resection group. However, no significant difference was noted in the 1 or 5 year progression free survival. In addition, there was a significant decrease in the incidence of adverse events in the surgical resection group and the local recurrence rate was significantly higher in the non-surgical group. The authors acknowledged that the number of trials of non-surgical ablation to be insufficient and that the number of cases undergoing PEI and TACE were also insufficient to compare the non-surgical modalities to each other. This publication illustrates the lack of sufficient evidence to suggest one non-surgical technique over another in the treatment of small HCC.

As seen above, there are only a few head to head studies of RFA vs. TACE and no RCT. However, due to available evidence, there are recommendations that for tumors that are non-resectable, RFA should be performed if the tumors are in early stages or smaller than 3 cm, and for intermediate tumors, TACE should be used as palliative treatment. From the few studies directly comparing the two treatment techniques above, it appears that for the patients within Milan criteria, there is survival advantage for patients undergoing RFA over TACE. However in one study this advantage is no longer seen in the propensity score model and is seen in only in the ECOG PS 0 group and not the PS 1 or greater group. For the study involving tumors less than 2 cm, there was no difference in overall survival though there was a difference in tumor response rate. However, in this study the results were not straightforward as there was significant crossover in terms of subsequent treatments [18].

What these studies suggest is that RFA is superior in survival advantage for patients with good performance status. Additionally, RFA appears to be more effective in terms of tumor response rate in early HCC and total tumor volume of less than 11 cm^3. TACE, though recommended as palliative therapy, should be considered in patients with tumors who might not qualify for RFA otherwise, due to contraindications, such as central tumors close to large bile ducts, or tumors adjacent to other organs [16–18].

Another treatment gaining acceptance in the treatment of HCC is combination therapy, TACE followed by RFA. This therapy makes use of the synergistic effect of TACE, which blocks blood flow the tumor and can extend the ablated area when followed by RFA soon after, among other potential effects.

A Personal View of the Data

For small tumors, RFA appears to be effective in achieving complete response. However, for tumors approaching 5 cm, the response rate and survival rate advantage diminish. With tumors 5 cm or larger, RFA results are rather poor and therefore TACE should really be used for palliation. When tumors qualify for possible RFA but due to contraindication to thermal ablation, TACE is a reasonable alternative. Combination of TACE followed by RFA appears to increase the effectiveness of

RFA over RFA alone and this treatment might very well be recommended in the future for intermediate size HCC if RCT can substantiate the preliminary results.

Recommendations

Loco-regional therapy is for patients who are not eligible for surgical resection and who are on transplant list with wait time longer than 6 months.

For patients with very early and no contraindication to RFA,

- RFA should be first line treatment.
- If RFA not possible, consider TACE as a reasonable alternative.

For patients with early HCC (within Milan)

- RFA if possible.
- Consider TACE/RFA combination if largest lesion approaching 5 cm to increase tumor response rate.
- TACE if RFA not possible.

References

1. Ferlay J, Shin HR, Bray F, et al. Estimates of worldwide burden of cancer in 2008: GLOBOCAN 2008. Int J Cancer. 2010;127:2893–917.
2. Altekruse SF, McGlynn KA, Reichman ME. Hepatocellular carcinoma incidence, mortality, and survival trends in the United States from 1975 to 2005. J Clin Oncol. 2009;27(9):1485–91.
3. CDC. Hepatocellular carcinoma—United States, 2001–2006. MMWR 2010. 59(17): 517–20. Reported by O'Connor S and Ward JW.
4. Bruix J, Sherman M. Management of heptocellular carcinoma: an update. AASLD practice guideline. Hepatology. 2011;53(3):1020–2.
5. Former A, Llovet JM, Bruix J. Hepatocellular carcinoma. Lancet. 2012;379(9822):1245–55.
6. McGlynn KA, London WT. The global epidemiology of hepatocellular carcinoma: present and future. Clin Liver Dis. 2011;15:223–43, vii–x.
7. Llovet JM, Lencioni R, Di Bisceglie AM, et al. EASL-EORTC Clinical practice guidelines: management of hepatocellular carcinoma. J Hepatol. 2012;56:908–43.
8. Llovet JM, Bru C, Bruix J. Prognosis of hepatocellular carcinoma: the BCLC staging classification. Semin Liver Dis. 1999;19:329–38.
9. Llovet JM, Fuster J, Bruix J. The Barcelona approach: diagnosis, staging, and treatment of hepatocellular carcinoma. Liver Transplant. 2004;10(Supp):S115–20.
10. Bruix J, Sherman M. Management of hepatocellular carcinoma: an update. Hepatology. 2011;53:1020–2.
11. Lencioni R. Loco-regional treatment of hepatocellular carcinoma. Hepatology. 2010;52:762–73.
12. Liang P, Wang Y, Yu X, Dong B. Malignant liver tumors: treatment with percutaneous microwave ablation—complications among cohort of 1136 patients. Radiology. 2009;251:933–40.

13. Georgiades CS, Hong K, Geschwind J. Radiofrequency ablation and chemoembolization for hepatocellular carcinoma. Cancer J. 2008;14:17–122.
14. Llovet JM, Real MI, Montana X, et al. Arterial embolization or chemoembolization versus symptomatic treatment in patients with unresectable hepatocellular carcinoma: a randomized controlled trial. Lancet. 2002;359:1734–9.
15. Lo CM, Ngan H, Tso WK, et al. Randomized controlled trial of transarterial Lipiodol chemoembolization for unresectable hepatocellular carcinoma. Hepatology. 2002;35:1164–71.
16. Hsu C, Huang Y, Chiou Y, et al. Comparison of radiofrequency ablation and transarterial chemoembolization for hepatocellular carcinoma within the Milan criteria: a propensity score analysis. Liver Transpl. 2011;17:556–66.
17. Kim JW, Kim JH, Sung K, et al. Transarterial chemoembolization vs. radiofrequency ablation for the treatment of single hepatocellular carcinoma 2 cm or smaller. Am J Gastroenterol. 2014;109:1234–40.
18. Liu P, Lee Y, Hsu C, et al. Survival advantage of radiofrequency ablation over transarterial chemoembolization for patients with hepatocellular carcinoma and good performance status within the Milan criteria. Am Surg Oncol. 2014;21(12):3835–43.
19. Liem M, Poon R, Lo C, Tso W, Fan S. Outcome of transarterial chemoembolization in patients with inoperable hepatocellular carcinoma eligible for radiofrequency ablation. World J Gastroenterol. 2005;11:4465–71.
20. Lu DS, Raman SS, Limanond P, et al. Influence of large peritumoral vessels on outcome of radiofrequency ablation of liver tumors. J Vasc Interv Radiol. 2003;14:1267–74.
21. Kapoor BS, Hunter DW. Injection of subphrenic saline during radiofrequency ablation to minimize diaphragmatic injury. Cardiovasc Interv Radiol. 2003;26:302–4.
22. Raman SS, Aziz D, Chang X, et al. Minimizing diaphragmatic injury during radiofrequency ablation: efficacy of intraabdominal carbon dioxide insufflation. Am J Roentgenol. 2004;183:197–200.
23. Bruix J, Sala M, Llovet JM. Chemoembolization for hepatocellular carcinoma. Gastroenterology. 2004;127 Suppl 1:S179–88.
24. Bouza C, Lopez-Cuadrado T, Alcazar R, Saz-Parkinson Z, Amate JM. Meta-analysis of percutaneous radiofrequency ablation versus ethanol injection in hepatocellular carcinoma. BMC Gastroenterol. 2009;9:31.
25. Boily G, Villeneuve J, Lacoursiere L, et al. Transarterial embolization therapies for the treatment of hepatocellular carcinoma: CEPO review and clinical recommendations. Int Hepatol-Pancreat-Biliary Assoc. 2014;17:52–65.
26. Llovet JM, Ricci S, Mazzaferro V, et al. SHARP investigators study group. Sorafenib in advanced hepatocellular carcinoma. N Engl J Med. 2008;359:378–90.
27. Liu Z, Goa F, Yang G, et al. Combination of radiofrequency ablation with transarterial chemoembolization for hepatocellular carcinoma: an up-to-date meta-analysis. Tumor Biol. 2014;35:7407–13.
28. Dong W, Zhang T, Wang Z, Liu H. Clinical outcome of small hepatocellular carcinoma after different treatments: a meta-analysis. World J Gastroenterol. 2014;20:10174–82.

Chapter 13
When Should Patients with Liver Metastases from Colorectal Cancer Receive Chemotherapy?

Malini D. Sur and Eugene A. Choi

Abstract Advances in hepatic resection techniques and cytotoxic therapy over the last 30 years have led to vast improvements in outcomes after hepatic resection in patients with colorectal liver metastases (CLM). Nonetheless, the optimal sequence of therapy for CLM remains a significant clinical challenge. This chapter will summarize the evidence-based literature that pertains to the timing of chemotherapy in relation to surgery for CLM in the absence of extra-hepatic metastases.

Keywords Colorectal liver metastases • Chemotherapy • Hepatectomy

Introduction

Hepatic metastases are the most common indication for liver resection in the United States [1]. For many aggressive primary cancers, there is no strong evidence to support surgery for secondary tumors in the liver. However, long-term survival after resection of colorectal liver metastases (CLM) in well-selected patients was observed as early as 1976 [2]. Significant advances in both hepatic resection techniques and chemotherapeutic agents over the last 30 years have led to vast improvements in outcomes after hepatic resection in patients with CLM, with a median survival currently estimated at 3.6 years [3]. Nevertheless, the management of CLM remains challenging in part due to the debate about the optimal sequence of treatments. This chapter will review the evidence-based literature about the timing of chemotherapy in relation to surgery for CLM in the absence of extra-hepatic metastases.

M.D. Sur
Department of Surgery, University of Chicago Medicine, Chicago, IL, USA

E.A. Choi (✉)
Department of Surgery, Baylor College of Medicine,
One Baylor Place MS: BCM390, Houston, TX 77030, USA
e-mail: eugene.choi@bcm.edu

J.M. Millis, J.B. Matthews (eds.), *Difficult Decisions in Hepatobiliary and Pancreatic Surgery*, Difficult Decisions in Surgery: An Evidence-Based Approach, DOI 10.1007/978-3-319-27365-5_13

Overall Risks and Benefits of Treatment Sequence Options

Historically, patients with clearly resectable CLM were quickly taken to the operating room to avoid tumor progression spread and conversion to unresectable disease. Adjuvant therapy was proposed as a way to reduce the rate of early recurrences [4], but there were concerns that administering systemic chemotherapy prior to surgery might increase the rate of post-operative complications. These concerns were heightened as the hepatotoxic effects of standard chemotherapeutic agents used against colorectal cancer, 5-fluorouracil, oxaliplatin, and irinotecan, were increasingly recognized [5]. Another disadvantage of upfront chemotherapy is significant tumor response that would make planning liver surgery difficult. The desire to maximize the functional liver remnant must be balanced with the risk of leaving behind radiographically undetectable but microscopic residual disease that may be present within the tissue occupied by the original lesion [6–8].

By 2001, it became apparent that a proportion of patients with CLM initially deemed unresectable would respond to chemotherapy to become surgical candidates [9]. The principle that neoadjuvant chemotherapy could reduce the extent of necessary hepatic resection to remove all metastatic disease was applicable to patients with resectable but bulky CLM. Prioritizing the administration of chemotherapy in the setting of metastatic disease reflects the desire to treat all disease (primary and metastatic) as quickly as possible. In addition, any occult or micrometastatic disease can be treated with chemotherapy. Although upfront chemotherapy delays surgery and might risk progression of disease, this approach may help select patients with favorable tumor biology for surgery. Those responding to treatment can undergo hepatectomy, while those with unfavorable tumor biology avoid high-risk surgery that is unlikely to be have significant long-term benefits. Patients who undergo resection after chemotherapy might also benefit from an increased likelihood of having margin negative resections [10]. Following surgery, an adjuvant chemotherapy regimen could be tailored to individual patients based on the pathologic response to the pre-operatively administered agent. Finally, neoadjuvant therapy avoids the risk of delays in systemic treatment after surgery due to post-operative complications that are frequent after major liver resections. The effect of hepatotoxicity of neoadjuvant agents on post-operative complication rates has also been raised, as the extent of liver resection and need for blood transfusion may be more influential factors [11]. Table 13.1 summarizes the proposed advantages and disadvantages of adjuvant versus neoadjuvant chemotherapy for CLM.

Search Strategy

A literature search of English language publications from 2004 to 2014 was conducted to identify published data addressing the timing of chemotherapy administration in relation to liver surgery for patients with potentially resectable liver

Table 13.1 Proposed advantages and disadvantages of adjuvant versus neoadjuvant chemotherapy for colorectal liver metastases

	Adjuvant chemotherapy	Neoadjuvant chemotherapy
Proposed advantages	Minimize risk of progression of resectable disease into disease that is unresectable or resectable with greater morbidity	Prioritize treatment of systemic disease, treating potentially occult micrometastases
	Avoid risk of increased surgical morbidity due to hepatotoxic effects of cytotoxic agents	Select patients with favorable tumor biology to undergo hepatectomy
	Optimize chances of resecting all disease by avoiding inadequate resection in areas of disappearing metastases	Allow time for portal vein embolization if needed
		Increase rates of margin-negative resection
		Adjust adjuvant therapy regimen based on response to neoadjuvant agent
Proposed disadvantages	Post-operative complications may substantially delay administration of systemic therapy	Risk progression of resectable disease into disease that is unresectable or resectable with greater morbidity
	Patients with unfavorable tumor biology may undergo major liver resection only to relapse very soon after	Hepatotoxicity of cytotoxic agents may increase morbidity of major liver resections

Table 13.2 PICO table for timing of chemotherapy for resectable colorectal liver metastases

P (Patients)	I (Intervention)	C (Comparator)	O (Outcomes)
Patients with resectable colorectal liver metastases	(a) Adjuvant chemotherapy	(a) Surgery alone	Progression-free survival, recurrence rate, recurrence-free survival, disease-free survival, overall survival, post-operative morbidity and mortality
	(b) Perioperative chemotherapy	(b) Surgery alone	
	(c) Neoadjuvant chemotherapy alone or perioperative chemotherapy	(c) Surgery alone or adjuvant chemotherapy	

metastases from primary colorectal cancer. The PICO outline was used, as demonstrated in Table 13.2. Databases searched were PubMed and Web of Science. Terms used in the search were "timing," "surgery," "chemotherapy," AND "liver metastatic colorectal cancer" OR "colorectal liver metastases." References cited within the resulting articles were carefully reviewed and included if they met inclusion and exclusion criteria.

Articles were included only if they compared adjuvant chemotherapy to surgery alone, perioperative chemotherapy to surgery alone, or adjuvant chemotherapy to perioperative chemotherapy. Articles were excluded if they primarily addressed chemotherapy for unresectable metastatic colorectal cancer, timing of colorectal surgery in relation to liver surgery alone, early versus delayed liver surgery alone, management of extrahepatic metastases, management of recurrent liver metastases, use of radiation, use of liver-directed ablative therapies, use of hepatic arterial infusion (HAI), or use of targeted therapy. Retrospective studies featuring fewer than 100 patients were excluded, as were case reports, chapters, comments, and nonsystematic review papers. Review papers focusing on the timing of chemotherapy and surgery were included. Three randomized control trials (RCT), one pooled analysis, and three retrospective cohort studies were included in our final analysis. The identified literature was classified using the GRADE system.

Results

No RCT has directly compared outcomes of CLM patients treated with adjuvant chemotherapy to those treated with perioperative chemotherapy. Our current understanding has therefore been largely shaped by trials comparing each modality to surgery alone as well as by cohort studies comparing the two modalities. While providing low-quality evidence, numerous single institution observational studies of patients undergoing a common sequence of treatments offer some additional insights. Table 13.3 summarizes the results of major studies comparing treatment options for CLM.

Two major RCTs examined the benefits of adjuvant chemotherapy after margin-negative resection of up to four synchronous or metachronous CLM compared to resection alone. Both used an adjuvant regimen involving only bolus 5-fluorouracil (5-FU) and leucovorin, which was standard at the time of enrollment. Unfortunately, this regimen is now known to be suboptimal compared to regimens combining 5-FU with oxaliplatin or irinotecan and therefore both studies have limited applicability today. Additionally, both trials were closed early and underpowered. The ENG (EORTC/NCIC-CTG/GVIVO) trial randomized 107 patients to fluorouracil and leucovorin or observation after surgery for CLM but also included patients undergoing surgery for lung metastases [12]. Data initially presented in 2002 showed that patients who received adjuvant therapy tended to have longer recurrence-free survival (RFS) and overall survival (OS). However, the results lacked statistical significance and were not fully published. The FFCD ACHBTH AURC 9002 trial randomized 171 patients who had undergone R0 resections of CLM to surgery alone or adjuvant therapy with fluorouracil and leucovorin as well [13]. No difference in 5-year OS was observed between the two groups, but the 5-year disease-free survival (DFS) rate was significantly greater among patients receiving adjuvant chemotherapy. Mitry et al. performed a pooled analysis of data from both trials and showed no difference in median OS but did demonstrate a trend towards longer median progression-free survival (PFS) in the chemotherapy group (62.2 months) compared to the surgery only group (47.3 months) [14]. Based on these data, resection of CLM without plans of administering additional cytotoxic therapy was abandoned.

Table 13.3 Studies comparing options for timing of chemotherapy for CLM

Study author and year	Study type	Number of patients	Outcome measures	Arm 1 results	Arm 2 results	Statistics	Quality of evidence
Surgery alone vs. adjuvant chemotherapy				Surgery alone	Adjuvant chemotherapy		
Langer 2002 (EORTC/NCIC-CTG/GIVO trial)	Randomized controlled trial	107	Median RFS	20 months	39 months	p=0.35	Low
			Median OS	43 months	53 months	p=0.39	
Portier 2006 (FFCD ACHBTH AURC 9002)	Randomized controlled trial	171	5-year DFS	26.7 %	33.5 %	OR=0.66 [0.46–0.96], p=0.028	Moderate
			5-year OS	41.1 %	51.1 %	OR=0.73 [0.48–1.10], p=0.13	
Mitry 2008	Pooled analysis of 2 randomized trials	278	Median PFS	18.8 months	27.9 months	HR=1.32 [1.00–1.76], p=0.058	Moderate
			Median OS	47.3 months	62.2 months	HR=1.32 [0.95–1.82], p=0.095	
Surgery alone vs. perioperative chemotherapy				Surgery alone	Perioperative chemotherapy		
Nordlinger 2008, 2013 (EORTC Intergroup Trial 40983)	Randomized controlled trial	364	3-year PFS	29.9 %	39.0 %	HR 0.78 [0.61–0.99], p=0.035	Moderate
			5-year OS	47.8 %	51.2 %	p=0.34	
			Median OS	54.3 months	61.3 months	p=0.34	
			Reversible complications	16 %	25 %	p=0.04	
Surgery alone or adjuvant chemotherapy vs. neoadjuvant chemotherapy alone or perioperative chemotherapy				Surgery alone or adjuvant chemotherapy	Neoadjuvant chemotherapy alone or perioperative chemotherapy		

(continued)

Table 13.3 (continued)

Study author and year	Study type	Number of patients	Outcome measures	Arm 1 results	Arm 2 results	Statistics	Quality of evidence
Pawlik 2007	Retrospective cohort	212	Complications	30.5 %	35.3 %	p=0.79	Low
			60-day mortality				
Scoggins 2009	Retrospective cohort	186	Median DFS	56 months	40 months	p=0.25	Low
			Median OS	65 months	56 months	p=0.30	
			Morbidity	47 %	49 %	p=0.81	
			90-day mortality	0.07 %	0 %	p=0.29	
Pinto Marques 2012	Retrospective cohort with matched pair analysis and propensity score analysis	676	Morbidity after minor hepatectomy	16.5 %	17.9 %	p=0.72	Moderate
			Morbidity after major hepatectomy	14.2 %	23.1 %	p=0.06	
			5-year OS	55 %	43 %	p=0.009	
		410 (matched-pair analysis)	Recurrence	41 %	51 %	p=0.03	
			5-year DFS	20 %	15 %	p=0.01	
			5-year OS	54 %	42 %	p=0.09	
		244 (propensity score analysis)	Median OS	69.6 months	56.8 months	p=0.12	
Scartozzi 2011	Retrospective cohort	104	Median OS	48 months	31 months	p=0.0358	Low
			Median PFS	25 months	16 months	p=0.031	
			Recurrence	52.5 %	75 %	p=0.0347	

Spelt 2012	Retrospective cohort	233	Complications	63.2 %	62.9 %	NS	Low
			90-day mortality	1.5 %	0 %	NS	
Araujo 2013	Retrospective cohort	411	3-year OS	78 %	74 %	p=0.48	Low
			5-year OS	60 %	56 %		
			3-year RFS	44 %	32 %	p=0.036; adjusting for CRS, p=0.42 (low CRS), p=0.74 (high CRS)	
			5-year RFS	38 %	31 %		
			Complications	39 %	38.3 %	p=0.92	
Zhu 2014	Retrospective cohort	466	5-year OS	48 %	52 %	NS	Low
			30-day morbidity	25.8 %	33.9 %	NS	
			30-day mortality	1.2 %	1.7 %	NS	

RFS recurrence-free survival, *DFS* disease-free survival, *PFS* progression-free survival, *OS* overall survival, *OR* odds ratio, *HR* hazard ratio, *NS* non-significant, *CRS* clinical risk score

In 2008, the same year that Mitry et al. published results of the pooled analysis, Nordlinger et al. published initial data from the EORTC Intergroup 40983 trial [15]. Long-term results were presented in 2013 [16]. In this landmark study, 364 patients with up to four synchronous or metachronous CLM were randomly assigned to "perioperative" chemotherapy consisting of 6 cycles of neoadjuvant 5-FU, leucovorin, and oxaliplatin (FOLFOX4) combined with six cycles of adjuvant chemotherapy or to surgery alone. Patients who underwent resection following chemotherapy did have a significantly higher rate of reversible postoperative complications (25 %). At 3 years, the rate of PFS among eligible patients was 39.0 % in those who received perioperative chemotherapy compared to 29.9 % in those who underwent surgery alone ($p=0.035$). However, no significant difference in OS was detected between the two groups, with mortality rates of 59 % of the perioperative chemotherapy group and 63 % of the surgery only group at a median follow-up of 8.5 years. A survival benefit may not have been identified because the study was underpowered to detect the predefined 5 % difference in 5-year OS or because only 63 % of the perioperative chemotherapy group went on to actually receive post-operative chemotherapy [17]. Although the study authors advocate for perioperative therapy based on the demonstrated improvement in PFS alone, others argue that the lack of a clear survival benefit challenges the routine use of neoadjuvant chemotherapy [17]. Moreover, the trial compared perioperative chemotherapy to surgery alone as opposed to surgery with adjuvant chemotherapy, and newer therapeutic agents were not studied.

The NSABP C-11 trial is a phase III RCT currently underway to investigate the difference in RFS between patients with resectable CLM receiving perioperative chemotherapy and those receiving adjuvant therapy alone. Patients who are oxaliplatin-naïve will receive FOLFOX and those who have been previously treated with oxaliplatin will receive 5-FU, leucovorin, and irinotecan (FOLFIRI). Randomization will be stratified according to the number of liver metastases, the planned chemotherapy regimen, and whether the disease is synchronous or metachronous. The results of this study will hopefully add critical insight into the optimal timing of cytotoxic agents in relation to surgery for CLM. The precise role of targeted therapy for CLM will need to be addressed in further investigations.

In the absence of additional data from RCTs, multidisciplinary decision-making about the treatment of CLM must rely on several relevant retrospective cohort studies published over the last 10 years. By design, these studies are inherently limited in their ability to control for all the clinicopathological variables that influence the choice of treatment modalities for individual patients, leading to a considerable risk of selection bias. For example, patients with signs of more aggressive disease may be more likely to be offered neoadjuvant therapy. Many of the retrospective reports are also based on relatively small numbers of patients and thus lack statistical power to detect significant differences in long-term outcomes. Finally, most of these studies demonstrate significant heterogeneity in the treatment protocols between the comparative arms. While the RCTs described above had a surgery alone arm, retrospective studies have generally compared patients who received neoadjuvant chemotherapy to those who did not. The latter group sometimes included patients who received adjuvant chemotherapy as well as those who did not. Multiple chemotherapeutic regimens, some consisting of targeted therapies, as well as local liver-directed therapies were sometimes included.

Despite these weaknesses, it is valuable to review the major retrospective cohort studies comparing different therapeutic sequence options for CLM. In 2009, Reddy et al. published a multi-institutional analysis of outcomes of 499 patients with CLM stratified into four groups based on the timing of chemotherapy that was ultimately delivered: pre-hepatectomy alone, post-hepatectomy alone, perioperative (i.e. pre- and post-hepatectomy), and none [18]. Not surprisingly, those treated with pre-hepatectomy chemotherapy were often associated with a larger number of liver tumors, a node-positive primary tumor, a major hepatectomy, and ablation procedures in addition to resection. After controlling for factors reflecting decisions to treat with upfront chemotherapy, multivariate analysis revealed that post-hepatectomy chemotherapy was significantly associated with RFS and OS but pre-hepatectomy chemotherapy was associated with no survival benefit. Because outcomes in those treated with perioperative chemotherapy were similar to those in the post-hepatectomy chemotherapy alone group, the investigators argued that chemotherapy administered after liver resection had the strongest oncologic benefit. The study was limited, however, by substantial variation in resectability criteria, resection techniques, choice of pre-operative imaging, and chemotherapeutic regimens across the participating institutions. In addition, given the retrospective nature, patients were grouped according to the chemotherapy schedule they ultimately received as opposed to the planned chemotherapy schedule. Patients treated with pre-hepatectomy chemotherapy who developed disease progression that precluded resection were not included.

Four years later, Pinto Marques et al. performed the largest of the retrospective studies known to date and also attempted to control for confounding through matched pair and propensity score analyses [19]. Among their 676 study patients, those who received neoadjuvant chemotherapy were more likely to have a lymph node positive primary tumor, synchronous disease, and a greater number of liver metastases. When all patients were considered, post-operative complications were significantly increased from 14.2 to 23.1 % with the addition of chemotherapy prior to major but not minor hepatectomy for CLM. Without controlling for baseline characteristics, 5-year OS was significantly worse in the patients treated with neoadjuvant therapy compared to patients who did receive chemotherapy prior to surgery (43 % vs. 55 %). A 1:1 matched-pair analysis was then undertaken using 205 pairs of patients with similar pathological characteristics. This still revealed a significantly higher rate of recurrence (51 % compared to 41 %, $p=0.03$) and lower rate of 5-year DFS (15 % compared to 20 %, $p=0.01$), but the difference in 5-year OS was not significant. Acknowledging the limitations of matched-pair analyses, the authors performed a third analysis based on propensity score matching using 244 patients that again revealed no significant difference in median OS. Thus, controlling for baseline characteristics demonstrated neither an advantage nor disadvantage in terms of long-term outcomes with the administration of pre-operative chemotherapy.

In 2013, Araujo et al. published another notable retrospective study based on their experience with 411 patients undergoing resection of CLM [20]. Once again, patients who received perioperative chemotherapy had generally less favorable disease as evidenced by higher clinical risk scores (CRS). CRS was established in 1999 as a strong marker for recurrence risk after resection of CLM and is determined by summing the presence of each of the following factors: a node-positive primary tumor, a disease-free interval from primary tumor to appearance of liver metastases under 12 months, more than one metastasis, pre-operative carcinoembryonic antigen (CEA) level above 200 ng/ml, and largest tumor size above 5 cm [21]. Scores of 2 or less are classified as low CRS while scores of 3 or greater are classified high CRS. Furthermore, a large number of patients in the adjuvant group received HAI, which is not routinely used at many institutions. Nonetheless, the authors detected no significant differences in the rates of post-operative complications, 3-year OS, or 5-year OS between patients who were treated with perioperative chemotherapy and those who received adjuvant therapy. Although a significantly higher rate of 3- and 5-year RFS among patients treated with adjuvant chemotherapy alone was found on univariate analysis, this was not observed once adjustments were made for clinicopathological and clinical risk scores (CRS).

Additional retrospective studies comparing outcomes between patients treated with and without neoadjuvant chemotherapy include investigations by Pawlik et al. Scoggins et al. Scartozzi et al. Spelt et al. and Zhu et al. [22–26]. Of these, all but one failed to detect major differences in post-operative morbidity and/or oncologic outcomes. Based on their analysis of 104 patients with CLM, Scartozzi et al. found a significantly longer median OS in those who did not receive neoadjuvant FOLFOX (48 months vs. 31 months, $p=0.0358$) [24]. However, patients treated with neoadjuvant chemotherapy more often had tumors larger than 5 cm and although CRS appeared similar in both groups, scores were only available in 69 % of patients. In addition, it was not clear if the neoadjuvant patients were also treated with adjuvant chemotherapy (i.e. a perioperative approach). Finally, data regarding surgical margins were not presented and could explain the poor survival among patients treated in the neoadjuvant setting, especially since the rate of recurrence was substantially higher in this group (75 % vs. 52.5 %, $p=0.0347$).

Additional Considerations

There are three additional considerations that are important in determining the optimal timing of chemotherapy in relation to hepatectomy for CLM. First, CLM may present in a synchronous or metachronous fashion. In synchronous cases, surgery may need to be prioritized if the primary colorectal cancer is symptomatic. In the face of life-threatening bleeding or perforation, the risks of delaying surgery for the administration of neoadjuvant chemotherapy are increased and should be avoided. Obstructing cancers can be treated surgically, but endoscopic stenting may theoretically allow symptom relief while reducing the time-delay to delivery of neoadjuvant chemotherapy. Although a combined colon and liver resection can be considered in stable symptomatic patients with easily resectable liver lesions, acutely ill patients should undergo the simplest operation that will treat the acute symptoms. In asymptomatic patients with synchronous disease, a decision must be made not only about the timing of chemotherapy but also about the timing of colorectal resection in relation to hepatectomy. There is evidence that the colorectal resection can be safely performed at the same time as the hepatectomy in well-selected patients [27, 28]. For CLM presenting in a metachronous manner, the presence of a long disease-free interval and an easily resectable solitary metastasis may support a decision to pursue upfront hepatectomy followed by adjuvant chemotherapy.

Second, although often grouped together in the discussion of CLM, colon cancer and rectal cancer have different treatment algorithms. The management of CLM in the setting of a rectal primary must account for local staging after assessment with endorectal ultrasound or pelvic magnetic resonance imaging. A patient with CLM in the setting of a locally advanced rectal cancer is an ideal candidate for upfront systemic chemotherapy, as the primary lesion will require neoadjuvant chemoradiation. A single- or two-stage resection may then be performed. In contrast, there is no clear role for neoadjuvant chemoradiation for primary colon cancers.

Third, the extent and anticipated morbidity of the planned hepatectomy must be considered. Criteria for resectability have changed significantly over time. Early in the surgical experience with CLM, bilobar disease was regarded as a contraindication to resection [4], but the current surgical paradigm classifies as resectable any patient with CLM that can be technically removed with negative margins and an adequate functional liver remnant [29]. Assessment of pre-operative liver function should include a history focusing on alcohol intake and risk factors for hepatitis along with liver enzymes, bilirubin, prothrombin time, and platelet levels. Percutaneous biopsy may be performed for confirmation of suspected chronic liver disease. Patients with pre-existing cirrhosis are poor candidates for resection of CLM. In general, upfront hepatectomy should be reserved for cases in which CLM can be completely resected with a minor liver resection and a low predicted risk of post-operative complications. When metastatic disease is technically resectable but requires a more extensive resection, portal vein embolization (PVE) of the lobe containing the bulk of the metastatic disease can be employed to encourage hypertrophy of the lobe that will remain after resection. Patients who require PVE are ideal candidates for neoadjuvant chemotherapy as hepatic regeneration occurs even as systematic cytotoxic agents are administered and complications do not appear to be increased [30]. However, in all patients receiving systemic therapy before surgery, the risk of post-operative liver failure after a major liver resection in the setting of potential chemotherapy-induced hepatotoxicity must be mitigated.

Recommendations Based on the Data

Given the limitations of the major relevant RCTs and retrospective studies, there is equipoise regarding the optimal timing of chemotherapy in relation to surgery for CLM. Nonetheless, a few general management recommendations can be made. First, in the absence of extrahepatic disease, patients with resectable colorectal liver metastases, if physiologically fit, should be treated with both resection and chemotherapy (evidence quality moderate; strong recommendation). Second, in patients who present with synchronous colorectal liver metastases and a symptomatic primary tumor requiring surgery, surgery should not be delayed for the administration of neoadjuvant chemotherapy (evidence quality low; weak recommendation). Third, in patients who present with synchronous colorectal liver metastases and an asymptomatic primary tumor, administration of neoadjuvant chemotherapy should be strongly considered by a multidisciplinary team prior to a one-stage or two-stage resection (evidence quality low; weak recommendation). Proceeding directly to hepatectomy with a plan for adjuvant therapy only may be reasonable when there is a solitary, small liver metastasis that can be safely resected at the time of the colectomy and there is low clinical suspicion of occult disease. Fourth, in patients who present with metachronous colorectal liver metastases, administration of neoadjuvant chemotherapy should be strongly considered by a multidisciplinary team prior to hepatectomy (evidence quality low; weak recommendation). Proceeding directly to hepatectomy with a plan for adjuvant therapy only may be reasonable when there is a solitary, small liver metastasis that can be safely resected with a low risk of complications, when the disease-free interval is greater than 12 months, and there is low suspicion for additional occult disease. Finally, in patients who present with synchronous colorectal liver metastases and a locally advanced primary rectal cancer, administration of neoadjuvant chemotherapy targeting the liver should be strongly considered in conjunction with neoadjuvant chemoradiation for the pelvis (evidence quality low; weak recommendation).

A Personal View of the Data

Advances in liver resection techniques and anti-cancer drugs over the past 20 years have greatly improved the ability to treat patients with CLM. Although there is insufficient evidence to make strong generalizable recommendations for the timing of chemotherapy in relation to hepatectomy in these patients, it is clear that a multidisciplinary approach should be pursued including medical oncologists, radiation oncologists when appropriate, and surgeons experienced in surgical oncology, colorectal surgery, and hepatobiliary surgery. Patients with CLM who have a high suspicion of aggressive or occult disease are likely the best candidates for neoadjuvant chemotherapy. Such suspicion should arise in the presence of a large tumor burden, a short disease-free interval, and a high CEA level. Patients with small, solitary CLM without suspicion of occult disease may be considered for an upfront surgical approach. Results of the NSABP C-11 trial are eagerly awaited, and further investigations into the timing of targeted therapy with respect to surgery are warranted as well.

> In the absence of extrahepatic disease, patients with resectable colorectal liver metastases, if physiologically fit, should be treated with both resection and chemotherapy. (evidence quality moderate; strong recommendation)

> In patients who present with synchronous colorectal liver metastases and a symptomatic primary tumor requiring surgery, surgery should not be delayed for the administration of neoadjuvant chemotherapy. (evidence quality low; weak recommendation)

> In patients who present with synchronous colorectal liver metastases and an asymptomatic primary tumor, administration of neoadjuvant chemotherapy should be strongly considered by a multidisciplinary team prior to a one-stage or two-stage resection. Upfront surgery may be considered when there is a solitary, small liver metastasis that can be safely resected at the time of the colectomy and there is low suspicion for occult disease. (evidence quality low; weak recommendation)

> In patients who present with metachronous colorectal liver metastases, administration of neoadjuvant chemotherapy should be strongly considered by a multidisciplinary team prior to hepatectomy. Upfront surgery may be considered when there is a solitary, small liver metastasis that can be safely resected with a low risk of complications, when the disease-free interval is greater than 12 months, and there is low suspicion for occult disease. (evidence quality low; weak recommendation)

> In patients who present with synchronous colorectal liver metastases and a locally advanced primary rectal cancer, administration of neoadjuvant chemotherapy targeting the liver should be strongly considered in conjunction with neoadjuvant chemoradiation for the pelvis. (evidence quality low; weak recommendation)

References

1. Dimick JB, Cowan Jr JA, Knol JA, Upchurch Jr GR. Hepatic resection in the United States: indications, outcomes, and hospital procedural volumes from a nationally representative database. Arch Surg. 2003;138(2):185–91.
2. Wilson SM, Adson MA. Surgical treatment of hepatic metastases from colorectal cancers. Arch Surg. 1976;111(4):330–4.
3. Kanas GP, Taylor A, Primrose JN, Langeberg WJ, Kelsh MA, Mowat FS, Alexander DD, Choti MA, Poston G. Survival after liver resection in metastatic colorectal cancer: review and meta-analysis of prognostic factors. Clin Epidemiol. 2012;4:283–301.
4. Nordlinger B, Quilichini MA, Parc R, Hannoun L, Delva E, Huguet C. Surgical resection of liver metastases from colo-rectal cancers. Int Surg. 1987;72(2):70–2.
5. Choti MA. Chemotherapy-associated hepatotoxicity: do we need to be concerned? Ann Surg Oncol. 2009;16(9):2391–4.
6. Benoist S, Brouquet A, Penna C, Julié C, El Hajjam M, Chagnon S, Mitry E, Rougier P, Nordlinger B. Complete response of colorectal liver metastases after chemotherapy: does it mean cure? J Clin Oncol. 2006;24(24):3939–45.
7. Tanaka K, Takakura H, Takeda K, Matsuo K, Nagano Y, Endo I. Importance of complete pathologic response to prehepatectomy chemotherapy in treating colorectal cancer metastases. Ann Surg. 2009;250(6):935–42.
8. Bischof DA, Clary BM, Maithel SK, Pawlik TM. Surgical management of disappearing colorectal liver metastases. Br J Surg. 2013;100(11):1414–20.
9. Adam R, Avisar E, Ariche A, Giachetti S, Azoulay D, Castaing D, Kunstlinger F, Levi F, Bismuth F. Five-year survival following hepatic resection after neoadjuvant therapy for nonresectable colorectal. Ann Surg Oncol. 2001;8(4):347–53.
10. Lordan JT, Karanjia ND. 'Close shave' in liver resection for colorectal liver metastases. Eur J Surg Oncol. 2010;36(1):47–51.
11. Wolf PS, Park JO, Bao F, Allen PJ, DeMatteo RP, Fong Y, Jarnagin WR, Kingham TP, Gönen M, Kemeny N, Shia J, D'Angelica MI. Preoperative chemotherapy and the risk of hepatotoxicity and morbidity after liver resection for metastatic colorectal cancer: a single institution experience. J Am Coll Surg. 2013;216(1):41–9.
12. Langer B, Bleiberg H, Labianca R, et al. Fluorouracil (FU) plus l-leucovorin (l-LV) versus observation after potentially curative resection of liver or lung metastases from colorectal cancer (CRC): results of the ENG (EORTC/NCIC CTG/GIVIO) randomized trial. Proc Am Soc Clin Oncol. 2002;21:149a (abstr 592).
13. Portier G, Elias D, Bouche O, et al. Multicenter randomized trial of adjuvant fluorouracil and folinic acid compared with surgery alone after resection of colorectal liver metastases. FFCD ACHBTH AURC 9002 trial. J Clin Oncol. 2006;24:4976–82.
14. Mitry E, Fields AL, Bleiberg H, et al. Adjuvant chemotherapy after potentially curative resection of metastases from colorectal cancer: a pooled analysis of two randomized trials. J Clin Oncol. 2008;26:4906–11.
15. Nordlinger B, Sorbye H, Glimelius B, Poston GJ, Schlag PM, Rougier P, Bechstein WO, Primrose JN, Walpole ET, Finch-Jones M, Jaeck D, Mirza D, Parks RW, Collette L, Praet M, Bethe U, Van Cutsem E, Scheithauer W, Gruenberger T, EORTC Gastro-Intestinal Tract Cancer Group; Cancer Research UK; Arbeitsgruppe Lebermetastasen und-tumoren in der Chirurgischen Arbeitsgemeinschaft Onkologie (ALM-CAO); Australasian Gastro-Intestinal Trials Group (AGITG); Fédération Francophone de Cancérologie Digestive (FFCD). Perioperative chemotherapy with FOLFOX4 and surgery versus surgery alone for resectable liver metastases from colorectal cancer (EORTC Intergroup trial 40983): a randomised controlled trial. Lancet. 2008;371(9617):1007–16.
16. Nordlinger B, Sorbye H, Glimelius B, Poston GJ, Schlag PM, Rougier P, Bechstein WO, Primrose JN, Walpole ET, Finch-Jones M, Jaeck D, Mirza D, Parks RW, Mauer M, Tanis E, Van Cutsem E, Scheithauer W, Gruenberger T, EORTC Gastro-Intestinal Tract Cancer Group;

Cancer Research UK; Arbeitsgruppe Lebermetastasen und–tumoren in der Chirurgischen Arbeitsgemeinschaft Onkologie (ALM-CAO); Australasian Gastro-Intestinal Trials Group (AGITG); Fédération Francophone de Cancérologie Digestive (FFCD). Perioperative FOLFOX4 chemotherapy and surgery versus surgery alone for resectable liver metastases from colorectal cancer (EORTC 40983): long-term results of a randomised, controlled, phase 3 trial. Lancet Oncol. 2013;14(12):1208–15.
17. Fong Y. Chemotherapy and resection for colorectal metastases. Lancet Oncol. 2013;14(12):1148–9.
18. Reddy SK, Zorzi D, Lum YW, Barbas AS, Pawlik TM, Ribero D, Abdalla EK, Choti MA, Kemp C, Vauthey JN, Morse MA, White RR, Clary BM. Timing of multimodality therapy for resectable synchronous colorectal liver metastases: a retrospective multi-institutional analysis. Ann Surg Oncol. 2009;16(7):1809–19.
19. Pinto Marques H, Barroso E, de Jong MC, Choti MA, Ribeiro V, Nobre AM, Carvalho C, Pawlik TM. Peri-operative chemotherapy for resectable colorectal liver metastasis: does timing of systemic therapy matter? J Surg Oncol. 2012;105(6):511–9.
20. Araujo R, Gonen M, Allen P, Blumgart L, DeMatteo R, Fong Y, Kemeny N, Jarnagin W, D'Angelica M. Comparison between perioperative and postoperative chemotherapy after potentially curative hepatic resection for metastatic colorectal cancer. Ann Surg Oncol. 2013;20(13):4312–21.
21. Fong Y, Fortner J, Sun RL, Brennan MF, Blumgart LH. Clinical score for predicting recurrence after hepatic resection for metastatic colorectal cancer: analysis of 1001 consecutive cases. Ann Surg. 1999;230(3):309–18; discussion 318–21.
22. Pawlik TM, Olino K, Gleisner AL, Torbenson M, Schulick R, Choti MA. Preoperative chemotherapy for colorectal liver metastases: impact on hepatic histology and postoperative outcome. J Gastrointest Surg. 2007;11(7):860–8.
23. Scoggins CR, Campbell ML, Landry CS, Slomiany BA, Woodall CE, McMasters KM, et al. Preoperative chemotherapy does not increase morbidity or mortality of hepatic resection for colorectal cancer metastases. Ann Surg Oncol. 2009;16(1):35–41.
24. Scartozzi M, Siquini W, Galizia E, Stortoni P, Marmorale C, Berardi R, Fianchini A, Cascinu S. The timing of surgery for resectable metachronous liver metastases from colorectal cancer: better sooner than later? A retrospective analysis. Dig Liver Dis. 2011;43(3):194–8.
25. Spelt L, Hermansson L, Tingstedt B, Andersson R. Influence of preoperative chemotherapy on the intraoperative and postoperative course of liver resection for colorectal cancer metastases. World J Surg. 2012;36(1):157–63.
26. Zhu D, Zhong Y, Wei Y, Ye L, Lin Q, Ren L, Ye Q, Liu T, Xu J, Qin X. Effect of neoadjuvant chemotherapy in patients with resectable colorectal liver metastases. PLoS One. 2014;9(1):e86543.
27. Martin 2nd RC, Augenstein V, Reuter NP, Scoggins CR, McMasters KM. Simultaneous versus staged resection for synchronous colorectal cancer liver metastases. J Am Coll Surg. 2009;208(5):842–50; discussion 850–2.
28. Abbott AM, Parsons HM, Tuttle TM, Jensen EH. Short-term outcomes after combined colon and liver resection for synchronous colon cancer liver metastases: a population study. Ann Surg Oncol. 2013;20(1):139–47.
29. Adams RB, Aloia TA, Loyer E, Pawlik TM, Taouli B, Vauthey JN, Americas Hepato-Pancreato-Biliary Association; Society of Surgical Oncology; Society for Surgery of the Alimentary Tract. Selection for hepatic resection of colorectal liver metastases: expert consensus statement. HPB (Oxf). 2013;15(2):91–103.
30. Covey AM, Brown KT, Jarnagin WR, Brody LA, Schwartz L, Tuorto S, Sofocleous CT, D'Angelica M, Getrajdman GI, DeMatteo R, Kemeny NE, Fong Y. Combined portal vein embolization and neoadjuvant chemotherapy as a treatment strategy for resectable hepatic colorectal metastases. Ann Surg. 2008;247(3):451–5.

Chapter 14
What Is the Best Way to Assess Hepatic Reserve Prior to Liver Resection in the Cirrhotic Patient?

Yilei Mao and Shunda Du

Abstract Postoperative liver failure still remains a major cause of mortality after partial hepatectomy, which results from an insufficient functional remnant liver. Therefore, the accurate evaluation of liver function is very important, particularly in cirrhotic patients who require hepatectomy. Traditional tests, such as serological indicators, Child-Pugh score, MELD score and ICG clearance test, are important in predicting and reducing the risks of hepatectomy. However, these tests only provide functional data on the entire liver, not on specific anatomic parts of the liver. Ideally, assessments of liver function should include both anatomical information and function of the whole and partial liver, providing reliable information for accurate evaluation of surgical risks. ^{99m}Tc-galactosyl serum albumin scintigraphy, can assess the liver function quantitatively. It combined with single photon emission computed tomography, CT and three-dimensional reconstruction, may be a better measure of liver function, especially of remnant liver function.

Keywords Hepatic reserve • Hepatectomy • Cirrhosis • Galactosyl serum albumin

Introduction

Liver resection is the accepted gold standard of treatment for liver tumors. Improvements in surgical methods and instruments have greatly reduced the perioperative mortality. However, the major cause of mortality after partial hepatectomy is liver failure, which results from an insufficient functional remnant liver mass [1]. Conversely, the erroneous results of liver function tests may mislead the surgeon to make a wrong decision such as precluding some patients with large liver tumors from undergoing surgery, even if surgery is beneficial. Therefore, the accurate

Y. Mao (✉) • S. Du
Department of Liver Surgery, Peking Union Medical College (PUMC) Hospital, 1# Shuai-Fu-Yuan, Wang-Fu-Jing, Beijing 100730, China
e-mail: yileimao@126.com; pumch-liver@hotmail.com

J.M. Millis, J.B. Matthews (eds.), *Difficult Decisions in Hepatobiliary and Pancreatic Surgery*, Difficult Decisions in Surgery: An Evidence-Based Approach, DOI 10.1007/978-3-319-27365-5_14

evaluation of liver function is very important, particularly in patients with damaged livers who require hepatectomy or liver transplantation [2].

Liver function includes the uptake, metabolism, conjugation and excretion. Among the methods used to evaluate liver function in practice are serological tests which are the earliest and most commonly used in determining whole liver function. Clinical scoring systems, such as Child-Pugh and model for end-stage liver disease (MELD) scores can roughly evaluate the risks of hepatectomy. The indocyanine green (ICG) clearance test is a widely used quantitative test of liver function in patients who scheduled for major hepatectomy. Although these tests can assess whole liver function, they cannot assess remnant liver function and predict the risk of liver failure post-operation. Computed tomography (CT) volumetry can provide anatomic information on remnant liver volume (RLV), but anatomic volume is not equal to functional volume, especially in patients with cirrhosis. In recent years, ^{99m}Tc-galactosyl serum albumin (^{99m}Tc-GSA) scintigraphy combined with single photon emission computed tomography (SPECT) and CT with three-dimensional imaging, is relatively accurate in measuring the whole and regional liver function. ^{99m}Tc-GSA scintigraphy may therefore be a promising method to plan surgical incisions and to predict operative risk. Based on a two-compartment kinetic model, a novel system was developed that provides 3D functional evaluation for any anatomical component of liver, and hepatectomy simulation with a freehand drawing tool. The result was showed by the parameter 'UI' which had high accuracy in predicting the risk of liver failure. In the future, many new methods will be established which can assess hepatic reserve accurately prior to liver resection in the cirrhotic patient.

Search Strategy

A literature search of English language publications since January, 2004 was used to identity published data on preoperative assessment of hepatic reserve in cirrhotic patients undergoing hepatectomy using the PICO outline (Table 14.1). Databases searched were PubMed, Embase, and Cochrane Evidence Based Medicine. Terms used in the search were "cirrhotic patients/cirrhosis", "liver resection/ hepatectomy", "liver function/hepatic reserve/Child-Pugh Score/indocyanine green clearance test (ICG)/model for end-stage liver disease (MELD) score/ Monoethylglycinexylidide (MEGX) test/galactose elimination capacity Test/computed tomography volumetry/galactosyl serum albumin (GSA)/transient elastography (TE)", "postoperative complications/postoperative hepatic failure/ascites/ hyperbilirubinemia /prolongedprothrombin time/length of stay/mortality/morbidity/ quality of life", and "preoperative/prior to liver resection". Eleven cohort studies, two systematic reviews and one meta-analysis, and four review articles were included in our analysis (Table 14.2). The other perspective cohort study [3] was enrolled about GSA which was accepted by the Annals of Surgical Oncology. The data was classified using the GRADE system.

Table 14.1 PICO table for perioperative assessment of hepatic reserve in the cirrhotic patient

P (Patients)	I (Intervention)	C (Comparator group)	O (Outcomes measured)
Cirrhotic patient undergoing liver resection	Novel preoperative liver function test, such as: indocyanine green(ICG) clearance test, model for end-stage liver disease (MELD) score, transient elastography, ^{99m}Tc-galactosyl serum albumin scintigraphy, *etc*	Classical preoperative liver function test, such as: Child-Pugh score, model for end-stage liver disease (MELD) score, indocyanine green(ICG)clearance test, computed tomography (CT) volumetry, *etc*	Postoperative complications, mortality

Results

Liver function includes the uptake, metabolism, conjugation and excretion. The serological tests are the earliest and most commonly used and still play important role. But any one serological indicator can show only one aspect not comprehensive function, and whole liver function not local. So different clinical scoring systems and metabolic quantitative liver function tests were developed to assess hepatic reserve.

The Child-Pugh Scoring System

The Child scoring system, first proposed in 1964, was originally developed to predict the outcome of cirrhotic patients undergoing surgical therapy for portal hypertension. This system was modified by Pugh et al. [4] in 1973, and called the Child-Pugh score. It includes total plasma bilirubin level, plasma albumin level, and prothrombin time together with the presence or absence of encephalopathy and ascites. Of all the tools for assessing liver function, the Child-Pugh system is simple but very useful [5]. It is widely used in hepatocellular carcinoma and cirrhosis patients, who will undergo resection or transplantation. Thus Child-Pugh is more relevant for liver resections, compared with MELD score system. A classification of grade A of the Child-Pugh grading system is a typical indication for liver resection. And liver transplantation is selected if oncological indications meets the established criteria [6]. Schneider showed that, for patients classified Child-Pugh A, the mortality is minimal at <5 % while for grade B cirrhotics the 1-year liver failure-related morality is almost 20 %, and for grade C cirrhosis is 55 %[7].

However, the Child-Pugh grading system only provides a rough evaluation for global liver function reserve, so more quantitative liver function tests may need for preoperative assessment.

Table 14.2 Incidence of different liver function assessments and clinical outcomes

Author (year)	N	Age	Child-Pugh score	MELD score	$ICGR_{15}$	TE (kPa)	GSA	LOS (d)	Ascites	Postoperative LF	Mortality	Study type (quality of evidence)
Matteo (2012)	90	64	A:90 % Other: 10 %	8.3	NR	16.2	NR	9	20 %	28.9 %	2.2 %	Prospective cohort (low)
Jeff (2013)	105	59	5	NR	4.2 %	9.4	NR	NR	NR	NR	1.9 %	Prospective cohort (low)
Scheingraber (2008)	95	60	NR	NR	ICG-PDR was used	NR	NR	NR	NR	24.2 %	3.2 %	Prospective cohort (low)
Ohwada (2006)	75	63	A: 96 % B: 4 %	NR	ICG-*k* and $ICGR_{15}$	NR	NR	NR	NR	11 %	1 %	Prospective cohort (low)
James (2013)	28	59	A: 96.4 % B: 3.6 %	7.2	11.8 %	10.2	NR	6	4/28	NR	/	Prospective cohort (low)
Hirohisa (2014)	548	66	NR	NR	12.5 %	NR	LHL15: 0.92	NR	NR	NR	0.89 %	Prospective cohort (low)
Cucchetti (2006)	200	64	5	8.8	NR	NR	NR	NR	5 %	7.5 %	NR	Prospective cohort (low)
Cescon (2009)	466	64	5.4	8.9	NR	NR	NR	NR	4.9 %	4.9 %	NR	Prospective cohort (low)
Kwon (2006)	178	62	A: 73 % B: 27 %	NR	GSA-Rmax and ICGR15 values correlate well	NR	GSA-RL	NR	13.5 %	NR	1.12	Retrospective cohort (low)
Kaibori (2008)	191	66.5	A: 86.4 % B: 13.6 %	NR	≥18.0 %: 9.7 %	NR	HA/ GSA-Rmax ratio	NR	NR	8.38 %	1.57 %	Prospective cohort (low)
Mao (2014)	142	53.3	A: 76.1 % B: 21.1 % C: 2.8 %	NR	Negative associate with UI	NR	UI	NR	UI can distinguish	UI can predict	NR	Prospective cohort (low)

MELD model for end-stage liver disease, *TE* transient elastography, *GSA* ^{99m}Tc-galactosyl serum albumin scintigraphy, *LOS* length of stay, *NR* not reported, *LHL* the ratio of uptake by the liver to that by the liver and the heart at 15 min in GSA, *LF*liver failure

The Model for End-Stage Liver Disease (MELD) Score

The limitations of the Child-Pugh score led to the development of MELD. MELD score was originally developed to evaluate the survival rate of patients undergoing transjugular intrahepatic portosystemic shunt procedures, and was thereafter modified to evaluate patients with liver disease undergoing surgery. MELD score is a constellation of serum bilirubin, creatinine concentration, INR and etiology of liver disease, and is calculated using the formula: 11.2 × Ln(INR) + 9.57 × Ln[creatinine(mg/dL)] + 3.78 × Ln [bilirubin(mg/dL)] + 6.43 × (etiology: 0 if cholestatic or alcoholic, 1 otherwise), with the score rounded to the nearest integer [8].

The MELD score is used to allocate organs for liver transplantation [9, 10]. The application of this system to determine organ allocation reduced 15 % of the mortality rate in liver transplant candidates [11]. Cholangitas et al. [9] stated that MELD score was shown to be useful for the prediction of long-term survival in patients with cirrhosis. Ascites, jaundice, prolonged prothrombin time, increase of serum creatinine and bilirubin levels, and decrease of albumin serum level are typical markers of impaired liver function. Cucchetti et al. has showed that MELD score can be used to predict the development of post-operative liver failure after hepatectomy for patients with cirrhosis undergoing resection of hepatocellular carcinoma, with a pre-operative score of ≥11 being associated with a poor outcome [12].

In subsequent clinical applications, outcomes were different in patients with the same score and different serum concentrations of sodium. So some modified MELD formulas that have been proposed to predict the prognosis of liver disease, such as MELD-Na score, integrated MELD (iMELD), MELD to sodium (MESO), United Kingdom end-stage liver disease (UKELD), etc. However, they cannot accurately predict the actual survival time of patients undergoing hepatectomy. At present, they are mainly used to assess the severity and prognosis of chronic liver diseases, and to evaluate the patients awaiting liver transplantation [13].

Computed Tomography (CT) Volumetry

At present, CT volumetry is the most often used imaging method to determine whether hepatectomy can be performed safely. Pre-operative estimations have been shown to correlate well with actual volumes resected. But the safety limit for the remnant liver volume in patients with normal liver remains controversial. Kubota et al. found that resections of 60 % of non-tumorous liver was possible in patients with normal livers [14]. Shoup et al. stated that a liver resection can be safely performed if the functional remnant liver volume(RLV) is larger than 25–30 % when using computed tomography volumetry [15, 16]. If the patients have underlying liver disease, then a margin of 40 % is taken into account [17]. Several studies found that in the presence of cirrhosis, a resection of >2 segments should only be performed of the estimated remnant functional liver was >40 %, while if it's <40 %, a pre-resection portal vein embolization (PVE) should be advised [18, 19].

However, if the patient has a compromised liver, then the liver volume does not truly reflect liver function [20]. CT volumetry is used for preoperative calculations of the volume of resected livers, but does not demonstrate the effects of diseased liver parenchyma on liver function. The evaluation of liver function before liver surgery is dependent on the combination of the results of CT volumetry with those of other liver function tests.

Transient Elastography

Recently, noninvasive measurements to assess the degree of liver fibrosis and cirrhosis before operation, like transient elastography, acoustic radiation force impulse imaging and magnetic resonance elastography, have been developed. The clinical studies are ongoing to validate the strength and the power of these novel approaches [21].

Transient elastography (TE) measured by FibroScan is a rapid, non-invasive, and reproducible method for measuring liver stiffness that is increasingly explored to assess liver fibrosis. It measures the velocity of a low-frequency (50 Hz) elastic shear wave propagating through the liver. This velocity is directly related to tissue stiffness, called the elastic modulus. The stiffer the tissue, the faster the shear wave propagates. TE measures liver stiffness in a volume that approximates a cylinder that is 1-cm wide and 4-cm long, 25–65 mm below skin surface. The results are expressed in kilopascals (kPa) and range from 2.5 to 75 kPa; a normal value is around 5 kPa [22].

Several advantages of TE have been reported, such as low invasiveness, a short procedure time (5 min), fast acquisition of results, and portability that enables testing at the bedside and in outpatient departments [50]. Although unreliable and unrepeatable measurements caused by host obesity, anatomical difficulties such as a narrow intercostal space, and inadequate operator experience have also been reported, the overall diagnostic accuracy for advanced liver fibrosis and early cirrhosis is up to 90 % in various liver diseases including chronic viral hepatitis and nonalcoholic fatty disease [23].

To evaluate the efficacy of preoperative assessment of liver fibrosis and cirrhosis using TE in predicting post-hepatectomy outcomes, several clinical studies has been carried out. In a prospective cohort [24], 90 patients undergoing hepatectomy for HCC were prospectively evaluated with FibroScan. Postoperative liver failure (PLF) occurred in 28.9 % of patients and receiver operating curves (ROC) analysis identified patients with liver stiffness value higher than or equal to 15.7 kPa as being at higher risk of PLF, while patients with liver stiffness value lower than 14.8 kPa had no PLF. Multivariate analysis showed that along with low preoperative serum sodium levels ($P=0.012$), histological cirrhosis ($P=0.024$), elevated liver stiffness ($P=0.005$) was an independent predictors of PLF. In a larger prospective cohort [25], 105 with a mean age of 59 years were included with both ICG retention rate at 15 min and TE were prospectively carried out. Using the calculated cutoff at 12.0 kPa, liver stiffness measurement was shown to have sensitivity of 85.7 % and specificity of 71.8 % in the prediction of major postoperative complications. On ROC, only liver stiffness measurement but not ICG showed significant correlation with major postoperative complications.

The Indocyanine Green (ICG) Clearance Test

ICG is a highly protein-bound, water-soluble, tricarbocyanine dye that bounds in plasma to albumin and β-lipoproteins and distributes uniformly in the blood within a few minutes after injection. It is selectively taken up by hepatocytes with a plasma extraction of 70–90 % and is excreted unchanged in the bile via a carrier-mediated mechanism. Therefore, it reflects several liver functions, including the blood flow-dependent clearance and transporter functions [26]. The standard procedure involves a bolus injection of 0.5 mg/kg of ICG following an overnight fast, and blood samples are collected at 5-min intervals for 20 min. ICG concentrations are measured using a spectrophotometer. The ICG clearance test can also be automatically calculated under a dye densito-graph (DDG) analyzer using an optical sensor placed on the finger pulse [27]. The machine expands the application of ICG clearance test in current clinical situation.

The results of ICG clearance test can be expressed in several ways, including the plasma disappearance rate (ICG-PDR), the ICG elimination rate constant (ICG-k) and the $ICGR_{15}$ which describes the percentage of circulatory retention of indocyanine green during the first 15 min after bolus injection [28]. In order to prospectively determine the efficacy of ICG-PDR in the clinical course, 95 patients undergoing liver resection were included in a cohort [29], with ICG-PDR, bilirubin and prothrombin time selected and prospectively measured. After hepatectomy, 3 patients died due to liver failure and 21 patients developed signs of liver dysfunction. ROC analysis revealed that ICG-PDR did significantly better indicate postoperative liver dysfunctions. Of date, pulse spectrophotometry was developed to noninvasively measure the ICG-k and a prospective clinical study was done [30]. Seventy five patients who underwent anatomical liver resection for hepatocellular carcinoma were enrolled and ICG-k was measured instantaneously using pulse spectrophotometry before surgery, during inflow occlusion and after hepatectomy. Eight patients suffered liver failure with one died in hospital. In a logistic regression model, the estimated remnant ICG-k was a significant predictor of postoperative liver failure and real-time monitoring of ICG-k was shown to be helpful for evaluating the remnant liver functional reserve before, during and after hepatectomy.

$ICGR_{15}$, as the most commonly determined value, has been extensively investigated in various kinds of clinical setting and incorporated into a number of test combinations or score systems. A decision tree for deciding the safe limit of hepatectomy was developed [31] basing on three variables: whether ascites is present, the serum total bilirubin level, and the $ICGR_{15}$. With strict application of this decision tree to 1,429 consecutive hepatectomy in 10 years, only one patient death was encountered. So $ICGR_{15}>15$ % is a high risk factor for serious post-hepatectomy complications [32], although a cutoff of 14 % has been suggested by Lau et al. [33]. $ICGR_{15}$, along with TE, was performed preoperatively in 44 patients with hepatocellular carcinoma [34]. $ICGR_{15}$ was found to correlate well with preoperative factors and postoperative outcome (peak AST level). A classification system for liver function using $ICGR_{15}$ and the ratio of uptake by the liver to that by the liver and heart at 15 min (LHL15) in ^{99m}Tc-galactosyl human serum albumin scintigraphy for hepatic resection, was created [35]. A total of 548 consecutive patients who underwent hepatectomy were enrolled in a prospective study to validate the ranking system and the result confirmed the usefulness of this system in predicting the safety of hepatic resection.

^{99m}Tc-Galactosyl Serum Albumin Scintigraphy

Molecular nuclear imaging techniques have developed these years. Some new agents, such as ^{99m}Tc-galactosyl serum albumin scintigraphy (GSA) and ^{99m}Tc-mebrofenin hepatobiliary scintigraphy, can measure both total and future remnant liver function and potentially identify patients at risk for postresectional liver failure.

GSA is an analogue of asialoglycoprotein, which binds to asialoglycoprotein receptors (ASGPR) on hepatocyte membranes, followed by receptor-mediated endocytosis. ASGPR density is closely related to hepatocyte function [36, 37]. The level of expression of receptor is significantly related to liver function and lower in diseased livers such as chronic hepatitis, cirrhosis and HCC [3]. Radio labeled ASGPR was developed originally by Vera et al. [38].^{99m}Tc-GSA is very stable and only distributes in the blood and liver after intravenous injection [36]. The liver is the only uptake site for ^{99m}Tc-GSA, making ^{99m}Tc-GSA an ideal agent for predicting hepatocyte mass and function by monitoring the functional status and distribution of ASGPR [39, 40].

After liver uptake, ^{99m}Tc-GSA remains trapped in the liver for at least 30 min, and there is practically no biliary excretion. Thus, SPECT can assess both liver function and functional volume at the same time [41]. The ^{99m}Tc-GSA liver uptake ratio (LHL15) and blood clearance ratio (HH15) are quantitative indices frequently used in planar dynamic ^{99m}Tc-GSA scintigraphy. LHL15 defined as 15 min after bullet injection of ^{99m}Tc-GSA and calculated by dividing the radioactivity in regions of interest (ROIs) of the liver by the radioactivity in the liver and heart, it represents the number of hepatocytes. HH15 is calculated by dividing the radioactivity in ROIs of the heart 15 min by the radioactivity 3 min after injection of ^{99m}Tc-GSA, it represents the rate of blood clearance [42]. Harada and his colleagues recently developed a simple software program to automatically calculate the pixel counts of the area between the hepatic curve and heart curve from 3 to 15 min [43]. Both LHL15 and HH15 reflect the liver function and the severity of liver disease [44]. For LHL15 and HH 15 measures preoperative total liver function, not the function of the remnant liver, postoperative liver failure has been observed in patients with normal LHL15 values [45].

LHL15 and HH15 are readily calculated from the radioactivity in the heart and liver ROIs, it may not reflect the actual liver function. So some complex and perfect compartmental models of ^{99m}Tc-GSA kinetics are developed for the assessment of liver function ([46] #174, [47] #30, [48] #149).

Many different parameters can be calculated from different kinetic models for the quantitative evaluation of liver function. The liver blood flow and maximal asialoglycoprotein receptor binding rate assessed by ^{99m}Tc-GSA are significantly correlated with other quantitative measures of liver function [48]. Total ASGPR amount are proportional to the number of viable hepatocytes and the correlation of total ASGPR amount with hepatocyte number was significantly higher than the correlation of ICG-k with total hepatocyte number [53].

Kwon etc. reported previously that the maximal removal rate of GSA(GSA-Rmax) values correlated well with the results from the transferrin, prealbumin, retinol binding protein, fibrinogen, prothrombin time, hepaplastin test, antithrombin III, and ICG tests [49]. In another retrospective study [50], this team reviewed 178 patients for elective hepatectomy. Preoperative estimation of the GSA-Rmax in the predicted remnant liver (GSA-RL) is used a parameter. In this study, seven patients postoperative hyperbilirubinemia were recorded with GSA-RL <0.15 mg/min. Two patients died of postoperative liver failure 1–2 months after surgery, the GSA-RL values were 0.078 and 0.090, respectively. They considered a margin of safety (0.05) and determined 0.15 as the cutoff value. Preoperative percutaneous transhepatic portal embolization should be performed for cases with a GSA-RL less than 0.15 to avoid postoperative hyperbilirubinemia or hepatic failure.

In another study, this team [51] followed 191 patients more than 1 year after hepatectomy with 16 patients suffered from liver failure and 3 of them died. Total 35 clinicopathologic factors were performed to identify independent predictors of postoperative liver failure after resection of HCC by univariate and multivariate analyses. In univariate analyse, elder, a lower serum albumin level, lower cholinesterase level, longer prothrombin time, lower platelet count, and lower GSA-Rmax, higher values of ICGR15, total bilirubin, AST, type IV collagen 7S, hyaluronate (HA), AFP, type IV collagen 7S/GSA-Rmax ratio, and HA/GSA-Rmax ratio, are the factors easy to the postoperative liver failure. Patients in the liver failure group had significantly more intraoperative blood loss and a longer postoperative hospital stay. Multivariate logistic regression analysis showed that HA/GSA-Rmax ratio ≥500 mg min/dl (OR 23.60; 95 % confidence interval (CI) 1.91–62.09; P=0.0138) was the only independent predictor of postoperative liver failure. An increase of the HA/GSA-Rmax ratio was associated with more severe liver dysfunction. The HA/GSA-Rmax ratio was also positively correlated with various conventional liver function tests, such as the $ICGR_{15}$, AST, total bilirubin, platelet count, albumin, cholinesterase, prothrombin time, type IV collagen 7S, HA and GSA-Rmax, etc. They conclude that the HA/GSA-Rmax ratio can predict postoperative liver failure, and a ratio ≥500 mg min/dl is a relative contraindication to liver resection with a sensitivity of 88 % and a specificity of 92 %, and its negative predictive rate was 99 %.

Recently, Mao and Du [52, 53] set up a computerized image system based on a two-compartment model, which could provide liver images, a freehand drawing tool for hepatectomy simulation, assess liver function and predict postoperative remnant liver function, using uptake index (UI) as a parameter. That study [54] recruited 71 pre-hepatectomy patients and 71 healthy volunteers. They found that median UI = 2.81 was the normal reference, lower UI values were associated with the more impaired liver functions. ROC analysis indicated that lower UI values could be used to predict the presence of ascites with high accuracy (AUC = 0.88, $P < 0.0001$). Preoperative UI values were also able to distinguish patients with and without elevated bilirubin (AUC = 0.86, $P < 0.0001$). Preoperative UI was also negatively associated with $ICGR_{15}$ values, i.e., the lower UI value was, the larger $ICGR_{15}$ value would be($r = -0.92$, $P < 0.0001$).

In this system, for each simulated liver resection plan, the corresponding anatomic and functional remnant liver volume, and the risk of postoperative liver failure were presented. There 33 patients had both preoperative and postoperative measures of UI values for the remnant liver via the system. Regression analysis using predicted UI as an explanatory variable showed a linear equation as: Post Surgery UI = −0.09 + 1.04(Predicted UI). It supported the accuracy of the preoperative prediction. To further evaluate the reliability of predicted UI values for the future remnant liver (FRL), predicted UIs were further compared with the parameters of the actual post operative liver functions tests. The results demonstrated that predicted UI negatively correlated with PT and total bilirubin level (Pearson's correlation coefficient $r = -0.67$ and −0.68 respectively, $P < 0.0001$). The AUC for predicted UI to distinguish patients with and without postoperative ascites was at 0.85, $P < 0.0001$. While Child score of 9 or larger was defined as high risk of liver failure, the ROC analysis results indicated that UI values had a high accuracy in predicting the risk of liver failure (AUC = 0.95, $P < 0.0001$). The threshold for very high risk was defined as $P = 0.05$ which corresponds to UI of 0.73 (FLVI = 26 %). In fact, there are some weak points in this study. Without Child C patients enrolled in the study might lead to conservative decision making rule. The small sample size also might affect the accuracy of the threshold to define the high risk region. Further improving the accuracy and validating the system in phase III clinical trial is needed before bring it to clinical practice.

Recommendations Based on the Data

The clinical methods to evaluate liver function including serological tests, various evaluation scoring systems, ICG clearance, 3D-CT volumetric calculation are all useful in clinical practice. They all have advantages and disadvantages, and cannot be replaced, currently.

The preoperative liver function evaluation must be a comprehensive process. In order to make a safe and thorough evaluation, multiple indices, as well as general condition of the patient, type of planned surgery, and proficiency of surgeons should be considered and combined. The maturation and application of new GSA based three-dimension imaging system may bring a new promising tool for the preoperative liver function evaluation.

References

1. Fujii Y, et al. Risk factors of posthepatectomy liver failure after portal vein embolization. J Hepatobiliary Pancreatol Surg. 2003;10(3):226–32.
2. Clavien PA, et al. Strategies for safer liver surgery and partial liver transplantation. N Engl J Med. 2007;356(15):1545–59.
3. Mao YL, et al. Application of technetium galactosyl human serum albumin diethylenetriamine pentaacetic acid injection on liver imaging in mouse models with different hepatic injuries. Zhongguo Yi Xue Ke Xue Yuan Xue Bao. 2008;30(4):404–8.
4. Pugh RN, et al. Transection of the oesophagus for bleeding oesophageal varices. Br J Surg. 1973;60(8):646–9.
5. Poon RT, Fan ST. Assessment of hepatic reserve for indication of hepatic resection: how I do it. J Hepatobiliary Pancreatol Surg. 2005;12(1):31–7.
6. Mizuguchi T, et al. Preoperative liver function assessments to estimate the prognosis and safety of liver resections. Surg Today. 2014;44(1):1–10.
7. Schneider PD. Preoperative assessment of liver function. Surg Clin N Am. 2004;84(2):355–73.
8. Malinchoc M, et al. A model to predict poor survival in patients undergoing transjugular intrahepatic portosystemic shunts. Hepatology. 2000;31(4):864–71.
9. Cholongitas E, et al. A systematic review of the performance of the model for end-stage liver disease (MELD) in the setting of liver transplantation. Liver Transpl. 2006;12(7):1049–61.
10. Huo TI, Lee SD, Lin HC. Selecting an optimal prognostic system for liver cirrhosis: the model for end-stage liver disease and beyond. Liver Int. 2008;28(5):606–13.
11. Dutkowski P, et al. The model for end-stage liver disease allocation system for liver transplantation saves lives, but increases morbidity and cost: a prospective outcome analysis. Liver Transpl. 2011;17(6):674–84.
12. Cucchetti A, et al. Impact of model for end-stage liver disease (MELD) score on prognosis after hepatectomy for hepatocellular carcinoma on cirrhosis. Liver Transpl. 2006;12(6):966–71.
13. Abradelo M, Jimenez C. Splitting liver grafts for two adults: suboptimal grafts or suboptimal matching? Hepatobiliary Surg Nutr. 2013;2(5):242–3.
14. Kubota K, et al. Measurement of liver volume and hepatic functional reserve as a guide to decision-making in resectional surgery for hepatic tumors. Hepatology. 1997;26(5):1176–81.
15. Shoup M, et al. Volumetric analysis predicts hepatic dysfunction in patients undergoing major liver resection. J Gastrointest Surg. 2003;7(3):325–30.
16. Vauthey JN, et al. Standardized measurement of the future liver remnant prior to extended liver resection: methodology and clinical associations. Surgery. 2000;127(5):512–9.
17. Clavien PA, et al. Protection of the liver during hepatic surgery. J Gastrointest Surg. 2004;8(3):313–27.
18. Azoulay D, et al. Percutaneous portal vein embolization increases the feasibility and safety of major liver resection for hepatocellular carcinoma in injured liver. Ann Surg. 2000;232(5):665–72.
19. Hemming AW, et al. Preoperative portal vein embolization for extended hepatectomy. Ann Surg. 2003;237(5):686–91; discussion 691–3.
20. de Graaf W, et al. Assessment of future remnant liver function using hepatobiliary scintigraphy in patients undergoing major liver resection. J Gastrointest Surg. 2010;14(2):369–78.
21. Castera L, et al. Biopsy and non-invasive methods for the diagnosis of liver fibrosis: does it take two to tango? Gut. 2010;59(7):861–6.
22. Sandrin L, et al. Transient elastography: a new noninvasive method for assessment of hepatic fibrosis. Ultrasound Med Biol. 2003;29(12):1705–13.
23. Tsochatzis EA, et al. Elastography for the diagnosis of severity of fibrosis in chronic liver disease: a meta-analysis of diagnostic accuracy. J Hepatol. 2011;54(4):650–9.

24. Cescon M, et al. Value of transient elastography measured with FibroScan in predicting the outcome of hepatic resection for hepatocellular carcinoma. Ann Surg. 2012;256(5):706–12; discussion 712–3.
25. Wong JS, et al. Liver stiffness measurement by transient elastography as a predictor on posthepatectomy outcomes. Ann Surg. 2013;257(5):922–8.
26. Morris-Stiff G, et al. Quantitative assessment of hepatic function and its relevance to the liver surgeon. J Gastrointest Surg. 2009;13(2):374–85.
27. Akita H, et al. Real-time intraoperative assessment of residual liver functional reserve using pulse dye densitometry. World J Surg. 2008;32(12):2668–74.
28. Sakka SG. Assessing liver function. Curr Opin Crit Care. 2007;13(2):207–14.
29. Scheingraber S, et al. Indocyanine green disappearance rate is the most useful marker for liver resection. Hepatogastroenterology. 2008;55(85):1394–9.
30. Ohwada S, et al. Perioperative real-time monitoring of indocyanine green clearance by pulse spectrophotometry predicts remnant liver functional reserve in resection of hepatocellular carcinoma. Br J Surg. 2006;93(3):339–46.
31. Imamura H, et al. Assessment of hepatic reserve for indication of hepatic resection: decision tree incorporating indocyanine green test. J Hepatobiliary Pancreatol Surg. 2005;12(1):16–22.
32. Das BC, Isaji S, Kawarada Y. Analysis of 100 consecutive hepatectomies: risk factors in patients with liver cirrhosis or obstructive jaundice. World J Surg. 2001;25(3):266–72; discussion 272–3.
33. Lau H, et al. Evaluation of preoperative hepatic function in patients with hepatocellular carcinoma undergoing hepatectomy. Br J Surg. 1997;84(9):1255–9.
34. Fung J, et al. Use of liver stiffness measurement for liver resection surgery: correlation with indocyanine green clearance testing and post-operative outcome. PLoS ONE. 2013;8(8), e72306.
35. Okabe H, et al. Rank classification based on the combination of indocyanine green retention rate at 15 min and (99 m)Tc-DTPA-galactosyl human serum albumin scintigraphy predicts the safety of hepatic resection. Nucl Med Commun. 2014;35(5):478–83.
36. Kudo M, et al. Functional hepatic imaging with receptor-binding radiopharmaceutical: clinical potential as a measure of functioning hepatocyte mass. Gastroenterol Jpn. 1991;26(6):734–41.
37. Shuke N, et al. Estimation of fractional liver uptake and blood retention of 99mTc-DTPA-galactosyl human serum albumin: an application of a simple graphical method to dynamic SPECT. Nucl Med Commun. 2003;24(5):503–11.
38. Vera DR, Stadalnik RC, Krohn KA. Technetium-99 m galactosyl-neoglycoalbumin: preparation and preclinical studies. J Nucl Med. 1985;26(10):1157–67.
39. Kokudo N, et al. Predictors of successful hepatic resection: prognostic usefulness of hepatic asialoglycoprotein receptor analysis. World J Surg. 2002;26(11):1342–7.
40. Kaibori M, et al. Usefulness of Tc-99 m-GSA scintigraphy for liver surgery. Ann Nucl Med. 2011;25(9):593–602.
41. Kudo M, et al. Synthesis and radiolabeling of galactosyl human serum albumin. Methods Enzymol. 1994;247:383–94.
42. Kwon AH, et al. Use of technetium 99 m diethylenetriamine-pentaacetic acid-galactosyl-human serum albumin liver scintigraphy in the evaluation of preoperative and postoperative hepatic functional reserve for hepatectomy. Surgery. 1995;117(4):429–34.
43. Harada K, et al. Area between the hepatic and heart curves of (99 m)Tc-galactosyl-human serum albumin scintigraphy represents liver function and disease progression for preoperative evaluation in hepatocellular carcinoma patients. J Hepatobiliary Pancreatol Sci. 2012;19(6):667–73.
44. Wu J, et al. The functional hepatic volume assessed by 99mTc-GSA hepatic scintigraphy. Ann Nucl Med. 1995;9(4):229–35.

45. Nanashima A, et al. Relationship between indocyanine green test and technetium-99 m galactosyl serum albumin scintigraphy in patients scheduled for hepatectomy: clinical evaluation and patient outcome. Hepatol Res. 2004;28(4):184–90.
46. Miki K, et al. Asialoglycoprotein receptor and hepatic blood flow using technetium-99m-DTPA-galactosylhuman serum albumin. J Nucl Med. 1997;38(11):1798–807.
47. Miki K, et al. Receptor measurements via Tc-GSA kinetic modeling are proportional to functional hepatocellular mass. J Nucl Med. 2001;42(5):733–7.
48. Ha-Kawa SK, et al. Compartmental analysis of asialoglycoprotein receptor scintigraphy for quantitative measurement of liver function: a multicentre study. Eur J Nucl Med. 1997;24(2):130–7.
49. Kwon AH, et al. Preoperative determination of the surgical procedure for hepatectomy using technetium-99mgalactosyl human serum albumin (99mTc-GSA) liver scintigraphy. Hepatology. 1997;25(2):426–9.
50. Kwon AH, et al. Preoperative regional maximal removal rate of technetium-99 m-galactosyl human serum albumin (GSA-Rmax) is useful for judging the safety of hepatic resection. Surgery. 2006;140(3):379–86.
51. Kaibori M, et al. HA/GSA-Rmax ratio as a predictor of postoperative liver failure. World J Surg. 2008;32(11):2410–8.
52. Du S, et al. A novel liver function evaluation system using radiopharmacokinetic modeling of technetium-99 m-DTPA-galactosyl human serum albumin. Nucl Med Commun. 2013;34(9):893–9.
53. Ge PL, Du SD, Mao YL. Advances in preoperative assessment of liver function. Hepatobiliary Pancreat Dis Int. 2014;13(4):361–70.
54. Mao Y, et al. Using dynamic 99mT c-GSA SPECT/CT fusion images for hepatectomy planning and postoperative liver failure prediction. Ann Surg Oncol. 2015;22(4):1301–7.

Chapter 15
Treatment Protocols for Small Hepatocellular Carcinoma (≤3 cm): RFA or Resection?

Yudong Qiu and Yilei Mao

Abstract Treatment selection for small hepatocellular carcinoma remains controversial. Although there are various studies showed different prognostic results in patients with small HCC by resection compared with RFA or LT, some other important factors, not only the tumor size, which may correlate with prognosis are still lack especially for gross classification. The identification of gross classification is crucial for the discrimination of small HCC and may play a great role for the final decision. Our results showed that not all the patients with small HCC are applicable for RFA treatment, so as to say, resection may be more beneficial for patients with the nonboundary type of small HCC.

Keywords Small hepatocellular carcinoma • RFA • Hepatic resection • Gross classification

Introduction

Hepatocellular carcinoma (HCC) is a major health problem worldwide and a prevalent tumor type in mainland China [1]. Progresses in diagnostic imaging have allowed detection of HCC at an early stage which can be curable by multiple treatment protocols. According to BCLC staging system, patients with very early or early-stage HCC should be considered for resection, ablation or transplantation [2, 3]. Also, the use of Milan Criteria to select patients for liver transplantation (LT) leads to good results for a solitary HCC up to 5 cm or for multiple HCC up to 3 in number and up to 3 cm for each tumor [4, 5]. In 2014, a new staging system called

Y. Qiu
Department of Hepatobiliary and Pancreas Surgery, Drum Tower Hospital, Medical School of Nanjing University, Nanjing, China

Y. Mao (✉)
Department of Liver Surgery, Peking Union Medical College Hospital, Peking Union Medical College & Chinese Academy of Medical Sciences,
1# Shuai-Fu-Yuan, Wang-Fu-Jing, Beijing 100730, China
e-mail: yileimao@126.com; pumch-liver@hotmail.com

J.M. Millis, J.B. Matthews (eds.), *Difficult Decisions in Hepatobiliary and Pancreatic Surgery*, Difficult Decisions in Surgery: An Evidence-Based Approach, DOI 10.1007/978-3-319-27365-5_15

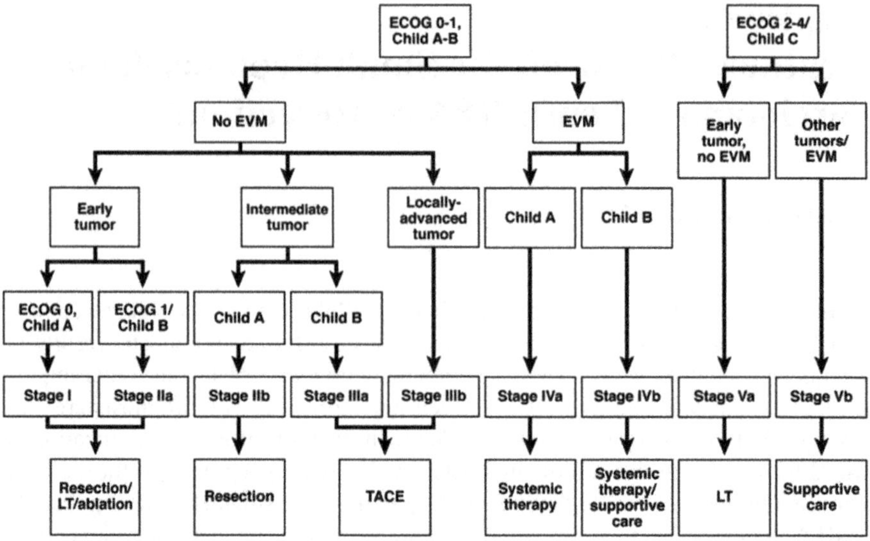

Fig. 15.1 The HKLC prognostic classification scheme. *EVM* extrahepatic vascular invasion/metastasis. Early tumor: ≤5 cm, ≤3 tumor nodules and no intrahepatic venous invasion; Intermediate tumor: (1) ≤5 cm, either >3 tumor nodules or with intrahepatic venous invasion, or (2) >5 cm, ≤3 tumor nodules and no intrahepatic venous invasion; and Locally-advanced tumor: (1) ≤5 cm, >3 tumor nodules and with intrahepatic venous invasion, or (2) >5 cm, >3 tumor nodules or/and with intrahepatic venous invasion, or (3) diffuse tumor

HKLC system was erected which may be more applicable to Asian patients (Fig. 15.1). For the HCC patients with stage I and IIa, resection, transplantation and ablation are all recommended [6]. Hence, three various therapies including resection, transplantation and ablation have been adopted in patients with small HCC although these three approaches have respective distinct indications which are not mentioned in the current staging systems.

Strategy Discussion

Hepatitis B is endemic in China and this results in a heavy burden of hepatocellular carcinoma (HCC) because hepatitis B virus is a major risk factor in the development of the disease [7, 8]. Most HCC patients with chronic infection with HCV have remarkable cirrhosis with impaired liver function, whereas patients with HBV-related HCC in general have better preserved liver function. Individuals would be considered for liver transplantation (LT) if they were with poor liver function reserve and especially small HCC within Milan Criteria (solitary tumour ≤5 cm and up to three nodules ≤3 cm) [9]. Nevertheless, this treatment which gives the potential to both resect the entire potentially tumor-bearing liver and eliminate the cirrhosis can be offered only to a minority of patients because of the shortage of donors and high cost [10]. Specifically, resection was more likely to be recommended over transplantation for patients with small solitary tumors, while patients with small multifocal lesion were much more likely to be referred for transplantation [11]. Pomfret EA et al. [12] also mentioned that the application of liver transplantation at very early stages of HCC development may be futile when treated in patients with well-compensated cirrhosis and very early HCC (single tumour of <2 cm in size; T1 stage [13, 14]). Due to the current issues about transplantation in China, this kind of therapy may be excluded from our first treatment of choice for small HCC.

Hepatectomy and ablation are another two treatment options available for small HCC that will potentially have a positive impact on survival. Not surprisingly, resection and ablation have achieved excellent survival outcomes in this setting, in the range of 60–70 % at 5 years [15, 16]. Resection has generally been accepted as the first treatment of choice for HCC in many centers. It is recommended by surgeons and allows for better local control, with an overall mortality rate less than 5 % in cirrhotic patients and long-term survival up to >50 % after adequate anatomical resections [17, 18]. Anatomical hepatectomy is defined to preliminarily make blood occlusion of hepatic segments and sectors where tumor located and then undergo liver resection according to anatomical range. This approach resected the whole tumor and the hepatic segments and sectors which its portal venous branches allocated. It may ensure the negative incisal margin and decrease the intrahepatic spread of the tumor. After reforming the operation skill, our new approach is probably able to precisely dissect the hepatic pedicle which the required resected segments are affiliated and not need to excessively dissect more fibrous connective tissues of hilar plate and gallbladder bed (Figs. 15.2 and 15.3), consequently, more normal liver are remained by the skill. Previous study also revealed that precise hemihepatectomy guided by middle hepatic vein resulted in fewer incidences of postoperative complications and had the potential to achieve more adequate tumor-free resection margin, which may result in higher tumor-free survival rate [19]. For the nodules in the left lateral lobe, laparoscopic hepatectomy may be another kind of surgical choice. In addition, when patients' performance status permitted, resection is still the first-line treatment for small nodules in right posterior and middle lobe. Therefore, surgical resection was regarded as a fantastic treatment option for small HCC.

However, less than 30 % of patients with small HCC are eligible for surgery, mainly because of the multiplicity and heterogeneity of the lesions that often occurs in a background of chronic liver disease, bad liver function, and deteriorating general condition [20, 21]. So, many nonsurgical ablative methods have been developed, such as cryoablation, percutaneous ethanol injection (PEI), acetic acid injection, radiofrequency ablation (RFA), microwave coagulation, and transcatheter arterial chemoembolization (TACE) [22]. Among these modalities, Radiofrequency (RFA) is now the first-line technique for ablation [23]. Treatment strategy for HCC is mainly decided according to the tumor size, tumor number, liver function and performance status. For small HCC, liver function, which is evaluated by three parts such as Child-Pugh grade, MELD score and the retention rate of ICG in 15 min (R15), may play a pivotal role in guiding decision making. If a patient is diagnosed as small HCC with bad liver function (MELD score >9 [24] or ICG-R15 >20 %

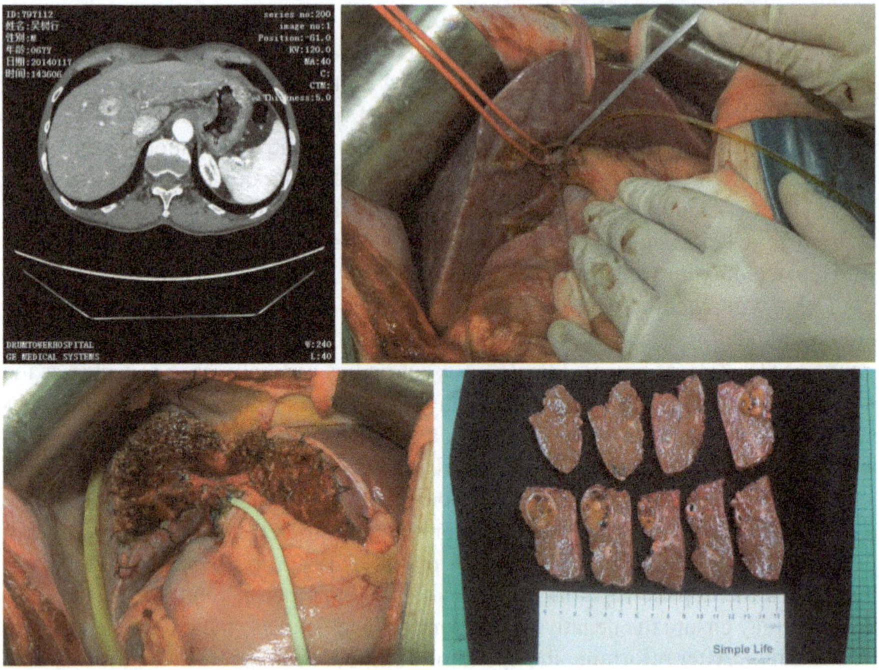

Fig. 15.2 Anatomical liver S4, 5, 8 resection. Boundary type of single nodular small HCC

[25]), RFA will be considered as first line probably. Nevertheless, there is still controversy regarding the treatment choices for small HCC [26] although recent advances in RFA technology have enabled clinicians to use RFA for larger tumors [27]. While a robust trial appropriately comparing resection and ablation is still not available [28], large case-control series and modelling studies support RFA as a non-inferior [29] and more cost-effective [30] treatment for very early HCCs. Wakai T et al. [31] proved that hepatectomy provides both similar local control and better long-term survival for patients with HCC ≤4 cm in comparison with percutaneous ablation. A nonrandomized prospective study suggested that resection is superior to RFA in long-term survival [29]. Moreover, a recently reported randomized trial confirmed that in patients with small HCC, percutaneous RFA showed similar local control and long-term survival compared with hepatectomy but are accompanied with a lower complication rate and shorter hospital stay day [32].

Results

As far as we know, there have been rare randomized trials to compare the efficacy of RFA with that of surgical resection for an operable early-stage HCC in terms of survival for HCCs ≤3 cm [33, 34]. In our opinion, a new risk factor like gross

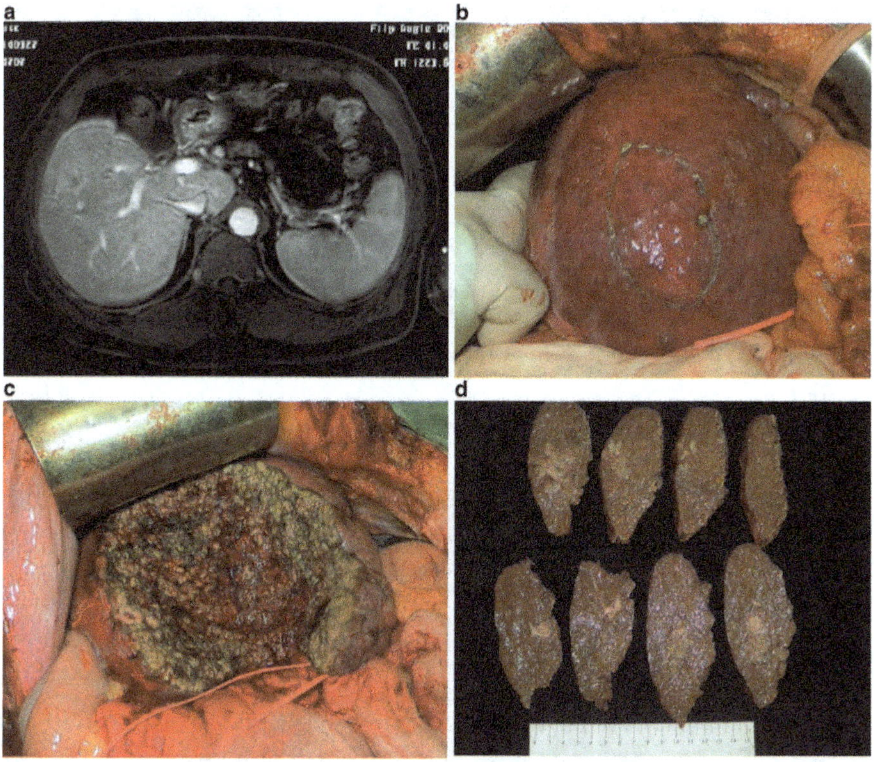

Fig. 15.3 Anatomical liver S5 resection. Infiltrating small HCC lesion

classification should be added in to further help make decision in treatment choice for small HCC. The concept of gross classification for HCC was first put forward in 1984 by Okuda K et al. [35]. According to those studies made by the Japanese scholars, HCC nodules were divided into four groups based on the classification in *The general rules for the clinical and pathological study of primary liver cancer, 4th ed.*, established by the Liver Cancer Study Group of Japan [36]: single nodular type (Fig. 15.4), single nodular type with extranodular growth, confluent multi-nodular type and invasive type (Fig. 15.5). In total, 88 patients with small HCC treated by RFA were divided into two groups on the basis of gross classification distinguished through preoperative imaging data. Our incipient results revealed that the single nodular type group (SN) had significantly better overall survival (OS) and recurrence-free survival (RFS) than the non-single nodular type group (non-SN) ($P < 0.05$) (Figs. 15.6 and 15.7). This significance indicated that not all the patients with small HCC are applicable for RFA treatment, so as to say, resection may be more beneficial for patients with the nonboundary type of small HCC.

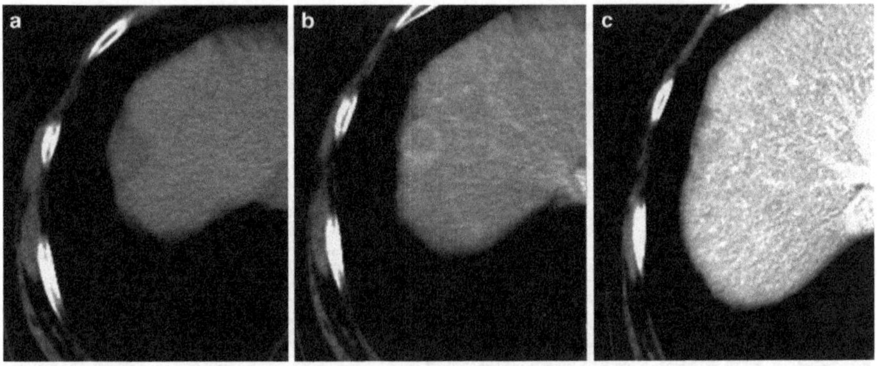

Fig. 15.4 Based on imaging examination, the macroscopic type was single nodular small HCC. (**a**) plain CT. (**b**) arterial phase. (**c**) portal phase *CT* computed tomography

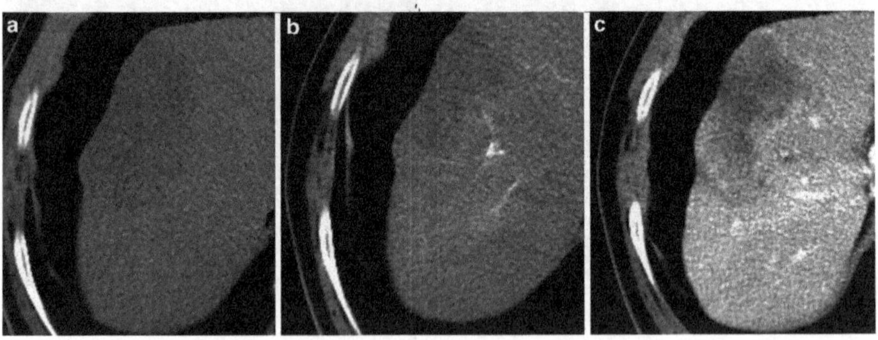

Fig. 15.5 Based on imaging examination, the macroscopic type was invasive small HCC. (**a**) plain CT. (**b**) arterial phase. (**c**) portal phase *CT*computed tomography

Risk of Recurrence

One of the greatest problems plaguing potential curative treatment for HCC is the high risk of recurrence (i.e., ablation and surgical resection). Whichever modality we choose to treat small HCC, recurrence and follow-up work should not be ignored. Early recurrence due to dissemination is likely to have poorer prognosis than late recurrence as it happens after resection. Tumor seeding due to tumor puncture for diagnosis or ablation is the most important, as it is associated with a poor prognosis among the patterns of recurrence [37, 38]. In current study, local recurrence was found to be more frequent after RFA than after HR. Local recurrences after RFA may be attributable to insufficient ablation of the primary tumor and/or the presence of tumor venous invasion in the adjacent liver [22]. Solving these problems,

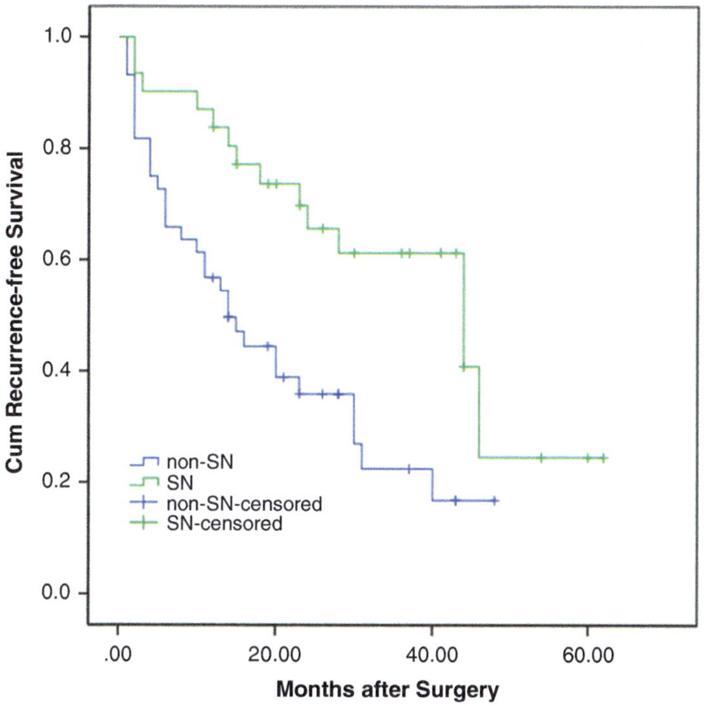

Fig. 15.6 Recurrence-free survival curves for patients with small HCC treated by RFA between SN and non-SN group ($P=0.21$)

prolongation of the follow-up time is needed and might be beneficial for the comparison of the disease-free and overall survival rates between RFA and hepatectomy. Resection or TACE when indicated would be the great treatment of choice against intrahepatic recurrences.

Conclusion

As previously stated, treatment decision in patients with small HCC should be individualized according to the parameters at first diagnosis. Combined with current research, three curative therapies (surgical resection, transplantation, RFA) are efficacious for small HCC. How to select an appropriate treatment seems to be a bit vague in order to achieve a better prognosis. Shown in our results, gross classification may play a pivotal role in therapy decision making for small HCC. In summary, comprehensive diagnosis and treatment is essential for future survival in patients with HCC. For these results to take place, all factors should be considered in

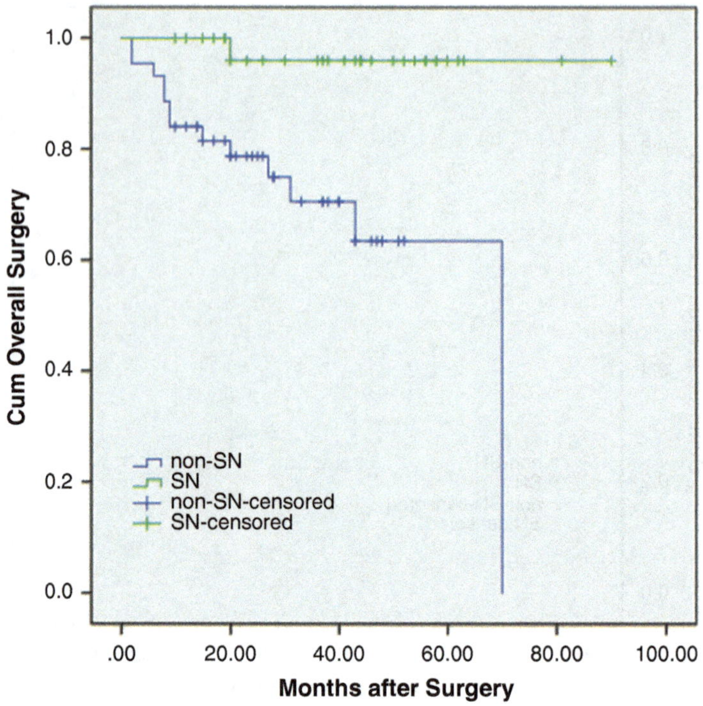

Fig. 15.7 Overall survival curves for patients with small HCC treated by RFA between SN and non-SN group ($P=0.19$)

treating small HCC. Only by combination of the past clinical experience, the current recommendations from guidelines and the latest research results will allow those patients to achieve benefits.

Recommendations

- For Asian patients with HBV-related small HCC, we recommend the use of RFA and resection to treat small HCC.
- For patients with Child-Pugh A and MELD score <9, resection should be considered. However, patients with MELD score >10, cirrhosis and portal hypertension are tending to be treated with RFA.
- There is evidence for RFA to treat those patients with the boundary type of small HCC in accordance with gross classification.
- Specifically, infiltrating hepatocellular carcinoma (iHCC) described as invasive type in gross classification was suggested to be treated with anatomical resection due to the high recurrence rate if managed with RFA.

References

1. Bruix J, Gores GJ, Mazzaferro V. Hepatocellular carcinoma: clinical frontiers and perspectives. Gut. 2014;63:844–55.
2. Llovet JM, Brú C, Bruix J. Prognosis of hepatocellular carcinoma: the BCLC staging classification. Semin Liver Dis. 1999;19:329–38.
3. Bruix J, Sherman M. Management of hepatocellular carcinoma: an update. Hepatology. 2011;53:1020–2.
4. Mazzaferro V, Regalia E, Doci R, et al. Liver transplantation for the treatment of small hepatocellular carcinomas in patients with cirrhosis. N Engl J Med. 1996;334:693–9.
5. Lau WY, Lai EC. Salvage surgery following downstaging of unresectable hepatocellular carcinoma – a strategy to increase resectability. Ann Surg Oncol. 2007;14:3301–9.
6. Yau T, Tang VY, Yao TJ, et al. Development of Hong Kong Liver Cancer staging system with treatment stratification for patients with hepatocellular carcinoma. Gastroenterology. 2014;146:1691–700.
7. Yin L, Li H, Li AJ, et al. Partial hepatectomy vs. transcatheter arterial chemoembolization for resectable multiple hepatocellular carcinoma beyond Milan Criteria: a RCT. J Hepatol. 2014;61:82–8.
8. Llovet JM, Bruix J. Novel advancements in the management of hepatocellular carcinoma in 2008. J Hepatol. 2008;48 Suppl 1:S20–37.
9. Bruix J, Sherman M. Management of hepatocellular carcinoma. Hepatology. 2005;42:1208–36.
10. Befeler AS, Hayashi PH, Di Bisceglie AM. Liver transplantation for hepatocellular carcinoma. Gastroenterology. 2005;128:1752–64.
11. Nathan H, Herlong HF, Gurakar A, et al. Clinical decision-making by gastroenterologists and hepatologists for patients with early hepatocellular carcinoma. Ann Surg Oncol. 2014;21:1844–51.
12. Pomfret EA, Washburn K, Wald C, et al. Report of a national conference on liver allocation in patients with hepatocellular carcinoma in the United States. Liver Transpl. 2010;16:262–78.
13. Vauthey JN, Lauwers GY, Esnaola NF, et al. Simplified staging for hepatocellular carcinoma. J Clin Oncol. 2002;20:1527–36.
14. OPTN U, editor. United network for organ sharing. Liver Transplant Candidates with hepatocellular carcinoma (HCC) Policy 3.6.4.4. http://optn.transplant.hrsa.gov/PoliciesandBylaws2/policies/pdfs/policy_8.pdf. Accessed 23 Jun 2013.
15. Livraghi T, Meloni F, Di Stasi M, et al. Sustained complete response and complications rates after radiofrequency ablation of very early hepatocellular carcinoma in cirrhosis: is resection still the treatment of choice? Hepatology. 2008;47:82–9.
16. Roayaie S, Obeidat K, Sposito C, et al. Resection of hepatocellular cancer </=2cm: results from two Western centers. Hepatology. 2012;57:1426–35.
17. Poon RT, Fan ST, Lo CM. Improving survival results after resection of hepatocellular carcinoma: a prospective study of 377 patients over 10 years. Ann Surg. 2001;234:63–70.
18. Makuuchi M, Sano K. The surgical approach to HCC: our progress and results in Japan. Liver Transpl. 2004;10:S46–52.
19. Qiu Y, Zhu X, Zhu R, et al. The clinical study of precise hemihepatectomy guided by middle hepatic vein. World J Surg. 2012;36:2428–35.
20. Verslype C, Van Cutsem E, Dicato M. The management of hepatocellular carcinoma. Current expert opinion and recommendations derived from the 10th World Congress on Gastrointestinal Cancer, Barcelona, 2008. Ann Oncol. 2009;20 Suppl 7:vii1–6.
21. Zhu AX. Molecularly targeted therapy for advanced hepatocellular carcinoma in 2012: current status and future perspectives. Semin Oncol. 2012;39:493–502.
22. Zhou Y, Zhao Y, Li B, et al. Meta-analysis of radiofrequency ablation versus hepatic resection for small hepatocellular carcinoma. BMC Gastroenterol. 2010;10:78.

23. Lencioni R. Loco-regional treatment of hepatocellular carcinoma. Hepatology. 2010;52:762–73.
24. Abdalla EK, Adam R, Bilchik AJ, et al. Improving resectability of hepatic colorectal metastases: expert consensus statement. Ann Surg Oncol. 2006;13:1271–80.
25. Kubota K, Makuuchi M, Kusaka K, et al. Measurement of liver volume and hepatic functional reserve as a guide to decision-making in resectional surgery for hepatic tumors. Hepatology. 1997;26:1176–81.
26. Earl TM, Chapman WC. Conventional surgical treatment of hepatocellular carcinoma. Clin Liver Dis. 2011;15:353–70.
27. Seror O, N'Kontchou G, Ibraheem M, et al. Large (>or=5.0-cm) HCCs: multipolar RF ablation with three internally cooled bipolar electrodes—initial experience in 26 patients. Radiology. 2008;248:288–96.
28. Majno PE, Mentha G, Mazzaferro V. Partial hepatectomy versus radiofrequency ablation for hepatocellular carcinoma: confirming the trial that will never be, and some comments on the indications for liver resection. Hepatology. 2010;51:1116–8.
29. Cho YK, Kim JK, Kim WT, et al. Hepatic resection versus radiofrequency ablation for very early stage hepatocellular carcinoma: a Markov model analysis. Hepatology. 2010;51:1284–90.
30. Roberts JP, Venook A, Kerlan R, et al. Hepatocellular carcinoma: ablate and wait versus rapid transplantation. Liver Transpl. 2010;16:925–9.
31. Wakai T, Shirai Y, Suda T, et al. Long-term outcomes of hepatectomy vs percutaneous ablation for treatment of hepatocellular carcinoma<or=4 cm. World J Gastroenterol. 2006;12:546–52.
32. Fang Y, Chen W, Liang X, et al. Comparison of long-term effectiveness and complications of radiofrequency ablation with hepatectomy for small hepatocellular carcinoma. J Gastroenterol Hepatol. 2014;29:193–200.
33. Chen MS, Li JQ, Zheng Y. A prospective randomized trial comparing percutaneous local ablative therapy and partial hepatectomy for small hepatocellular carcinoma. Ann Surg. 2006;243:321–8.
34. Arii S, Yamaoka Y, Futagawa S, et al. Results of surgical and nonsurgical treatment for small-sized hepatocellular carcinomas: a retrospective and nationwide survey in Japan. The Liver Cancer Study Group of Japan. Hepatology. 2000;32:1224–9.
35. Okuda K, Peters RL, Simson IW. Gross anatomic features of hepatocellular carcinoma from three disparate geographic areas. Proposal of new classification. Cancer. 1984;54:2165–73.
36. Liver Cancer Study Group of Japan. The general rules for the clinical and pathological study of primary liver cancer. 4th ed. Tokyo: Kanehara; 2001.
37. Nicoli N, Casaril A, Abu Hilal M, et al. A case of rapid intrahepatic dissemination of hepatocellular carcinoma after radiofrequency thermal ablation. Am J Surg. 2004;188:165–7.
38. Forner A, Llovet JM, Bruix J. Hepatocellular carcinoma. Lancet. 2012;379:1245–55.

Chapter 16
Which Is the Better Predictor of Hepatic Reserve Prior to Liver Resection: MELD or the Child-Pugh Score?

Trevor W. Reichman and Humberto Bohorquez

Abstract Critical assessment of the hepatic reserve is essential prior to liver resection especially in patients with chronic liver disease. Development of liver dysfunction post resection can result in a significant increase in associated complications resulting in prolonged length of hospital stay and increased hospital costs. In addition, the development of liver failure is almost universally fatal unless the patient can undergo liver transplantation. Several scoring systems have been identified which assess the degree of liver disease including the Child-Turcotte-Pugh scoring system (CTP) and the Model for End Stage Liver Disease (MELD). Both of these scoring systems have been used to predict mortality post liver resection. Based on the current available literature, MELD appears to be the best predictor of postoperative liver dysfunction/failure in patients with cirrhosis, and patients with MELD scores ≥9 should not be considered for hepatic resection. Other factors not included in MELD such as platelet count, presence of portal hypertension, extent of liver resection (and the resulting residual liver volume) and the presence of ascites should also be considered when selecting patients with chronic liver disease to undergo liver resection.

Keywords Hepatectomy • Liver resection • MELD • Child-Pugh Score • Liver failure • Cirrhosis

Introduction

Recent surgical advances in liver resections have improved the safety and complication rates from this complex operation, and a hepatectomy is now a well-accepted treatment for patients with both benign and malignant liver tumors and metastatic

T.W. Reichman (✉) • H. Bohorquez
Multi-Organ Transplant Institute, Department of Surgery, Ochsner Medical Center, 1514 Jefferson Highway, New Orleans, LA 70121, USA
e-mail: treichman@ochsner.org

J.M. Millis, J.B. Matthews (eds.), *Difficult Decisions in Hepatobiliary and Pancreatic Surgery*, Difficult Decisions in Surgery: An Evidence-Based Approach, DOI 10.1007/978-3-319-27365-5_16

cancers to the liver. The presence of an adequate, healthy remnant liver is essential in order to prevent postoperative liver dysfunction and/or liver failure after liver resection and is especially critical in patients with known chronic liver disease. In the case of hepatocellular cancer (HCC), >80 % of the patients diagnosed have chronic liver disease [1]. With donor shortages across the globe, not all patients with chronic liver disease can undergo transplantation for HCC [2]. Appropriate assessment of the hepatic reserve is essential to avoiding post-operative liver dysfunction and liver failure.

Liver Failure Following Liver Resection

Progression of liver dysfunction to liver failure is almost universally fatal unless the patient can undergo liver transplantation. Post-hepatectomy liver failure was recently defined by the International Study Group of Liver Surgery (ISGLS) as the inability of the liver to maintain its synthetic, excretory, and detoxifying functions, which is manifested by an increased INR and hyperbilirubinemia on or after postoperative day 5 [3]. The reported rate of liver failure varies between 1.2 and 32 % depending on the study population [3]. Liver dysfunction post liver resection ultimately results in increased length of stay and increased hospital costs. Recently, post operative liver dysfunction was also linked to post resection disease-free survival in patients undergoing resection for HCC [4].

Evaluation of the Degree of Chronic Liver Disease

It is well established that there is an increased risk performing surgery on patients with chronic liver disease and cirrhosis. This increased risk derives from both factors associated with chronic liver disease (e.g. portal hypertension, ascites, thrombocytopenia, and coagulopathy) and also the potential exacerbation of liver dysfunction secondary to general anesthesia and a laparotomy incision. Based on several studies, mortality can be as high as 70–80 % in patients with advanced cirrhosis [5, 6].

Based on this knowledge, it is not surprising that there is also an increased risk in performing liver resections on patients with chronic liver disease. Accurate assessment of the functional reserve is critical prior to liver resection especially in patients with chronic liver disease. Two well-known scoring systems are the Model for End Stage Liver Disease (MELD) and the Child-Turcotte-Pugh (CTP) scoring system. The accuracy of these tests in predicting hepatic dysfunction post liver resection is still debated.

The CTP score was initially reported in 1964 as a way to assess liver function in patients with chronic liver disease and was later modified by Pugh in 1973 [7, 8]. The current scoring system utilizes the serum bilirubin, serum albumin, prothromin time (PT)/ international normalized ratio (INR), degree of ascites and degree of hepatic encephalopathy assigning 1–3 points for each variable. Patients are divided into three classes based on total points with ≤6, 7–9, and ≥10 points representing Child's class A, B, and C, respectively. Unlike the CTP score which contain variables that are somewhat subjective, the MELD score, a linear regression model based on patient's serum creatinine, total bilirubin and INR, was initially designed to predict mortality in cirrhotic patients who were undergoing transjugular intrahepatic portosystemic shunts (TIPS) [9]. Subsequently, the model has been validated prospectively as a prognostic tool in patients awaiting liver transplantation [10]. This model also effectively predicts mortality in patients who underwent non-transplant surgery [11].

Search Strategy

A literature search of the English language publications from 1990 to 2014 was used to identify published data on the use of Child Class and/or MELD score as a predictor of hepatic reserve prior to liver resection using the PICO outline (Table 16.1). The databases searched included PubMed, Science Citation Index/ Social Sciences Citation index, Embase, and Cochran Evidence Based Medicine. Keywords used for the search included "MELD score," Child score/classification," "Child-Pugh score/classification," "Child-Turcotte-Pugh score/classification," "cirrhosis," AND "liver resection," OR "hepatectomy." Articles were classified using the GRADE system.

Liver Resections and the Childs-Turcotte-Pugh Score

CTP score has been applied to liver resection in an attempt to predict hepatic reserve and mortality post liver resection. It is fairly well established that patients with Class C cirrhosis poorly tolerate resection. An early study by Nagasue et al. documented their experience with 63 patients (46 Class B and 17 Class C cirrhotics). In their series, they had a 17.6 % overall peri-operative mortality (30 days from surgery) for their class C patients and a 23.5 % in-hospital death rate [12].

Table 16.1 PICO table for assessment of hepatic reserve prior to liver resection

P (Patients)	I (Intervention)	C (Comparator group)	O (Outcomes measured)
Patients with cirrhosis undergoing hepatic resection	Use of MELD scoring system preoperatively to assess hepatic reserve	Use of the Child-Turcotte-Pugh classification to assess hepatic reserve prior to liver resection	Incidence of liver dysfunction/ failure post liver resection resulting in increased length of stay, hospital cost, morbidity, and mortality

Few studies also focus on class B cirrhotics with even fewer giving a detailed analysis of peri-operative morbidity. Two studies were identified which focused on outcomes following resection of class B cirrhotics. The first series by Nakahara et al. examined 119 patients with HCC who underwent resection that were identified as class B cirrhotics [13]. Of these patients, >75 % of them underwent a limited resection (less then a segmentectomy). In this series, the in-hospital mortality was 5 %, with two patients suffering from liver failure in the immediate postoperative setting. Multivariate analysis revealed risk factors for poor outcome which included elevated bilirubin (>1.5 mg/dl) and the presence of ascites [13]. Similarly, Kuroda et al. studied 150 class B cirrhotics. Although the risk of immediate post-operative liver failure appears to be low in these patients, many patients ultimately die of liver failure (15 %) [14]. Based on these studies, limited resection can be performed on patients with CTP Class B cirrhosis with caution but major resections should be avoided.

One would predict that class A cirrhotics would have less post-operative liver dysfunction and liver failure based on the fact that Class A patients by definition have minimal symptoms (if any) of chronic liver disease. The majority of large published studies focus on patients with class A cirrhosis and HCC. However, studies have clear bias and show improvement in outcomes over time but little change in the number of patients with cirrhosis [15]. Even for patients with class A cirrhosis, the range of liver function appears to vary widely as judged by ICG retention studies performed on Class A patients [16]. In a series of 625 patients resected for HCC, CTP was not found to be an independent predictor of perioperative morbidity [17]. In contrast, Nagasue et al. reported their outcomes of 229 patients and found that CTP was predictive of post-operative complications. In this series, only patient with cirrhosis were at risk for developing post-operative liver failure [18]. In a large European study, all patient resected were considered Class A but they noted a 32 % incidence of post-operative liver failure in patients with stage 4 fibrosis (cirrhosis) [19].

The extent of liver resection is obviously an important predictor of post-operative liver dysfunction and liver failure. Two studies were identified which focused on major hepatic resections and CTP classification. Yang et al. specifically examined outcomes of patients with cirrhosis following major hepatic resection [20]. In this series, 270 patients had class A cirrhosis versus 35 with class B cirrhosis. Risk factors for preoperative morbidity were the presence of portal hypertension, Child class B, and platelet count $<100\times10^9$/l. However, independent risk factors for postoperative hepatic dysfunction were a prothrombin time >14 s and a platelet count $<100\times10^9$/l, not CTP score. In addition, four patients died of post-operative liver failure of which two were Class A cirrhotics. Similarly, Zhou et al. examined their experience after major hepatectomy in 81 patients of which 6 (7.4 %) had class B cirrhosis and only one patient suffered perioperative hepatic failure [21].

Based on the current available literature, Class C cirrhosis should be an absolute contraindication to resection. On the other hand, resection in Class A and B cirrhosis is not an absolute contraindication, but these patients should be selected carefully in order to minimize post-operative complications. In addition, the magnitude of resection required for cure should be carefully considered when selecting suitable patients for hepatic resection.

Liver Resections and the Meld Score

MELD has been applied to cirrhotic patients who underwent liver resection for hepatocellular carcinoma (HCC) for more than a decade. Marrero et al. in a subgroup of ten patients first reported that MELD score correlates with post-operative survival in patients who underwent liver resection for HCC and found that a MELD score >10 was indicative of poor prognosis [22]. Similarly, Teh et al. retrospectively analyzed 82 cirrhotic patients who underwent liver resection for HCC [23]. A MELD score ≥9 was an independent predictor of perioperative mortality (0 % in patients with MELD score ≤8 vs. 29 % with MELD score ≥9). In another study with 154 liver resections, Cuchetti et al. demonstrated that MELD score not only predicts accurately postoperative liver failure, complications, and survival but that is also helpful stratifying the risk [24]. When the patients were analyzed in three groups according to their MELD score, <9, 9–10 and ≥11, postoperative liver failure occurred in 0, 3.6 and 37.5 % respectively. A MELD score cut-off of <9 for mortality-morbidity for liver resections in cirrhotic patients has been confirmed by others [25–27].

AASLD and EASL guidelines recommend liver resection for HCC patients with solitary tumors and well-preserved liver function defined as normal bilirubin, platelets >100,000/mm^3 and hepatic pressure <10 mmHg [28, 29]. Cuchetti reviewed this concept in 241 cirrhotic patients that underwent liver resections and were divided in two groups according to the presence or absence of portal hypertension [30]. The study showed lower survival in those patients with portal hypertension because of greater liver impairment; however, after propensity score matching of 78 patients, the overall survival was similar in patients with and without portal hypertension. In this subgroup of patients, the only predictors of postoperative liver failure were MELD score and the extent of hepatectomy. They concluded that when other prognostic variables were appropriately handled, the presence of portal hypertension had no impact on peri-operative outcomes and that the presence of portal hypertension alone should not be considered a contraindication for hepatic resection.

MELD score has been reported to have low prognostic power in non-cirrhotic or well preserve hepatic function patients. Schroeder et al. in a review of 587 hepatectomies found no correlation between MELD score and post-operative outcomes [31]. However, the majority of the study population (91 %) had minimal or no evidence of liver disease (MELD score 5.7 ± 3.3). A similar smaller study of 46 patients (21 without cirrhosis vs. 25 with cirrhosis) with HCC who underwent liver resection demonstrated that MELD score failed to predict perioperative outcomes in the non-cirrhotic patients [32]. By contrast, in the cirrhotic group, the model was able to predict poor outcomes when MELD was calculated preoperatively and on postoperative day 5 (MELD score >9 and >15, respectively).

Extent of resection, a major limitation for hepatectomies especially in cirrhotic patients, also correlates with the MELD score. In a report by Cescon et al., 341 cirrhotic patients were retrospectively evaluated to determine the incidence and factors that affect irreversible post-operative liver failure (IPLF). In this study, MELD score and extent of hepatectomy were identified as independent factors of IPLF [33]. For analysis, patients were stratified according to their MELD score. In patients with MELD <9, IPLF occurred in one patient (0.4 %) with four segments resected; in MELD scores 9–10, IPLF occurred in 1.2 % of patients that underwent resection of less than one segment, in 5.1 % for ≥1 or 2 segments resected and in 11 % for ≥3 segments. In patients with a MELD score >10, IPLF occurred in >15 % of the patients regardless of the degree of resection. Interestingly, in the group with MELD scores 9–10, all IPLF cases occurred in patients with a sodium level <140 mEq/L; a level that seems to define high/low risk groups for liver resection.

The MELD-Sodium (MELD-Na) model, a revised MELD formula that incorporates serum sodium levels, is superior at predicting outcomes in liver transplantation especially in those patients with lower MELD scores. Recently, a study successfully applied the MELD-Na score in predicting morbidity and mortality following elective colon cancer surgery irrespective of underlying liver disease [34]. Studies are needed to define whether this parameter could be applied to patients who underwent liver resection.

The MELD score has also been evaluated against other prognostic tests and scores to test their ability to determine the functional hepatic reserve in cirrhotic patients undergoing liver resection. In a study from the University of Toronto, the MELD score was compared against the use of ICG retention at 15 min (ICG15), a dynamic test for hepatic functional reserve [35]. In this study of 129 patients who underwent liver resection for HCC, ICG15 ≥15 % and MELD score ≥14 were independent factors to predicts length of stay >10 days. However, MELD score failed to predict liver failure at post-operative day 3 while ICG15 did. Postoperative survival was not analyzed. Likewise, in a prospective study that included 40 patients, ICG15 and MELD score correlated with prognosis; however, ICG15 had a higher sensitivity and specificity than the MELD score, 85 % and 90 % vs. 60 and 80 %, respectively [36].

Child-Turcotte-Pugh vs. MELD Score

Although the CTP score is easy to use and evaluates major elements of liver function, it has several limitations. Two of the components of the score, ascites and encephalopathy, are subjective measurements; the score factors are weighted equally and use arbitrary cut-off. Therefore, CTP score calculation is not always reliable, and since patients within the same CTP class are not necessarily homogeneous, discrimination of the risk is limited. As a consequence, patients could erroneously be classified and either be exposed unnecessarily to high risk procedures or excluded from beneficial therapeutic interventions.

By contrast, MELD score is objective, reproducible, weighs its components differently and does not depend on arbitrary cut-offs providing a very useful tool to predict outcomes in cirrhotic patients. In patients with cirrhosis who underwent liver resection, preoperative MELD score has been able to not only predict outcomes but also to stratify the risk. Moreover, in patients within the same CTP class or same level of portal hypertension, the MELD score was able to successfully discriminate the risk and identify appropriate candidates for liver resection. In addition, delta MELD, variations in MELD score at different points of the perioperative time, is also predictive of morbidity and mortality.

MELD score, however, seems to be limited to cirrhotic patients and fails to predict outcomes in non-cirrhotic patients. In this population, a combination of the serum sodium level and/or MELD-Na seems to improve accuracy but further studies are required to validate this observation.

There are several limitations to the studies that use CTP and MELD score to stratify patients for liver resection. First, there is a lack of prospective randomized control trials. Second, the majority the patients evaluated in different studies were cirrhotic patients with CTP class A (88–100 %), indicating a selection bias where liver resection is offered to patients with minimal liver disease. Third, minimal information is available comparing these scoring systems in non-cirrhotic patients. Table 16.2 compares major studies examining MELD vs. CTP.

A Personal View of the Data

The currently available literature has a large selection bias and lacks large amounts of patients with advanced cirrhosis. In our practice, MELD has been found to be the most predictive of hepatic reserve. However, we rarely use the MELD score in isolation to determine a patient's candidacy for resection. Other factor not accounted for in MELD such as the presence of ascites, evidence of portal hypertension on imaging or endoscopic gastroduodenoscopy (EGD), and the platelet count (<100) are also used in determining the ability of patient to tolerate resection. Detailed volumetric analysis is performed to determine the residual liver volume and also to aid in planning the resection. If the residual volume appears to be marginal, portal vein embolization is performed to increase the remnant volume but also to test the regenerative capacity of the remaining liver. Biopsy of the remnant segment is also performed liberally to determine the degree of fibrosis/cirrhosis. For patients with HCC, if there is any question as to the hepatic reserve of the liver and the patient is within Milan or close to being within Milan, many of these patients are referred for transplant evaluation.

Table 16.2 Studies which compare CTP to MELD

Study	Patients	Patients with cirrhosis	CTP A/B/C class (%)	MELD score	Extent of resection	Mortality prognostic factor	Quality of evidence
Teh (2005)	82	100 %	97.5/2.5/0	≤8 = 37; ≥9 = 43 range (6–17)	<3 seg = 72 %≥ 3 seg = 28 %	MELD score (≥9)	Low
Cuchetti (2006)	154	100 %	92.9/7.1	9 (range 6–15)	Minor = 146 (94.8 %)	MELD score (<9, ≥11)	Low
					Major 8 (5.2 %)		
Schroeder (2006)	587	N/M	88.2/7.8/0.7	6.51 ± 4.5 range (6–38)	≤2 seg = 61.4 %	CTP score (6.2 ± 1.9) MELD score = not significant	Low
					Total R/L = 31.7		
					Triseg = 6.5 %		
Cuchetti (2009)	241	100 %	PH = 88.8/11.2/0	PH = 9.5 ± 1.8	≤1 segment = 81 %	MELD score >10	Low
			noPH = 98/2/0	noPH = 8.4 ± 1.3	2 seg = 14.1 %	Extent of hepatectomy	
					Major hepatectomy 4.9 %		
Cescon (2009)	466	100 %	94.2/5.8/0	8.9 ± 1.8	<1 Segment = 45 %	CTP B MELD <9, 9–10,>10	Low
				>10 (17 %)			
					1-segmen = 29.6 %	Na <140 mEq/L	
					2 seg = 2.4 Major hepatectomy 12.4	Extent of hepatectomy	

CTP Child-Turcotte-Pugh, *MELD* Model for End Stage Liver Disease, *N/M* not measured, *N/S* not specified, *PH* portal hypertension, *noPH* no portal hypertension

Recommendations

- The MELD scoring system is the best at predicting preoperative liver dysfunction and liver failure with a MELD score of 9 acting as a cutoff (evidence quality low, weak recommendation)
- Other factors such as extent of resection, presence of portal hypertension, absolute platelet count, and the serum sodium should also be taken into account when selecting patients with chronic liver disease for resection (evidence quality low, weak recommendation)

References

1. Mittal S, El-Serag HB. Epidemiology of hepatocellular carcinoma: consider the population. J Clin Gastroenterol. 2013;47(Suppl):S2–6.
2. Smith JM, Biggins SW, Haselby DG, Kim WR, Wedd J, Lamb K, et al. Kidney, pancreas and liver allocation and distribution in the United States. Am J Transplant. 2012;12(12):3191–212.
3. Rahbari NN, Garden OJ, Padbury R, Brooke-Smith M, Crawford M, Adam R, et al. Posthepatectomy liver failure: a definition and grading by the International Study Group of Liver Surgery (ISGLS). Surgery. 2011;149(5):713–24.
4. Fukushima K, Fukumoto T, Kuramitsu K, Kido M, Takebe A, Tanaka M, et al. Assessment of ISGLS definition of posthepatectomy liver failure and its effect on outcome in patients with hepatocellular carcinoma. J Gastrointest Surg. 2014;18(4):729–36.
5. Garrison RN, Cryer HM, Howard DA, Polk Jr HC. Clarification of risk factors for abdominal operations in patients with hepatic cirrhosis. Ann Surg. 1984;199(6):648–55.
6. Mansour A, Watson W, Shayani V, Pickleman J. Abdominal operations in patients with cirrhosis: still a major surgical challenge. Surgery. 1997;122(4):730–5; discussion 5–6.
7. Child C, Turcotte JG. Surgery and portal hypertension. In: Child C, editor. The liver and portal hypertension. Philadelphia: Saunders; 1964. p. 50–64.
8. Pugh RN, Murray-Lyon IM, Dawson JL, Pietroni MC, Williams R. Transection of the oesophagus for bleeding oesophageal varices. Br J Surg. 1973;60(8):646–9.
9. Malinchoc M, Kamath PS, Gordon FD, Peine CJ, Rank J, ter Borg PC. A model to predict poor survival in patients undergoing transjugular intrahepatic portosystemic shunts. Hepatology. 2000;31(4):864–71.
10. Kamath PS, Wiesner RH, Malinchoc M, Kremers W, Therneau TM, Kosberg CL, et al. A model to predict survival in patients with end-stage liver disease. Hepatology. 2001;33(2):464–70.
11. Befeler AS, Palmer DE, Hoffman M, Longo W, Solomon H, Di Bisceglie AM. The safety of intra-abdominal surgery in patients with cirrhosis: model for end-stage liver disease score is superior to Child-Turcotte-Pugh classification in predicting outcome. Arch Surg. 2005;140(7):650–4; discussion 5.
12. Nagasue N, Kohno H, Tachibana M, Yamanoi A, Ohmori H, El-Assal ON. Prognostic factors after hepatic resection for hepatocellular carcinoma associated with Child-Turcotte class B and C cirrhosis. Ann Surg. 1999;229(1):84–90.
13. Nakahara H, Itamoto T, Katayama K, Ohdan H, Hino H, Ochi M, et al. Indication of hepatectomy for cirrhotic patients with hepatocellular carcinoma classified as Child-Pugh class B. World J Surg. 2005;29(6):734–8.

14. Kuroda S, Tashiro H, Kobayashi T, Oshita A, Amano H, Ohdan H. Selection criteria for hepatectomy in patients with hepatocellular carcinoma classified as Child-Pugh class B. World J Surg. 2011;35(4):834–41.
15. Fan ST, Lo CM, Liu CL, Lam CM, Yuen WK, Yeung C, et al. Hepatectomy for hepatocellular carcinoma: toward zero hospital deaths. Ann Surg. 1999;229(3):322–30.
16. Lau H, Man K, Fan ST, Yu WC, Lo CM, Wong J. Evaluation of preoperative hepatic function in patients with hepatocellular carcinoma undergoing hepatectomy. Br J Surg. 1997;84(9):1255–9.
17. Taketomi A, Kitagawa D, Itoh S, Harimoto N, Yamashita Y, Gion T, et al. Trends in morbidity and mortality after hepatic resection for hepatocellular carcinoma: an institute's experience with 625 patients. J Am Coll Surg. 2007;204(4):580–7.
18. Nagasue N, Kohno H, Chang YC, Taniura H, Yamanoi A, Uchida M, et al. Liver resection for hepatocellular carcinoma. Results of 229 consecutive patients during 11 years. Ann Surg. 1993;217(4):375–84.
19. Farges O, Malassagne B, Flejou JF, Balzan S, Sauvanet A, Belghiti J. Risk of major liver resection in patients with underlying chronic liver disease: a reappraisal. Ann Surg. 1999;229(2):210–5.
20. Yang T, Zhang J, Lu JH, Yang GS, Wu MC, Yu WF. Risk factors influencing postoperative outcomes of major hepatic resection of hepatocellular carcinoma for patients with underlying liver diseases. World J Surg. 2011;35(9):2073–82.
21. Zhou L, Rui JA, Wang SB, Chen SG, Qu Q, Chi TY, et al. Outcomes and prognostic factors of cirrhotic patients with hepatocellular carcinoma after radical major hepatectomy. World J Surg. 2007;31(9):1782–7.
22. Marrero JA, Fontana RJ, Barrat A, Askari F, Conjeevaram HS, Su GL, et al. Prognosis of hepatocellular carcinoma: comparison of 7 staging systems in an American cohort. Hepatology. 2005;41(4):707–16.
23. Teh SH, Christein J, Donohue J, Que F, Kendrick M, Farnell M, et al. Hepatic resection of hepatocellular carcinoma in patients with cirrhosis: Model of End-Stage Liver Disease (MELD) score predicts perioperative mortality. J Gastrointest Surg. 2005;9(9):1207–15; discussion 15.
24. Cucchetti A, Ercolani G, Cescon M, Ravaioli M, Zanello M, Del Gaudio M, et al. Recovery from liver failure after hepatectomy for hepatocellular carcinoma in cirrhosis: meaning of the model for end-stage liver disease. J Am Coll Surg. 2006;203(5):670–6.
25. Delis SG, Bakoyiannis A, Biliatis I, Athanassiou K, Tassopoulos N, Dervenis C. Model for end-stage liver disease (MELD) score, as a prognostic factor for post-operative morbidity and mortality in cirrhotic patients, undergoing hepatectomy for hepatocellular carcinoma. HPB (Oxf). 2009;11(4):351–7.
26. Hsu KY, Chau GY, Lui WY, Tsay SH, King KL, Wu CW. Predicting morbidity and mortality after hepatic resection in patients with hepatocellular carcinoma: the role of Model for End-Stage Liver Disease score. World J Surg. 2009;33(11):2412–9.
27. Rahbari NN, Reissfelder C, Koch M, Elbers H, Striebel F, Buchler MW, et al. The predictive value of postoperative clinical risk scores for outcome after hepatic resection: a validation analysis in 807 patients. Ann Surg Oncol. 2011;18(13):3640–9.
28. Bruix J, Sherman M, American Association for the Study of Liver D. Management of hepatocellular carcinoma: an update. Hepatology. 2011;53(3):1020–2.
29. European Association For The Study Of The L, European Organisation For R, Treatment Of C. EASL-EORTC. EASL-EORTC clinical practice guidelines: management of hepatocellular carcinoma. J Hepatol. 2012;56(4):908–43.
30. Cucchetti A, Ercolani G, Vivarelli M, Cescon M, Ravaioli M, Ramacciato G, et al. Is portal hypertension a contraindication to hepatic resection? Ann Surg. 2009;250(6):922–8.
31. Schroeder RA, Marroquin CE, Bute BP, Khuri S, Henderson WG, Kuo PC. Predictive indices of morbidity and mortality after liver resection. Ann Surg. 2006;243(3):373–9.

32. Teh SH, Sheppard BC, Schwartz J, Orloff SL. Model for End-stage Liver Disease score fails to predict perioperative outcome after hepatic resection for hepatocellular carcinoma in patients without cirrhosis. Am J Surg. 2008;195(5):697–701.
33. Cescon M, Cucchetti A, Grazi GL, Ferrero A, Vigano L, Ercolani G, et al. Indication of the extent of hepatectomy for hepatocellular carcinoma on cirrhosis by a simple algorithm based on preoperative variables. Arch Surg. 2009;144(1):57–63; discussion.
34. Causey MW, Nelson D, Johnson EK, Maykel J, Davis B, Rivadeneira DE, et al. The impact of Model for End-Stage Liver Disease-Na in predicting morbidity and mortality following elective colon cancer surgery irrespective of underlying liver disease. Am J Surg. 2014;207(4):520–6.
35. Greco E, Nanji S, Bromberg IL, Shah S, Wei AC, Moulton CA, et al. Predictors of peri-opertative morbidity and liver dysfunction after hepatic resection in patients with chronic liver disease. HPB (OXf). 2011;13(8):559–65.
36. Gupta S, Chawla Y, Kaur J, Saxena R, Duseja A, Dhiman RK, et al. Indocyanine green clearance test (using spectrophotometry) and its correlation with model for end stage liver disease (MELD) score in Indian patients with cirrhosis of liver. Trop Gastroenterol. 2012;33(2):129–34.

Chapter 17
Early (<24 h) or Delayed Cholecystectomy for Acute Cholecystitis?

Stephan G. Wyers

Abstract The optimal timing for operation for acute calculous cholecysitis remains controversial. Two courses of surgical management have traditionally been pursued: (1) early laparoscopic cholecystectomy (within the first 72 h of onset of symptoms) or (2) initial conservative management with administration of intravenous antibiotics until inflammation resolves followed by delayed laparoscopic cholecystectomy (generally greater than 6 weeks after presentation). There is a growing body of evidence from both retrospective reviews of large clinical databases and prospective randomized controlled trials to recommend early laparoscopic cholecystectomy (ELC) over delayed laparoscopic cholecystectomy (DLC).

Keywords Acute cholecystitis • Laparoscopic cholecystectomy • Management • Timing

The question of optimal timing of any operation necessarily involves an understanding of the natural history of the disease and reference time points in its clinical course. Acute calculous cholecystitis begins with cystic duct obstruction by a gallstone. Persistence of the obstruction leads to distension of the gallbladder, edema in the gallbladder wall, inflammation in the gallbladder wall and adjacent tissues. After 72 h the inflamed tissue becomes thickened, more vascular and adherent to surrounding structures making dissection in the hepatocystic triangle more difficult. Delaying cholecystectomy for a period of 6 weeks or longer results in the formation of fibrotic adhesions in the hepatocystic triangle distorting the anatomy and complicating dissection. The question of timing of operation also requires agreement about a specific clinical event that defines the start of the disease process. Various studies use different clinical events, such as the onset of symptoms reported by the patient

S.G. Wyers (✉)
Section of General Surgery, University of Chicago Medicine, MC5031, 5841 S. Maryland Avenue, Chicago, IL 60637, USA
e-mail: swyers@surgery.bsd.uchicago.edu

J.M. Millis, J.B. Matthews (eds.), *Difficult Decisions in Hepatobiliary and Pancreatic Surgery*, Difficult Decisions in Surgery: An Evidence-Based Approach, DOI 10.1007/978-3-319-27365-5_17

or admission to the hospital, as surrogate starting points for comparison. This variability complicates comparison of the available studies and limits the ability to make recommendations for optimal timing of laparoscopic cholecystectomy.

The rationale for delayed surgery is based on the observation that acute inflammation may lead to increased risk of surgical complications. This rationale was reinforced in the early years after laparoscopic cholecystectomy was developed. While the benefits of laparoscopic cholecystectomy (decreased hospital stay, decreased overall morbidity, earlier return to full activity etc.) were obvious in comparison to open surgery [1], surgery in the setting of acute inflammation led to higher rates of conversion to open operation [2] and rates of common bile duct injury greater than those in the era of open cholecystectomy for acute cholecystitis [3]. In the early years of laparoscopic cholecystectomy, acute cholecystitis was considered a relative contraindication [4]. While later prospective trials showed early laparoscopic cholecystectomy to be as safe as open cholecystectomy for acute cholecystitis [5], most surgeons continued to opt for initial conservative treatment and delayed laparoscopic cholecystectomy. As late as 2004 surveys of practice patterns in Britain and the United States showed that only 20–30 % of patients with acute cholecystitis were operated on in the early phase [6, 7]. While the rate of bile duct injury has decreased with time, it has not fallen to the rates reported in the open era [8]. Common bile duct injury remains the most significant surgical complication of laparoscopic cholecystectomy.

Retrospective Studies

The rationale for early laparoscopic cholecystectomy for acute cholecystitis is supported by a growing amount of evidence from retrospective studies. First, early surgery avoids the risks to the patient of gallstone related complications that the wait for a delayed operation assumes. Cheruvu and Eyre-Brook showed that 18.5 % of patients with acute cholecystitis required readmission to the hospital in the first 6 weeks after their initial presentation [9]. These risks only grow with the longer operation is postponed. A recent Canadian study [10] followed a cohort of over 10,000 patients who did not undergo cholecystectomy on their first admission for acute cholecystitis. The probability of a gallstone related complication at 6 weeks, 12 weeks, and 1 year after discharge was 14 %, 19 %, and 29 % respectively. Of these 30 % were for biliary tract obstruction or pancreatitis. Second, retrospective studies from large databases have indicated that early laparoscopic cholecystectomy is as safe and effective as delayed surgery. In a retrospective cohort study of over 14,000 patients [11] early cholecystectomy was associated with a lower risk of common bile duct injury and of common bile duct injury or death than delayed cholecystectomy. The rate of conversion from laparoscopic to open operation was no different in the early group (11 %) and in the delayed group (10 %). Furthermore, hospital stay was 2 days shorter for the early surgery group. Third, retrospective studies suggest that the sooner laparoscopic cholecystectomy is performed during

Table 17.1 Characteristics of prospective randomized controlled trials comparing Early Laparoscopic Cholecystectomy (ELC) to Delayed Laparoscopic Cholecystectomy (DLC)

Authors (Ref.)	Year	Single or multicenter	Number patients total (ELC:DLC)	Average age (years)	Female (%)
Gutt et al. [14]	2013	Multicenter	618 (304:314)	56.2	58.7
Macafee et al. [15][a]	2009	Single	72 (36:36)	52.5	65.2
Yadav et al. [16]	2009	Single	50 (25:25)	41	76
Kolla et al. [17]	2004	Single	40 (20:20)	40	80
Johannson et al.[18]	2003	Single	145 (74:71)	57	60
Davila et al. [19]	1999	Single	63 (27:36)	56	71.4
Lai et al. [20]	1998	Single	104 (53:51)	56	63.5
Lo et al. [21]	1998	Single	86 (45:41)	60	43.3

[a]The study by Macafee et al. does not furnish outcomes of interest for this review

the initial hospitalization the more favorable the outcomes. In a recent retrospective analysis from Switzerland of 4,113 patients [12] immediate surgery was found to have statistically significant advantages in conversion and reoperation rates, postoperative complications, and length of hospital stay compared to delayed cholecystectomy 1–6 days after hospital admission. Brooks et al. reviewed the course of 5,268 patients in the American College of Surgeons National Surgical Quality Improvement Program database [13]. Patients who underwent operation later in the course of admission (>24 h) had greater risk of open operation and longer postoperative and overall lengths of hospitalization.

Prospective Studies

A search of the Medline database from 1987 to the present as well as a review of the recent literature produces eight prospective randomized controlled clinical trials which compare early laparoscopic cholecystectomy (ELC) to delayed laparoscopic cholecystectomy (DLC) in the setting of calculous acute cholecystitis [14–21]. All of prospective surgical trials reviewed here suffer from the inability to blind participants and investigators (Table 17.1).

The ACDC (Acute Cholecystitis-early laparoscopic surgery versus antibiotic therapy and Delayed elective Cholecystectomy) trial by Gutt et al. [14] is larger than the remaining studies combined. It specifically addresses the question of immediate (<24 h) laparoscopic cholecystectomy vs. delayed (>7 days) laparoscopic cholecystectomy.

The variable criteria used by the studies to define the timing of early and delayed cholecystectomy are given in Table 17.2.

Not all of the studies measured the same primary and secondary outcomes. All studies (except Macafee [15]) reported quantitative outcome data for mortality, morbidity, conversion to open operation and hospital stay. Bile duct injury was

Table 17.2 Timing of Early Laparoscopic Cholecystectomy (ELC) and Timing of Delayed Laparoscopic Cholecystectomy (DLC)

Study	Year	Timing of ELC	Timing of DLC
Gutt	2013	<24 h from admission	7–45 days
Macafee	2009	<4 days from admission	3 months
Yadav	2009	<4 days	6–8 weeks
Kolla	2004	<4 days	6–12 weeks
Johannson	2003	<7 days	6–8 weeks
Davila	1999	<4 days	8 weeks
Lai	1998	<7 days	6–8 weeks
Lo	1998	<7 days	13 weeks

Table 17.3 Outcomes measured in the prospective randomized trials of ELC vs. DLC

Study	Mor-tality	Morbi-dity	CBD injury	Conversion to open	Operative time	Failure of conservative therapy	Hospital stay	Hospital costs
Gutt	x	x	x	x		x	x	x
Yadav	x	x		x	x		x	
Kolla	x	x		x	x		x	
Johannson	x	x		x	x		x	
Davila	x	x		x			x	
Lai	x	x		x	x		x	
Lo	x	x		x	x		x	

included in the morbidity for all studies and as a primary outcome in one. Most studies reported outcomes for operative time. Only one [14] examined hospital cost (Table 17.3).

Mortality The only deaths reported in the seven trials were in the largest trial [14]. There was one death in both the ELC (.3 %) and DLC (.3 %) groups. There were no deaths reported in the smaller trials.

Common Bile Duct Injury In total in the seven trials above, there were three common bile duct injuries. One was in the ELC group (1/523, .2 %) and two were in the DLC groups (2/533, .4 %). In a recent meta-analysis of these seven trials [22] these small rates did not achieve statistical significance.

Other Morbidity The ACDC trial [14] showed significantly lower morbidity scores at 75 days and fewer adverse events in the ELC group compared to the DLC group. When combined with the other studies in a meta-analysis there was a trend, albeit not statistically significant, toward decreased morbidity favoring the ELC group [22].

Conversion to Open Operation The ACDC trial [14] showed no significant difference between the two groups with respect to conversion to open operation (ELC 30/304, 9.9 %: DLC 33/314, 11.9 % p=.44). A Cochrane meta-analysis of five of the six smaller trials also showed no significant difference in conversion rates between ELC and DLC [23].

Operation Time There was considerable heterogeneity in the six smaller trials. A meta-analysis of the six smaller studies showed a trend toward longer operating times in the ELC group [23]. This trend was not statistically significant.

Failure of Conservative Therapy (DLC) In the ACDC trial [14] change of antibiotics was necessary in 31 of 314 (9.9 %) patients; and, of these 31 patients premature surgery was necessary in 17 (54.8 %).

Hospital Length of Stay All seven of the trials showed significant reduction in total length of stay in the hospital. In the ACDC trial [14] the mean length of stay was 4.6 days less in the ELC group. This was a 50 % reduction in hospital stay.

Hospital Cost In the ACDC trial [14] the reduced hospital stay for the ELC group (<24 h) translated directly into reduced cost (approximately 3000€/case). This was the only prospective trial to evaluate cost.

Return to Work and Normal Activity Only one trial examined return to work and normal activity. The study by Lo et al. [21] showed that patients in the ELC group had shorter average total recuperation periods (7 days) and shorter average periods of time off work (11 days).

Summary and Recommendations

Early (<24 h) laparoscopic cholecystectomy has significant medical and socioeconomic benefits and is the recommended approach for low risk patients with acute cholecystitis. Recommendation Grade 1C. Both ELC and DLC have very low rates of mortality and common bile duct injury and, as a result, the prospective studies cited here are insufficiently powered to show superiority with regard to these outcomes. Given these low rates it has been estimated that prospective studies would require thousands to tens of thousands of patients in each arm in order to show significant differences in bile duct injury and mortality. The overall morbidity of ELC compared to DLC is not greater and in the ACDC trial is shown to be significantly less than DLC. The prospective studies demonstrate that ELC dramatically reduces the length of hospital stay and total hospital cost. For a disease as common as acute cholecystitis ELC offers significant reduction in direct hospital costs and improvement in hospital efficiency. Though only one trial demonstrated earlier return to work and normal activity with ELC, it stands to reason that the patients who avoid DLC have a shorter time to resolution of their illness overall given that morbidity does not increase with ELC. Further prospective studies may improve the strength of this recommendation.

A Personal View of the Data

It has been my practice to operate within 24 h on all patients with acute cholecystitis whose symptoms are of less than 72 h duration and who are candidates for general anesthesia. A more difficult decision is the management of patients whose symptoms have been present for more than 3–4 days prior to admission. (Most of the prospective studies cited above used symptoms of greater than 7 days duration prior to admission as an exclusion criterion.) For this group of patients a more nuanced approach is in order. The presence of other known high risk factors (male sex, a palpable inflammatory mass on physical exam, extensive upper abdominal surgery, morbid obesity or findings on imaging) would warrant a conservative approach in my view. The Tokyo Guidelines for the surgical management of acute cholecystitis is based on a clinical grading scale of the severity of the acute cholecystitis and endorses this nuanced approach in this group with Grade II (moderate) acute cholecystitis [24].

The studies reviewed above argue strongly that a policy of early laparoscopic cholecystectomy should be adopted more broadly in acute cholecystitis. This should be undertaken with renewed dedication to what Strasberg has called a "culture of safety" [25]. Whether operating for biliary colic or acute cholecystitis, I dissect the hepatocystic triangle to "the critical view of safety" which has been well defined in the literature [26]. If inflammation prohibits dissection to the "critical view of safety", cholangiography under fluoroscopy is my next step. If this fails to clarify the anatomy or reveals an injury I convert to open operation. Conversion to open operation should never be viewed as a complication but rather a triumph of good judgment over technical ability. Given the marked improvement in laparoscopic cameras, angled lenses, and monitors in the past 25 years, visualization does not necessarily improve with conversion – except in one very important respect; there is improved ability to appreciate three dimensional anatomic relationships. Way reviewed common bile duct injuries by experienced surgeons and attributed them to cognitive visual spatial errors [27]. Most bile duct injuries are not recognized in the operating room; therefore, most are due to misidentification. In a difficult laparoscopic or open case I don't hesitate to get a "second set of eyes" from an experienced colleague if one is available. Conversion to open operation allows direct palpation to assist the dissection in densely inflamed tissue. After conversion I will use these advantages to dissect to a critical view of safety. Only if this is unsuccessful do I use "top down" or "fundus first" approach. This also entails risk since the normal plane between the liver and gallbladder is frequently obliterated by the inflammation. Getting into the hepatic parenchyma from this approach can produce significant hemorrhage. This is the setup for coupling a bile duct injury with a vascular injury. Much better options to avoid this most severe combination of injures would be placement of an open cholecystostomy tube or partial cholecystectomy with extraction of stones and placement of a drain.

Other than the high risk situations described above, I reserve delayed laparoscopic cholecystectomy for patients whose comorbidities place them at high risk for general anesthesia (e.g. ASA class 4 or 5) or whose symptoms are of greater than 7 days duration. In addition to intravenous antibiotics percutaneous cholecystomy tubes may be used in this group of patients. While there are still clinical situations which warrant delayed laparoscopic cholecystectomy, in my experience, this often results in the performance of a difficult operation 6 weeks later in a patient who is better prepared for the operating room.

References

1. The Southern Surgeons Club. A prospective analysis of 1518 laparoscopic cholecystectomies. The Southern Surgeons Club. N Engl J Med. 1991;324(16):1073–8.
2. Cheema S, Brannigan AE, Johnson S, Delaney PV, Grace PA. Timing of laparoscopic cholecystectomy in acute cholecystitis. Ir J Med Sci. 2003;172(3):128–31.
3. Richardson MC, Bell G, Fullarton GM. Incidence and nature of bile duct injuries following laparoscopic cholecystectomy an audit of 5913 cases. West of Scotland Laparoscopic Cholecystectomy Audit Group. Br J Surg. 1996;83(10):1356–60.
4. Wilson P, Leese T, Morgan WP, Kelly JF, Brigg JK. Elective laparoscopic cholecystectomy for "all comers". Lancet. 1991;338(8770):795–7.
5. Kiviluoto J, Siren P, Luukkonen P, Kivilaakso E. Randomised trial of laparoscopic versus open cholecystectomy for acute and gangrenous cholecystitis. Lancet. 1998;351(9099):321–5.
6. Livingston EH, Rege RV. A nationwide study of conversion from laparoscopic to open cholecystectomy. Am J Surg. 2004;188(3):205–11.
7. Senapati PS, Bhattarcharya D, Harinath G, Ammori BJ. A survey of the timing and approach to the surgical management of cholelithiasis in patients with acute biliary pancreatitis and acute cholecystitis in the UK. Ann R Coll Surg Engl. 2003;85(3):306–12.
8. Dolan JP, Diggs BS, Sheppard BC, Hunter JG. Ten-year trend in the national volume of bile duct injuries requiring operative repair. Surg Endosc. 2005;19(7):967–73.
9. Cheruvu CV, Eyre-Brooke IA. Consequences of a prolonged wait before gallbladder surgery. Ann R Coll Surg Engl. 2002;84(1):20–2.
10. deMestral C, Rotstein OD, Laupacis A, Hoch JS, Zagorski B, Nathens AB. A population-based analysis of the clinical course of 10,304 patients with acute cholecystitis, discharged without cholecystectomy. J Trauma Acute Care Surg. 2013;74(1):26–30; discussion 30–1.
11. deMestral C, Rotstein OD, Laupacis A, Hoch JS, Zagorski B, Alali AS, Nathens AB. Comparative outcomes of early and delayed cholecystectomy for acute cholecystitis: a population-based propensity score analysis. Ann Surg. 2014;259(1):10–5.
12. Banz V, Gsponer T, Candinas D, Guller U. Population based analysis of 4113 patients with acute cholecystitis: defining the optimal time point for laparoscopic cholecystectomy. Ann Surg. 2011;254(6):964–70.
13. Brooks KR, Scarborough JE, Vaslef SN, Shapiro ML. No need to wait: an analysis of the timing of cholecystectomy during admission for acute cholecystitis using the American College of Surgeons National Quality Improvement Program database. J Trauma Acute Care Surg. 2013;74(1):167–73.
14. Gutt CN, Enke J, Koninger J, Harnoss JC, Weigand K, Kipfmuller, Schunter O, Gotze T, Golling MT, Menges M, Klar E, Feilhauer K, Zoller WG, Ridwelski K, Ackmann S, Baron A, Schon MR, Seitz HK, Daniel D, Stremmel W, Buchler MW. Acute Cholecystitis: early versus delayed cholecystectomy, a multicenter randomized trial (ACDC study NCT00447304). Ann Surg. 2013;258(3):385–93.
15. Macafee DA, Humes DJ, Bouliotis G, Beckingham IJ, Whynes DK, Lobo DN. Prospective randomized trial using cost-utility analysis of early versus delayed laproscopic cholecystectomy for acute gallbladder disease. Br J Surg. 2009;96(9):1031–40.

16. Yadav RP, Adhikary S, Agrawal CS, Bhattarai B, Gupta RK, Ghimire A. A comparative study of early vs. delayed laparoscopic cholecystectomy in acute cholecystitis. Kathmandu Univ Med J (KUMJ). 2009;7(25):16–20.
17. Kolla SB, Aggarwal S, Kumar A, Kumar R, Chumber S, Parshad R, et al. Early v. delayed laparoscopic cholecystectomy for acute cholecystitis. Surg Endosc. 2004;18:1323–7.
18. Johannson M, Thune A, Blomquist LN, Lundell L. Management of acute cholecystitis in the laparoscopic era: results of a prospective, randomized clinical trial. J Gastrointest Surg. 2003;7(5):642–5.
19. Davila D, Manares C, Picho ML, Albors P, Cardenas E, Fuster E, et al. Experience in treatment (early vs. delayed) of acute cholecystitis via laparoscopy. Cir Esp. 1999;66 Suppl 1:233.
20. Lai PBS, Kwong KH, Leung KL. Randomized trial of early versus delayed laparoscopic cholecystectomy for acute cholecystitis. Br J Surg. 1998;85(6):764–7.
21. Lo C, Liu C, Fan S, Lai ECS, Wong J. Prospective randomized trial of early versus delayed laparoscopic cholecystectomy for acute cholecystitis. Ann Surg. 1998;227(4):461–7.
22. Zhou MW, Gu XD, Xiang JB, Chen ZY. Comparison of clinical safety and outcomes of early versus delayed laparoscopic cholecystectomy for acute cholecystitis: a meta-analysis. Sci World J. 2014:274516.
23. Gurusamy KS, Davidson C, Gluud C, Davidson BR. Early versus delayed laparoscopic cholecystectomy for people with acute cholecystitis. Cochrane Database Syst Rev. 2013;6, CD005440.
24. Yamashita Y, Takada T, Strasberg SM, Pitt HA, Gouma DJ, Buchler MW, Gomi H, Dervenis C, Windsor JA, Kim SW, deSantibanes E, Padbury R, Chen XP, Chan AC, Fan ST, Jagannath P, Mayumi T, Yoshida M, Miura F, Tsuyuguchi T, Itoi T, Supe AN, Tokyo Guidelines Revision Committee. J Hepatobiliary Pancreatol Sci. 2013;20(1):89–96.
25. Strasberg SM. Biliary injury in laparoscopic surgery: part 2. Changing the culture of cholecystectomy. J Am Coll Surg. 2005;201(4):604–11.
26. Strasberg SM, Brunt LM. Rationale and use of the critical view of safety in laparoscopic cholecystectomy. J Am Coll Surg. 2010;211(1):132–8.
27. Way LW, Stewart L, Gantert W, Liu K, Lee CM, Whang K, Hunter JG. Causes and prevention of laparoscopic bile duct injuries: analysis of 252 cases from a human factors and cognitive psychology perspective. Ann Surg. 2003;237(4):460–9.

Chapter 18
Primary Closure or T-Tube Drainage After Open or Laparoscopic Common Bile Duct Exploration?

Ezra N. Teitelbaum, Anthony D. Yang, and David M. Mahvi

Abstract Common bile duct exploration (CBDE) is an operation that can be performed either laparoscopically or open in order to treat choledocholithiasis by removing stones from the common bile duct. CBDE can be performing via either a transcystic approach or a transcholedochal one, in which an incision (or choledochotomy) is made directly into the common bile duct in order to access the stones within it. Traditionally this cholecdochotomy have been closed around an external drain, or "T-tube", at the end of CBDE operations, in order to drain the biliary system and allow access for future interventions should the need arise. However, recent data suggesting that primary closure of the choledochotomy may in fact be a superior technique have challenged the surgical dogma of routine T-tube placement after CBDE.

In this chapter we summarize and evaluate the available evidence comparing T-tube drainage with primary choledochotomy closure after CBDE. Six randomized trials have compared these strategies after open CBDE, and four such trials have been performed for laparoscopic CBDE. The existing literature mostly examines perioperative and short-term postoperative outcomes, such as operative time, 30-day postoperative morbidity and mortality, hospital length of stay, and need for re-interventions during the immediate postoperative period. Long-term implications of using or foregoing T-tube drainage have not been as well studied.

Based on these studies, there is a high level of evidence that primary choledochotomy closure after CBDE (both open and laparoscopic) results in shorter operative times and shorter hospital length of stay when compared with t-tube drainage. There is moderate evidence that primary closure and t-tube drainage after CBDE result in equivalent rates of serious complications in the perioperative period. Due to insufficient data, there is a very low level of evidence that the two techniques result in equivalent rates of long-term recurrent choledocholithiasis and biliary stricture. Based on the sum of this evidence, we make a moderate strength recom-

---

E.N. Teitelbaum • A.D. Yang • D.M. Mahvi (✉)
Department of Surgery, Northwestern University,
251 E. Huron St., Galter Room 3-710, Chicago, IL 60611, USA
e-mail: dmahvi@nm.org

J.M. Millis, J.B. Matthews (eds.), *Difficult Decisions in Hepatobiliary and Pancreatic Surgery*, Difficult Decisions in Surgery: An Evidence-Based Approach, DOI 10.1007/978-3-319-27365-5_18

mendation that primary choledochotomy closure should be the preferred technique in uncomplicated cases of both open and laparoscopic CBDE.

Keywords Common bile duct exploration • Choledocholithiasis • T-tube • Choledochotomy closure • Bile duct surgery • Hepatobiliary

Introduction

Choledocholithiasis, or stones within the common bile duct, occurs in between 3.4 and 17 % of patients with symptomatic gallstone disease [1, 2]. Currently, two standard-of-care approaches exist for treating patients with choledocholithiasis. The first involves performing an endoscopic retrograde cholangiopancreatography (ERCP) in order to remove the stone or stones from the common bile duct. However, with this approach, a cholecystectomy must also be subsequently performed in order to eliminate the source of the stones and thus prevent disease recurrence. Alternatively, a surgical common bile duct exploration (CBDE) can be performed in either an open or laparoscopic fashion at the time of cholecystectomy, in order treat the patient's current problem and prevent future episodes, all with a single procedure. CBDE was first performed in 1890 by Courvoisier and in the early 1990s with the widespread adoption of laparoscopic cholecystectomy, CBDE was first performed in a laparoscopic, minimally invasive fashion. CBDE at the time of cholecystectomy, especially when performed laparoscopically, has been shown to result in a shorter hospital length of stay, less hospital costs, and possibly fewer complications, when compared with the two-stage approach of ERCP and cholecystectomy [3, 4].

Two primary methods exist for performing CBDE: transcystic and transcholedochal. In the transcystic approach, a flexible choledochoscope or fluoroscopically-directed instruments are inserted through a ductotomy in the cystic duct (similar to that through which a standard intraoperative cholangiogram is performed). In the transcholedochal method, a longitudinal ductotomy is made into the common duct itself, through which a choledochoscope and/or other instruments are passed in order to capture the stones within. At the conclusion of a *transcholedochal* CBDE, the choledochotomy can be dealt with in two ways: (1) it can be closed primarily or (2) a "T-tube" can be placed into the choledochotomy, the ductomy then closed around the tube, and opposite end of the tube externalized to bag drainage (Fig. 18.1).

Placing a T-tube drain after CBDE offers several theoretical advantages and is still considered to be the standard of care by many surgeons. A T-tube allows for external drainage of the biliary system in the case of residual biliary obstruction from retained stones, ampullary edema, or stenosis. Additionally, the biliary system can be instrumented through the T-tube under fluoroscopic guidance, in order to treat the postoperative conditions mentioned previously without the need for additional procedures or operations. Finally, a T-tube is thought to prevent stricture of

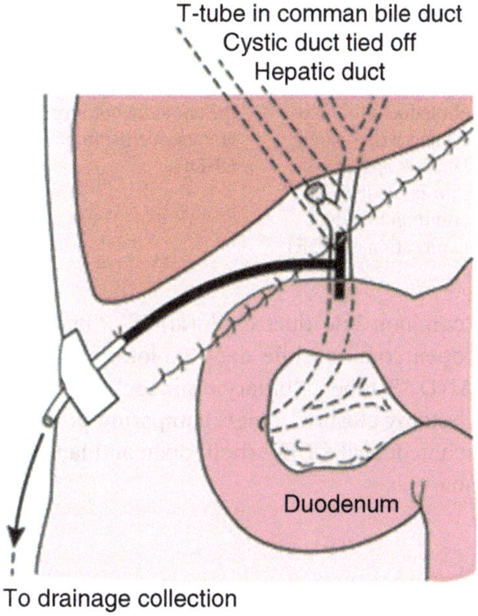

Fig. 18.1 A cartoon depicting the anatomy of placement of a T-tube after open transcholedochal CBDE and concurrent cholecystectomy for treatment of choledocholithiais. The opposite end of the tube exits through a stab-incision in the abdominal wall and is placed either to bag drainage or occluded (Figure used with permission from O'Toole MT [21])

the common bile duct, although this is a theoretical advantage without comparative data to either support or refute it.

Conversely, T-tube placement at the conclusion of an otherwise successful CBDE carries its own set of risks. The tube offers an avenue for infection of the biliary system and it can become dislodged prematurely in the postoperative period, resulting in a biliary leak. A leak can also occur when the T-tube is eventually removed intentionally, if an adequate tract to the skin has not formed.

Since T-tube drainage after CBDE confers both potential advantages and disadvantages, this operative strategy has been compared with primary choledochotomy closure in several well-designed studies. This chapter will deal exclusively with the clinical decision of whether to place a T-tube or perform a primary choledocotomy closure after transcholedochal CBDE. We will discuss the results of trials examining these alternative operative strategies, summarize the existing evidence, make recommendations regarding the evidence supporting the best answer to this clinical question, and discuss the limitations to those recommendations.

Search Strategy

A search of English language publications was performed to assess existing evidence comparing the use of T-tube drainage and primary closure after CBDE using the PICO outline shown in Table 18.1. Databases searched were PubMed, Ovid MEDLINE, and Cochrane Evidence Based Medicine. Search terms used were

Table 18.1 PICO terms used in defining the clinical question and search strategy

P (Patients)	I (Intervention)	C (Comparator)	O (Outcomes)
Patients with choledocholithiasis treated with open or laparoscopic transcholedochal common bile duct exploration (CBDE)	Primary closure of the choledochotomy at the conclusion of CBDE	T-tube placement through the choledochotomy for postoperative biliary drainage at the conclusion of CBDE	Operative time, mortality, serious morbidity, hospital length of stay, recurrent choledocholithiasis, biliary stricture

"common bile duct exploration", "laparoscopic common bile duct exploration", "open common bile duct exploration", "choledocholithiasis", "transcholedochal" AND "T-tube", "biliary drainage", "tube drainage", "primary closure", "choledochotomy closure". Trials comparing primary closure and T-tube drainage after transcholedochal CBDE (both open and laparoscopic) were included in the subsequent analysis.

Results

Six randomized trials including a total of 359 patients have compared the strategies of primary closure versus T-tube drainage after open CBDE [5–10]. Four such trials with 399 total patients have been performed for laparoscopic CBDE [11–14]. Additionally two Cochrane Group meta-analyses have been performed which aggregated and analyzed these studies (one for open CBDE [15] and one for laparoscopic [16]). The existing literature mostly examines perioperative and short-term postoperative outcomes, such as operative time, 30-day postoperative morbidity and mortality, hospital length of stay, and need for re-interventions during the immediate postoperative period. Long-term implications of using or foregoing T-tube drainage have not been as well studied. The following sections discuss the available evidence with respect to specific outcomes after both open and laparoscopic CBDE. Tables 18.2 and 18.3 summarize these quantitative comparison data comparing primary closure to T-tube drainage for open and laparoscopic CBDE respectively.

Operative Time

Placement of a T-tube after CBDE, whether open or laparoscopic, requires several discrete steps: the limbs of the t-tube are fashioned into the proper lengths and configuration, the tube is inserted into the common ductotomy, the ductotomy is partially sutured closed so that the T-tube is secured in position but not so tightly that it cannot eventually be removed, and the external portion of the tube must be brought

Table 18.2 Comparison of compiled data from randomized trials comparing primary closure versus T-tube drainage for *open* CBDE [15]

Outcomes	Primary closure	T-tube drainage
Operative time (mins)	88*	117
Mortality (%)	0.6	1.2
Serious morbidity (%)	6.6	14.5
Hospital stay (days)	9.1*	13.8

*p<0.05 in favor of primary closure

Table 18.3 Comparison of compiled data from randomized trials comparing primary closure versus T-tube drainage for *laparoscopic* CBDE [16]

Outcomes	Primary closure	T-tube drainage
Operative time (mins)	106*	127
Mortality (%)	0	0
Serious morbidity (%)	6.1	9.7
Hospital stay (days)	3.9*	7.2

*p<0.05 in favor of primary closure

out through to the skin. This is opposed to the strategy of primary closure, during which the common ductotomy is simply sutured closed in order to conclude the procedure.

Accordingly, it seems intuitive that primary closure should result in shorter operative times, and this appears to have been borne out in the randomized studies that have compared the two approaches for both laparoscopic and open CBDE. Of the randomized trails performed for open CBDE, only one compared operative times, and found primary closure to be faster by 28 min [5]. The evidence for laparoscopic CBDE is more robust, with all four randomized trials comparing operative times. All of these studies demonstrated shorter operative times in their primary closure patients, with similar mean differences between the groups ranging from 17 to 26 min [11–14].

Perioperative Mortality and Morbidity

When performed in experienced hands, both open and laparoscopic CBDE carry a very low risk of perioperative mortality. As such, it is not surprising that even when the results of all randomized trials are aggregated, there are no differences in mortality between primary closure and T-tube drainage. In studies of open CBDE the aggregate perioperative mortality with t-tube drainage was 1.2 %, as opposed to 0.6 % with primary closure [15], and this difference was not statistically significant. In the four randomized trials comparing these techniques for laparoscopic CBDE, there were no perioperative deaths among the 399 patients, which speaks to both the safety and physiologic benefits of a laparoscopic approach.

Serious morbidity has also not been conclusively shown to differ between primary ductotomy closure and T-tube drainage, although there may be an advantage to primary closure in this regard. A meta-analysis of trials comparing the approaches after open CBDE, found a serious morbidity rate of 14.5 % after T-tube drainage, as opposed to 6.6 % after primary closure, although this difference narrowly missed obtaining statistical significance. Similarly, when the trials comparing the approaches during laparoscopic CBDE were analyzed, the overall serious complication rate was 11.3 % in the T-tube group versus 6.1 % in the primary closure patients; however, this difference was also not statistically significant.

A closer examination of the results of these trials reveals that a number of these serious complications were directly related to use of the T-tube, and thus these trials may simply not be adequately powered to detect the added risk that T-tube placement confers (i.e., a Type II statistical error is present). For example, patients in several trials required reoperation for replacement of prematurely dislodged T-tubes, in some cases leading to bile peritonitis. Also, bile leakage after T-tube removal occurred in approximately 1–2 % of patients, which usually required either replacement of another tube through the existing tract, percutaneous drainage of a bile collection, or reoperation for drainage and tube replacement. This is in contrast to the primary closure group, in which bile leakage from the choledochotomy closure occurred in less than 1 % of patients, and could almost uniformly be treated with ERCP sphincterotomy and/or stenting without the need for reoperation [15]. Therefore, even when a "serious morbidity" occurs after CBDE with primary closure, it appears to result in less severe consequences for the patient when contrasted with complications directly related to the use of a T-tube.

Hospital Length of Stay

The use of a T-tube adds another clinical variable, as the drain outputs must be tracked, the decision to place the tube to drainage versus clamping is weighed, and routine and/or clinically-prompted T-tube cholangiograms are often obtained in order to evaluate for biliary obstruction and/or leakage. Additionally, patients must be educated regarding the self-care and management of the tube at home prior to leaving the hospital. All of these factors can potentially lead to longer hospital length of stay in the perioperative period, and this has been reflected in the literature examining both open and laparoscopic CBDE. In trials comparing approaches for open CBDE, primary closure resulted in a marked advantage over T-tube drainage, with a mean difference in hospital length of stay of 4.7 days [15]. This superiority of primary closure was also present to a lesser extent in the trials involving laparoscopic CBDE, with a mean difference of 3.3 days. The smaller difference in length of stay after laparoscopic CBDE is likely due to the overall decreased length of stay after laparoscopic, when compared with open, surgery then to a less significant advantage of primary closure over t-tube drainage. Additionally, one study compared time to return to work, and found patients undergoing primary closure did so 8 days earlier than those with T-tubes [13].

Long-Term Outcomes

Most trials have focused on perioperative outcomes when comparing the strategies of primary closure and T-tube drainage after CBDE, but some longer-term outcomes data does exist. One of the theoretical reasons behind the use of a T-tube is to facilitate biliary access in the case of retained stones and/or prevent biliary stricture. However, in the limited outcomes data available, neither of these potential complications appear to be either frequent or lessened in severity by the use of T-tube drainage at the time of initial CBDE. In experienced hands, the rate of a retained common duct stones is less than 5 % for both open and laparoscopic CBDE. Additionally, missed stones are usually small, and thus are almost universally retrievable via ERCP, obviating the need for T-tube access to the biliary system in the rare instance that they do occur. In the three open and one laparoscopic trials that evaluated longer-term outcomes at 6-months to 2.5 years, no patients in either arm (primary closure or t-tube drainage) had either recurrence of choledocholithiasis or new-onset of biliary stricture [5, 6, 10, 11]. There are no studies examining outcomes beyond 2.5 years.

Recommendations Based on the Data

1. Primary choledochotomy closure after CBDE (both open and laparoscopic) results in shorter operative times and shorter hospital length of stay when compared with t-tube drainage – *HIGH level of evidence*
2. Primary closure and t-tube drainage after CBDE result in equivalent rates of serious complications in the perioperative period – *MODERATE level of evidence*
3. Primary closure and t-tube drainage after CBDE result in equivalent rates of long-term recurrent choledocholithiasis and biliary stricture – *VERY LOW level of evidence*
4. Primary choledochotomy closure should be the preferred technique in uncomplicated cases of both open and laparoscopic CBDE – *MODERATE strength recommendation*

Potential Exceptions to Recommendations

As with any surgical disease and operation, each patient undergoing CBDE for choledocholithiasis must be evaluated individually, and various factors must be taken into account when determining the most beneficial approach to their condition. That is to say, despite our moderate strength recommendation of the use of primary closure, there are many instances in which T-tube drainage might be the superior option for a given patient. For example, if a completion cholangiogram at the conclusion of a CBDE procedure demonstrates poor flow of contrast into the duodenum despite an absence of stones in the common bile duct, edema or stricture at the Ampulla of Vater may be present. In this case, placing a T-tube would be the best option, as both drainage and instrumentation of the biliary system will likely be necessary in the immediate postoperative period. Alternatively, if a patient undergoing CBDE has a prior Roux-en-Y gastric bypass that precludes future ERCP, the safest option may be to place a T-tube, so that the biliary system can be accessed easily in the case of a retained stone or bile leakage. Finally, the lack of data regarding the incidence of biliary stricture beyond 2.5 years should also be taken into account when making the decision for or against T-tube placement at the time of CBDE.

Utilization of CBDE and Future Directions for Training

While it is important to study technical considerations such as T-tube drainage versus primary closure, CBDE still remains an extremely underutilized method for treating common bile duct stones. This remains true despite the advantages of CBDE (particularly laparoscopic CBDE) compared to ERCP [3, 4]. For example, a study examining data from the United States National Inpatient Sample found that of patients admitted to hospitals with a diagnosis of choledocholithiais, 93 % were treated with ERCP as opposed to 7 % with CBDE [17].

Several reasons likely exist for this disparity including: lack of CBDE instrument availability, lack of familiarity with the procedure on the part of surgeons and support staff, and relatively poor financial reimbursement for surgeons. The lack of exposure to, and training in, CBDE during surgical residency is almost certainly a central barrier to more widespread adoption of CBDE for treatment of choledocholithiasis. A review of residents' operative case logs showed that graduating chief residents had performed a mean of 1.7 open and 0.7 laparoscopic CBDE procedures during their entire residency, with a mode of 1 and 0 respectively [18]. This limited experience is not sufficient for gaining competency with either primary choledochotomy closure or T-tube placement, let alone the remainder of the skills required to perform CBDE.

In order to address this lack of exposure to CBDE during residency and hopefully increase the utilization of procedure at our institution, we have developed a laparoscopic CBDE simulator for training and evaluation purposes [19]. The simulator recreates the three visualization modalities involved in the operation (laparoscopic, endoscopic, and fluoroscopic), and trainees are able to perform a complete simulated procedure via either a transcystic or transcholedochal approach. We have been able to demonstrate that a technical curriculum based around practice on the simulator is able to consistently train senior surgery residents to the level of a predetermined "mastery standard" over the course of a two-month rotation [20]. Hopefully, similar training initiates can be developed nationally, with the goal of increasing the utilization of CBDE and ultimately improving patient outcomes. If CBDE becomes more commonly used by surgeons for the treatment of choledocholithisis, the question of whether to perform a primary choledochotomy closure or leave a T-tube for biliary drainage will become even more clinically relevant and important.

References

1. Houdart R, Perniceni T, Darne B, Salmeron M, Simon JF. Predicting common bile duct lithiasis: determination and prospective validation of a model predicting low risk. Am J Surg. 1995;170:38–43.
2. Collins C, Maguire D, Ireland A, Fitzgerald E, O'Sullivan GC. A prospective study of common bile duct calculi in patients undergoing laparoscopic cholecystectomy: natural history of choledocholithiasis revisited. Ann Surg. 2004;239:28–33.
3. Cuschieri A, Lezoche E, Morino M, et al. E.A.E.S. multicenter prospective randomized trial comparing two-stage vs single-stage management of patients with gallstone disease and ductal calculi. Surg Endosc. 1999;13:952–7.
4. Rogers SJ, Cello JP, Horn JK, et al. Prospective randomized trial of LC+LCBDE vs ERCP/S+LC for common bile duct stone disease. Arch Surg. 2010;145:28–33.
5. Marwah S, Singh I, Godara R, Sen J, Marwah N, Karwasra RK. Evaluation of primary duct closure vs T-tube drainage following choledochotomy. Indian J Gastroenterol. 2004;23:227–8.
6. Ambreen M, Shaikh AR, Jamal A, Qureshi JN, Dalwani AG, Memon MM. Primary closure versus T-tube drainage after open choledochotomy. Asian J Surg/Asian Surg Assoc. 2009;32:21–5.
7. Lygidakis NJ. Choledochotomy for biliary lithiasis: T-tube drainage or primary closure. Effects on postoperative bacteremia and T-tube bile infection. Am J Surg. 1983;146:254–6.
8. Makinen AM, Matikainen M, Nordback I. T-tube drainage is needed after routine common bile duct closure: results of a randomized trial. Surg Res Commun. 1989;6:299–302.
9. Payne RA, Woods WG. Primary suture or T-tube drainage after choledochotomy. Ann R Coll Surg Engl. 1986;68:196–8.
10. Williams JA, Treacy PJ, Sidey P, Worthley CS, Townsend NC, Russell EA. Primary duct closure versus T-tube drainage following exploration of the common bile duct. Aust N Z J Surg. 1994;64:823–6.
11. Dong ZT, Wu GZ, Luo KL, Li JM. Primary closure after laparoscopic common bile duct exploration versus T-tube. J Surg Res. 2014;189:249–54.
12. Zhang WJ, Xu GF, Wu GZ, Li JM, Dong ZT, Mo XD. Laparoscopic exploration of common bile duct with primary closure versus T-tube drainage: a randomized clinical trial. J Surg Res. 2009;157:e1–5.
13. Leida Z, Ping B, Shuguang W, Yu H. A randomized comparison of primary closure and T-tube drainage of the common bile duct after laparoscopic choledochotomy. Surg Endosc. 2008;22:1595–600.
14. El-Geidie AA. Is the use of T-tube necessary after laparoscopic choledochotomy? J Gastrointest Surg. 2010;14:844–8.
15. Gurusamy KS, Koti R, Davidson BR. T-tube drainage versus primary closure after open common bile duct exploration. Cochrane Database Syst Rev. 2013;6, CD005640.
16. Gurusamy KS, Koti R, Davidson BR. T-tube drainage versus primary closure after laparoscopic common bile duct exploration. Cochrane Database Syst Rev. 2013;6, CD005641.
17. Poulose BK, Arbogast PG, Holzman MD. National analysis of in-hospital resource utilization in choledocholithiasis management using propensity scores. Surg Endosc. 2006;20:186–90.
18. Helling TS, Khandelwal A. The challenges of resident training in complex hepatic, pancreatic, and biliary procedures. J Gastrointest Surg. 2008;12:153–8.

19. Santos BF, Reif TJ, Soper NJ, Nagle AP, Rooney DM, Hungness ES. Development and evaluation of a laparoscopic common bile duct exploration simulator and procedural rating scale. Surg Endosc. 2012;26:2403–15.
20. Teitelbaum EN, Soper NJ, Santos BF, et al. A simulator-based resident curriculum for laparoscopic common bile duct exploration. Surgery. 2014;156:880–7, 90–3.
21. O'Toole MT, editor. Miller-Keane encyclopedia and dictionary of medicine, nursing and allied health. 7th ed. Philadelphia: Saunders; 2003.

Chapter 19
Single-Incision or Multiport Laparoscopic Cholecystectomy

Bill Ran Luo and Nathaniel J. Soper

Abstract This chapter reviews the current body of literature comparing multi-port laparoscopic cholecystectomy versus single incision laparoscopic cholecystectomy; specifically differences between complications, conversion rates, pain, cosmesis, quality of life, cost, and rate of hernia formation.

Keywords Laparoscopic cholecystectomy • Single-incision • Multi-port • Morbidity • Pain • Cosmesis • Cost

Introduction

Laparoscopic cholecystectomy is one of the most common operations performed in the western world today. The standard of care for gallbladder removal prior to the 1980s was an open cholecystectomy, but with the acceptance of laparoscopic cholecystectomy as a standard technique in the 1990s, the world of minimally invasive surgery for gallbladder pathology expanded [2]. After an initial learning curve, laparoscopic cholecystectomy was demonstrated to have an overall complication rate of less than 5 % with an established rate of common bile duct injury between 0.3 and 0.5 % [1]. Given the drive for surgeons to continue to innovate and create less invasive surgical techniques, single incision laparoscopic cholecystectomies have developed a large base of support. However, as standard multi-port laparoscopic cholecystectomy (MPLC) has such proven and safe results, single incision cholecystectomy naturally must be analyzed and dissected critically, to ensure that outcomes are cost effective, efficient, and, most importantly, safe for patients. These single incision approaches have multiple eponyms; including single incision

B.R. Luo • N.J. Soper (✉)
Department of Surgery, Northwestern Medicine,
251 E. Huron St. Galter 3-150, Chicago, IL 60611, USA
e-mail: nsoper@nmh.org

J.M. Millis, J.B. Matthews (eds.), *Difficult Decisions in Hepatobiliary and Pancreatic Surgery*, Difficult Decisions in Surgery: An Evidence-Based Approach, DOI 10.1007/978-3-319-27365-5_19

laparoscopic surgery (SILS), single port access (SPA), and laparo-endoscopic single site (LESS). In this chapter, we will abbreviate the single-incision laparoscopic cholecystectomy as SILC.

Search Strategy

A literature search of English language publications from 2000 to 2014 was used to identify published data on single incision and multi-port laparoscopic cholecystectomy comparative results in the adult population using the PICO outline. Databases searched were PubMed, Embase, Science Citation Index/Social sciences Citation Index and Cochrane Evidence Based Medicine. Terms used in the search were "single incision cholecystectomy", "SILS" "single access cholecystectomy", "SPA", "single port cholecystectomy", "laparoendoscopic single site cholecystectomy", "LESS", "multi-port laparoscopic cholecystectomy", "standard laparoscopic cholecystectomy", "conventional cholecystectomy", "conventional laparoscopic cholecystectomy" AND "cost" OR "pain" OR "morbidity" OR "mortality" OR "conversion" OR "conversion rate" OR "effectiveness" OR "operative time" OR "cosmesis" OR "hernia" OR "hernia rates" OR "complications" OR "admission" OR "re-admission" OR "outcomes" OR "randomized trials" OR "randomised trials" OR "prospective trials". Articles were excluded if they exclusively addressed open cholecystectomy, natural orifice (NOTES) cholecystectomy, robotic cholecystectomy, or pediatric patients. Ten randomized controlled trials, 11 retrospective studies, and 6 systematic reviews were included in our analysis. The data were classified using the GRADE system.

Results of Single Incision Laparoscopic Cholecystectomy Compared with Standard Multi-port Laparoscopic Cholecystectomy

Peri-operative Morbidity and Mortality

Laparoscopic cholecystectomy has evolved to be an operation that is safe for patients for both acute cholecystitis and in the elective setting, with low morbidity (3.1 %) and mortality (0.3 %) [1]. There have been no reported mortalities following SILC in any published studies [3–7, 10–25, 27, 30]. With analysis of all adverse events, the data favored MPLC, with an odds ratio of 1.14 (0.69–1.91) [27]. One meta-analysis that stratified expertise bias showed a difference in complications for SILC (5.35 %) versus conventional (3.79) in non-expert hands [31]. However, other studies showed either no difference or an improved overall complication rate for SILC [20, 30]. There were no differences for major biliary complications, which for SILC ranged from 0.3 to 0.5 % [8, 15, 28, 29, 31]. Bleeding risks appear to be equivalent between the two techniques, about 1 % in these studies [16, 20, 26], with one study showing a minimal favorability toward MPLC [27]. Periumbilical port site infections for SILC trended higher in some studies, but failed to reach statistical significance [20, 26]. **Based on the available randomized trials and meta-analyses – there is high level evidence that there is no difference in mortality, major complications, or biliary complications (Grade 1A recommendation that either SILC or MPLC are safe approaches), but there is low level evidence which suggests that there may be a small increase in adverse events and port site infections in SILC patients (Grade 2C recommendation in favor of MPLC).**

Conversion Rates

There were no differences between conventional and SILC in conversion rates to a laparotomy, with rates as low as 0.2 % [26, 31]. More likely is the conversion from SILC to MPLC, with variable rates of 0.2 % up to 8 %, but these conversions were proven to be safe in multiple studies [24, 27, 30]. **There is high level evidence that conversion from SILC to MPLC is safe, as well as high level evidence that rates of conversion to a laparotomy for both procedures are negligible and comparable in the elective setting. (Grade 1A recommendation that either SILC or MPLC are safe modalities).**

Cost

One of the largest prospective randomized trials comparing MPLC and SILC found significant increases in charges for SILC, specifically increased total hospital charges of $2,100, surgical equipment $1,700, operating room costs $913, and anesthesia costs $241 [19]. There were no differences in pharmacy, laboratory, recovery room, observation or ICU costs. These increases in costs were consistently higher for SILC in several other studies, although the increased costs ranged from $400 to 964 with some variability in significance [9, 12, 26]. Only one retrospective study analyzed cost, showing a slight increase in SILC patients, but only those that converted to MPLC. The rest of the large prospective randomized trials did not analyze the cost differences between the two. **There is moderate level evidence that SILC incurs more hospital costs when compared with MPLC. (Grade 1B recommendation in favor of MPLC.)**

Pain

Leung et al. demonstrated significantly higher level of pain in SILC group at post-operative day 1 and day 3. However, by post-operative week 1 the pain score became comparable [19]. Marks et al. demonstrated no difference in pain scores at 1 day, 1 week, and 2 weeks, but on day 3 and day 5 there was a statistically significant increase in pain scores in the SILC group [20]. Lai et al. reported no difference between the two groups 6 h postoperatively, but 7 days later the SILC group had significantly more pain [16]. Milas et al. showed high heterogeneity, with no statistical significance when it came to pain scores, but had a trend toward higher scores in SILC patients [31]. Trasuli et al. showed no significant difference in pain scores in the pooled data at any of the early time points out to 48 h. However, there was a small increase in conventional laparoscopy patients without statistical significance after 72 h [27]. Pisanu et al. found no statistical significance between pain scores at 6 h and 24 h post-operatively [26]. **There is moderate level evidence that there are higher pain scores in patients that undergo SILC (Grade 2B recommendation in favor of MPLC). There is also variability in the post-operative interval at which the difference in pain scores are reported.**

Cosmesis, Patient Satisfaction, and Quality of Life Scores

There is high variability between studies looking at patient satisfaction, cosmetic scores, and quality of life scores. Leung et al. showed equivalent quality of life scores at 1 week, 3 weeks and 6 months, and satisfaction scores were similar at 3 weeks and 6 months post-operatively [19]. Trasulli et al. found no significant difference in cosmetic scores in the early post-operative period, but at 3 months and 6 months there was a trend toward improved cosmetic scores in SILC [27]. Several other studies found slight differences in favor of SILC for cosmetic outcomes [26, 31]. **There is moderate level evidence demonstrating equivalent results for cosmetic outcomes, patient satisfaction scores, and quality of life scores when comparing SILC with MPLC. (Grade 1B recommendation that the modalities are similar.)**

Hernia Rates

There are no studies that compare the specific outcome variable of incisional hernia rates between SILC and MPLC. Most of the patients are small subsets from randomized studies, with inadequate power to reach statistical significance, even in pooled meta-analysis data. However, there are a few studies demonstrating a significant trend toward an increase in incisional hernia rates following cholecystectomy in the

SILC population [20, 27]. There are also other studies that show no significant differences between the two groups, but there may not be adequate long term followup to demonstrate a difference [18, 19, 21, 23]. **There is low level evidence suggesting that there may be an increased risk of incisional hernia formation after SILC cholecystectomy; however, long-term studies are necessary**. (**Grade 2C recommendation in favor of MPLC**.)

Recommendations

When compared with multi-port laparoscopic cholecystectomy, SILC has similar morbidity, conversion rates to open surgery, cosmesis, and quality of life. There are small increases in SILC for pain, cost, and possibly rates of post-operative incisional hernia formation. The current recommendation is that MPLC is still the standard of care for patients undergoing elective cholecystectomy.

1. In experienced hands, SILC and MPLC are equivalent with respect to mortality, major complications, and biliary complications (evidence quality high, strong recommendation).
2. SILC is associated with a small increase in minor adverse events, postoperative pain, port site infection, and hernia compared to MPLC (evidence quality low, weak recommendation).
3. Because SILC is more expensive without demonstrable improvement in safety, cosmesis, quality of life, or patient satisfaction, MPLC remains the preferred minimally invasive approach for routine cholecystectomy (evidence quality moderate, strong recommendation).

A Personal View of the Data

One of the major limitations of all of these studies is the state of the gallbladder pathology itself. To achieve homogenous patients the randomized trials have included only elective gallbladder pathology, usually symptomatic cholelithiasis or gallbladder polyps, without evidence of acute cholecystitis or other more complex conditions. Additional data need to be collected to establish the safety profile of SILC in acute cholecystitis. Cosmesis is difficult to interpret; patients that are more concerned with cosmetic appearance are more likely to seek out a SILC and may be more likely to enroll in a study where they could potentially be randomized to the SILC group, whereas patients who do not place a large emphasis on cosmesis might be more likely to opt out of the randomization. Costs may eventually become more in favor of SILC as dedicated SILS instrumentation is becoming more cost-effective to produce. Post-operative incisional hernia rates can only be truly studied if there is a standardization of technique for SILC platforms, conventional laparoscopic access (Hasson versus Veress), and extraction sites (umbilical versus epigastric), and be powered appropriately for this specific outcome variable. All of these are variables that can create bias or confounding factors. There also would need to be long term follow-up, but as demonstrated by most of the studies, the drop-out rates can reach up to 20 % even at 1 year post-operatively [20].

References

1. Ingrahm AM, Cohen ME, Ko CY, Hall BL. A current profile and assessment of North American cholecystectomy: results from the American College of Surgeons National Surgical Quality Improvement Program. J Am Coll Surg. 2010;211:176–86.
2. Soper NJ. Cholecystectomy: from Langenbuch to natural orifice transluminal endoscopic surgery. World J Surg. 2011;35(7):1422–7.
3. Brody F, Vaziri K, Kasza J, Edwards C. Single incision laparoscopic cholecystectomy. J Am Coll Surg. 2010;210(2):e9–13.
4. Valverde A. Single incision laparoscopic cholecystectomy using the SILS monotrocar. J Visc Surg. 2012;149:e38–43.

Retrospective Review

5. Podolsky ER, Currillo PG. Single port access (SPA) surgery – a 24 month experience. J Gastrointest Surg. 2010;14:759–67.
6. Rawlings A, Hodgett SE, Matthews BD, et al. Single incision laparoscopic cholecystectomy: initial experience with critical view of safety dissection and routine intraoperative cholangiography. J Am Coll Surg. 2010;211:1–7.
7. Love KM, Durham CA, Meara MP, Mays AC, Bower CE. Single-incision laparoscopic cholecystectomy: a cost comparison. Surg Endosc. 2011;25(5):1553–8.
8. Antoniou SA, Pointner R, Granderath FA. Single-incision laparoscopic cholecystectomy: a systematic review. Surg Endosc. 2011;25:367–77.
9. Beck C, Eakin J, Dettorre R, Renton D. Analysis of perioperative factors and cost comparison of single-incision and traditional multi-incision laparoscopic cholecystectomy. Surg Endosc. 2013;27(1):104–8.
10. Joseph S, Moore BT, Sorensen GB, et al. Single-incision laparoscopic cholecystectomy: a comparison with the gold standard. Surg Endosc. 2011;25:3008–15.
11. Vemulapalli P, Agaba EA, Camacho D. Single incision laparoscopic cholecystectomy: a single center experience. Int J Surg. 2011;9:410–3.
12. Chekan E, Moore M, Hunter TD, Gunnarsson C. Costs and clinical outcomes of conventional single port and micro-laparoscopic cholecystectomy. JSLS. 2013;17(1):30–45.
13. Feinberg EJ, Agaba E, Feinberg ML, Camacho D, Vemulapalli P. Single-incision laparoscopic cholecystectomy learning curve experience seen in a single institution. Surg Laparosc Endosc Percutan Tech. 2012;22:114–7.
14. Hwang HK, Choi SH, Kang CM, Lee WJ. Single-fulcrum laparoscopic cholecystectomy in uncomplicated gallbladder diseases: a retrospective comparative analysis with conventional laparoscopic cholecystectomy. Yonsei Med J. 2013;54(6):1471–7.
15. Hodgett SE, Hernandez JM, Morton CA, et al. Laparoendoscopic single site (LESS) cholecystectomy. J Gastrointest Surg. 2009;13:188–9.

Randomized Trials

16. Lai EC, Yang GP, Tang CN, et al. Prospective randomized comparative study of single incision laparoscopic cholecystectomy versus conventional four-port laparoscopic cholecystectomy. Am J Surg. 2011;202(3):254–8.
17. Aprea G, Coppola BE, Guida F, Masone S, Persico G. Laparoendoscopic single site (LESS) versus classic video-laparoscopic cholecystectomy: a randomized prospective study. J Surg Res. 2011;166(2):e109–12.
18. Vilallonga R, Barbaros U, Sumer A, et al. Single-port transumbilical laparoscopic cholecystectomy: a prospective randomized comparison of clinical results of 140 cases. J Minim Access Surg. 2012;8(3):74–8.
19. Leung D, Yetasook AK, Carbray J, et al. Single-incision surgery has higher cost with equivalent pain and quality-of-life scores compared with multiple-incision laparoscopic cholecystectomy: a prospective randomized blinded comparison. J Am Coll Surg. 2012;215(5):702–8.
20. Marks JM, Phillips MS, Tacchino R, et al. Single-incision laparoscopic cholecystectomy is associated with improved cosmesis scoring at the cost of significantly higher hernia rates: 1-year results of a prospective randomized, multicenter, single-blinded trial of traditional multiport laparoscopic cholecystectomy vs single-incision laparoscopic cholecystectomy. J Am Coll Surg. 2013;216(6):1037–47.
21. Pan MX, Jiang ZS, Cheng Y, et al. Single-incision vs three-port laparoscopic cholecystectomy: prospective randomized study. World J Gastroenterol. 2013;19(3):394–8.
22. Deveci U, Barbaros U, Kapakli MS, et al. The comparison of single incision laparoscopic cholecystectomy and three port laparoscopic cholecystectomy: prospective randomized study. J Korean Surg Soc. 2013;85(6):275–82.
23. Garg P, Thakur JD, Singh I, et al. A prospective controlled trial comparing single-incision and conventional laparoscopic cholecystectomy: caution before damage control. Surg Laparosc Endosc Percutan Tech. 2012;22:220–5.
24. Kurpiewski W, Pesta W, Kowalczyk M, et al. The outcomes of SILS cholecystectomy in comparison with classic four-trocar laparoscopic cholecystectomy. Videosurg Miniinv. 2012;7(4):286–93.
25. Lirici MM, Califano AD, Angelini P, Corcione F. Laparo-endoscopic single site cholecystectomy versus standard laparoscopic cholecystectomy: results of a pilot randomized trial. Am J Surg. 2011;202:45–52.

Meta-analysis/Systematic Reviews

26. Pisanu A, Reccia I, Porceddu G, Uccheddu A. Meta-analysis of prospective randomized studies comparing single-incision laparoscopic cholecystectomy (SILC) and conventional multiport laparoscopic cholecystectomy (CMLC). J Gastrointest Surg. 2012;16:1790–801.
27. Trastulli S, Cirocchi R, Desiderio J, et al. Systematic review and meta-analysis of randomized clinical trials comparing single-incision versus conventional laparoscopic cholecystectomy. Br J Surg. 2013;100(2):191–208.
28. Qiu J, Yuan H, Chen S, et al. Single-port versus conventional multiport laparoscopic cholecystectomy: a meta-analysis of randomized controlled trials and nonrandomized studies. J Laparoendosc Adv Surg Tech A. 2013;23(10):815–31.

29. Arezzo A, Scozzari G, Famiglietti F, Passero R, Morino M. Is single-incision laparoscopic cholecystectomy safe? Results of a systematic review and meta-analysis. Surg Endosc. 2013;27(7):2293–304.
30. Gurusamy KS, Vaughan J, Rossi M, Davidson BR. Fewer-than-four ports versus four ports for laparoscopic cholecystectomy (Review). Cochrane Database Syst Rev. 2014;2:CD007109.
31. Milas M, Devedija S, Trkulja V. Single incision versus standard multiport laparoscopic cholecystectomy: up-dated systematic review and meta-analysis of randomized trials. Surgeon. 2014;pii:S1479-666X(14)00015-8.

Chapter 20
Management of Recurrent Cholangitis

Steven C. Stain and Ankesh Nigam

Abstract Recurrent cholangitis is inevitably due to biliary obstruction, and the most frequent causes are either: stones in the common or hepatic bile duct; or intrinsic stricture(s) of the biliary tract or narrowing at previously constructed bilioenteric anastomoses. The initial treatment is straightforward, and includes fluid resuscitation and antibiotic therapy, and is followed by biliary decompression using any means necessary. Depending upon the etiology and available expertise, this is generally accomplished by retrograde endoscopic or percutaneous transhepatic drainage. Emergent operative therapy is a rare event in current practice. Definitive therapy is dependent upon the etiology, and may utilize endoscopic or percutaneous dilation of strictures. However, hepatic resection of diseased segments or operative correction of biliary or anastomotic strictures may be required, with the goal of reestablishing uninterrupted flow of bile to the gastrointestinal tract to prevent recurrent infection.

Keywords Biliary obstruction • Endoscopic • Percutaneous • Hepaticojejunostomy

Introduction

Cholangitis, the most serious manifestation of biliary tract bacterial infection in the setting of biliary obstruction, is associated with pain, fever, jaundice, hypotension and mental status change. The initial treatment is antibiotics and fluid resuscitation. Biliary sepsis resolves in most patients with conservative therapy, and this allows the use of noninvasive imaging (CT scan or MRI) in order to determine the cause and level of obstruction. However, in the 15 % of patients who fail to respond to conservative treatment, emergent biliary decompression is necessary to avoid the high mortality from cholangitis in this group. With success rates of 90–98 %,

S.C. Stain (✉) • A. Nigam
Department of Surgery, Albany Medical College,
50 New Scotland Ave, MC 194, Albany, NY 12208, USA
e-mail: stains@mail.amc.edu

J.M. Millis, J.B. Matthews (eds.), *Difficult Decisions in Hepatobiliary and Pancreatic Surgery*, Difficult Decisions in Surgery: An Evidence-Based Approach, DOI 10.1007/978-3-319-27365-5_20

endoscopic biliary drainage was established as the preferred method of decompression over surgical drainage in the randomized clinical trial by Lai et al. in 1992, in which the mortality in the endoscopic arm was 10 % vs 32 % in surgical group [1, 2]. When the endoscopic route is not available due to anatomic considerations or available expertise, percutaneous transhepatic biliary decompression provides reliable acute treatment of cholangitis. Emergent treatment of cholangitis by operative techniques is seldom necessary in current surgical practice.

Recurrent cholangitis occurs in two distinct clinical settings. The first is in patients with recurrent pyogenic cholangitis characterized by biliary strictures located in the common bile duct or, more frequently, involving the intrahepatic ducts causing biliary stasis and pigmented stones resulting in choledocholithiasis or hepatolithiasis. This disease entity is more common in East Asia, although it has been reported in other populations. The second common clinical presentation of recurrent cholangitis results from strictures following previous interventions, either after bilioenteric anastomosis or endoscopic biliary procedures. There are several options for treating these patients with recurrent cholangitis and include endoscopic, percutaneous or operative techniques.

Search Strategy

A literature search of English language publications from 2003 to 2014 was used to identity published data on recurrent cholangitis using the PICO outline (Table 20.1). Databases searched were PubMed, Cochrane Evidence Based Medicine, American College of Physicians Journal Club, Trip Database. Terms used in the search were "recurrent cholangitis", "endoscopic treatment recurrent cholangitis", "percutaneous treatment recurrent cholangitis", "randomized clinical trial and cholangitis", "randomized clinical trial and choledocholithiasis", "recurrent bile duct stones", "choledochoduodenostomy, hepaticojejunostomy and stricture". Articles were excluded if they specifically addressed patients treated after malignancy, liver transplantation, or sclerosing cholangitis. There were hundreds of citations related to these search terms, and 28 articles were included in our analysis. There were no randomized control trials or multicenter studies, and all reviewed articles were

Table 20.1 PICO table for treatment of management of recurrent cholangitis

P (Patients)	I (Intervention)	C (Comparator group)	O (Outcomes measured)
Patients who develop recurrent cholangitis after:	Hepatic resection percutaneous therapy	No intervention	Morbidity and mortality
			Recurrent symptoms
1. Hepatolithiasis	Endoscopic therapy		Recurrent stone formation
2. Prior Intervention			Need for further intervention

single institution series with varied lengths of follow up. The data was classified using the GRADE system.

Results

Recurrent Cholangitis from Hepatolithiasis

Recurrent pyogenic cholangitis is associated with hepatolithiasis, and is characterized by intra and extrahepatic biliary strictures, the formation of stones, and repeated biliary infections. It is predominantly a disease of the Far East, although there have been several North American series reported. Primary hepatolithiasis refers to stones that are formed de novo in the intrahepatic ducts, and secondary hepatolithiasis results from retrograde migration of stones from the common bile duct and gallbladder into the intrahepatic ducts due to distal obstruction [3]. Chronic proliferative cholangitis, which consists of extensive proliferation of fibrous connective tissue, moderate-to-severe infiltration by inflammatory cells, and the proliferation of mucus-producing peribiliary glands in the ductal was has been suggested as a fundamental histologic lesion of stone-bearing intrahepatic bile ducts [4]. Patients with either primary or secondary hepatolithiasis have recurrent cholangitis, with recurrent episodes of abdominal pain, fever and or jaundice. Primary treatments include hepatic resection of the disease liver segment, with or without bilioenteric bypass, percutaneous transhepatic cholangioscopic lithotomy (PTCSL), or peroral cholangioscopic lithotripsy [5, 6]. These procedures can be combined at the time of initial treatment, or utilized in sequence for the frequent recurrence of stones in the biliary tract common in these patients. Even after seemingly effective treatment, patients often suffer from long term complications of recurrent cholangitis, hepatic cirrhosis and cholangiocarcinoma.

The traditional treatment of hepatic resection, most frequently applied in patients with predominantly unilobar hepatic stones, is most appropriate for patients with lobar atrophy. Chen et al. reported that 103 of the 487 patients treated from 1989 to 2001 in their series (21 %) underwent partial hepatectomy [7]. It is worthwhile to note that hepaticojejunostomy was added to the liver resection in 62 of their 103 patients (60 %). With a mean follow-up of 56 months (range 6–158) only eight patients developed recurrent stones. Ten patients had coexisting cholangiocarcinoma, and three additional patients developed cholangiocarcinoma 7–36 months after the initial procedure. The total of 13 patients who develop cholangiocarcinoma (12.6 %) underscores the long term risk of patients with recurrent pyogenic cholangitis associated with hepatolithiasis. Three other reports from Hong Kong, Taiwan and Japan focused on the outcome of hepatectomy for hepatolithiasis and recurrent cholangitis were included in our analysis in Table 20.2 and showed comparable results [8–10]. Cheung emphasized the importance of flexible choledochoscopy at the time of resection to ensure stone clearance, and added biliary drainage by

Table 20.2 Outcomes after treatment of hepatolithiasis

Author (Year)	N	Intervention	Morbidity	Mortality	Recurrent stones (%)	Recurrent symptoms	Need for further intervention	Study type (quality of evidence)
Chen (2004)	103	Hepatic resection with hepaticojejunostomy in 62 patients 60 %	28 %	2 %	9 %	8 %	5 %	Retrospective cohort (low)
Cheung (2005)	52	Hepatic resection with biliary drainage in 5 patients (9.6 %)	44 %	3.8 %	13.5 %	13.3 %	11.5 %	Retrospective cohort (low)
	149	Percutaneous choledochoscopy	Not reported	Not reported	Not reported	22.2 %	21.5 %	Retrospective cohort (low)
Lee (2007)	123	Hepatic resection and T-Tube placement	33.3 %	1.6 %	5.7 %	13 %	Indicated in 8.9 %, but 7 of the 11 refused treatment	Retrospective cohort (low)
Ueneshi (2009)	87	Hepatic resection and T-tube placement	Not reported	3.5 %	20.6 %	32.2 %	20 %: 10 % immediately post op, and additional 10 % long term	Retrospective cohort (low)
Al-Sukhani (2008)	10	CBDE, choledochojejunostomy and Hutson loop	30 %	0	33 %	36 %	21 %	Prospective cohort (low)
	17	Hepatic resection; 10 with Huston loop and 17 without Hutson loop	35 %	0	33 %	36 %	21 %	Retrospective cohort (low)
Kassem (2014)	42	Hepaticojejunostomy with Hutson loop; including 5 with hepatic resection	28.6 %	0	67 %	52 %	67 %	Prospective cohort (moderate)
Tian (2013)	90	Laparoscopic hepatic resection with CBDE in 81	21 %	0	27.8 %	17 %	17 %	Retrospective cohort (low)

Tan (2014)	46	ERCP	34.8 %	4.3 %	37 %	36.9 %	Not reported	Retrospective cohort (low)
	37	Laparoscopic hepatectomy	32.4 %	0	27 %	10.8 %	Not reported	Retrospective cohort (low)
	41	Laparoscopic intrahepatic duct exploration	26.8 %	0	41.5 %	21.9 %	Not reported	Retrospective cohort (low)
Huang (2003)	245	Percutaneous transhepatic cholangioscopic lithotomy	1.6 % procedure related	0.8 % procedure related	50 %	52 %	100 %	Prospective cohort (low)

hepaticojejunostomy or sphincteroplasty in only five patients [8]. All six patients with cholangiocarcinoma died during their median follow-up of 40.3 months.

Moderate sized series of hepatolithiasis and recurrent pyogenic cholangitis have been published from hepatobiliary surgical centers in the North America and Middle East [11, 12]. These two series both advocate the use of subcutaneous hepaticojejunal access loops (Hutson loop) as a means to treat removal of recurrent stones. In the Toronto General Hospital series, the majority of patients (67 %) had East Asian ethnicity [11]. Twenty seven of their 42 patients underwent surgery after failed endoscopic or percutaneous intervention, and 20 patients had Hutson loops. Only 4 of their 27 patients had stone-related symptoms requiring percutaneous intervention compared to 4 of the 11 surviving nonoperative patients. The series from Kassem et al., from Egypt was the only surgical series with a post intervention prospective follow up protocol [12]. All patients were reviewed at 6 weeks after surgery, at 3 month intervals for the first year, and a 6 month intervals thereafter. Accordingly, they had the highest incidence of postoperative symptoms, recurrent stones, and interventions. All patients with suspicion of residual or recurrent stones were investigated, which may explain their high rates. Symptom free was defined as patients who were symptom free 1 year after last intervention. However, after their repeat interventions, only seven patients (17 %) failed to benefit from the access loop.

Three included series focused on the laparoscopic technique for treating recurrent hepatolithiasis associated with recurrent pyogenic cholangitis Table 20.2 [13–15]. Tian reported laparoscopic hepatic resection in 90 patients which consisted of 67 left hepatic resections and 23 right hepatic resections [15]. This was combined with common bile duct exploration for 81 of their patients with extrahepatic stones.

Nonoperative approaches have also been employed for treatment of hepatolithiasis. In a series of 124 patients, Tan reported the results of 46 patients with intrahepatic stones treated by ERCP [16]. The mortality was 4.3 %, and the stones recurred in 17 of the 46 patients (37.0 %). Percutaneous transhepatic cholangioscopic lithotomy is another approach for primary treatment of hepatolithiasis or for those patients with recurrent stones after prior operation. Huang reported a large series of 245 patients with a mean follow up of 10.3 year [17]. These were patients that were either considered poor surgical risks, refused surgery, or had previous biliary operations. Initial complete stone clearance was achieved in 209 patients (85.3 %), but required a mean of 4.7 sessions (range 1–20). Even after complete stone clearance, 52 % of the patients developed symptoms and 50 % had recurrent stones. Over the duration of their follow up, the overall recurrence rate of hepatolithiasis and/or symptoms was 63.2 %. Twenty-seven patients died (cirrhosis – 18, cholangiocarcinoma – 5 or other causes – 4), highlighting the long term complications of recurrent biliary obstruction.

Recurrent Cholangitis from Choledocholithiasis

Experienced hepatobiliary surgeons are proficient at performing bilioenteric anastomoses for a variety of indications, including pancreaticoduodenectomy, repair of bile duct injuries, or transplantation. Biloenteric bypass (hepaticojejunostomy, cholechochojejunostomy or choledochoduodenostomy) was the standard treatment for patients with primary common bile duct stones or for patients who failed endoscopic stone removal. Advances in laparoscopic and endoscopic techniques have made open operation infrequently necessary. It was difficult to find a recent reference of open cholechoenterostomy for common bile duct stones. The title, *Open Choledocho-Enterostomy for Common Bile Duct Stones: Is it Out of Date in Laparo-Endosocopic Therapy*, indicates the infrequency that open surgical biliary bypass is performed for retained or recurrent bile duct stones in the absence of bile duct stricture [18]. Abdelmajid et al., performed 51 biliary enteric bypasses with excellent results between 2005 and 2009 for elderly patients, most of whom had multiple stones (at least five), or unextractable calculi (Table 20.3). Li studied the results of 193 patients treated by open cholecholithotomy and T-tube drainage – 81, cholechoduodenostomy – 41, or choledochojejunsotomy – 71 [19]. This series include patients with primary common bile duct stones – 81, and those with secondary bile stones that presumably originated in the gallbladder – 112. The authors found a significantly lower rate of recurrent symptoms in patients treated by choledochoduodenostomy than those with either T-tube drainage or choledochojejuonostomy. This difference was more pronounced in those patients with primary common bile duct stones (cholechochoduodenostomy – 2.6 %; choledochojejunostomy – 14.7 %; T-tube drainage – 36.4 %). Small series have been reported using laparoscopic choledochoduodenostomy for biliary obstruction [20, 21]. The paper by Chander had 27 patients with dilated common bile ducts (>15 mm) with multiple stones, recurrent stones or primary common bile duct stones. Details of patient follow up are limited, but they report no deaths, with minimal morbidity and no recurrence of symptoms [21]. For historical purposes, we have included a paper from Johns Hopkins during the open cholecystectomy era, in our analysis [22]. The authors treated 30 patients with primary common bile duct stones, defined as patients with a 2 year symptom free interval following cholecystectomy in the absence of a long cystic duct remnant or biliary stricture. Most patients presented with acute cholangitis, and the mean interval to developing symptoms was 12 years. Twenty six of the 30 patients had simple stone extraction and T-Tube placement, with no recurrent stones in 82 %. Four patients had biliary drainage by choledochoduodenostomy (3) or sphincteroplasty (1) without recurrent symptoms or stones.

Due to advances in therapeutic endoscopy, there are a multitude of techniques to remove persistent common bile duct stones by endoscopic sphincterotomy, papillary large balloon dilatation of the papilla, or lithotripsy. It is infrequent that the most patients are even evaluated by surgeons [23–25]. The results of endoscopic treatment are reasonably good, and although not quite comparable to surgical series, large or multiple calculi can usually be removed by endoscopic means [24–26]. The

Table 20.3 Recurrent cholangitis due to choledocholithiasis

Author (Year)	N	Intervention	Morbidity	Mortality	Recurrent stones (%)	Recurrent symptoms	Need for further intervention	Study type (quality of evidence)
Abdelmajid (2014)	51	Choledochoduodenostomy (50) Hepaticojejunostomy (1)	11.7 %	3.9 %	0	0	0	Retrospective cohort (low)
Li (2007)	81	CBDE with T-tube	Not reported	Not reported	8.6 %	8.6 %	Not reported	Retrospective cohort (moderate)
	41	Choledochoduodenostomy	Not reported	Not reported	2.4 %	2.4 %	Not reported	Retrospective cohort (moderate)
	71	Choledochojejunostomy	Not reported	Not reported	8.5 %	8.5 %	Not reported	Retrospective cohort (moderate)
Chander (2012)	27	Laparoscopic choledochochoduodenostomy	3.7 %	0	0	0	0	Retrospective cohort (very low quality)
Kajanchee (2012)	20	Laparoscopic choledochoduodenostomy	35 %	5 %	0	5 %	0	Retrospective cohort (low)
Saharia (1977)	30	CBDE with T-tube (26) Choledochoduodenostomy (3) Sphincteroplasty (1)	Not reported	0	13 %	13 %	13 %	Retrospective cohort (low)
Sugiyama (2004)	84	Endoscopic transpapillary stone extraction using basket, balloon or lithotripsy	2 %	0	30.9 %	41.6 %	42.8 %	Retrospective cohort (low)
Swahn (2010)	44	Endoscopic intraductal electrohydraulic or laser lithotripsy	9 %	2.3 %	29.5 %	36.3 %	56.8 %	Retrospective cohort (low)
Yoon (2014)	52	Endoscopic papillary balloon dilation with mechanical, electrohydraulic or laser lithotripsy	7.6 %	0	30 %	7.7 %	30 %	Retrospective cohort (low)

2004 article by Sugiyama reported 84 patients who had initial successful clearance of common bile duct stones after endoscopic sphincterotomy a median of 4.4 years earlier (range 0.9–17.2 years) [26]. Bile duct clearance was achieved in 74 patients, and 10 patients required 2–3 procedures. Twenty six patients had stone recurrence, but 25 of these 26 were successfully treated by transpapillary stone extraction, and only one patient required choledochojejunostomy. The referral for subsequent surgery (14 %) was higher in the paper from Swahn et al., which employed endoscopic intraductal electrohydraulic and laser lithotripsy for difficult bile duct stones in octogenarians [25]. The results of endoscopic treatment reflect that additional sessions to remove stones were considered a reintervention (Table 20.3).

Recurrent Cholangitis Following Biliary-Enteric Anastomosis for Benign Disease

Major bile duct injuries are generally treated successfully by hepaticojejunostomy. In an analysis of 144 patients with bile duct injuries at the Cleveland Clinic, 84 major bile duct injuries required a biliary enteric reconstruction (hepaticojejunostomy – 73; hepatoduodenostomy – 11) [27]. Eleven of these patients (13 %) had long term major biliary complications, and all occurred after high bile duct injuries (Strasberg E3, E4 or E5) and were the focus of our analysis. Eight of the 11 patients were treated by transhepatic stenting of biliary anastomotic stenting for a mean of 10 weeks, and five required repeat treatment, only one of which eventually had operative revision. Another study looked at patients who developed biliary strictures after pancreaticoduodenectomy [28]. Anastomotic strictures occurred in 10 of 392 patients (2.6 %) who had Whipple resections for benign disease and all were treated with percutaneous catheters and balloon dilation. Only one patient required operative revision of the bile duct anastomosis. A large series of 110 patients treated by percutaneous balloon dilation of benign bilioenteric anastomotic strictures was successful in most patients, but required multiple sessions (mean 5; range 2–30) [29]. Only 13 patients (15 %) developing recurrent biliary obstruction, that were treated by repeat dilation (4), lithotripsy (3), or surgery (4). However, a high number of patients were lost to follow up (21 %). These results are summarized in Table 20.4.

Recommendations for Treatment of Recurrent Cholangitis

There have been no randomized clinical trials for the treatment of recurrent cholangitis. Recommendations are based on observational cohort studies that report experience at single institutions, primarily with a single therapy. A few series do report their results using two or three different treatment options.

Table 20.4 Recurrent cholangitis after biliary-enteric anastomosis for benign disease

Author (Year)	N	Intervention	Morbidity	Mortality	Recurrent stones (%)	Recurrent symptoms	Need for further intervention	Study type (quality of evidence)
Walsh (2007)	8	Transhepatic stenting of biliary anastomosis	Not reported	0	None	87.5 %	62.5 %	Retrospective cohort (low)
House (2006)	10	Transhepatic stenting of biliary anastomosis	Not reported	0	None	100 %	100 %	Retrospective cohort (moderate)
Bonnel	110	Transhepatic stenting of biliary anastomosis	10 %	0	None	15 %	100 %	Retrospective cohort (moderate)

Recommendations

1. Recurrent cholangitis from hepatolithiasis
   (a) Hepatic resection for patients with unilateral hepatic stones and lobar atrophy (evidence quality low; strong recommendation)
   (b) Bilioenteric anastomosis for patients with recurrent disease and consideration of hepaticojejunal access loop (evidence quality low; strong recommendation)
   (c) Patients considered high risk for surgery may be treated percutaneous cholangioscopy or repeat endoscopic treatment. Either modality may be combined with lithotripsy. (evidence quality low; weak recommendation)
2. Recurrent cholangitis from choledocholithiasis
   (a) Transpapillary endoscopic treatment using available techniques such as sphincterotomy, papillary balloon dilation and/or lithotripsy. Surgical bilioenteric anastomosis is reserved for patients that have failed multiple endoscopic attempts. (evidence quality high; strong recommendation)
3. Recurrent Cholangitis Following Biliary-enteric Anastomosis for Benign Disease
   (a) Balloon dilation of the anastomosis with temporary stenting, including a second attempt, especially for a short stricture (evidence quality low; weak recommendation)
   (b) Operative revision of failed anastomotic balloon dilation (evidence quality low; strong recommendation)

A Personal View of the Data

Recurrent cholangitis secondary to hepatolithiasis should be considered a surgical disease, and the best outcomes result from hepatic resection of involved segments (especially when there is lobar atrophy) with biliary enteric anastomoses above intrahepatic strictures after surgical clearance of the biliary tree, with consideration of a hepatojejunal access loop. In the modern era of minimally invasive medicine with highly effective nonoperative techniques of managing recurrent cholangitis in the setting of common bile duct or hepatic duct strictures with resulting choledocholithiasis, there has been a growing tendency to use endoscopic or percutaneous methods to manage this disease process. This is certainly appropriate given the high success rate of these procedures that can be done with less morbidity and mortality compared to operative techniques. Although frequently requiring repeated episodes of treatment, the long-term results of these nonsurgical options have been found to be comparable to surgical procedures. However, if these techniques are unsuccessful, the options of surgical management involving biliary enteric anastomosis should be considered. Moreover, the possibility of underlying malignancy must always be remembered so as not to lose the patient to unsuspected cancer. Similarly, in the patients presenting with recurrent cholangitis after previous biliary interventions, nonoperative techniques are appropriate and useful. However, when such interventions fail or when suspicion of malignancy rises, surgical options must be entertained.

References

1. Lai EC, Mok FP, Tan ES, Lo CM, Fan ST, You KT, Wong J. Endoscopic biliary drainage for severe acute cholangitis. N Engl J Med. 1992;326(24):1582–6.
2. Yusoff IF, Barkun JS, Barkun AN. Diagnosis and management of cholecystitis and cholangitis. Gastroenterol Clin N Am. 2003;32(4):1145–68.
3. Tsui WM, Chan YK, Wong CT, Lo YF, Yeung YW, Lee YW. Hepatolithiasis and the syndrome of recurrent pyogenic cholangitis: clinical, radiologic, and pathologic features. Semin Liver Dis. 2011;31(1):33–48.
4. Li FY, Cheng NS, Mao H, Jiang LS, Cheng JQ, Li QS, Munireddy S. Significance of controlling chronic proliferative cholangitis in the treatment of hepatolithiasis. World J Surg. 2009;33(10):2155–60.
5. Chen C, Huang M, Yang J, Yang C, Yeh Y, Wu H, Chou D, Yueh S, Nien C. Reappraisal of percutaneous transhepatic cholangioscopic lithotomy for primary hepatolithiasis. Surg Endosc. 2005;19(4):505–9.
6. Tsuyuguchi T, Miyakawa K, Sugiyama H, Sakai Y, Nishikawa T, Sakamoto D, Nakamura M, Yasui S, Mikata R, Yokosuka O. Ten-year long-term results after non-surgical management of hepatolithiasis, including cases with choledochoenterostomy. J Hepatobiliary Pancreat Sci. 2014;21(11):795–800. doi:10.1002/jhbp.134.
7. Chen DW, Tung-Ping Poon R, Liu CL, Fan ST, Wong J. Immediate and long-term outcomes of hepatectomy for hepatolithiasis. Surgery. 2004;135(4):386–93.
8. Cheung MT, Kwok PC. Liver resection for intrahepatic stones. Arch Surg. 2005;140(10):993–7.
9. Lee TY, Chen YL, Chang HC, Chan CP, Kuo SJ. Outcomes of hepatectomy for hepatolithiasis. World J Surg. 2007;31(3):479–82.
10. Uenishi T, Hamba H, Takemura S, Oba K, Ogawa M, Yamamoto T, Tanaka S, Kubo S. Outcomes of hepatic resection for hepatolithiasis. Am J Surg. 2009;198(2):199–202.
11. Al-Sukhni W, Gallinger S, Pratzer A, Wei A, Ho CS, Kortan P, Taylor BR, Grant DR, McGilvray I, Cattral MS, Langer B, Greig PD. Recurrent pyogenic cholangitis with hepatolithiasis – the role of surgical therapy in North America. J Gastrointest Surg. 2008;12(3):496–503.
12. Kassem MI, Sorour MA, Ghazal AH, El-Haddad HM, El-Riwini MT, El-Bahrawy HA. Management of intrahepatic stones: the role of subcutaneous hepaticojejunal access loop. A prospective cohort study. Int J Surg. 2014;12(9):886–92.
13. Tang CN, Tai CK, Siu WT, Ha JP, Tsui KK, Li MK. Laparoscopic treatment of recurrent pyogenic cholangitis. J Hepatobiliary Pancreat Surg. 2005;12(3):243–8.
14. Han HS, Yi NJ. Laparoscopic treatment of intrahepatic duct stone. Surg Laparosc Endosc Percutan Technol. 2004;14(3):157–62.
15. Tian J, Li JW, Chen J, Fan YD, Bie P, Wang SG, Zheng SG. The safety and feasibility of reoperation for the treatment of hepatolithiasis by laparoscopic approach. Surg Endosc. 2013;27(4):1315–20.

16. Tan J, Tan Y, Chen F, Zhu Y, Leng J, Dong J. Endoscopic or laparoscopic approach for hepatolithiasis in the era of endoscopy in China. Surg Endosc. 2015;29(1):154–62.
17. Huang MH, Chen CH, Yang JC, Yang CC, Yeh YH, Chou DA, Mo LR, Yueh SK, Nien CK. Long-term outcome of percutaneous transhepatic cholangioscopic lithotomy for hepatolithiasis. Am J Gastroenterol. 2003;98(12):2655–62.
18. Abdelmajid K, Houssem H, Rafik G, Jarrar MS, Fehmi H. Open choldecho-enterostomy for common bile duct stones: is it out of date in laparo-endoscopic era? N Am J Med Sci. 2013;5(4):288–92.
19. Li ZF, Chen XP. Recurrent lithiasis after surgical treatment of elderly patients with choledocholithiasis. Hepatobiliary Pancreat Dis Int. 2007;6(1):67–71.
20. Chander J, Mangla V, Vindal A, Lal P, Ramteke VK. Laparoscopic choledochoduodenostomy for biliary stone disease: a single-center 10-year experience. J Laparoendosc Adv Surg Technol A. 2012;22(1):81–4.
21. Khajanchee YS, Cassera MA, Hammill CW, Swanström LL, Hansen PD. Outcomes following laparoscopic choledochoduodenostomy in the management of benign biliary obstruction. J Gastrointest Surg. 2012;16(4):801–5.
22. Saharia PC, Zuidema GD, Cameron JL. Primary common duct stones. Ann Surg. 1977;185(5):598–604.
23. Hong WD, Zhu QH, Huang QK. Endoscopic sphincterotomy plus endoprostheses in the treatment of large or multiple common bile duct stones. Dig Endosc. 2011;23(3):240–3.
24. Yoon HG, Moon JH, Choi HJ, Kim DC, Kang MS, Lee TH, Cha SW, Cho YD, Park SH, Kim SJ. Endoscopic papillary large balloon dilation for the management of recurrent difficult bile duct stones after previous endoscopic sphincterotomy. Dig Endosc. 2014;26(2):259–63.
25. Swahn F, Edlund G, Enochsson L, Svensson C, Lindberg B, Arnelo U. Ten years of Swedish experience with intraductal electrohydraulic lithotripsy and laser lithotripsy for the treatment of difficult bile duct stones: an effective and safe option for octogenarians. Surg Endosc. 2010;24(5):1011–6.
26. Sugiyama M, Suzuki Y, Abe N, Masaki T, Mori T, Atomi Y. Endoscopic retreatment of recurrent choledocholithiasis after sphincterotomy. Gut. 2004;53(12):1856–9.
27. Walsh RM, Henderson JM, Vogt DP, Brown N. Long-term outcome of biliary reconstruction for bile duct injuries from laparoscopic cholecystectomies. Surgery. 2007;142(4):450–6.
28. House MG, Cameron JL, Schulick RD, Campbell KA, Sauter PK, Coleman J, Lillemoe KD, Yeo CJ. Incidence and outcome of biliary strictures after pancreaticoduodenectomy. Ann Surg. 2006;243(5):571–6.
29. Bonnel DH, Fingerhut AL. Percutaneous transhepatic balloon dilatation of benign bilioenteric strictures: long-term results in 110 patients. Am J Surg. 2012;203(6):675–83.

Chapter 21
Management of Postoperative Bile Duct Stricture

Nicholas J. Zyromski and James R. Butler

Abstract Postoperative bile duct strictures are relatively rare, but challenging problems to manage. Multiple techniques to treat bile duct strictures exist, including endoscopic, percutaneous, and surgical approaches. The optimal technique for individual patients is best determined by a multidisciplinary team composed of experienced endoscopists, interventional radiologists, and hepatobiliary surgeons. The location and type of injury (i.e. Bile leak, bile duct transection, etc.) dictate therapeutic approach. The underlying hepatic artery anatomy must be understood. Excellent outcomes are expected from experienced centers; these patients are ideally followed life-long, as a small percentage will develop late recurrent stricture.

Keywords Bile duct stricture • Bile duct injury • Bile duct • Stricture • Bile leak • Cholangitis • ERCP

Introduction

Postoperative bile duct stricture (PBDS) occurs most commonly after cholecystectomy [1], but may also complicate other complex hepatobiliary operations including liver transplant, pancreatoduodenectomy, hepatectomy, and resection of the extrahepatic biliary tree (i.e. for choledochal cyst, cholangiocarcinoma, or primary sclerosing cholangitis) [2–5].

Bile duct strictures represent a broadly heterogeneous pathology; a major challenge when attempting to collate and summarize best therapeutic practice lies in segregating and comparing treatment outcomes of similar strictures. Perhaps the most widely accepted classification of PBDS was proposed by Strasberg [6].

N.J. Zyromski (✉) • J.R. Butler
Department of Surgery, Indiana University School of Medicine,
545 Barnhill Dr EH 519, Indianapolis, IN 46202, USA
e-mail: nzyromsk@iupui.edu

J.M. Millis, J.B. Matthews (eds.), *Difficult Decisions in Hepatobiliary and Pancreatic Surgery*, Difficult Decisions in Surgery: An Evidence-Based Approach, DOI 10.1007/978-3-319-27365-5_21

Importantly, this classification recognizes more than simple anatomic level of injury, and also includes factors such as partial versus complete bile duct transection, presence of ongoing bile leak, and presence of complete bile duct occlusion.

Multiple treatment strategies have been applied to postoperative bile duct stricture, including surgical repair (hepaticojejunostomy, choledochoduodenostomy) [2, 7–27], percutaneous dilation and/or stenting [28–31], and endoscopic dilation (most commonly with stenting) [32–41]. The location (level) of bile duct injury is obviously of major importance when choosing treatment strategy. Therapy of PBDS also depends on many other factors including timing of injury recognition [42, 43], presence of ongoing bile leak or biliary sepsis, presence of concomitant vascular (hepatic artery) injury, and availability of local expertise and experience. In many patients, multiple therapeutic approaches (or repeated application of a single therapeutic approach) may be required to achieve durable resolution.

Further complicating analysis of PBDS treatment is the fact that no one consistent outcome measure has been accepted to define treatment failure or success. Recurrent stricture is typically apparent on imaging studies (cholangiography or cross sectional images); however, patients with modest strictures may remain asymptomatic. Similarly, while liver chemistry biochemical abnormality (particularly alkaline phosphatase) may be the first sign of impending stricture, abnormal liver chemistry may be observed without obvious morphologic stricture. The occurrence of cholangitis is somewhat subjective, difficult to accurately compile retrospectively, and inconsistently reported. Repeated percutaneous and endoscopic interventions are commonly necessary; the question of how many interventions defines success or failure remains unanswered. In addition, the use of surgical, percutaneous, or endoscopically placed biliary stents is common in PBDS treatment. The timing and number of stent exchanges, however, is widely variable. Finally, it has been recognized that as many as 10 % of post-operative biliary strictures may develop 10 years or more after the original operation; however, very few studies have the appropriate length of follow up (some authorities suggest 20 years) to document all strictures [2, 23].

With all of the above in mind, the goal of this review is to compare the success of PBDS treatment strategies (surgical versus percutaneous and endoscopic) based on the outcomes of recurrent stricture and cholangitis. The review will focus primarily on bile duct injury/strictures sustained after cholecystectomy. Many studies highlight one specific treatment approach; a few series compare surgical repair with endoscopic and/or percutaneous treatment [21, 44–55], and importantly, no prospective trials comparing different treatment strategies have been performed.

Search Strategy

The MEDLINE, EMBASE, and Cochrane Library were searched from 1946 to September 2014, using the following strategy: bile duct stricture*, bile duct leak*, bile duct injury* (where * retrieves word variants such as plurals and other variations). These terms were combined with the medical subject headings "postoperative complications" and "treatment outcomes," which were 'exploded' to also include specific variants of these terms. These terms were also combined with specific operative procedures (i.e. "pancreatoduodenectomy," "hepatectomy," etc.). Results were limited to human subjects and English language, case reports and letters were eliminated. Reference lists of high impact results were queried to identify additional results.

Results

PBDS After Complex Hepatobiliary Procedures

Systematic review of biliary strictures following orthotopic liver transplant (OLT), extrahepatic biliary tree resection (EBR), and pancreatoduodenectomy (PD) are beyond the scope of this chapter; however, a few salient points are noteworthy. Stricture is a significant complication of OLT, occurring in up to 20 % of cases [4, 56, 57]. This problem is commonly associated with hepatic artery complications. In patients with end-to-end biliary reconstruction, most biliary strictures are amenable to endoscopic therapy (with stenting), while those with Roux-en-Y hepaticojejunostomy are commonly approached by percutaneous transhepatic methods.

The incidence of PBDS after PD is approximately 3 % [3, 58, 59], though given the increasing frequency of pancreatic surgery, surprisingly few data are available specific to postoperative bile duct stricture. The time to stricture formation after PD averages 13–16 months, and most patients present with cholangitis and/or jaundice. Recurrent malignancy should be considered as a cause of PBDS in patients having PD for diagnosis of cancer. Percutaneous therapy is successful in most patients (95 % in one series [59]), though depending on local expertise, some authors have chosen to address these patients surgically with equally good outcomes [58].

Even fewer data on PBDS are available specific to resection of the extrahepatic biliary tree (for example, for choledochal cyst) [5, 60]. As the reconstruction in these cases is almost universally by Roux-en-Y hepaticojejunostomy, the primary treatment modality is percutaneous intervention. Most authorities recommend lifelong follow up for these patients, as strictures may present very late (decades) after definitive surgical treatment.

PBDS After Cholecystectomy

Cholecystectomy, both in the pre-laparoscopic era as well as in contemporary time represents by far and away the most common cause of PBDS. National estimates suggest as many as 0.5 % of all cholecystectomies have associated bile leak or bile duct injury, both of which may lead to PBDS [1]. Treatment of PBDS depends on a number of variables. First and foremost is the anatomic level of injury. Additional considerations include local availability of specialty treatment (i.e. interventional radiology, endoscopy, and specialized hepatobiliary surgical units), timing of repair, and presence of major vascular injury [11, 12]. Comparison of PBDS treatment outcomes by different techniques is limited significantly by small sample sizes, retrospective analyses, and most importantly, difficulty comparing similar types of injuries/strictures. For example, injuries of Strasberg type A (consisting simply of bile leak, either from the cystic duct stump or from a peripheral bile duct in the gallbladder bed) are easily and durably managed with endoscopic stenting more than 95 % of the time. On the other hand, type E injuries, including those proximal to the hepatic bifurcation, those with major vascular injury, and those with complete hepatic duct occlusion or transection involve an exponentially greater degree of complexity and in extreme cases may even require major hepatectomy for definitive treatment [61]. Nevertheless, patients with both of these types of injuries are often included in the same analysis and even in comparison studies. No prospective study exits comparing similar types of PBDS treated by different techniques. Based on existing retrospective data, however, several general treatment recommendations may be observed.

Surgical Repair

Select studies reviewing surgical repair of PBDS are shown in Table 21.1. The larger series number in the hundreds of patients, though these series often span several decades. Advances in surgical technique (as well as endoscopic and percutaneous techniques) that have evolved over the time of the study should be considered. Reasonable follow up is measured in multiples of years; most PBDS will manifest with some combination of pain, jaundice, and cholangitis within the first 5 years of operation, though as many as 10 % of PBDS may present quite late (decades) [2]. Lifelong follow up of patients after surgical repair of PBDS therefore seems quite prudent.

Most surgical series document excellent (>90 %) durable long-term success when following basic tenets of repair: utilizing a tension-free anastomosis of healthy, well-perfused bile ducts to similarly well-perfused intestine. Most authorities recommend repair either very early (within 48 h of the injury, particularly if no major hepatic artery injury is coincident) or waiting for 4–6 weeks to permit patient optimization [2, 15, 42]. Optimizing patient physiology includes controlling biliary sepsis, supplementing nutrition as necessary, and defining the level of biliary injury and presence of hepatic arterial injury. Many studies have shown less than optimal outcomes for PBDS repaired in the 2–4 week time period post injury; these poor outcomes have been attributed to poor bile duct perfusion in the presence of evolving ischemia.

Several technical considerations are worth discussion. First, the level of repair has been debated: some authorities suggest that routine use of the Hepp-Couinaud

Table 21.1 Surgical repair of postoperative bile duct strictures

Author (ref)	Year	N	F/U	Success
Addeo [24]	2013	46	97	93 %
Perera [22]	2011	200	60	77 %
Mercado [23]	2011	312	52	96 %
Pottakrat [21]	2010	364	61	92 %
Sahaspal [20]	2010	69	[a]	86 %
Jablunsca [19]	2009	94	62	85 %
Stewart [18]	2009	307	40	91 %
Walsh [17]	2007	84	67	89 %
DeReuver [16]	2007	151	63	91 %
Thompson [15]	2006	47	n/s	89 %
Sicklick [14]	2005	208	[b]	[b]
Schmidt [13]	2005	54	62	81 %
Stewart [11]	2004	261	[b]	[b]
Alves [12]	2004	55	59	97 %
Mercado [10]	2003	30	56	87 %
Johnson [9]	2000	27	55	95 %
Lillemoe [8]	2000	156	58	91 %
Murr [7]	1999	59	42	91 %

n/s not stated
[a]"Long-term"
[b]Immediate postoperative outcomes

Table 21.2 Surgical repair of postoperative bile duct strictures by choledochoduodenostomy

Author (ref)	Year	N	F/U	Success
Luu [27]	2013	55	29	98 %
Rose [26]	2013	59	28	88 %
Leppard [25]	2011	79	74	98 %[a]

[a]Included patients with chronic pancreatitis bile duct strictures

technique may be associated with improved outcomes [7, 10, 63]. Second, while most biliary surgeons prefer Roux-en-Y hepaticojejunostomy, some have advocated choledochoduodenostomy as definitive repair [25–27]. Table 21.2 summarizes outcomes of choledochoduodenostomy for repair of PBDS. Potential advantages of choledochoduodenostomy include subjecting the patient to a less complex operation (fewer anastomoses) and maintenance of continuity with the upper gut, permitting endoscopic biliary evaluation if necessary. Detractors of this technique impugn the sump syndrome (foodstuffs lodged in the distal/intrapancreatic common bile duct) as a cause of recurrent cholangitis and liver abscess. Dividing the bile duct completely and performing end-to-side choledochoduodenostomy may avoid the sump syndrome. Most post-cholecystectomy biliary injuries are high, and therefore Roux-en-Y hepaticojejunostomy may be the preferable approach in these situations.

Table 21.3 Percutaneous treatment of postoperative bile duct strictures

Author	Year	N	F/U	Success
Cantwell [31]	2008	75	96	52 %
Kocher [30]	2007	21	12	94 %
Mesra [29]	2004	51	76	59 %
Bonnell [28]	1997	25	55	72 %

Most would agree that preoperative placement of transhepatic biliary stents greatly facilitates operative conduct. In contrast, the issue of transhepatic stenting in the postoperative period is a topic of ongoing debate. Historically, two camps have included routine stenters and routine non-stenters. Many experienced biliary surgeons have come to a middle ground, maintaining transhepatic stents in the situation of a small caliber bile duct or high reconstruction, while avoiding stents in the case of large diameter biliary-enteric anastomoses. The duration of stenting postoperatively is not consistent; however, a time period of 3–6 months at minimum seems reasonable to attenuate stricture formation. Over-the-wire transhepatic cholangiography with either manometry or a "clinical trial" may be used before removing stents. Biliary manometry (the Whittaker test) is used infrequently; the alternative, "clinical trial" involves maintaining the transhepatic stent at a level proximal to the anastomosis for a short period of time while monitoring the patient for symptoms of pain or cholangitis.

Percutaneous Therapy

Exclusive percutaneous management of PBDS has been used at select centers with experienced interventional radiology groups [28–31]. Table 21.3 summarizes results of these studies, and Table 21.5 includes patients with percutaneous transhepatic stenting reported in trials that include surgical repair and/or endoscopic treatment. In general, fewer studies of percutaneous biliary stenting as definitive treatment for PBDS have been reported when compared to the surgical or endoscopic approaches. This observation perhaps highlights the rarity of expertise in biliary interventional radiology nationwide. Studies of percutaneous biliary stenting for PBDS are all hampered by small sample sizes and relatively short follow up. Most of these series count patients who have required multiple stent exchanges and prolonged duration of stenting as successfully treated. The duration of stenting is variable, but may last more than 1–2 years. Most of these series document success rates significantly lower than those reported in surgical series, though the definition of success (i.e. radiological vs clinical) varies considerably. Noteworthy is the fact that most of these series contain at least some patients who have failed either surgical or endoscopic treatment. Also noteworthy in the big picture is the substantial technical expertise necessary to access a non-dilated biliary system by the percutaneous transhepatic approach.

Table 21.4 Endoscopic treatment of postoperative bile duct strictures

Author	Year	N	F/U-mos	Success
Canena [41]	2014	20	44	100 %
Ghazanfar [40]	2012	97	N/S	88 %
Artifon [39]	2012	31	N/S	72 %
Draganon [34]	2012	14	48	62 %
Kuroda [38]	2010	21	121	95 %
Sakai [37]	2009	24	N/S	94 %
Katsinelos [36]	2008	63	N/S	95 %
DeReuver [35]	2007	203	54	84 %
Constamanga [33]	2001	45	49	89 %
Dumonceau [32]	1998	48	50	73 %

N/S not stated

Endoscopic Therapy

Table 21.4 documents select series of patients with PBDS treated exclusively by endoscopic dilation and stenting. Follow up in these series is on par with surgical series. Success rates generally range above 90 % overall, with the caveat that patients with Type A injuries (i.e. bile leaks) are included in many of these series. Improved outcomes have been observed over time, as may be expected with advances in endoscopic technology, technique, and experience. More recently, trials of multiple plastic versus larger caliber metallic endobiliary stents have been undertaken; some authorities feel that covered metallic endobiliary stents may provide the most expeditious and durable treatment.

Again, it is important to reiterate that no one technique is suitable to treat all PBDS. A good practice for hepatobiliary surgeons interested in managing these patients is to work closely with their endoscopy (and interventional radiology) colleagues, reviewing the imaging studies early in the treatment course. With experience, one is often able to get a sense of which PBDS will respond to endotherapy alone, and which may require earlier surgical intervention (avoiding protracted periods of stent changes).

Studies with Multiple Treatment Techniques

Table 21.5 lists studies in which patients have been treated by multiple techniques. These studies span the broadest time frame of the current review, and also represent the most heterogeneous group of patients in terms of injury level, treatment selection, and outcome definitions. While many of these studies purport comparison of two groups of patients, great care must be taken drawing conclusions regarding superiority of any one technique.

Table 21.5 Reports including multiple treatment modalities applied to postoperative bile duct strictures

Author	Year	N	F/U-mos	Surgery (success)	Endo (success)	Perc (success)
Pitt [2]	2013	45	58	25 (88 %)	–	20 (55 %)
Benkabbou [55]	2013	528	60	(88 %)	(76 %)	(50 %)
Pottakrt [53]	2010	57	27	25 (N/S)	5 (N/S)	–
Abel-Raouf [52]	2010	260	N/S	16 (NS)	234 (82 %)	–
Fatima [51]	2010	159	45	63 (95 %)	92 (95 %)	–
Ozturk [30]	2009	31	[a]	24 (67 %)	5 (100 %)	–
Nuzzo [50]	2008	77	N/S	41 (78 %)	17 (74 %)	6 (74 %)
DeSantibanes [49]	2006	142	78	106 (86 %)	–	36 (47 %)
Depalma [48]	2003	157	N/S	77 (73 %)	80 (54 %)	–
Tucchi [47]	2000	42	91	22 (77 %)	20 (80 %)	–
Born [46]	1999	40	44	21 (43 %)	31 (90 %)	–
Davids [45]	1993	101	46	35 (83 %)	66 (83 %)	–
Pitt [44]	1989	42	58	25 (88 %)		20 (55 %)

N/S not stated

[a]"Long-term"

In general, treatment outcomes in this group of reports mirror those observed in studies of individual treatment modality: relatively less durable success by percutaneous approach, with approximately 90+ percent success seen in both endoscopic and surgical treatment groups. Reasonable follow up has been achieved in many of these groups. Again, many studies of endoscopic treatment include patients with Strasberg type A injuries (bile leaks), in whom excellent results are expected.

The paper reported by Pitt and his colleagues from Indiana University is noteworthy [2]. This large series is the only report to date to include surgical, percutaneous, and endoscopic treatment of PBDS in a large number of patients. The outcomes achieved by these experienced hepatobiliary surgeons, interventional radiologists, and endoscopists essentially mirrors outcomes described above: moderates success with transhepatic stenting, excellent success with surgical and endoscopic (including type A injury) therapy. Better success in more recent years was attributed to increased experience and stent maintenance for more than 6 months (all treatment modalities). An important observation corroborating prior surgical studies was the poorer outcomes in those patients repaired surgically during "intermediate" time period (i.e. 2–4 weeks post injury) compared to immediate (<48 h) or delayed (>4 week) repair.

Recommendations Based on the Data

- Patients with Strasberg type A injury/PBDS (i.e. bile leak alone) are best treated by endoscopic therapy with stenting (evidence quality moderate, strong recommendation)

- Surgical therapy appears to be the most durable treatment modality overall for patients with Strasberg type B-E injury/PBDS (evidence quality moderate, strong recommendation)
- Timing of surgical repair should be either immediate (<48 h) or delayed for >4–6 weeks from the time of injury (evidence quality moderate, strong recommendation)
- Hepaticojejunostomy Roux-en-Y may be preferable to choledochoduodenostomy for repair of high PBDS (evidence quality weak, weak recommendation).

A Personal View of the Data

Multidisciplinary evaluation of patients with PBDS including experienced endoscopists, interventional radiologists, and hepatobiliary surgeons is ideal to determine the best technique with which to approach specific clinical situations, and therefore achieve optimal outcomes in these complex patients. The location and type of injury/PBDS dictates therapeutic approach (i.e. surgical, percutaneous, endoscopic). In real practice, multiple approaches often provide complimentary information and therapeutic benefit for individual patients.

Surgical management of PBDS demands knowledge of biliary anatomy and the presence of concomitant hepatic artery injury. Timing of repair should be based on the clinical situation, and in most cases delayed 4–6 weeks to control biliary sepsis and permit physical and nutritional optimization. While specific techniques such as high repair (Hepp-Couinaud technique) [62], choledochoduodenostomy, and duration of transhepatic stenting may be debated, it appears clear that the best surgical outcomes come in the hands of experienced biliary units. In patients with PBDS after Roux-en-Y repair, percutaneous stenting is a very reasonable first approach when local expertise is available.

Patient quality of life, time lost from work, overall cost of treatment, and litigation were not addressed in this review; however, each of these issues plays an important role in managing PBDS patients. Long-term (lifetime) follow up of these patients after PBDS repair is ideal.

In this era of evidence-based medicine, it is highly unlikely that a prospective, randomized trial will ever be performed comparing surgical repair to endoscopic or percutaneous treatment of a specific PBDS. Nevertheless, as in other practical medical practice, reasonably solid retrospective analyses inform rational management of this problem [63].

References

1. Flum DR, Cheadle A, Prela C, Dellinger EP, Chan L. Bile duct injury during cholecystectomy and survival in medicare beneficiaries. JAMA. 2003;290(16):2168–73.
2. Pitt HA, Sherman S, Johnson MS, Hollenbeck AN, Lee J, Daum MR, Lillemoe KD, Lehman GA. Improved outcomes of bile duct injuries in the 21st century. Ann Surg. 2013;258:490–9.

3. House MG, Cameron JL, Schulick RD, et al. Incidence and outcome of biliary strictures after pancreaticoduodenectomy. Ann Surg. 2006;243(5):571–6.
4. Tector AJ, Mangus RS, Chestovich P, et al. Use of extended criteria livers decreases wait time for liver transplantation without adversely impacting posttransplant survival. Ann Surg. 2006;244:493–50.
5. Ziegler KM, Pitt HA, Zyromski NJ, et al. Choledochoceles: are they choledochal cysts? Ann Surg. 2010;25(4):683–90.
6. Strasberg SM, Hertl M, Soper NJ, et al. An analysis of the problem of biliary injury during laparoscopic cholecystectomy. J Am Coll Surg. 1995;180(1):101–25.
7. Murr MM, Gigot JF, Nagorney DM, Harmsen WS, Ilstrup DM, Farnell MB. Long-term results of biliary reconstruction after laparoscopic bile duct injuries. Arch Surg. 1999;134:604–9; discussion 609–10.
8. Lillemoe KD, Melton GB, Cameron JL, Pitt HA, Campbell KA, Talamini MA, Sauter PA, Coleman J, Yeo CJ. Postoperative bile duct strictures: management and outcome in the 1990s. Ann Surg. 2000;232:430–41.
9. Johnson SR, Koehler A, Pennington LK, Hanto DW. Long-term results of surgical repair of bile duct injuries following laparoscopic cholecystectomy. Surgery. 2000;128:668–77.
10. Mercado MA, Chan C, Orozco H, Tielve M, Hinojosa CA. Acute bile duct injury. The need for a high repair. Surg Endosc. 2003;17:1351–5.
11. Stewart LG, Robinson TN, Lee CM, et al. Right hepatic artery injury associated with laparoscopic bile duct injury: incidence, mechanism, and consequences. J Gastrointest Surg. 2004;8(5):523–30.
12. Alves A, Farges O, Nicolet J, Watrin T, Sauvanet A, Belghiti J. Incidence and consequence of an hepatic artery injury in patients with postcholecystectomy bile duct strictures. Ann Surg. 2003;238:93–6.
13. Schmidt SC, Langrehr JM, Hintze RE, Neuhaus P. Long-term results and risk factors influencing outcome of major bile duct injuries following cholecystectomy. Br J Surg. 2005;92:76–82.
14. Sicklick JK, Camp MS, Lillemoe KD, Melton GB, Yeo CJ, Campbell KA, Talamini MA, Pitt HA, Coleman J, Sauter PA, Cameron JL. Surgical management of bile duct injuries sustained during laparoscopic cholecystectomy: perioperative results in 200 patients. Ann Surg. 2005;241:786–92; discussion 793–5.
15. Thomson BN, Parks RW, Madhavan KK, Wigmore SJ, Garden OJ. Early specialist repair of biliary injury. Br J Surg. 2006;93:216–20.
16. de Reuver PR, Grossmann I, Busch OR, Obertop H, van Gulik TM, Gouma DJ. Referral pattern and timing of repair are risk factors for complications after reconstructive surgery for bile duct injury. Ann Surg. 2007;245:763–70.
17. Walsh RM, Henderson JM, Vogt DP, Brown N. Long-term outcome of biliary reconstruction for bile duct injuries from laparoscopic cholecystectomies. Surgery. 2007;142:450–6; discussion 456–7.
18. Stewart L, Way LW. Laparoscopic bile duct injuries: timing of surgical repair does not influence success rate. A multivariate analysis of factors influencing surgical outcomes. HPB (Oxf). 2009;11:516–22.
19. Jablonska B, Lampe P, Olakowski M, Gorka Z, Lekstan A, Gruszka T. Hepaticojejunostomy vs. end-to-end biliary reconstructions in the treatment of iatrogenic bile duct injuries. J Gastrointest Surg. 2009;13:1084–93.
20. Sahajpal AK, Chow SC, Dixon E, Greig PD, Gallinger S, Wei AC. Bile duct injuries associated with laparoscopic cholecystectomy timing of repair and long-term outcomes. Arch Surg. 2010;145:757–63.
21. Pottakkat B, Vijayahari R, Prakash A, Singh RK, Behari A, Kumar A, Kapoor VK, Saxena R. Factors predicting failure following high bilio-enteric anastomosis for post-cholecystectomy benign biliary strictures. J Gastrointest Surg. 2010;14:1389–94.
22. Perera MT, Silva MA, Hegab B, Muralidharan V, Bramhall SR, Mayer AD, Buckels JA, Mirza DF. Specialist early and immediate repair of post-laparoscopic cholecystectomy bile duct injuries is associated with an improved long-term outcome. Ann Surg. 2011;253:553–60.

23. Mercado MA, Franssen B, Dominguez I, Arriola-Cabrera JC, Ramirez-Del Val F, Elnecave-Olaiz A, Aramburo-Garcia R, Garcia A. Transition from a low: to a high-volume centre for bile duct repair: changes in technique and improved outcome. HPB (Oxf). 2011;13:767–73.
24. Addeo P, Oussoultzoglou E, Fuchshuber P, Rosso E, Nobili C, Souche R, Jaeck D, Bachellier P. Reoperative surgery after repair of postcholecystectomy bile duct injuries: is it worthwhile? World J Surg. 2013;37:573–81.
25. Leppard WM, Shary TM, Adams DB, Morgan KA. Choledochoduodenostomy: is it really so bad? J Gastrointest Surg. 2011;15(5):754–7.
26. Rose JB, Bilderback P, Raphaeli T, Traverso W, Helton S, Ryan Jr JA, Biehl T. Use the duodenum, it's right there: a retrospective cohort study comparing biliary reconstruction using either the jejunum or the duodenum. JAMA Surg. 2013;148:860–5.
27. Luu C, Lee B, Stabile BE. Choledochoduodenostomy as the biliary-enteric bypass of choice for benign and malignant distal common bile duct strictures. Am Surg. 2013;79:1054–7.
28. Bonnell DH, Liguory CL, Lefgebvre JF, Cornud FE. Placement of metallic stents for treatment of postoperative biliary strictures: long term outcome in 25 patients. AJR. 1997;169(6):1517–22.
29. Misra S, Melton GB, Geschwind JF, Venbrux AC, Cameron JL, Lillemoe KD. Percutaneous management of bile duct strictures and injuries associated with laparoscopic cholecystectomy: a decade of experience. J Am Coll Surg. 2004;198:218–26.
30. Kocher M, Cerna M, Havlik R, Kral V, Gryga A, Duda M. Percutaneous treatment of benign bile duct strictures. Eur J Radiol. 2007;62:170–4.
31. Cantwell CP, Pena CS, Gervais DA, et al. Thirty years' experience with balloon dilation of benign postoperative biliary strictures: long term outcomes. Radiology. 2008;249(3):1050–7.
32. Dumonceau JM, Deviere J, Delhaye M, Baize M, Cremer M. Plastic and metal stents for postoperative benign bile duct strictures: the best and the worst. Gastrointest Enosc. 1998;47(1):8–17.
33. Costamagna G, Pandolfi M, Mutignani M, Spada C, Perri V. Long-term results of endoscopic management of postoperative bile duct strictures with increasing numbers of stents. Gastrointest Endosc. 2001;54:162–8.
34. Draganov P, Hoffman B, Marsh W, Cotton P, Cunningham J. Long-term outcome in patients with benign biliary strictures treated endoscopically with multiple stents. Gastrointest Endosc. 2002;55:680–6.
35. de Reuver PR, Rauws EA, Vermeulen M, Dijkgraaf MG, Gouma DJ, Bruno MJ. Endoscopic treatment of post-surgical bile duct injuries: long term outcome and predictors of success. Gut. 2007;56:1599–605.
36. Katsinelos P, Kountouras J, Paroutoglou G, Chatzimavroudis G, Germanidis G, Zavos C, Pilpilidis I, Paikos D, Papaziogas B. A comparative study of 10-Fr vs. 7-Fr straight plastic stents in the treatment of postcholecystectomy bile leak. Surg Endosc. 2008;22:101–6.
37. Sakai Y, Tsuyuguchi T, Ishihara T, et al. The usefulness of endoscopic transpapillary procedure in post-cholecystectomy bile duct stricture and post-cholecystectomy bile leakage. Hepatogastroenterology. 2009;56(92):978–83.
38. Kuroda Y, Tsuyuguchi T, Sakai Y, et al. Long-term follow-up evaluation for more than 10 years after endoscopic treatment for postoperative bile duct strictures. Surg Endosc. 2010;24(4):834–40.
39. Artifon EL, Coelho F, Frazao M, et al. A prospective randomized study comparing partially covered metal stent versus plastic multistent in the endoscopic management of patients with postoperative benign bile duct strictures: a follow up above 5 years. Rev Gastroenterol Peru. 2012;32(1):26–31.
40. Ghazanfar S, Qureshi S, Leghari A, Taj MA, Niaz SK, Quraishy MS. Endoscopic management of post operative bile duct injuries. J Pak Med Assoc. 2012;62:257–62.
41. Canena J, Liberto M, Coutinho AP, et al. Predictive value of cholangioscopy after endoscopic management of early postcholecystectomy bile duct strictures with an increasing number of plastic stents: a prospective study. Gastrointest Endosc. 2014;79(2):279–88.
42. Iannelli A, Paineau J, Hamy A, Schneck AS, Schaaf C, Gugenheim J. Primary versus delayed repair for bile duct injuries sustained during cholecystectomy: results of a survey of the Association Francaise de Chirurgie. HPB (Oxf). 2013;15:611–6.

43. Stewart L, Way LW. Bile duct injuries during laparoscopic cholecystectomy. Factors that influence the results of treatment. Arch Surg. 1995;130:1123–8; discussion 1129.
44. Pitt HA, Kaufman SL, Coleman JA, et al. Benign postoperative biliary strictures: operate or dilate? Ann Surg. 1989;210:417–25.
45. Davids PH, Tanka AK, Rauws EA, van Gulik TM, van Leeuwen DJ, de Wit LT, Verbeek PC, Huibregtse K, van der Heyde MN, Tytgat GN. Benign biliary strictures. Surgery or endoscopy? Ann Surg. 1993;217:237–43.
46. Born P, Rosch T, Bruhl K, Sandschin W, Allescher HD, Frimberger E, Classen M. Long-term results of endoscopic and percutaneous transhepatic treatment of benign biliary strictures. Endoscopy. 1999;31:725–31.
47. Tocchi A, Mazzoni G, Liotta G, Costa G, Lepre L, Miccini M, De Masi E, Lamazza MA, Fiori E. Management of benign biliary strictures: biliary enteric anastomosis vs endoscopic stenting. Arch Surg. 2000;135:153–7.
48. De Palma GD, Persico G, Sottile R, Puzziello A, Iuliano G, Salvati V, Donisi M, Persico F, Mastantuono L, Persico M, Masone S. Surgery or endoscopy for treatment of postcholecystectomy bile duct strictures? Am J Surg. 2003;185:532–5.
49. de Santibanes E, Palavecino M, Ardiles V, Pekolj J. Bile duct injuries: management of late complications. Surg Endosc. 2006;20:1648–53.
50. Ozturek E, Can MF, Yagci G, et al. Management and mid-to long-term results of early referred bile duct injuries during laparoscopic cholecystectomy. Hepatogastroenterology. 2009;56(89):17–25.
51. Nuzzo G, Giuliante F, Giovannini I, Murazio M, D'Acapito F, Ardito F, Vellone M, Gauzolino R, Costamagna G, Di Stasi C. Advantages of multidisciplinary management of bile duct injuries occurring during cholecystectomy. Am J Surg. 2008;195:763–9.
52. Fatima J, Barton JG, Grotz TE, Geng Z, Harmsen WS, Huebner M, Baron TH, Kendrick ML, Donohue JH, Que FG, Nagorney DM, Farnell MB. Is there a role for endoscopic therapy as a definitive treatment for post-laparoscopic bile duct injuries? J Am Coll Surg. 2010;211:495–502.
53. Abdel-Raouf A, Hamdy E, El-Hanafy E, El-Ebidy G. Endoscopic management of postoperative bile duct injuries: a single center experience. Saudi J Gastroenterol. 2010;16:19–24.
54. Fathy O, Wahab MA, Hamdy E, et al. Post-cholecystectomy biliary injuries: one center experience. Hepatogastroenterology. 2011;58(107–08):719–24.
55. Benkabbou A, Castaing D, Salloum C, Adam R, Azoulay D, Vibert E. Treatment of failed Roux-en-Y hepaticojejunostomy after post-cholecystectomy bile ducts injuries. Surgery. 2013;153:95–102.
56. Kobayashi N, Kubota K, Shimamura T, Watanabe S, Kato S, Suzuki K, Uchiyama T, Maeda S, Takeda K, Nakajima A, Endo I. Complications of the treatment of endoscopic biliary strictures developing after liver transplantation. J Hepatobiliary Pancreat Sci. 2011;18:202–10.
57. Gaman G, Geley F, Doros A, et al. Biliary complications after orthotopic liver transplantation: the Hungarian experience. Transplant Proc. 2013;45(10):3695–7.
58. Prawdzik C, Belyaev O, Chromik AM, et al. Surgical revision of hepaticojejunostomy strictures after pancreatectomy. Langembecks Arch Surg. 2015;400(1):67–75.
59. Ammori BJ, Joesph S, Attia M, et al. Biliary strictures complicating pancreaticoduodenectomy. Int J Pancreatol. 2000;28(1):15–21.
60. Kim JH, Choi TY, Han JH, et al. Risk factors for postoperative anastomotic stricture after excision of choledochal cysts with hepaticojejunostomy. J Gastrointest Surg. 2008;243(5):571–6.
61. Laurant A, Sauvant A, Farges O, et al. Major hepatectomy for the treatment of complex bile duct injury. Ann Surg. 2008;248(1):77–83.
62. Hepp J. Hepaticojejunostomy using the left biliary trunk for iatrogenic biliary lesions: the French connection. World J Surg. 1985;9:507–11.
63. Smith GCS, Pell JP. Parachute use to prevent death and major trauma related to gravitational challenge: systematic review of randomised controlled trials. BMJ. 2003;327:1459–61.

Chapter 22
Immediate or Delayed Repair for Bile Duct Injury Recognized Postoperatively?

Zhi Ven Fong and Keith D. Lillemoe

Abstract Bile duct injuries occurring during laparoscopic cholecystectomy are rare, but result in considerable morbidity, rare mortality and major health care costs. Significant debate and controversy, however, remains regarding the optimal timing of repair of bile duct injury recognized in the postoperative period. Delayed bile duct injury repair has been associated with superior clinical outcomes when compared to immediate repair. Repair via a Roux-en-Y hepaticojejunostomy approach has been shown to have higher success rates when compared to direct repair of these injuries. Repair of bile duct injuries is feasible with no long-term physical quality of life impairments, but with deterioration in mental health that improves over time after repair.

Keywords Bile duct injury • Cholecystectomy • Immediate repair • Delayed repair • Success rate

Introduction

Since the introduction of laparoscopic cholecystectomy (LC) for symptomatic gallstones in the 1980s, the procedure has evolved into one of the most common operations performed in Europe and the US [1]. Although less morbid than its open approach [2, 3], the incidence of a major complication, bile duct injury (BDI), is higher, ranging from 0.15 to 0.6 % (1 per 200) [1, 4–8] versus 0.1–0.3 % (1 per 500 cases) [9] as observed in the open approach cohort (OC). Additionally, BDIs associated with LC tends to be more complex (more proximal injuries involving bifurcation) when compared to injuries sustained during OC [10–12]. It is now accepted that the majority of bile duct injuries occur due to a misidentification of the bile duct

Z.V. Fong • K.D. Lillemoe (✉)
Department of Surgery, Massachusetts General Hospital, Harvard Medical School, 15 Parkman Street, Boston, MA 02114-3117, USA
e-mail: klillemoe@partners.org

J.M. Millis, J.B. Matthews (eds.), *Difficult Decisions in Hepatobiliary and Pancreatic Surgery*, Difficult Decisions in Surgery: An Evidence-Based Approach, DOI 10.1007/978-3-319-27365-5_22

often due to visual-perception illusion and/or inadequate visualization [13]. Irrespective of etiology, bile duct injury represents a significant health and financial burden to both the patient and the healthcare industry [8, 14–16].

In the recent decade, increased experience and regionalization have led to the improved outcomes of BDIs [17, 18]. Multidisciplinary teams comprising of interventional radiologists, gastrointestinal endoscopists and hepatopancreaticobiliary surgeons enable successful repair of BDIs at varying levels of injury and treatment of its long-term sequelaes [4, 17, 19]. While the majority of bile leaks can be managed successfully by endoscopists, the long-term outcomes for major bile duct injuries are still best with surgical intervention, with long-term success rates in excess of 80 % [4, 20, 21]. Questions, however, remain regarding the optimal timing of surgical intervention in BDIs. This chapter compares the outcomes of immediate versus delayed repair for BDIs recognized postoperatively, specifically addressing long-term success rates, mortality, health-related quality of life (HRQoL) and cost. It is important to emphasize, however, that the ultimate decision to delay or undergo repair is based on the surgeon's clinical judgment, weighing in variables such as the presence of vascular injury, biliary leak and local/systemic inflammation.

Search Strategy

A systematic literature search of the English language publications from 2000 to 2014 was performed to identify studies analyzing the outcomes of immediate versus delayed BDI repairs using the PICO outline (Table 22.1. The databases searched were PubMed, EMBASE and Cochrane Review. Terms used in the search were "bile duct injury/immediate repair", "bile duct injury/early repair", "bile duct injury/delayed repair", "laparoscopic cholecystectomy injury/immediate repair", "laparoscopic cholecystectomy/delayed repair" AND ("postoperative morbidity" OR "postoperative mortality" OR "biliary stricture" OR "reintervention"). Articles were excluded if they addressed bile leaks from cystic stump or accessory hepatic ducts rather than common bile duct injury or if intervention focused on endoscopy and interventional therapy rather than surgical. Articles analyzing BDIs discovered intraoperatively were also excluded. Nine retrospective cohort studies were included in our analysis. The data was classified using the GRADE system.

Table 22.1 PICO table for immediate versus delayed repair of bile duct injuries recognized postoperatively

P (Patients)	I (Intervention)	C (Comparator group)	O (Outcomes measured)
Patients with bile duct injuries from cholecystectomies	Immediate surgical repair	Delayed surgical repair	Postoperative morbidity, stricture rate, mortality, quality of life, cost and return to work

Results

Long-Term Success Rate

Long-term success rate, defined as not needing subsequent interventions after the index reconstructive procedure (most commonly for strictures) is the most commonly utilized metric to define the success of the restorative operation. There were nine retrospective cohort studies identified that compared immediate versus delayed repair of postoperatively found BDIs. There were no prospective, randomized controlled trial performed and will likely not be feasible given the rarity and complexity of BDIs. Given the lack of level I data, our current understanding and clinical algorithm for managing postoperatively discovered BDIs are based on retrospective cohort studies, which heavily favors delayed repair of these injuries (all quality of evidence: low, Table 22.2).

Of the nine studies, six demonstrated higher long-term success rates when delayed repair was undertaken versus immediate repair of BDIs diagnosed postoperatively. In the largest cohort study, Iannelli and colleagues conducted a national French survey involving 47 surgical centers encompassing 543 patients and reported that delayed repair (≥45 days) of BDIs was associated with a higher success rate when compared to immediate repair (<45 days, 93.2 % vs 59.3 %, $p<0.001$) [22]. However, long-term follow-up is required to accurately evaluate success rate of the intervention and none was reported in the study. In the study with the longest follow-up of 72 months, Sahajpal et al. reported that success rates was higher when delayed repair was undertaken (>6 weeks, 100 %) as compared to repair in the intermediate period (72 h to 6 weeks, 91 %, $p=0.03$) [23].

The limitation to this review is that all studies utilize different time thresholds when comparing immediate versus delayed repair of postoperatively diagnosed BDIs. The summary in Table 22.2 suggests that a delayed repair of at least >6 weeks is ideal to achieve long-term success rates ranging from 90 to 100 %, and that repair anytime before that was associated with a higher rate of the need for reintervention.

There were no studies reporting superior outcomes with immediate repair of BDIs. Of the three studies that reported no difference between both approaches, Sicklick et al. dichotomized the timing interval to <1 month, 1–12 months and >12 months [24]. Another compared outcomes when repair was undertaken <2 weeks from BDI versus 2 weeks to 6 months after injury [25]. Assuming the above review holds true that a higher success rate is achieved if postoperatively found BDI repairs were delayed for at least 6 weeks, the aforementioned time frames will not appropriately portray an accurate comparison of immediate versus delayed repair of postoperatively diagnosed BDIs.

Table 22.2 Long-term success and mortality rate of immediate versus delayed repair of postoperatively recognized bile duct injury after cholecystectomy

1st author, year	n	Follow-up (months)	Timing definition	Level of injury	Method of repair	Success rate (%)[a]	Mortality (%)
Pitt, 2013	98	54	<2 weeks	Strasberg:	RYBE, 98 %	<2 weeks: 90	–
			2–4 weeks	B–C, 3 %	End-to-end, 1 %	2–4 weeks: 43*	
			6–8 weeks	D, 3 %	Transplant, 1 %	6–8 weeks: 100	
				E1–E5, 93 %			
Iannelli, 2013	543	–	<45 days	All defined as extrahepatic injuries	RYBE, 48 %	<45 days: 59*	<45 days: 3.9
			≥45 days		End-to-end, 52 %	≥45 days: 93.2	≥45 days: 0.8*
Sahajpal, 2010	69	72	0–72 h	Strasberg:	RYBE: 94 %	0–72 h: 98	0–72 h: 0
			72 h to 6 weeks	A–C, 1 %	Hepatectomy: 4 %	72 h to 6 weeks: 91*	72 h to 6 weeks: 1
			>6 weeks	D–E5, 99 %	End-to-end: 1 %	>6 weeks: 100	>6 weeks: 0
Stewart, 2009	137	40	1 week	Stewart-Way:	–	1 week: 90	–
			2 weeks	I, 5 %		2 weeks: 93	
			3–6 weeks	II, 24 %		3–6 weeks: 91	
			>6 weeks	III, 61 %		>6 weeks: 95	
				IV, 10 %			
Goykhman, 2008	29	24	24–72 h	CHD, 55 %	RYBE: 100 %	24–72 h: 0*	–
			>8 weeks	RHD, 17 %		>8 weeks: 90	
				RPHD, 10 %			
Walsh, 2007	144	67	<7 days	Strasberg:	RYBE: 87 %	<7 days: 81*	–
			>79 days	B–C, 12 %		>79 days: 92	
				E1–E2, 27 %			
				E3, 38 %			
				E4, 20 %			
				E5, 1 %			

De Reuver, 2007	151	54	<6 weeks	Amsterdam:	–	<6 weeks: 67*	<6 weeks: 0
			≥6 weeks	A, 0.7		≥6 weeks: 95	≥6 weeks: 0
				B, 8.6			
				C, 9.9			
				D, 80.7			
Thomson, 2005	68	33	<2 weeks	Strasberg:	RYBE: 85 %	<2 weeks: 86	<2 weeks: 8*
			2 weeks to 6 months	B, 1 %	End-to-end: 9 %	2 weeks to 6 months: 88	2 weeks to 6 months: 0
				D, 2 %			
				E1, 8 %			
				E2, 30 %			
				E3, 25 %			
				E4, 18 %			
				E5, 3 %			
Sicklick, 2005	175	–	<1 month	Bismuth:	RYBE: 98 %	p>0.05	p>0.05
			1–12 months	1, 6 %	End-to-end: 2 %		
			>12 months	2, 31 %			
				3, 26 %			
				4, 12 %			
				5, 22 %			

RYBE roux-en y biliary-enteric, *CHD* common hepatic duct, *RHD* right hepatic duct, *RPHD* right posterior hepatic duct

*Denotes statistical significance at the $p<0.05$ level

[a]Success defined as no need for further intervention after primary repair

Method of Repair

The most common methods of repairing BDI are direct repair with primary anastomosis (DR) and a Roux-en-Y hepaticojejunostomy (RYHJ). Historically, DR outside of the immediate setting if BDI was discovered intraoperatively has been associated with poor outcomes, with failure rates ranging from 64 to 78 % [22, 25, 26]. Thermal injuries that jeopardizes the microvascular supply to the biliary tree and right hepatic artery injury have all been theorized to lead to the ultimate failure of DR. Additionally, DR is difficult to perform in a tension-free fashion secondary to retraction of the proximal transected bile duct proximally if repair is delayed. Ianelli et al. demonstrated that the timing of surgical repair was a stronger predictor of success than the method of repair: DR was associated with success rates of 36 % when performed at the time of LC, and 57 % when performed within 45 days (none reported >45 days); RYHJ was associated with success rates of 37 % when performed at time of LC, but improved to 54 % and 93 % when performed within 45 days and >45 days post-BDI respectively [22].

Mortality

Of the nine cohort studies analyzed, only four studies provided mortality data. Of the four studies, three reported a higher mortality rate in the immediate repair (<6 weeks) group but only two achieved statistical significance (Table 22.2). The studies are likely underpowered for a mortality analysis, and the discrepancy between mortality rates in both groups would likely be more apparent favoring delayed repair of postoperatively found BDIs if the sample size were larger.

Health-Related Quality of Life and Cost

While clinical outcomes of BDI repair have been well described and compared, patient reported outcomes like HRQoL arguably plays a larger role in defining the success of the index repair. The Vanderbilt group recently performed a meta-analysis of six studies (581 patients), which compared the HRQoL of patients with BDIs with patients who underwent an uncomplicated LC. After controlling for follow-up time, BDI patients were not more likely to have a reduced physical HRQoL than LC patients ($p=0.993$), but were about 38 times more likely to have a reduced mental HRQoL (OR=38.4, 95 % C.I. 19.14–77.10, $p<0.001$) [14]. More recently, the Hopkins group assessed patients after BDI repair with a median follow-up of 169 months. Their study corroborated the findings of the aforementioned meta-analysis, with 49 % of patients reporting a depressed mood and 40 % reporting low energy level but unchanged levels of physical activity and general health [27].

Unique to their study, however, was a pre- versus post-intervention analysis, which showed that the detrimental effect on mental health significantly improved over time after BDI repair (49 % depressed mood before repair, vs 18 % after repair, $p<0.001$; 40 % low energy before repair, vs 18 % after repair, $p=0.01$).

The impact of BDI on healthcare cost, on the other hand, is dramatic secondary to the need for complex repair and long-term multidisciplinary management of complications (i.e. endoscopic balloon dilatation, interventional radiology guided biliary drains). The cost of repair of BDIs can run 5–26 times the cost of an uncomplicated LC, costing over $50,000 for all its related care. These increased cost are especially apparent in postoperatively discovered BDIs versus those recognized intraoperatively, with the former group's care costing 43–83 % less than the latter group [8, 28]. The tremendous expenses incurred holds true in Europe as well, with a Swedish group reporting costs from 473,690 EUR to 608,789 EUR per million inhabitants annually [29]. When discussing the financial burden of BDIs, cost associated with litigation should be considered as well. Up to 19–31 % of patients suffering BDIs seek litigation [15, 30], with half of them settling out of court (mean payment $469,711). Of those that proceeded to trial, about 20 % concludes with plaintiff jury verdicts with mean payment of $188,772 [31].

A Personal View of the Data

The incidence of BDI after LC is uncommon, but results in significant added morbidity, mortality and represents a financial burden on healthcare cost. While there are no level I evidence in the BDI literature, considerable retrospective data indicate that delayed repair of postoperatively found BDIs have been found to result in superior outcomes when compared to immediate repair, achieving a significantly higher long-term success rate and lower mortality rates. The decision to perform or delay repair of BDI must also be driven by the surgeon's clinical judgment (eradication of local and systemic sepsis and inflammation). Repair via a RYHJ reconstruction is associated with a higher success rate when compared to DR, with DR likely anatomically impossible to perform secondary to traction of the transected bile ducts. Patients suffering BDIs have no long-term impairment in physical HRQoL but experienced worse mental health as compared to patients undergoing uncomplicated LC. However, this impairment in mental HRQoL improves over time after BDI repair.

Recommendation Based on the Data

- For patients with postoperatively found BDI, we recommend delayed repair of up to 6 weeks after the index injury to achieve optimal long-term success rates (evidence quality low; strong recommendation).

- Postoperatively found BDIs should be repaired via a RYHJJ approach, as DR results in a higher failure rate (evidence quality low; strong recommendation).

References

1. Flum DR, Dellinger EP, Cheadle A, et al. Intraoperative cholangiography and risk of common bile duct injury during cholecystectomy. JAMA. 2003;289(13):1639–44.
2. Kiviluoto T, Siren J, Luukkonen P, et al. Randomised trial of laparoscopic versus open cholecystectomy for acute and gangrenous cholecystitis. Lancet. 1998;351(9099):321–5.
3. Steiner CA, Bass EB, Talamini MA, et al. Surgical rates and operative mortality for open and laparoscopic cholecystectomy in Maryland. N Engl J Med. 1994;330(6):403–8.
4. Pitt HA, Sherman S, Johnson MS, et al. Improved outcomes of bile duct injuries in the 21st century. Ann Surg. 2013;258(3):490–9.
5. Walsh RM, Henderson JM, Vogt DP, et al. Long-term outcome of biliary reconstruction for bile duct injuries from laparoscopic cholecystectomies. Surgery. 2007;142(4):450–6; discussion 456–7.
6. Nuzzo G, Giuliante F, Giovannini I, et al. Bile duct injury during laparoscopic cholecystectomy: results of an Italian national survey on 56 591 cholecystectomies. Arch Surg. 2005;140(10):986–92.
7. Schwaitzberg SD, Scott DJ, Jones DB, et al. Threefold increased bile duct injury rate is associated with less surgeon experience in an insurance claims database: more rigorous training in biliary surgery may be needed. Surg Endosc. 2014;28:3068–73.
8. Savader SJ, Lillemoe KD, Prescott CA, et al. Laparoscopic cholecystectomy-related bile duct injuries: a health and financial disaster. Ann Surg. 1997;225(3):268–73.
9. Roslyn JJ, Binns GS, Hughes EF, et al. Open cholecystectomy. A contemporary analysis of 42,474 patients. Ann Surg. 1993;218(2):129–37.
10. Lillemoe KD, Melton GB, Cameron JL, et al. Postoperative bile duct strictures: management and outcome in the 1990s. Ann Surg. 2000;232(3):430–41.
11. Chuang KI, Corley D, Postlethwaite DA, et al. Does increased experience with laparoscopic cholecystectomy yield more complex bile duct injuries? Am J Surg. 2012;203(4):480–7.
12. Slater K, Strong RW, Wall DR, et al. Iatrogenic bile duct injury: the scourge of laparoscopic cholecystectomy. ANZ J Surg. 2002;72(2):83–8.
13. Chen G, Wang H, Chen L, et al. Living donor liver transplantation using a left lobe graft from a donor with severe liver trauma: a 7-year follow-up. Liver Transpl. 2009;15(10):1370–3.
14. Landman MP, Feurer ID, Moore DE, et al. The long-term effect of bile duct injuries on health-related quality of life: a meta-analysis. HPB (Oxf). 2013;15(4):252–9.
15. Melton GB, Lillemoe KD, Cameron JL, et al. Major bile duct injuries associated with laparoscopic cholecystectomy: effect of surgical repair on quality of life. Ann Surg. 2002;235(6):888–95.
16. Boerma D, Rauws EA, Keulemans YC, et al. Impaired quality of life 5 years after bile duct injury during laparoscopic cholecystectomy: a prospective analysis. Ann Surg. 2001;234(6):750–7.
17. Walsh RM, Vogt DP, Ponsky JL, et al. Management of failed biliary repairs for major bile duct injuries after laparoscopic cholecystectomy. J Am Coll Surg. 2004;199(2):192–7.
18. Mercado MA, Franssen B, Dominguez I, et al. Transition from a low: to a high-volume centre for bile duct repair: changes in technique and improved outcome. HPB (Oxf). 2011;13(11):767–73.
19. Nuzzo G, Giuliante F, Giovannini I, et al. Advantages of multidisciplinary management of bile duct injuries occurring during cholecystectomy. Am J Surg. 2008;195(6):763–9.

20. Lillemoe KD, Martin SA, Cameron JL, et al. Major bile duct injuries during laparoscopic cholecystectomy. Follow-up after combined surgical and radiologic management. Ann Surg. 1997;225(5):459–68; discussion 468–71.
21. Johnson SR, Koehler A, Pennington LK, et al. Long-term results of surgical repair of bile duct injuries following laparoscopic cholecystectomy. Surgery. 2000;128(4):668–77.
22. Iannelli A, Paineau J, Hamy A, et al. Primary versus delayed repair for bile duct injuries sustained during cholecystectomy: results of a survey of the Association Francaise de Chirurgie. HPB (Oxf). 2013;15(8):611–6.
23. Sahajpal AK, Chow SC, Dixon E, et al. Bile duct injuries associated with laparoscopic cholecystectomy: timing of repair and long-term outcomes. Arch Surg. 2010;145(8):757–63.
24. Sicklick JK, Camp MS, Lillemoe KD, et al. Surgical management of bile duct injuries sustained during laparoscopic cholecystectomy: perioperative results in 200 patients. Ann Surg. 2005;241(5):786–92; discussion 793–5.
25. Thomson BN, Parks RW, Madhavan KK, et al. Early specialist repair of biliary injury. Br J Surg. 2006;93(2):216–20.
26. Stewart L, Way LW. Bile duct injuries during laparoscopic cholecystectomy. Factors that influence the results of treatment. Arch Surg. 1995;130(10):1123–8; discussion 1129.
27. Ejaz A, Spolverato G, Kim Y, et al. Long-term health-related quality of life after iatrogenic bile duct injury repair. J Am Coll Surg. 2014;219:923–32.
28. Bass EB, Pitt HA, Lillemoe KD. Cost-effectiveness of laparoscopic cholecystectomy versus open cholecystectomy. Am J Surg. 1993;165(4):466–71.
29. Andersson R, Eriksson K, Blind PJ, et al. Iatrogenic bile duct injury – a cost analysis. HPB (Oxf). 2008;10(6):416–9.
30. de Reuver PR, Sprangers MA, Rauws EA, et al. Impact of bile duct injury after laparoscopic cholecystectomy on quality of life: a longitudinal study after multidisciplinary treatment. Endoscopy. 2008;40(8):637–43.
31. Kern KA. Malpractice litigation involving laparoscopic cholecystectomy. Cost, cause, and consequences. Arch Surg. 1997;132(4):392–7; discussion 397–8.

Chapter 23
Management of Suspected Choledocholithiasis on Intraoperative Cholangiography

B. Fernando Santos and Eric S. Hungness

Abstract Choledocholithiasis is a frequently encountered problem on intraoperative cholangiography at the time of laparoscopic cholecystectomy. While numerous strategies have been described for dealing with this intraoperative scenario, most surgeons employ laparoscopic common bile duct exploration (LCBDE), open common bile duct exploration, or postoperative endoscopic retrograde cholangiopancreatography (ERCP) in this situation. It is important to understand the relative outcomes of each of these strategies in terms of stone clearance rates, morbidity, the need for secondary procedures, and other outcomes such as hospital length of stay. Although the data are limited, the initial procedure of choice may be LCBDE through a transcystic approach, followed by either transcholedochal exploration (laparoscopic or open) or postoperative ERCP depending on anatomic factors and available expertise.

Keywords Choledocholithiasis • Bile duct exploration • Open • Laparoscopic • Sphincterotomy • Endoscopic retrograde cholangiopancreatography • Cholangiography

Introduction

Choledocholithiasis is a common problem, occurring in approximately 10–15 % of all patients undergoing cholecystectomy [1]. In the "open" surgical era, the standard of care for choledocholithiasis was open cholecystectomy with concurrent common bile duct exploration. The introduction of laparoscopic cholecystectomy, however,

B.F. Santos (✉)
Geisel School of Medicine at Dartmouth, White River Junction Veterans Affairs Medical Center, 215 N. Main Street, Building 31-269, White River Junction, Hartford, VT 05009, USA
e-mail: Byron.Santos-Aleman@va.gov

E.S. Hungness
Northwestern University, Chicago, IL, USA
e-mail: ehungnes@nmh.org

J.M. Millis, J.B. Matthews (eds.), *Difficult Decisions in Hepatobiliary and Pancreatic Surgery*, Difficult Decisions in Surgery: An Evidence-Based Approach, DOI 10.1007/978-3-319-27365-5_23

made conversion to open common bile duct exploration in the setting of choledocholithiasis discovered intraoperatively a less attractive option, leading to the increased utilization of endoscopic retrograde cholangiopancreatography (ERCP) for the diagnosis and management of choledocholithiasis. The eventual development of laparoscopic common bile duct exploration, while expanding the available therapeutic options for choledocholithiasis, has made the algorithm for the management of choledocholithiasis more complex. This evidence-based chapter seeks to identify and analyze the best available evidence for the management of a frequently encountered scenario: choledocholithiasis discovered intra-operatively during laparoscopic cholecystectomy. While numerous options have been described for dealing with this scenario, the chapter will focus on the three main options of laparoscopic common bile duct exploration (LCBDE), open common bile duct exploration (OCBDE), and postoperative ERCP.

Search Strategy

A systematic search of the English language literature was conducted using PubMed and the PICO methodology (Table 23.1). The "filter" function was used to select articles classified as "Randomized Controlled Trial" in order to obtain the highest quality comparative studies. The search terms used included "laparoscopic bile duct exploration," "open bile duct exploration," "bile duct exploration", "ERCP," "endoscopic sphincterotomy," "choledocholithiasis," and "common bile duct stones." Studies that directly compared at least two of the three interventions (OCBDE, LCBDE, or ERCP) were included. Studies that compared two different variations of a single intervention (e.g. LCBDE with choledochoscopy versus LCBDE with fluoroscopy alone) were excluded, as were studies involving intraoperative ERCP. Treatment outcomes of interest included stone clearance rate, morbidity including bile duct injury, and the need for secondary procedures. Event rates were reported as percentages or total numbers of patients, with means reported as mean ± standard deviation unless otherwise noted.

Table 23.1 PICO table – management strategies for patients with choledocholithiasis discovered on intraoperative cholangiography

P (Patients)	I (Intervention)	C (Comparator)	O (Outcomes)
Patients with choledocholithiasis on intraoperative cholangiogram	Laparoscopic common bile duct exploration	Open common bile duct exploration or postoperative ERCP	Stone clearance rate, morbidity, need for secondary procedures, and hospital length of stay

Results

A literature search was conducted and included articles published prior to September 17th, 2014. A total of 590 articles were screened with a total of 16 randomized controlled trials (RCT) meeting the inclusion and exclusion criteria. Seven of these articles compared OCBDE to preoperative ERCP plus cholecystectomy [2–8], six articles compared LCBDE to preoperative ERCP plus cholecystectomy [9–14], one article compared OCBDE to LCBDE [15], and two articles compared LCBDE to laparoscopic cholecystectomy with postoperative ERCP [16, 17].

The most relevant RCTs to help determine the best evidence-based strategy for the management of choledocholithiasis found on intraoperative cholangiography are those that compare LCBDE to postoperative ERCP (Rhodes 1998; Nathanson 2005) [16, 17], and LCBDE to OCBDE (Grubnik 2012) [15] (Table 23.2). Unfortunately, there are no RCTs that have compared open cholecystectomy with OCBDE versus open cholecystectomy with postoperative ERCP.

LCBDE Versus Postoperative ERCP

'The study by Rhodes et al. recruited 480 patients undergoing laparoscopic cholecystectomy [17]. Eighty patients (17 %) in the study group had cholangiograms demonstrating common bile duct (CBD) stones. The patients with choledocholithiasis were randomized intraoperatively to LCBDE or postoperative ERCP. For patients in the LCBDE group, a transcystic approach was attempted for patients with small CBD stones (<9 mm). A transcholedochal approach was instead used for patients with larger stones, proximal stones, a failed transcystic approach, and as long as the CBD was at least 6 mm to decrease the risk of postoperative stricture. Inability to clear the ducts with LCBDE led to postoperative ERCP. Patients randomized to postoperative ERCP underwent cholecystectomy followed by ERCP within 48 h of surgery. Inability to clear the duct with postoperative ERCP was followed by repeat ERCP attempt (s) 1 week later. The initial stone clearance rate for both groups was equivalent (75 %). Morbidity was similar between groups (18 % for LCBDE versus 20 % for postoperative ERCP). Morbidity for LCBDE included conversion to open surgery (2.5 %), urinary retention (2.5 %), readmission for pain of unclear etiology (5 %), and bile leak related to transcholedochal exploration (7.5 %). Morbidity for the postoperative ERCP group included hemorrhage requiring laparoscopic re-operation (2.5 %), bile leak while waiting for ERCP (2.5 %), bleeding from sphincterotomy site (7.5 %), and inability to clear CBD after repeated ERCP attempts (7.5 %). The need for postoperative ERCP was 25 % in the LCBDE group. Ten patients in the LCBDE group required additional procedures (nine ERCPs and one conversion to OCBDE). Ten patients randomized to postoperative ERCP required a second ERCP, with five of these patients requiring a third ERCP for a total of 15 additional ERCPs. Final stone clearance rate was 100 % for LCBDE patients and 93 % for

Table 23.2 Results of trials comparing LCBDE, OCBDE, and/or postoperative ERCP for patients with choledocholithiasis discovered on intraoperative cholangiography

Study	N	Arm	Stone clearance (initial)	Stone clearance (final)	Morbidity	Common bile duct injury	Number of additional procedures	Length of stay	Study quality
Rhodes (1998)	40	LCBDE	75 %	100 %	18 %	0 %	10	1 day[a]	Low
	40	ERCP	75 %	93 %	20 %	0 %	15	3.5 days	
Nathanson (2005)	41	LCBDE	98 %	100 %	29 %	2.4 %	1	6.4 days	Low
	45	ERCP	96 %	100 %	20 %	2.2 %	2	7.7 days	
Grubnik (2012)	138	LCBDE	94 %	100 %	6.5 %	0 %	4	4.2 days[a]	Low
	118	OCBDE	97 %	100 %	12.7 %	0 %	5	12.6 days	

[a]Statistically significant difference

postoperative ERCP patients. Median hospital length of stay was significantly shorter for the LCBDE group (1 day, range 1–26 days) versus the postoperative ERCP group (3.5 days, range 1–11 days, p=0.0001). The conclusions of this study were that LCBDE can be performed with equivalent stone clearance rates, similar morbidity, but a shorter hospital stay compared to postoperative ERCP.

Martin et al. reported on the technical evolution of a laparoscopic approach to patients with choledocholithiasis, achieving successful stone clearance in 90 % of patients using a combination of transcystic or transcholedochal exploration [18]. Given the higher morbidity with transcholedochal versus transcystic exploration in their series, however, the same investigators (Nathanson et al.) then sought to study whether patients who had failed transcystic stone clearance were better off with immediate transcholedochal LCBDE or postoperative ERCP [16]. They enrolled 372 patients undergoing an attempt at transcystic LCBDE. The 23 % of patients (n=86) who failed transcystic LCBDE were randomized intraoperatively to transcholedochal LCBDE versus postoperative ERCP. Initial stone clearance rates were similar (98 % for transcholedochal and 96 % for postoperative ERCP). One patient in the LCBDE group required postoperative ERCP for a retained stone, while two postoperative ERCP patients required LCBDE for retained stones. Overall morbidity was similar between groups and included bile leak (six patients for transcholedochal LCBDE, none for ERCP), clinical pancreatitis (one patient in each group), severe sepsis (one patient in each group), retained stone (two patients for postoperative ERCP and one patient for LCBDE), gastrointestinal bleeding (two patients for postoperative ERCP), early re-operation (two for transcholedochal LCBDE, and two for postoperative ERCP), and late re-operation for a biliary stricture (one patient in each group) possibly representing a bile duct injury from the procedure (s). Hospital length of stay was similar (mean of 6.4 versus 7.7 days for transcholedochal LCBDE and postoperative ERCP, respectively). The conclusions of this study were that either transcholedochal LCBDE or postoperative ERCP could be performed with similar results for patients who had failed attempted transcystic LCBDE. The authors recommended that transcholedochal LCBDE be avoided in patients with a CBD less than 7 mm or in the setting of severe inflammation. They advocated the use of transcholedochal LCBDE in patients with a history of a Billroth II reconstruction, in those who failed ERCP, or in those who otherwise would experience long delays in being transferred to other centers for ERCP.

The results of these studies suggest that for patients found to have choledocholithiasis on intraoperative cholangiography, LCBDE can achieve similar stone clearance rates and morbidity compared to postoperative ERCP, and yet result in a shorter length of stay and a decreased number of procedures.

LCBDE Versus OCBCE

How does LCBDE compare to OCBDE, the gold standard for choledocholithiasis during the "open era," in patients found to have choledocholithiasis on intraoperative cholangiography? A single, randomized controlled trial from Eastern Europe addresses this question (Grubnik 2012) [15]. This trial enrolled 256 patients with suspected choledocholithiasis, confirmed on intraoperative cholangiography, and randomized them to LCBDE (n = 138) or OCBDE (n = 118). Bile duct exploration was performed using an initial transcystic approach followed by a transcholedochal approach if unsuccessful. Stone clearance rates for LCBDE were 71 % with an initial transcystic approach and 94 % with a subsequent transcholedochal approach. Stone clearance rate with a transcystic approach was 10 % for OCBDE and 96.6 % with a subsequent transcholedochal or transduodenal (one patient) approach. Four patients (6.5 %) in the LCBCE group required postoperative ERCPs for stone clearance, resulting in a 100 % final stone clearance rate. In the OCBDE group four patients (3.3 %) required ERCP with one patient requiring an additional open re-exploration., for a final stone clearance rate of 100 %. Overall morbidity was similar between groups, with the exception of wound infections, which were more frequent in OCBDE (6 % versus 0.7 % for LCBDE). Bile leak was similar in both groups (1.4 % in LCBDE patients versus 0.8 % in OCBDE patients). Blood loss (20 ± 12 ml versus 285 ± 27 ml) and length of stay were significantly less in the LCBDE group (4.2 ± 1.8 days versus 12.6 ± 4.5 days for OCBDE, $p < 0.01$). The conclusions of this study were that LCBDE could be performed with similar efficacy and morbidity but with a shortened length of stay compared to OCBDE.

There are several limitations of these studies including unclear preoperative selection criteria and unclear length of follow-up. In addition, the use of non-choledochoscopic methods for LCBDE in the study by Rhodes et al., and the use of various methods for closing the choledochotomy (primary closure versus T-tube versus primary closure with ampullary stent) introduce additional heterogeneity to these studies. Finally, it is unclear from the studies how experienced the ERCP operators were. The study by Rhodes has the potential for bias, as the surgeon performing the LCBDEs also performed a majority of the ERCPs, with an initial stone clearance rate of 75 %. This low rate of clearance with postoperative ERCP seems relatively low compared to clearance rates published in the literature of greater than 95 % in some large series [19].

Recommendations Based on the Data

1. Patients with choledocholithiasis discovered on intraoperative cholangiography, should undergo an initial attempt at transcystic LCBDE if feasible (distal stone, stone diameter <9 mm). (Evidence quality low, weak recommendation).
2. Patients with choledocholithiasis in whom transcystic LCBDE is unsuccessful, should undergo either transcholedochal exploration (laparoscopic or open, depending on surgeon experience) if the bile duct is greater than 7 mm, or postoperative ERCP if feasible (available skilled endoscopist and favorable anatomy). (Evidence quality low, weak recommendation).

A Personal View of the Data

The available data show that LCBDE compared to postoperative ERCP has comparable safety and efficacy for the management of choledocholithiasis found on intraoperative cholangiography, and on average results in a shorter hospital stay and fewer numbers of postoperative procedures. The data also show that the efficacy of LCBDE is comparable to that of OCBDE, but with decreased morbidity related to wound complications and a shorter hospital length of stay. These data are consistent with data showing the benefits of both LCBDE and OCBDE compared to ERCP performed in the preoperative setting, which have been previously well-established [2–8, 14]. Transcystic LCBDE appears to have fewer complications compared to transcholedochal LCBDE and may be the most reasonable option to attempt initially, with transcholedochal LCBE or postoperative ERCP reserved as second-line options depending on surgeon experience and access to ERCP. Although not used in the study by Rhodes et al., flexible choledochoscopy is a valuable adjunct that may increase the efficacy of transcystic LCBDE. Future studies with larger numbers of patients are needed to confirm these benefits of LCBDE versus postoperative ERCP, and would be most applicable if they limited LCBDE to a transcystic approach which is a technique that is more likely to be a adopted by surgeons compared to transcholedochal LCBDE.

Despite the evidence for its safety and efficacy, LCBDE continues to remain largely underutilized for the treatment of choledocholithiasis compared to ERCP in the United States, especially in urban settings [20, 21]. Among the many reasons for this may be that LCBDE is viewed by some surgeons as too technically challenging, time-consuming, logistically difficult, unnecessary in the setting of access to skilled endoscopists in some centers, and the fact that LCBDE currently lacks a strong training paradigm. Current training for LCBDE is largely dependent on operative experience alone, which even for experienced surgeons can be infrequent. Simulation-based LCBDE training curricula have recently been developed and may have the potential to improve training for this relatively infrequent clinical scenario [22, 23]. Such training could not only address surgeon skill but also could be applied to improve familiarity of the operating room staff with the procedure and its equipment needs, ultimately improving utilization of LCBDE in practice.

References

1. Tranter SE, Thompson MH. Spontaneous passage of bile duct stones: frequency of occurrence and relation to clinical presentation. Ann R Coll Surg Engl. 2003;85:174–7.
2. Hammarstrom LE, Holmin T, Stridbeck H, Ihse I. Long-term follow-up of a prospective randomized study of endoscopic versus surgical treatment of bile duct calculi in patients with gallbladder in situ. Br J Surg. 1995;82:1516–21.
3. Kapoor R, Kaushik SP, Saraswat VA, Choudhuri G, Sikora SS, Saxena R, Kapoor VK. Prospective randomized trial comparing endoscopic sphincterotomy followed by surgery

with surgery alone in good risk patients with choledocholithiasis. HPB Surg World J Hepatic Pancreat Biliary Surg. 1996;9:145–8.

4. Neoptolemos JP, Carr-Locke DL, Fossard DP. Prospective randomised study of preoperative endoscopic sphincterotomy versus surgery alone for common bile duct stones. Br Med J (Clin Res Ed). 1987;294:470–4.
5. Stain SC, Cohen H, Tsuishoysha M, Donovan AJ. Choledocholithiasis. Endoscopic sphincterotomy or common bile duct exploration. Ann Surg. 1991;213:627–33; discussion 633–624.
6. Stiegmann GV, Goff JS, Mansour A, Pearlman N, Reveille RM, Norton L. Precholecystectomy endoscopic cholangiography and stone removal is not superior to cholecystectomy, cholangiography, and common duct exploration. Am J Surg. 1992;163:227–30.
7. Suc B, Escat J, Cherqui D, Fourtanier G, Hay JM, Fingerhut A, Millat B. Surgery vs endoscopy as primary treatment in symptomatic patients with suspected common bile duct stones: a multicenter randomized trial. French Associations for Surgical Research. Arch Surg. 1998;133:702–8.
8. Targarona EM, Ayuso RM, Bordas JM, Ros E, Pros I, Martinez J, Teres J, Trias M. Randomised trial of endoscopic sphincterotomy with gallbladder left in situ versus open surgery for common bileduct calculi in high-risk patients. Lancet. 1996;347:926–9.
9. Bansal VK, Misra MC, Garg P, Prabhu M. A prospective randomized trial comparing two-stage versus single-stage management of patients with gallstone disease and common bile duct stones. Surg Endosc. 2010;24:1986–9.
10. Cuschieri A, Lezoche E, Morino M, Croce E, Lacy A, Toouli J, Faggioni A, Ribeiro VM, Jakimowicz J, Visa J, Hanna GB. E.A.E.S. multicenter prospective randomized trial comparing two-stage vs single-stage management of patients with gallstone disease and ductal calculi. Surg Endosc. 1999;13:952–7.
11. Koc B, Karahan S, Adas G, Tutal F, Guven H, Ozsoy A. Comparison of laparoscopic common bile duct exploration and endoscopic retrograde cholangiopancreatography plus laparoscopic cholecystectomy for choledocholithiasis: a prospective randomized study. Am J Surg. 2013;206:457–63.
12. Noble H, Tranter S, Chesworth T, Norton S, Thompson M. A randomized, clinical trial to compare endoscopic sphincterotomy and subsequent laparoscopic cholecystectomy with primary laparoscopic bile duct exploration during cholecystectomy in higher risk patients with choledocholithiasis. J Laparoendosc Adv Surg Tech A. 2009;19:713–20.
13. Rogers SJ, Cello JP, Horn JK, Siperstein AE, Schecter WP, Campbell AR, Mackersie RC, Rodas A, Kreuwel HT, Harris HW. Prospective randomized trial of LC+LCBDE vs ERCP/S+LC for common bile duct stone disease. Arch Surg. 2010;145:28–33.
14. Iranmanesh P, Frossard JL, Mugnier-Konrad B, Morel P, Majno P, Nguyen-Tang T, Berney T, Mentha G, Toso C. Initial cholecystectomy vs sequential common duct endoscopic assessment and subsequent cholecystectomy for suspected gallstone migration: a randomized clinical trial. JAMA. 2014;312:137–44.
15. Grubnik VV, Tkachenko AI, Ilyashenko VV, Vorotyntseva KO. Laparoscopic common bile duct exploration versus open surgery: comparative prospective randomized trial. Surg Endosc. 2012;26:2165–71.
16. Nathanson LK, O'Rourke NA, Martin IJ, Fielding GA, Cowen AE, Roberts RK, Kendall BJ, Kerlin P, Devereux BM. Postoperative ERCP versus laparoscopic choledochotomy for clearance of selected bile duct calculi: a randomized trial. Ann Surg. 2005;242:188–92.
17. Rhodes M, Sussman L, Cohen L, Lewis MP. Randomised trial of laparoscopic exploration of common bile duct versus postoperative endoscopic retrograde cholangiography for common bile duct stones. Lancet. 1998;351:159–61.
18. Martin IJ, Bailey IS, Rhodes M, O'Rourke N, Nathanson L, Fielding G. Towards T-tube free laparoscopic bile duct exploration: a methodologic evolution during 300 consecutive procedures. Ann Surg. 1998;228:29–34.

19. Tantau M, Mercea V, Crisan D, Tantau A, Mester G, Vesa S, Sparchez Z. ERCP on a cohort of 2,986 patients with cholelitiasis: a 10-year experience of a single center. J Gastrointest Liver Dis. 2013;22:141–7.
20. Poulose BK, Arbogast PG, Holzman MD. National analysis of in-hospital resource utilization in choledocholithiasis management using propensity scores. Surg Endosc. 2006;20:186–90.
21. Poulose BK, Phillips S, Nealon W, Shelton J, Kummerow K, Penson D, Holzman MD. Choledocholithiasis management in rural America: health disparity or health opportunity? J Surg Res. 2011;170:214–9.
22. Santos BF, Reif TJ, Soper NJ, Nagle AP, Rooney DM, Hungness ES. Development and evaluation of a laparoscopic common bile duct exploration simulator and procedural rating scale. Surg Endosc. 2012;26:2403–15.
23. Teitelbaum EN, Soper NJ, Santos BF, Rooney DM, Patel P, Nagle AP, Hungness ES. A simulator-based resident curriculum for laparoscopic common bile duct exploration. Surgery. 2014;156:880–93.

Chapter 24
Management of Incidentally Discovered Gallbladder Cancer

May Chen Tee and KMarie Reid-Lombardo

Abstract The management of incidentally discovered gallbladder cancer, identified either intra-operatively or post-operatively, is still hotly debated. Surgical management options for incidentally discovered gallbladder cancer include observation after simple cholecystectomy (open or laparoscopic) or radical surgical re-excision of the gallbladder fossa with hilar lymphadenectomy. Adjuvant therapy after diagnoses remains controversial and is often individualized. Evidence to date strongly favors radical re-excision in cases of T1a tumors with positive margins or lymph nodes and T1b-T3 tumors without evidence of distant nodal (N2) or metastatic (M1) disease. The role of adjuvant therapy appears to be one that complements definitive surgical resection and is advised for increased stage, residual disease after surgical resection (R1/R2 resection), and/or the presence of lymph node metastasis (N1 disease). Improved overall survival and disease-free recurrence has been demonstrated for radical surgical re-excision with consideration of adjuvant therapy for the aforementioned indications.

Keywords Gallbladder cancer • Gall bladder adenocarcinoma • Simple cholecystectomy • Radical cholecystectomy • Surgical re-excision • Adjuvant therapy • Cholecystectomy

---

M.C. Tee
Department of Surgery, Mayo Clinic, 200 First Street S.W., Rochester, MN 55905, USA

K. Reid-Lombardo (✉)
Division of Subspecialty General Surgery, Department of Surgery, Mayo Clinic, 200 First Street S.W., Rochester, MN 55905, USA
e-mail: reidlombardo.kmarie@mayo.edu

J.M. Millis, J.B. Matthews (eds.), *Difficult Decisions in Hepatobiliary and Pancreatic Surgery*, Difficult Decisions in Surgery: An Evidence-Based Approach, DOI 10.1007/978-3-319-27365-5_24

Introduction

Epidemiology

Gallbladder cancer is a rare and highly aggressive malignancy [1, 2]. It is the most common malignant neoplasm of the biliary tract and is the sixth most common gastrointestinal malignancy worldwide [2]. Data from a nationally maintained, prospective database of 10,925 Swiss patients undergoing laparoscopic cholecystectomy identified the incidence of undiagnosed gallbladder cancer to be 0.34 % [3]. Most gallbladder cancers are adenocarcinomas (classified as papillary, tubular, or nodular) that arise from the mucosa, often within a background of chronic inflammation, which represents an important risk factor [1, 2]. Additional risk factors include: female gender, cholelithiasis, ethnicity (Central/Northern European, American Indian, Indian, and Chilean populations), chronic bacterial infections (*Salmonella typhi*), anomalous junction of the pancreaticobiliary ductal system, occupational exposures (petroleum refining), and environmental exposures such as cigarette smoking [2]. Additional surrogates for either chronic inflammation or cholestasis predisposing individuals to the formation of gallstones have also been associated with increased risk, namely gallbladder polyps, porcelain gallbladder, and postmenopausal state [1, 2]. The pathogenesis of gallbladder cancer is multifactorial with genetic influences and generally involves a dysplasia-carcinoma sequence [1].

Clinical Presentation

In many patients, gallbladder cancer presents at an advanced stage, often at the time of cholecystectomy for presumed chronic cholecystitis [1]. The clinical presentation is often non-specific and may include abdominal pain (73 %), nausea/vomiting (43 %), jaundice (37 %), anorexia (35 %), or weight loss (35 %) [1]. Constitutional symptoms, ascites, duodenal obstruction, gastrointestinal bleeding/hemobilia, and a palpable mass on physical exam generally indicate advanced disease that belies a poor prognostic outcome [1].

The staging of gallbladder cancer is defined by the 7th edition of the American Joint Committee on Cancer (AJCC) 2010 TNM classification [2], which is summarized in Table 24.1. Stages I disease represents early gallbladder cancer and is managed by either simple or radical cholecystectomy (Fig. 24.1), depending on depth of tumor invasion. Stage II disease is managed by radical cholecystectomy. Stage III disease represents locally advanced and/or regional nodal disease, which is managed by en bloc oncologic resection of adjacent and involved organs with hilar lymphadenectomy. Stage IV disease is characterized by nodal metastases outside the regional lymph node basin and/or distant metastatic disease, both of which preclude curative surgical resection and warrant appropriate palliation.

Table 24.1 American Joint Committee on Cancer (AJCC) 7th edition staging for gallbladder cancer

Stage	T	N	M
0	Tis	N0	M0
I	T1	N0	M0
II	T2	N0	M0
III A	T3	N0	M0
III B	T1–3	N1	M0
IV A	T4	N0-1	M0
IV B	Any T	N2	M0
	Any T	Any N	M1

Management of gallbladder cancer is often dictated by the presumed clinical (or pathological) stage of the cancer as suggested by the National Comprehensive Cancer Network (NCCN) [4]. These treatment recommendations by stage and depth of invasion are summarized in Table 24.2 [4]. However, with the increasing incidence of elective cholecystectomies, the issue on how to treat incidentally diagnosed gallbladder cancer (i.e. gallbladder cancer that is not identified pre-operatively and only suspected intra-operatively or confirmed post-operatively after submission of the specimen for pathological evaluation) is hotly debated. The options for management include observation, systemic chemotherapy, or surgical management. This chapter will focus on the controversies and difficulties in therapeutic decision-making for patients diagnosed with incidental gallbladder cancer.

Literature Search

A literature search was conducted with the assistance of a Mayo Clinic reference librarian. English language publications from the inception of each database to August 2014 were evaluated to identify published data on the management of incidentally discovered gallbladder cancer using a PICO outline, Table 24.3. The patients of interest were incidentally detected gallbladder cancer as defined previously. We compared surgical management as the primary intervention of interest to observation and/or chemoradiation therapy. The outcomes of interest were recurrence-free survival, overall survival, and morbidity/mortality. Databases searched included: Ovid MEDLINE, PubMed, Embase, Cochrane Central Register of Controlled Trials, and Cochrane Database of Systematic Reviews. Terms used in the search were "gallbladder neoplasm" AND "incidental, accidental, unplanned, or unsuspected."

A total of 251 articles were retrieved that were published up to August 2014. A review of the title and abstract eliminated papers whose content did not appear relevant to the PICO question at hand or if conference data from an abstract were unavailable. Articles (n = 86) were reviewed if they addressed the topic of incidentally

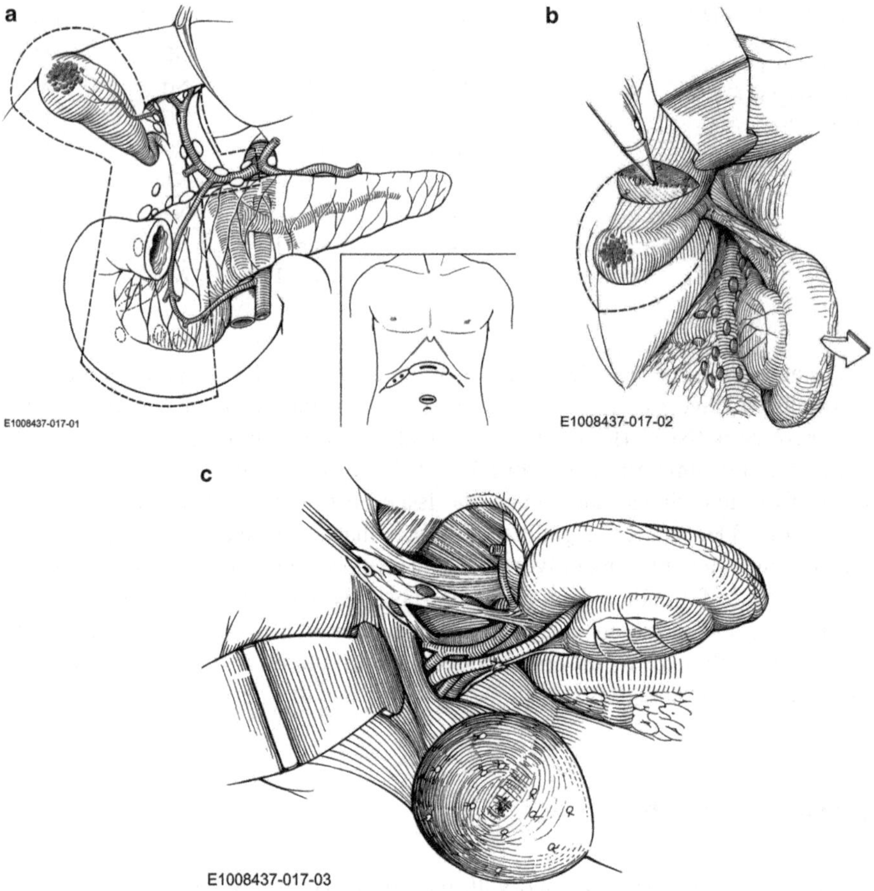

Fig. 24.1 Radical cholecystectomy. (**a**) The *lower right* inset illustrates the typical right subcostal incision used for radical cholecystectomy, with inclusion of the port sites. The main drawing shows the borders of a radical cholecystectomy that includes resection of segment 4B and 5 of the gallbladder bed, along with the extent of the regional lymphadenectomy. (**b**) Division of the hepatic parenchyma with an ultrasonic dissector. The duodenum has been mobilized (*arrow*) revealing the retroduodenal and retropancreatic lymph nodes posteriorly. The nodes are part of the N2 dissection that will be performed later. (**c**) The gallbladder and liver surrounding the gallbladder have been resected, and the hepatoduodenal nodes have been freed from all surfaces but the anteromedial side of the portal triad (Permission to reprint grant from Journal of Gastrointestinal Surgery)

detected gallbladder cancer and either: surgical management, chemo or radiation therapy, or observation alone. A total of 60 articles were reviewed in full text with 26 articles further excluded due to small case series (N ≤10) or lack of pathological data. Bibliographies from these reviewed articles served as a source of additional papers for analysis based on title and citation (n = 10) for a total of 70 articles. Data quality from these articles was classified using the GRADE system [5, 6]. Table 24.4 provides a summary of the most relevant articles reviewed.

Table 24.2 AJCC 7th edition TNM classification with NCCN guidelines for management based on TNM stage

TMN stage	Descriptions	Suggested management
Primary tumor invasion (T)	Depth of invasion to histology layer:	Surgical procedure:
Tis	Carcinoma in situ	Simple cholecystectomy
T1a	Lamina propria	Simple cholecystectomy[a]
T1b	Muscular layer	Radical cholecystectomy[b]
T2	Perimuscular connective tissue	Radical cholecystectomy[b]
T3	Serosa and/or liver/adjacent organ	Radical en bloc resection[c]
T4	Main PV/HA or $\geq$ 2 extrahepatic organs	Palliation or neoadjuvant chemo/radiation therapy for down-staging and re-consideration of resection
Regional lymph nodes (N)	Lymph node metastasis to:	Surgical procedure:
N0	None	Portal lymphadenectomy[d]
N1	CD, CBD, HA, and/or PV	Portal lymphadenectomy[d]
N2	Peri-aortic, peri-caval, superior mesenteric artery and/or celiac artery nodes	Palliation
Metastatic disease (M)	Evidence of metastasis to:	Surgical procedure
M0	No distant metastasis	As above for T1–3, N0-1 disease
M1	Distant metastasis	Palliation

Legend *PV* portal vein, *HA* hepatic artery, *CD* cystic duct, *CBD* common bile duct
[a]Cholecystectomy alone is adequate if pathological margins are histologically negative (R0)
[b]Radical cholecystectomy involves excision of the gallbladder, partial liver resection ($\geq$2 cm of the gallbladder bed), portal lymphadenectomy, bile duct excision (if the cystic duct margins are positive), and consideration of port site excision. Routine port site excision has not consistently shown survival benefit
[c]Radical en bloc resection involves radical cholecystectomy with segmental liver resection and en bloc resection of all adjacent structures involved with the primary malignancy
[d]Portal lymphadenectomy involves clearance of all peri-portal (hepatoduodenal) fibro-fatty tissue. The median number of lymph node harvest is three. Extended lymphadenectomy does not confer survival advantage and may be associated with increased peri-operative morbidity

Table 24.3 PICO table for outcomes following management of incidentally discovered gallbladder cancer

P (Patients)	I (Intervention)	C (Comparator group)	O (Outcomes)
Adult patients undergoing abdominal surgery with incidentally detected gallbladder cancer (intra-op/post-op findings)	Surgical management (radical re-excision) with or without adjunctive therapy	Chemo-radiation therapy or observation	Recurrence-free survival, overall survival, morbidity/mortality

Table 24.4 Summary of important studies evaluating the management of incidental gallbladder cancer

Study	Design	N	Patients	Intervention	Control	Outcome	Grade of evidence quality
Wakai [9]	Retrospective	25	T1b gallbladder adenocarcinoma	Radical re-resection	Simple cholecystectomy	Median survival 95 mon (simple) vs. 90 mon (radical), $p=0.16$	Low-moderate
Toyonaga [16]	Retrospective	73	T2 gallbladder adenocarcinoma	Radical re-resection for in T2 tumors	Simple cholecystectomy for T2 tumors	5-year survival 54 % (radical) versus 35 % (simple), $p=0.05$	Low-moderate
Tanner [34]	Retrospective	131	T1–T4 gallbladder adenocarcinoma	Radical cholecystectomy	Simple cholecystectomy	Median survival 24 months (radical) vs. 6 months (simple), $p<0.0001$	Moderate
Foster [17]	Retrospective	64	T1–T3 gallbladder adenocarcinoma	Radical cholecystectomy	Simple cholecystectomy	5-year survival 78 % (radical) vs. 10 % (simple), $p<0.0001$	Low-moderate
Goetz [13]	Prospective	103	T1 gallbladder carcinoma (incidental)	Radical cholecystectomy	Simple cholecystectomy	5-year survival T1b: 79 % (radical) vs. 42 % (simple), $p=0.03$ T1a: no significant difference between radical and simple cholecystectomy, $p=0.10$	Moderate

Coburn [19]	Retrospective (SEER data)	2,835	T1–T3 gallbladder adenocarcinoma	En bloc re-resection +/− lymphadenectomy	Simple cholecystectomy	Survival by stage	Moderate
						T1: HR = 0.54 (0.31–0.97), p = 0.04 (en bloc versus simple)	
						T3: HR = 0.70 (0.48–1.00), p = 0.05 (lymphadenectomy versus none)	
Chan [35]	Retrospective	86	T1–T4 gallbladder adenocarcinoma	Curative resection	Palliative resection or bypass	Overall survival	Low-moderate
						3-year: 55 % (curative) vs. 0 % (palliative), p = 0.01	
						Median: 33.9 mon (curative) vs. 3 mon (palliative), p < 0.0001	
Abramson [8]	Retrospective decision analysis	199	T1b gallbladder adenocarcinoma	Radical cholecystectomy	Simple cholecystectomy	Life expectancy after resection	Moderate
						9.85 years (radical) versus 6.42 years (simple)	
Downing [18]	Retrospective (SEER data)	2,495	Tis-T2 gallbladder adenocarcinoma	Radical cholecystectomy	Simple cholecystectomy	Survival by stage	Moderate
						T1b: HR = 1.51 (0.78–2.90), p = 0.22 (radical versus simple)	
						T2: HR = 0.64 (0.46–0.90), p = 0.01 (radical versus simple)	
Fuks [21]	Retrospective	218	T1–T4 gallbladder adenocarcinoma	Radical re-resection	Simple cholecystectomy	5-year survival by stage	Moderate
						T2: 62 % (radical) versus 0 % (simple), p = 0.0001	
						T3: 19 % (radical) versus 0 % (simple), p = 0.04	

(continued)

Table 24.4 (continued)

Study	Design	N	Patients	Intervention	Control	Outcome	Grade of evidence quality
Clemente [36]	Retrospective	34	All incidental gallbladder cancer	Radical re-resection	Simple cholecystectomy	5-year overall survival 78.3 % (radical) versus 38.5 % (simple)	Low-moderate
Hari [14]	Retrospective (SEER data)	2,788	T1a/T1b gallbladder adenocarcinoma	Radical cholecystectomy	Simple cholecystectomy	5-year survival by operation 50 % (simple chole) vs. 79 % (radical chole), $p<0.0001$	Moderate
Yi [37]	Retrospective	38	All incidental gallbladder cancer	Radical re-resection	Simple cholecystectomy	Median survival by stage T1b: 62 mon (radical) vs. 24 mon (simple), $p=0.131$ T3: 22 mon (radical) vs. 5 mon (simple), $p=0.02$	Low

Low: further research is very likely to have an impact on the estimate of effect and is likely to change the estimate [5]
Moderate: further research is likely to have an impact on the estimate of effect and may change the estimate [5]
High: further research is unlikely to change the estimate of effect [5]

Results

Treatment of Tis and T1a Tumors

Management of early (Tis and T1a) gallbladder cancers whether they are incidentally or pre-operatively discovered can generally consist of simple cholecystectomy alone [4, 7]. In-situ (Tis) disease does not harbor invasive tendencies and thus, simple cholecystectomy should be adequate. Lymph node metastasis in T1a gallbladder cancer is reported to be 1.8 % and 5-year survival following either simple or extended cholecystectomy approaches 100 %. Survival benefit is not demonstrated with radical cholecystectomy for Tis and T1a gallbladder cancers. Thus, current recommendations for T1a gallbladder cancer in the absence of positive margins or suspected and/or confirmed lymph node metastasis are for simple cholecystectomy alone [4, 7].

Treatment of T1b Tumors

Of the manuscripts reviewed, there was an overwhelming survival benefit with radical re-resection for incidentally discovered T1b tumors when compared to observation alone. Abramson et al. evaluated this benefit in a decision analysis study [8]. Twenty six studies with a combined total of 199 patients who underwent laparoscopic cholecystectomy with a final pathologic diagnosis of T1b gallbladder adenocarcinoma were identified. Of those, 158 patients underwent observation alone while 41 patients were offered a radical re-resection. The two groups were compared regarding 5-year survival and peri-operative mortality. Simple cholecystectomy alone resulted in a 61.3 % 5-year survival compared to 87.5 % for patients who underwent radical re-resection for T1b disease. The median survival following simple cholecystectomy was 6.42 years compared to 9.85 years in the group that underwent radical re-resection. Peri-operative mortality associated with radical re-resection was found to be 2 % (range: 0–6 %). Decision analysis was invoked to show that peri-operative mortality greater or equal to 36 % for radical re-resection would favor observation alone. Thus, the results demonstrate improved survival following radical re-resection for T1b gallbladder cancers, without unreasonably increased peri-operative risks [8]. In contrast, a smaller, retrospective case series evaluating T1b gallbladder cancers suggested no survival benefit to radical re-resection over observation following simple cholecystectomy; however, the study may not have been sufficiently powered to detect such a difference [9].

Other studies have reported survival benefit for patients with T1b tumors who undergo extended surgical resection, compared to observation after simple cholecystectomy alone [7, 10–15]. In a prospectively maintained German registry of all gallbladder cancers, 103 patients with incidentally detected T1 gallbladder cancer patients were identified [13]. The overall 5-year survival for T1 gallbladder cancers did not show a significant difference in survival between patients who underwent re-resection (72 %) versus those who did not (40 %), p=0.06 [13]. However, stratification by T1 stage demonstrated improved 5-year survival with re-resection for T1b tumors (42 % without re-resection and 79 % with re-resection, p=0.03) but not T1a tumors (p=0.10) [13]. These findings are supported by a retrospective review of clinico-pathological features of T1 gallbladder cancers from South Korea [15]. This study demonstrated no lymphatic or lymphovascular invasion in T1a tumors but a 3.8 % rate of lymph node metastasis and 1.9 % rate of lymphatic infiltration in T1b tumors, leading to the recommendation of hilar lymphadenectomy for all T1b tumors and simple cholecystectomy alone for T1a tumors [15].

A systematic review of management for T1 gallbladder cancers similarly recommended simple cholecystectomy for T1a tumors, given the localized disease process and negligible rate of lymphatic involvement [7]. Given an aggregated 10.9 % rate of lymph node metastases across several studies, T1b tumors should be considered for radical cholecystectomy, although the strength of the evidence available (much of which were retrospective case series) precluded the authors from making this a formal recommendation [7].

Treatment Options for Stage T2/T3

A case series (n=73) from Japan has demonstrated that the most significant prognostic factor is depth of tumor invasion, assessed by both univariate and multivariate analysis [16]. This group examined incidentally detected gallbladder adenocarcinoma following laparoscopic cholecystectomy and stratified patients by T1, T2, and T3 stage. There was no difference in overall and median survival for patients with T1 disease who underwent simple cholecystectomy versus radical re-resection; however, this group did not stratify T1 lesions by T1a versus T1b depth of invasion. There was improved 5-year survival demonstrated for re-resection of T2 tumors and this benefit was particularly significant for initially positive surgical margins at the time of cholecystectomy (54 % versus 35 %, p=0.05). There was a trend towards improved survival for re-resection of T3 tumors (median survival improved with T3 re-resection from 7 months to 15 months). A statistically significant survival benefit of T3 lesions may not have been evident due to issues of underpowered subgroup analysis (n=7) [16].

Radical re-resection also demonstrated survival benefit for T2/T3 gallbladder cancers when compared to simple cholecystectomy alone [17]. This retrospective, single-institution study reported improved 5-year survival for patients with T2/T3 tumors who underwent radical re-resection (78 %) versus patients with T2/T3 tumors who underwent simple cholecystectomy alone (10 %) [17]. In addition, there was no difference in overall survival if patients underwent surgical re-resection following an incidental diagnosis when compared to patients who were resected based on pre-operative suspicion at the index operation [17]. Cho et al. reported similar findings of T2 and greater gallbladder cancers in that there is no difference in survival following a two-stage re-resection or single-stage resection for incidental gallbladder cancer.

Hilar Lymphadenectomy: Is It Beneficial?

A larger epidemiologic study using the Surveillance, Epidemiology, and End Results (SEER) database analyzed whether Tis/T1/T2 incidentally found gallbladder cancers reported similar survival in patients who underwent extended surgical resection and lymphadenectomy versus simple cholecystectomy at the time of diagnosis [18]. Increased survival was demonstrated in patients who underwent extended surgical resection compared with simple cholecystectomy alone, especially for patients with T2 tumors ($p=0.01$) [18]. Poor prognostic survival factors included older patient age, increased T stage, and positive lymph nodes [18]. Moreover, patients who underwent resection of five or more lymph nodes, especially for T2 tumors, demonstrated improved survival over no lymph nodes or only 1–4 lymph nodes excised ($p<0.001$) [18].

In contrast to this, another SEER database study showed improved survival of radical resection for T2 tumors ($p=0.03$) and T1 tumors ($p=0.02$) [19]. The hazard ratio for death in a Cox multi-variable model for T1 tumors undergoing radical re-resection was 0.54 (95 % CI: 0.31–0.97, $p=0.04$) [19]. Lymphadenectomy was also associated with improved survival for T2 ($p<0.001$) and T3 ($p<0.001$) tumors but not T1 tumors ($p=0.55$) [19]. The hazard ratio for death in a Cox multi-variable model for T3 tumors undergoing lymphadenectomy was 0.70 (95 % CI: 0.48–1.00, $p=0.05$) [19]. This data is supported by a large review from the Memorial Sloan-Kettering Cancer Center, that demonstrated residual disease risk of 50 % for T1 tumors, 61 % for T2 tumors, 85 % for T3 tumors, and 100 % for T4 tumors [20].

Common Bile Duct Resections

Results from a French multi-center database of incidentally detected gallbladder cancer demonstrate that re-resection compared to observation significantly increased survival in patients with T2 (overall 5-year survival 62 % versus 0 %, $p=0.0001$) and T3 (overall 5-year survival 19 % versus 0 %, $p=0.04$) tumors [21]. Common bile duct re-excision was not associated with improved survival ($p=0.06$) but was associated with increased risk of postoperative complications (60 % versus 23 %, $p=0.0001$) [21]. A similar study from Johns Hopkins reported no additional survival benefit or facilitation of lymphadenectomy [22]. In this study, the median lymph node harvest was three, both in patients who underwent bile duct excision and those who did not [22]. Routine common bile duct resection was also not found to be associated with improved survival in a study evaluating extent of radical re-resection but may instead contribute to unnecessary patient morbidity [23].

Port Site Resections

The earliest study that demonstrated a series of port site recurrences following laparoscopic cholecystectomy for gallbladder cancer was in 1995 by Wibbenmeyer et al. [24]. Subsequent reports of port site recurrence following laparoscopic cholecystectomy for gallbladder cancer ensued, with a combined port site recurrence rate of 14–16 % [3, 24, 25]. More recently, in a Swiss database of over 10,000 patients undergoing laparoscopic cholecystectomy containing 37 patients with incidental gallbladder adenocarcinoma, port site recurrence was identified in 14 % of these patients at a median time to recurrence of 10 months (range: 6–16 months) [3]. All patients with port site recurrence died within 3 years of their initial operation [3].

In another national database study from Sweden, 55 gallbladder carcinomas were identified from a total of 11,976 laparoscopic cholecystectomies for which 16 % developed port site metastasis [25]. The same study did not identify any evidence of port site recurrence in patients who had laparoscopic cholecystectomies converted to open procedures, which prompted a recommendation to perform open cholecystectomy in cases of suspected gallbladder cancer [25].

A multi-institution French study addressed the question of need for port-site excision by identifying 254 patients over a 10-year period with incidentally discovered gallbladder cancer during laparoscopic cholecystectomy. Of these 254 patients, 148 underwent resection with curative intent (54 patients had port site excision and 94 patients did not have port site excision) [26]. Overall survival was not different at 1, 3, and 5 years in the group that underwent the port site excision versus the group that did not ($p=0.37$) [26]. The recurrence rate for gallbladder cancer and incidence of peritoneal carcinomatosis between the two groups also did not differ [26]. There was only one instance of port site recurrence and death from peritoneal carcinomatosis in a patient who underwent port site re-excision; this was attributed to the presence of occult peritoneal disease identified following radical re-excision [26]. Port site involvement may instead be an indication of occult advanced disease and may not warrant aggressive measures of radical resection, given the dubious survival benefit and associated surgical morbidity. Notably, the incidence of port site hernia was 8 % in the group undergoing port site re-excision with the incidence of ventral hernia from the subcostal incision being similar between the two groups [26]. A single-institution review demonstrated similar results, that the excision of port sites did not improve overall or recurrence free survival, after controlling for stage and R0 resection [27].

Data from MD Anderson ($n=79$) did not demonstrate any difference in 5-year overall survival or abdominal wall recurrences in patients with gallbladder cancer who underwent laparoscopic versus open cholecystectomy [28]. A case series ($n=20$) from Italy also did not show increased risk of abdominal wall recurrence following laparoscopic cholecystectomy for gallbladder cancer [29]. These results were further corroborated by a temporal analysis of gallbladder cancer prognosis in the pre and post laparoscopic cholecystectomy era [30]. Whalen et al. reviewed data from the Connecticut tumor registry and compared a cohort of 194 patients (1985–

1988) to 208 patients (1992–1995) and did not find any differences in survival ($p=0.54$) between the two time periods [30].

Adjuvant Chemotherapy

Adjuvant therapy following curative intent resection of gallbladder cancer was queried in a recent meta-analysis [31]. This meta-analysis pooled 20 studies for a total of 6,712 patients who underwent surgical resection of gallbladder cancer and cholangiocarcinoma [31]. Sub-group analyses were conducted for gallbladder cancer resections comparing patients who underwent adjuvant therapy (chemotherapy or chemo-radiation therapy) and patients who were treated with surgery alone [31]. Overall, there was a non-statistically significant trend toward improved survival with adjuvant therapy compared to surgery alone (pooled $OR=0.74$; $p=0.06$) [31]. Stratified meta-analysis did suggest improved survival with adjuvant therapy for lymph node positive disease ($OR=0.49$, $p=0.004$) and R1 resection ($OR=0.36$, $p=0.002$) [31]. Thus, adjuvant therapy should be recommended in lymph node positive or R1 resected gallbladder cancer [31]. A SEER database analysis from another study provided similar recommendations for adjuvant therapy in cases of node-positive disease and consideration for patients with T2 tumors [32].

The Mayo Clinic experience of multi-disciplinary management for gallbladder cancer is in line with reports from other institutions [33, 34]. A retrospective review of all surgical procedures performed for gallbladder cancer ($n=131$) demonstrated a median overall survival of 24 months for patients who underwent radical cholecystectomy compared to 6 months for simple cholecystectomy and 4 months for palliative surgery ($p<0.0001$) [34]. Overall 5-year survival was demonstrated to be 21 % for patients undergoing radical cholecystectomy compared to 6 % for patients undergoing simple cholecystectomy ($p<0.0001$) [34]. When stratifying by stage of cancer, all stages (except Stage I) demonstrated improved survival with radical cholecystectomy over simple cholecystectomy [34]. There were 48 patients from this cohort who received adjuvant therapy (37 %) [34]. In a separate study by the same institution, the benefits of adjuvant chemo-radiation therapy following surgical resection were demonstrated with a 5-year overall survival of 64 % compared to a historical control of 33 % [33].

Evidence-Based Recommendations

1. Gallbladder cancer is a highly aggressive malignancy and complete surgical resection to histologically negative margins (R0 resection) remains the standard for potential cure. (Strong recommendation based on high grade evidence).
2. Any incidentally detected gallbladder cancer that is beyond T1a in the absence of distant nodal (N2) or metastatic (M1) disease should be managed with further surgical resection. T1a tumors with any positive margins or positive lymph nodes in the cholecystectomy specimen should also be managed with further surgical resection. (Strong recommendation based on moderate to high grade evidence).

3. Multi-disciplinary referral for consideration of chemotherapy with or without radiation therapy after surgical resection should be offered to patients with evidence of lymph node metastases, R1 resection, and/or T2 or greater tumor. (Strong recommendation based on moderate to high grade evidence).

Expert View of the Data

Poor prognostic indicators for gallbladder cancer include incomplete surgical resection (R1/R2 resection), lymph node metastases, and tumor characteristics (grade and stage). Patients with incidentally discovered gallbladder cancer generally have more favorable prognosis due to the early nature of their disease. Given the aggressiveness of gallbladder cancer, we would recommend complete surgical re-resection for any tumor that demonstrates a T stage greater than T1a, positive margins, or lymph node involvement. Controversy in the literature regarding management of T1 tumors is likely due to lack of stratification of T1a from T1b tumors, the former of which represents primarily localized disease.

The type of surgical re-resection depends on the stage and positivity of the margins. For T1b/T2 tumors, radical cholecystectomy with resection of at least 2 cm of liver bed at the gallbladder fossa and hilar lymphadenectomy are sufficient. The re-excision of the bile duct would be indicated for a positive cystic duct margin on the original specimen but should not be done routinely, as there is no survival benefit to a procedure that is associated with increased postoperative morbidity. Involvement of adjacent organs (T3) tumors mandates en bloc resection of all involved organs should this be technically feasible in the absence of prohibitive patient co-morbidities.

Controversy still exists regarding port site excision. Recurrence at the port site is more a harbinger of carcinomatosis or aggressive disease rather than a technical factor for incomplete excision. Our institutional bias is not to resect port sites following laparoscopic cholecystectomy, as definitive survival benefit has not been demonstrated and it may be associated with increased long-term morbidity, such as the development of abdominal wall hernias.

The role of chemo and/or radiation therapy should be considered primarily as an adjunctive measure to maximize cure in patients who have undergone appropriate surgical resection for gallbladder cancer. Chemo-radiation therapy should be considered following surgical resection in instances of R1 resection, presence of lymph node metastasis, and/or T2 or greater stage. It may also be considered as a palliative measure in the patient who has incidentally discovered gallbladder cancer following a laparoscopic cholecystectomy whose physiologic or functional status would make radical re-resection prohibitive. In patients who are staged following discovery of incidental gallbladder cancer with potentially unresectable disease, chemo-radiation therapy in the neoadjuvant setting may also be beneficial for tumor down-staging and eventual resection.

In summary, the primary treatment of any resectable (T1–T3) gallbladder cancer in the absence of distant metastatic disease (N2 or M1) remains complete surgical resection with curative intent. This includes radical re-resection for any T1a tumor with residual disease or any tumor greater or equal to T1b stage. A potential role for postoperative observation is the completely excised T1a tumor that has no evidence of lymph node metastasis after simple cholecystectomy. Chemo-radiation therapy would be indicated in the adjuvant setting for incomplete excision, lymph node metastasis, more advanced stage (T2 or greater), or inability to undergo further surgical resection (due to technical or patient factors).

References

1. Reid KM, Ramos-De la Medina A, Donohue JH. Diagnosis and surgical management of gallbladder cancer: a review. J Gastrointest Surg. 2007;11(5):671–81.
2. Wernberg JA, Lucarelli DD. Gallbladder cancer. Surg Clin N Am. 2014;94(2):343–60.
3. Z'Graggen K, Birrer S, Maurer CA, Wehrli H, Klaiber C, Baer HU. Incidence of port site recurrence after laparoscopic cholecystectomy for preoperatively unsuspected gallbladder carcinoma. Surgery. 1998;124(5):831–8.
4. Network NCC. Hepatobiliary Cancers. 2014.
5. Brozek JL, Akl EA, Alonso-Coello P, Lang D, Jaeschke R, Williams JW, et al. Grading quality of evidence and strength of recommendations in clinical practice guidelines. Part 1 of 3. An overview of the GRADE approach and grading quality of evidence about interventions. Allergy. 2009;64(5):669–77.
6. Brozek JL, Akl EA, Compalati E, Kreis J, Terracciano L, Fiocchi A, et al. Grading quality of evidence and strength of recommendations in clinical practice guidelines part 3 of 3. The GRADE approach to developing recommendations. Allergy. 2011;66(5):588–95.
7. Lee SE, Jang JY, Lim CS, Kang MJ, Kim SW. Systematic review on the surgical treatment for T1 gallbladder cancer. World J Gastroenterol. 2011;17(2):174–80. PMCID: 3020370.
8. Abramson MA, Pandharipande P, Ruan D, Gold JS, Whang EE. Radical resection for T1b gallbladder cancer: a decision analysis. HPB. 2009;11(8):656–63.
9. Wakai T, Shirai Y, Yokoyama N, Nagakura S, Watanabe H, Hatakeyama K. Early gallbladder carcinoma does not warrant radical resection. Br J Surg. 2001;88(5):675–8.
10. Bartlett DL, Fong Y, Fortner JG, Brennan MF, Blumgart LH. Long-term results after resection for gallbladder cancer. Implications for staging and management. Ann Surg. 1996;224(5):639–46. PMCID: 1235441.
11. Dixon E, Vollmer Jr CM, Sahajpal A, Cattral M, Grant D, Doig C, et al. An aggressive surgical approach leads to improved survival in patients with gallbladder cancer: a 12-year study at a North American Center. Ann Surg. 2005;241(3):385–94. PMCID: 1356976.
12. Fong Y, Jarnagin W, Blumgart LH. Gallbladder cancer: comparison of patients presenting initially for definitive operation with those presenting after prior noncurative intervention. Ann Surg. 2000;232(4):557–69. PMCID: 1421188.
13. Goetze TO, Paolucci V. Immediate re-resection of T1 incidental gallbladder carcinomas: a survival analysis of the German Registry. Surg Endosc. 2008;22(11):2462–5.
14. Hari DM, HJ, Chiu CG, Leung AM, Sim M, Bilchik AJ. A 21-year analysis of T1 gallbladder carcinoma: Is cholecystectomy alone adequate? HPB. 2012; Conference: 12th Annual Americas Hepato-Pancreato-Biliary Congress Miami Beach, FL United States. Conference Start: 20120307 Conference End: 11. Conference Publication: (var.pagings). 14 (pp 33).
15. You DD, Lee HG, Paik KY, Heo JS, Choi SH, Choi DW. What is an adequate extent of resection for T1 gallbladder cancers? Ann Surg. 2008;247(5):835–8.

16. Toyonaga T, Chijiiwa K, Nakano K, Noshiro H, Yamaguchi K, Sada M, et al. Completion radical surgery after cholecystectomy for accidentally undiagnosed gallbladder carcinoma. World J Surg. 2003;27(3):266–71.
17. Foster JM, Hoshi H, Gibbs JF, Iyer R, Javle M, Chu Q, et al. Gallbladder cancer: defining the indications for primary radical resection and radical re-resection. Ann Surg Oncol. 2007;14(2):833–40.
18. Downing SR, Cadogan K-A, Ortega G, Oyetunji TA, Siram SM, Chang DC, et al. Early-stage gallbladder cancer in the surveillance, epidemiology, and end results database: effect of extended surgical resection. Arch Surg. 2011;146(6):734–8.
19. Coburn NG, Cleary SP, Tan JC, Law CH. Surgery for gallbladder cancer: a population-based analysis. J Am Coll Surg. 2008;207(3):371–82.
20. Duffy A, Capanu M, Abou-Alfa GK, Huitzil D, Jarnagin W, Fong Y, et al. Gallbladder cancer (GBC): 10-year experience at Memorial Sloan-Kettering Cancer Centre (MSKCC). J Surg Oncol. 2008;98(7):485–9.
21. Fuks D, Reqimbeau JM, Le Treut YP, Bachellier P, Raventos A, Pruvot FR, Chiche L, Farges O. Incidental gallbladder cancer by the AFC-GBC-2009 Study Group. World J Surg. 2011;35(8):1887–97.
22. Pawlik TM, Gleisner AL, Vigano L, Kooby DA, Bauer TW, Frilling A, et al. Incidence of finding residual disease for incidental gallbladder carcinoma: implications for re-resection. J Gastrointest Surg. 2007;11(11):1478–86; discussion 86–7.
23. D'Angelica M, Dalal KM, DeMatteo RP, Fong Y, Blumgart LH, Jarnagin WR. Analysis of the extent of resection for adenocarcinoma of the gallbladder. Ann Surg Oncol. 2009;16(4):806–16.
24. Wibbenmeyer LA, Wade TP, Chen RC, Meyer RC, Turgeon RP, Andrus CH. Laparoscopic cholecystectomy can disseminate in situ carcinoma of the gallbladder. J Am Coll Surg. 1995;181(6):504–10.
25. Lundberg O, Kristoffersson A. Port site metastases from gallbladder cancer after laparoscopic cholecystectomy. Results of a Swedish survey and review of published reports. Eur J Surg. 1999;165(3):215–22.
26. Fuks D, Regimbeau JM, Pessaux P, Bachellier P, Raventos A, Mantion G, et al. Is port-site resection necessary in the surgical management of gallbladder cancer? J Visceral Surg. 2013;150(4):277–84.
27. Maker AV, Butte JM, Oxenberg J, Kuk D, Gonen M, Fong Y, et al. Is port site resection necessary in the surgical management of gallbladder cancer? Ann Surg Oncol. 2012;19(2):409–17.
28. Ricardo AE, Feig BW, Ellis LM, Hunt KK, Curley SA, MacFadyen Jr BV, et al. Gallbladder cancer and trocar site recurrences. Am J Surg. 1997;174(6):619–22; discussion 22–3.
29. Sarli L, Contini S, Sansebastiano G, Gobbi S, Costi R, Roncoroni L. Does laparoscopic cholecystectomy worsen the prognosis of unsuspected gallbladder cancer? Arch Surg. 2000;135(11):1340–4.
30. Whalen GF, Bird I, Tanski W, Russell JC, Clive J. Laparoscopic cholecystectomy does not demonstrably decrease survival of patients with serendipitously treated gallbladder cancer. J Am Coll Surg. 2001;192(2):189–95.
31. Horgan AM, Amir E, Walter T, Knox JJ. Adjuvant therapy in the treatment of biliary tract cancer: a systematic review and meta-analysis. J Clin Oncol. 2012;30(16):1934–40.
32. Wang SJ, Lemieux A, Kalpathy-Cramer J, Ord CB, Walker GV, Fuller CD, et al. Nomogram for predicting the benefit of adjuvant chemoradiotherapy for resected gallbladder cancer. J Clin Oncol. 2011;29(35):4627–32. PMCID: 3236647.
33. Kresl JJ, Schild SE, Henning GT, Gunderson LL, Donohue J, Pitot H, et al. Adjuvant external beam radiation therapy with concurrent chemotherapy in the management of gallbladder carcinoma. Int J Radiat Oncol Biol Phys. 2002;52(1):167–75.
34. Taner CB, Nagorney DM, Donohue JH. Surgical treatment of gallbladder cancer. J Gastrointest Surg. 2004;8(1):83–9; discussion 9.

35. Chan SY, Poon R, Lo CM, Ng KK, Fan ST. Management of carcinoma of the gallbladder: a single-institution experience in 16 years. J Surg Oncol. 2008;97(2):156–64.
36. Clemente G, Nuzzo G, de Rose AM, Giovannini I, la Torre G, Ardito F, Giuliante F. Unexpected gallbladder cancer after laparoscopic cholecystectomy for acute cholecystitis: a worrisome picture. J Gastrointest Surg. 2012;16(8):1462–8.
37. Yi X, Long X, Zai H, Xiao D, Li W, Li Y. Unsuspected gallbladder carcinoma discovered during or after cholecystectomy: focus on appropriate radical re-resection according to the T-stage. Clin Transl Oncol. 2013;15(8):652–8.

Chapter 25
Gallstone Ileus

Pierre F. Saldinger and Alexander Itskovich

Abstract Gallstone ileus is a rare form of bowel obstruction caused by an impacted gallstone. It requires two critical elements: a cholecysto-enteric fistula and a gallstone of sufficient diameter to migrate and obstruct the intestinal lumen. Classically, gallstone ileus was addressed by relieving the blockage and closing the fistula. However, because the typical presentation involves elderly patients with numerous comorbidities, lengthy, complex procedures are often poorly tolerated. Obviating the exploration of the fistula has been proposed as a means of decreasing postoperative morbidity and mortality. Although no prospective trials have performed on the subject, several retrospective reviews support this conclusion.

Keywords Gallstone ileus • Cholecystoduodenal fistula • Cholecystointestinal fistula • Cholecystosigmoid fistula • Bouveret syndrome

Introduction

Gallstone ileus represents approximately 1 % of all patients presenting with small bowel obstruction. Greater than 70 % of patients are women. The majority of cases affect patients older than 65. The location of the fistula represents the entry point of the gallstone into the alimentary tract. The most common sites (in descending order) include the duodenum, stomach, colon, and small intestine. The stone will subsequently migrate and lodge in the narrowest point of the intestine that is distal to the fistula [1, 2].

The area of stone impaction may represent an anatomic narrowing (e.g., ileocecal valve) or the result of a previous pathologic process (strictures, adhesions). Greater than 60 % of stones lodge in the vicinity of the ileocecal valve. Other sites

P.F. Saldinger (✉)
Department of Surgery, New York Presbyterian Queens, Weill Cornell Medical College, 56-45 Main Street, Flushing, NY 11355, USA
e-mail: Pfs9003@med.cornell.edu

A. Itskovich
Department of Surgery, The Brooklyn Hospital Center, 121 Dekalb Ave, Brooklyn, NY, USA

J.M. Millis, J.B. Matthews (eds.), *Difficult Decisions in Hepatobiliary and Pancreatic Surgery*, Difficult Decisions in Surgery: An Evidence-Based Approach, DOI 10.1007/978-3-319-27365-5_25

of obstruction include the jejunum (16 %), stomach (14 %), colon (4 %) and duodenum (3.5 %) [1, 2].

Presentation varies largely depending on the level of obstruction. Patients most commonly complain of nausea, vomiting and abdominal pain. A careful history will often suggest prior episodes of biliary colic or acute cholecystitis. Most patients will present with abdominal distention. Vital signs and laboratory work often reveal a systemic inflammatory response and evidence of dehydration.

Rigler's classic X-ray findings of pneumobilia, small bowel obstruction and a right iliac fossa gallstone is only present in 30–35 of cases. CT is the diagnostic study of choice. It is a highly accurate method of establishing the diagnosis. Three criteria must be met. The CT must show (1) evidence of bowel obstruction with (2) the presence of an ectopic gallstone (rim calcified or totally calcified) and an (3) abnormal gallbladder with the presence of an irregular wall or an air fluid level. With all three elements present, the sensitivity and specificity of CT are 93 % and 100 % respectively. For a stone to become impacted, it typically has to measure at least 2 cm in diameter [1, 3, 4].

Preoperative management begins with immediate crystalloid resuscitation, nasogastric tube drainage and the correction of electrolyte abnormities. In the setting of hemodynamic instability secondary to severe sepsis or septic shock, patients may require invasive hemodynamic monitoring. Once resuscitated, patients are expeditiously taken to the operating room where they undergo general endotracheal anesthesia.

The abdomen is entered and the small bowel evaluated. The transition zone is noted and the bowel proximal to the obstruction is assessed for additional stones. A longitudinal incision is made on the small bowel proximal to the site of obstruction. The stone is milked into the enterotomy which is subsequently closed in a transverse fashion. If the segment affected has evidence of bowel ischemia, a resection with primary anastomosis is performed.

Electing to perform a resection of the cholecystoenteric fistula is controversial. The planes are often obscured secondary to chronic inflammation and exploration often substantially increases operative time. In the open approach, the gallbladder is dissected in a top down fashion until the structures in the Triangle of Calot are identified. The cystic duct and artery are dissected and clipped. The fistula is dissected from the involved structure (usually the duodenum). The area of the fistula is debrided and the enterotomy repaired in a transverse fashion. Multiple critical structures may be at risk during the dissection.

Search Strategy

A search of the English literature was conducted to identify data on the management of Gallstone Ileus published between 1994 and 2014 utilizing the PICO outline (Insert Table 25.1). PubMed was utilized to conduct all queries. Terms used in the search were "Gallstone Ileus", "Cholecystoduodenal fistula", "Cholecystogastric fistula", "Cholecystosigmoid fistula" and "Bouveret Syndrome". No randomized

Table 25.1 Literature search outline utilizing the PICO method

P (patients)	I (intervention)	C (comparator)	O (outcomes)
Patients with gallstone ileus	Enterolithotomy with cholecystectomy and cholecystoenteric fistula closure	Enterolithotomy alone	Morbidity and mortality

trials were identified. Three large retrospective reviews were identified. The remainder of the literature is primarily small case series and case reports. All data was evaluated based on the GRADE system.

Results

Enterolithotomy vs Enterolithotomy with Cholecystectomy and Cholecysto-Enteric Fistula Closure

In a 2014 retrospective review (largest to date), Halabi et al. queried the national inpatient sample and identified 3,268 cases of Gallstone Ileus occurring between 2005 and 2009. Stone extraction alone occurred in 62 % of patients. Nineteen percent of patients underwent closure of their cholecysto-enteric fistula. Nineteen percent of patients required small bowel resection. The most common complication was acute renal failure (30 %) and the perioperative mortality rate was 6.67 %. On multivariate analysis, closure of the enteric fistula was associated with a higher mortality rate (odds ratio 2.86).

In a 2013 retrospective review of the NSQIP Database, Mallipeddi et al. evaluated 127 patients that presented with gallstone ileus from 2005 to 2010. They noted an overall morbidity and mortality rate of 35.4 % and 5.5 % respectively. No difference in mortality was noted in patients that underwent fistula closure. However, the fistula closure group did experience longer operative times, postoperative hospitalization times and minor complications. The most common complications were urinary tract infections and surgical site infections [5].

In their 1994 review, Reisner et al. present 1001 reported cases of gallstone ileus. They reported a mortality rate of 16.9 % for the fistula closure group and an 11.7 mortality rate for the enterotomy group alone. In addition, they report a gallstone ileus recurrence rate of less than 5 %. They conclude that simple enterolithotomy is both safe and effective in dealing with Gallstone Ileus [1, 2, 4].

Recurrent Gallstone Ileus

The literature for recurrent gallstone ileus is made up largely of case reports. Reisner et al. published the largest series with 1001 patients and reports a recurrence rate of 5 %. Additionally, they report that approximately 10 % of patients require reoperation [1].

Minimally Invasive Techniques

The feasibility of laparoscopic approach has been demonstrated in several case reports. Potential limiting factors include patient stability, capacity to tolerate pneumoperitoneum, restricted working space, and the surgeons laparoscopic comfort level. Both intracorporeal and extracorporeal anastomotic methods have been described. It is critical that the surgeon be comfortable fully examining the bowel laparoscopically as up to 5 % of patients will have additional stones present proximal to the obstruction.

Several reports have demonstrated the feasibility of endoscopic extraction and fragmentation in selected cases. Specifically, extraction may be successful in the setting of Bouveret syndrome (gallstone ileus causing gastric outlet obstruction). The role of endoscopy and criteria for its utilization have not been clearly defined [6–11].

Recommendations

Although limited in terms of quality of evidence, the literature to date suggests that enterolithotomy alone is sufficient in the management of gallstone ileus (level of recommendation; weak). This is supported by both retrospective data showing a higher incidence of complications with fistula closure and the low rates of reported recurrence with enterolithotomy alone.

The limited literature to date suggests a low recurrence rate after enterolithotomy alone. However, no conclusion can be based on the available data and the question of whether the cholecysto-enteric fistula should be addressed in an interval fashion remains unanswered.

Multiple case reports have demonstrated the feasibility of both the laparoscopic and endoscopic approach in selected cases. Bouveret Syndrome in particular seems amenable to endoscopy. Both the enterolithotomy and repair of a cholecystoduodenal fistula have been performed laparoscopically. No study evaluating the laparoscopic versus open approach has been published to date.

A Personal View of the Data

Gallstone Ileus affects primarily elderly patients with multiple comorbidities. Addressing the small bowel obstruction should be the surgeon's priority. Exploring the area of fistulization is usually unnecessary and is best avoided. Although the available data cannot be used to make any definitive conclusions, it supports enterolithotomy alone.

Even in experienced hands, the obliteration of anatomical planes in the right upper quadrant makes safe resection of a cholecysto-enteric fistula challenging. In a patient population that is often in extremis with poor physiologic reserve, the consequences of lengthy, complex operations may be considerable.

Summary of Recommendations

- Patients with gallstone ileus should be managed with enterolithotomy alone (evidence quality low; weak recommendation)

References

1. Reisner RM, Cohen JR. Gallstone ileus: a review of 1001 reported cases. Am Surg. 1994;60(6):441–6.
2. Halabi WJ, Kang CY, Ketana N, Lafaro KJ, Nguyen VQ, Stamos MJ, Imagawa DK, Demirijian AN. Surgery for gallstone ileus: a nationwide comparison of trends and outcomes. Ann Surg. 2014;259(2):329–35.
3. Rigler LG, Borman CN, Noble JF. Gallstone obstruction. Pathogenesis and roentgen manifestations. JAMA. 1941;117:1753–9.
4. Yu CY, Lin CC, Shyu RY, Hsieh CB, Wu HS, Tyan YS, Hwan JL, Liou CH, Chang WC, Chen CY. Value of CT in the diagnosis and management of gallstone ileus. World J Gastroenterol. 2005;11(14):2142–7.
5. Mallipeddi MK, Pappas TN, Shapiro ML, Scarborough JE. Gallstone Ileus: revisiting surgical outcomes using National Surgical Quality Improvement Program Data. J Surg Res. 2013;184(1):84–8.
6. Rodriguez-Sanjuan JC, Casado F, Fernandez MJ, Morales DJ, Naranjo A. Cholecystectomy and fistula closure versus enterolithotomy alone in gallstone ileus. Br J Surg. 1997;84(5):634–7.
7. Allen JW, McCurry T, Rivas H, Cacchione RN. Totally laparoscopic management of gallstone ileus. Surg Endosc. 2003;17(2):353.
8. Sesti J, Okoro C, Parikh M. Laparoscopic enterolithotomy for gallstone ileus. J Am Coll Surg. 2013;217(2):e13–5.
9. Kim YG, Byeon JS, Lee SK, Yang DH, Ye BD, Kim KJ, Myung SJ, Yang SK, Kim JH. Gallstone ileus successfully treated with endoscopic fragmentation by using double balloon endoscopy. Gastrointest Endosc. 2011;74(1):228–30.
10. Muratori R, Cennamo V, Menna M, Cecinato P, Eusebi LH, Mazzella G, Bazzoli F. Colonic gallstone ileus treated with radiologically guided extracorporeal shock wave lithotripsy followed by endoscopic extraction. Endoscopy. 2012;44 Suppl 2:e88–9. UCTN.
11. Reinhardt SW, Jin LX, Pitt SC, Earl TM, Chapman WC, Doyle MB. Bouveret syndrome complicated by classic gallstone ileus: progression of disease or iatrogenic. J Gastrointest Surg. 2013;17(11):2020–4.

Chapter 26
Surgery or Endoscopy for Bile Duct Strictures Secondary to Chronic Pancreatitis?

Katherine A. Morgan, Gregory A. Cote, and David B. Adams

Abstract A terminal benign biliary stricture (BBS) is a common complication of chronic pancreatitis (CP). Historically, BBS was a surgical disease, treated with operative biliary bypass. With the advent of endoscopic retrograde cholangiopancreatography and endoscopic stenting, therapeutic endoscopy has become the primary approach to BBS. Endoscopic management has limitations, however, including unsatisfactory long term durability. Improvements in stent technology and technique are promising. Surgery can often concomitantly best address other CP related complications including pain. Surgery has higher short term morbidity but may be more durable long-term. Minimally invasive techniques in biliary bypass are feasible.

Keywords Chronic pancreatitis • Biliary stricture • Bile duct stricture • Jaundice • ERCP • Endoscopic stent • Choledochoduodenostomy • Choledochojejunostomy

K.A. Morgan
Department of Surgery, Medical University of South Carolina,
114 Doughty Street, Ste 249, MSC 295, Charleston, SC 29425, USA
e-mail: morganka@musc.edu

G.A. Cote
Division of Gastroenterology and Hepatology, Medical University of South Carolina,
25 Courtenay Drive, Charleston, SC 29425, USA
e-mail: cotea@musc.edu

D.B. Adams (✉)
Department of Surgery, Medical University of South Carolina,
114 Doughty Street, Ste 249, MSC 295, Charleston, SC 29425, USA
e-mail: adamsdav@musc.edu

J.M. Millis, J.B. Matthews (eds.), *Difficult Decisions in Hepatobiliary and Pancreatic Surgery*, Difficult Decisions in Surgery: An Evidence-Based Approach, DOI 10.1007/978-3-319-27365-5_26

Introduction

Chronic pancreatitis (CP) is a debilitating and morbid disease marked by the progressive replacement of healthy pancreatic parenchyma with fibrotic tissue. In severe disease, 10–30 % of patients will develop a symptomatic benign biliary stricture (BBS). At greatest risk are those patients with an inflammatory pseudotumor in the head of the pancreas due to extrinsic compression of the intrapancreatic portion of the bile duct. Timely and effective treatment of a BBS in CP is essential to avoid the significant consequences of chronic cholestasis, recurrent cholangitis, and secondary biliary cirrhosis. Patients with a persistent symptomatic stricture despite resolution of acute inflammation do well with intervention. A stricture is considered symptomatic when it causes jaundice, pain, or cholangitis.

Historically, BBS in CP was a surgical disease. Surgical options include primarily choledochoduodenostomy (side-to-side or end-to side) and choledochojejunostomy (Roux-en-Y), but also reinsertion of the common bile duct into the resection bed after local resection of the pancreatic head. With the advent of endoscopic retrograde cholangiopancreatography (ERCP) and endobiliary stents, endoscopic drainage has been increasingly utilized as a first-line intervention for patients with a symptomatic BBS secondary to CP, as it is less morbid than the surgical approach. Endoscopic drainage is traditionally accomplished by performance of a biliary sphincterotomy, dilation of the stricture using graduated catheters or hydrostatic balloons, and placement of multiple plastic stents in parallel. The short-term efficacy of endoscopic drainage is high, but its durability is suboptimal and requires an average of 3–4 ERCPs to achieve maximal dilation. The advent of fully covered, self-expanding metallic stents (SEMS)—not currently FDA approved for BBS—may improve the short- and long-term efficacy of endoscopic therapy by providing sustained radial expansion of the stricture during stent indwell. Additionally, SEMS may reduce the resource intensity of endoscopic therapy by lowering the number of ERCPs required to treat a BBS. There have been no randomized, comparative effectiveness trials of endoscopy versus surgery for CP-induced BBS, so the decision to proceed with either alternative is often based on local expertise and additional clinical factors (e.g., medical comorbidities, concomitant pancreatic pathology). The available evidence is worth consideration.

Search Strategy

A systematic review of the literature for pertinent studies was undertaken utilizing Ovid/Medline databases from 1990 to present. Search terms included: chronic pancreatitis (as a Medical Subject Heading, MeSH) AND biliary stricture OR bile duct stricture OR jaundice OR ERCP OR biliary bypass OR choledochoduodenostomy OR choledochojejunostomy OR hepaticojejunostomy. Search was restricted to articles written in English. We only included clinical trials and cohort studies; case reports or series were excluded. In addition, the references from relevant studies were reviewed to identify any potential studies missed using this method.

Patients	Surgical intervention	Endoscopic intervention	Outcomes
Patients with chronic pancreatitis and associated biliary stricture	Choledochoduodenostomy, choledochojejunostomy, or Frey procedure	Endoscopic stenting	Therapeutic success (stricture resolution), stricture recurrence, morbidity, number of procedures, length of hospitalization

Results

Studies Comparing Endoscopic and Surgical Intervention

There are no randomized trials comparing the efficacy of endoscopic and surgical therapies for BBS in CP. Multiple single institution cohort studies of endoscopic and surgical approaches and few prospective trials of endoscopic therapy are available for review.

Regimbeau and colleagues compared the outcomes of endoscopy and surgery in 39 patients undergoing management for CP-related BBS. Thirty-three patients underwent endoscopic therapy (ET) initially and six surgery (ST). Patients undergoing ET required a mean of three ERCPs, including SEMS (35 %) and multiple plastic stents (65 %) for a mean duration of 11 months. ST included choledochoduodenostomy (CDD, 4), choledochojejunostomy (CDJ, 1), and insertion of the CBD into the pancreatic head [1], combined with Frey [5] and pancreaticojejunostomy [1]. The complication rate was high in the surgical group (83 % vs. 21 %, $p=0.01$), although much of the morbidity was related to the associated pancreatic procedure. Length of stay was similar. Initial success was similar between groups, obtained in 74 % of ST and 75 % of ET, but long-term success (24 months) was significantly greater in the ST group as compared to the ET group (65 % vs 12 %, $p=0.01$). Seventeen of 33 patients (52 %) initially treated with ET ultimately underwent surgery for recurrent BBS [1].

Outcomes of Surgical Intervention

Multiple retrospective single institution reports of surgical outcomes in management of CP BBS have been undertaken. Notably, R.L. Sanders reported his experience with 25 patients undergoing CDD to the Southern Surgical Association in 1946. There were two (8 %) perioperative deaths and the remaining patients did well long-term [2]. Many other similar and important series are reported. We limit our review to the more modern era since 1990, as endoscopic stent therapy was widely available at that point. In 2011, our group reported experience with 79 patients undergoing CDD for CP related BBS, with a morbidity rate of 19 % and long-term success in 77/79 patients, with one requiring endoscopic management of anastomotic stricture (Fig. 26.1). "Sump syndrome," which refers to a clinical diathesis of fever, elevated hepatic chemistries, cholangitis, or hepatic abscess due to biliary stasis in the terminal bile duct and reflux of duodenal contents, is a reported complication after CDD. With adequate anastomotic size, however, sump syndrome is a rare event, occurring in 2.5 % of patients in the authors' series [3]. Several other retrospective series of CDD for CP related BBS have been reported over the past two decades with morbidity rates of 9.8–28 %, mortality rates of 0–6 %, and long-term success rates of 90–100 % [4–6].

While CDD has been the classic operative approach to biliary bypass in CP in order to avoid circumferential dissection of the bile duct in an inflammatory field, CDJ is a reasonable alternative approach. CDJ can be undertaken particularly when a fibrotic duodenum is not suitable for anastomosis and is some surgeons' preference to avoid the sump syndrome. Blankensteijn and Terpstra presented 113 patients who underwent operative biliary bypass (64 CDD and 49 CDJ). Perioperative morbidity and mortality following CDD were 10.9 % and 4.7 % and following CDJ were 28.6 % and 12.2 % respectively. Recurrent cholangitis was not seen after CDD but occurred in three patients after CDJ (6.1 %) [7]. Nealon and Urrutia described their series of 64 patients undergoing CDJ for CP associated BBS. Length of stay was 12 days and long-term outcomes were excellent with no episodes of clinically apparent jaundice or cholangitis [8].

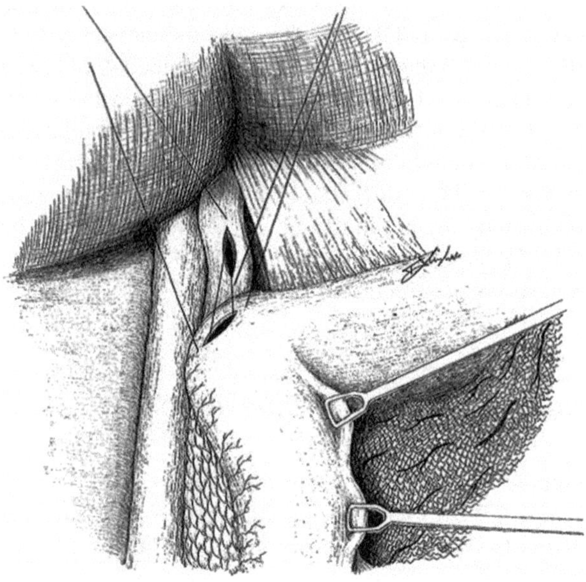

Fig. 26.1 A side to side choledochoduodenostomy is performed with generous mobilization of the duodenum to allow for a tension free anastomosis at least 2 cm in length

Minimally invasive surgical approaches to CP related BBS have more recently been reported. In 2012, Khajanchee and colleagues reported on 20 cases of laparoscopic CDD, with 25 % conversion to open surgery, morbidity of 30 %, and long-term success in 95 % [9]. Jeyapalan and colleagues described their experience with laparoscopic CDD in six patients in 2002. Length of stay was 6 days, and one patient died. No patient required re-intervention at short-term follow-up [10].

In patients with other complications of CP in addition to BBS such as debilitating pain, surgery is often the primary approach in the physiologically fit patient. In patients with dilated duct pancreatitis (main duct diameter >6 mm), drainage with a lateral pancreaticojejunostomy, combined with a CDD, may be undertaken. Alternatively, in these patients with typically head-dominant inflammatory disease, pancreatic head resection is a therapeutic option. In patients with biliary obstruction and duodenal stenosis a pancreatoduodenectomy (PD) is indicated [11]. In patients with biliary stricture and CP related pain, a PD or a duodenal preserving pancreatic head resection can be beneficial. Frey suggested in 1990 that his local pancreatic head resection combined with lateral pancreaticojejunostomy (LR-LPJ) could often relieve biliary obstruction by releasing the constrictive fibrotic tissue in the pancreatic head [12]. In 1994, Izbicki and colleagues described a similar effect with their duodenal preserving pancreatic head resection (DPPHR) in 37 patients, with excellent long-term results [13]. In 1997 the same group reported on a subset of patients with persistent biliary obstruction despite DPPHR. They described successful management of seven such patients with reinsertion of the common bile duct into the pancreatic head resection cavity [14]. In 2008, the group described their experience with now 82 such patients, with 30 % morbidity (similar to DPPHR without biliary reinsertion), but significant biliary anastomotic stricture rate of 18 % [15]. Recently, in 2013, Rebibo and colleagues presented their experience with LR-LPJ and biliary bypass, performing concomitant CDD in eight patients, CDJ in four patients and reinsertion of the CBD into the pancreatic head resection cavity in three patients. The perioperative morbidity was high (73 %) but primarily related to pancreatic head resection. Two of the three patients with biliary reinsertion did develop strictures in long-term follow-up [16].

Outcomes of Endoscopic Intervention

The basic principal of endoscopic treatment of chronic pancreatitis-induced biliary stricture is to maximally dilate the stricture using graduated catheters or hydrostatic balloons, followed by placement of multiple plastic (typically polyethylene) stents in parallel (Figs. 26.2 and 26.3). Since stent occlusion rates begin to rise after 3–4 months, patients typically return for repeat ERCP and upsizing of stents to the extent possible. Most experts advocate maintaining patency of the stricture for up to 12 months after embarking upon endoscopic treatment, so patients can assume an average of 3–4 ERCPs and up to 1 year of therapy in order to achieve stricture resolution. This “aggressive stenting” approach evolved from high recurrence rates

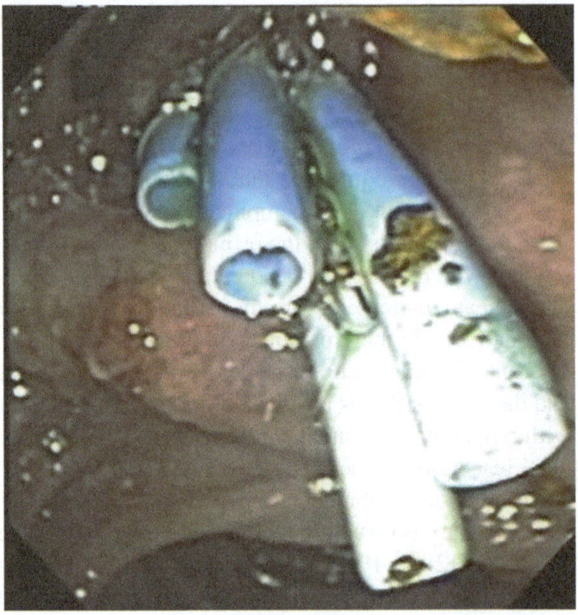

Fig. 26.2 Endoscopic image of multiple parallel endoscopically placed plastic transampullary biliary stents

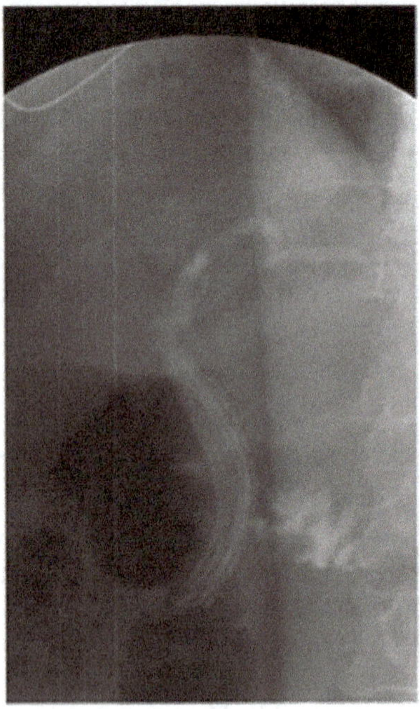

Fig. 26.3 Fluoroscopic image of multiple parallel endoscopically placed plastic transampullary biliary stents

(nearly 20 %), predominantly in the setting of postoperative strictures, when treatment was limited to dilation alone or with placement of only two plastic stents in parallel [17, 18].

The short-term efficacy of endoscopic biliary drainage is well established, but most experts would agree that the long-term durability (typically defined, albeit arbitrarily, of >1 year follow-up after all stents have been removed) of endoscopic treatment in the setting of chronic pancreatitis is approximately 65 %. This is significantly lower than postoperative biliary strictures, where long-term resolution rates of >80 % are considered the norm [19].

Given the need for multiple procedures and the poor long-term efficacy of plastic stents, there is substantial interest in using removable, fully-covered, self-expandable metallic stents (SEMS) to treat benign biliary strictures. SEMS have superior patency to plastic stents, and so may require fewer ERCPs to resolve a stricture. Furthermore, SEMS radially expand within the duct, potentially achieving a more sustained dilation of the stricture and lower recurrence rates; there are no data confirming this hypothesis to date. Potential negatives of SEMS include difficulty with removal and SEMS-specific complications such as acute pancreatitis (via compression of the pancreatic orifice), cholecystitis (via occlusion of the cystic duct insertion), and secondary bile duct injury usually when the stent is oversized (larger than the diameter of the bile duct itself). There are no comparative effectiveness studies of SEMS and plastic stents for treating benign biliary strictures, but a growing body of literature favors their safety and efficacy of SEMS in appropriately selected patients.

Comparative study of surgery and endoscopy for chronic pancreatitis related biliary strictures

First author year	Design	N	Outcome	Surgery	Endoscopy	P	Quality of evidence
Regimbeau [1]	Retrospective review	39	Initial success	74 %	75 %	NS	Low
			Success at 24 months	65 %	12 %	0.01	
			Morbidity	83 %	21 %	0.01	
			Length of stay, days	16	24	NS	

Results of surgery for chronic pancreatitis related biliary strictures

First author year	Design	N	Type of surgery	Morbidity	Long-term success	Quality of evidence
Blankenstein 1990 [7]	Retrospective	113	CDD (64), CDJ (49)	CDD 10.9 %, CDJ 28.6 %	CDD 100 %, CDJ 94 %	Low
Escuadera Fabre 1991 [6]	Retrospective	71	CDD	28 %	96 %	Low
Mendes de Almeida 1996 [5]	Retrospective	125	CDD	NR	90 %	Low

(continued)

First author year	Design	N	Type of surgery	Morbidity	Long-term success	Quality of evidence
Leppard 2011 [3]	Retrospective	79	CDD	19 %	99 %	Low
Cataldegirmen 2008 [15]	Retrospective	82	Frey + CBD resertion	15 %	82 %	Low
Rebibo 2013 [16]	Retrospective	15	Frey + CDD [8], Frey + CDJ [4], Frey + CBD reinsertion [3]	73 %	80 %	Low
Jeyapalan 2002 [10]	Retrospective	6	Lap CDD			Low
Bosanquet 2012	Retrospective	37	CDD	14 %		Low
Khajanchee 2012 [9]	Retrospective	20	Laparoscopic CDD	30 %	95 %	Low
Nealon 1996 [8]	Retrospective	64	CDJ	NR	100 %	Low

Results of endoscopy for chronic pancreatitis associated biliary strictures (Adapted and modified from Dumonceau et al. (2012) [40])

First author, year	n	Long-term success, %	Stenting duration, months	Stent dysfunction of any cause per patient, %	Follow-up post stent removal, months	Patients who underwent surgical drainage, %	Quality of evidence
Single plastic stent							
Deviere 1990 [20]	25	12	n.a.	72	14	24	Low
Barthet 1994 [21]	19	10	10	NA	18	21	Low
Smits 1996 [22]	58	28	10	64	49	28	Low
Vitale 2000 [23]	25	80	13	20	32	8	Low
Farnbacher 2000 [24]	31	32	10	52	28	6	Low
Eickoff 2001 [25]	39	31	9	43	58	28	Low
Kahl 2003 [26]	61	26	12	34	40	49	Low
Catalano 2004 [27]	34	24	21	41	50	41	Low
Cahen 2005 [28]	58	38	9	48	45	28	Low
Multiple plastic stents							
Draganov 2002 [29]	9	44	14	n.a.	48	n.a.	Low
Pozsar 2004 [30]	29	60	21	n.a.	12	13	Low
Catalano 2004 [27]	12	92	14	8	47	8	Very low
Weber 2014 [31]	61 (89 % plastic)	31	12	n.a.	n.a.	28	Very low

(continued)

First author, year	n	Long-term success, %	Stenting duration, months	Stent dysfunction of any cause per patient, %	Follow-up post stent removal, months	Patients who underwent surgical drainage, %	Quality of evidence
Covered, self-expandable metallic stents							
Cahen 2008 [32]	6	50	5	33	28	17	Low
Behm 2009 [33]	20	80	5	5	22	0	Low
Mahajan 2009 [34]	19	n.a.	3	11	4	n.a.	Low
Poley 2012 [35]	13	46	4–8	n.a.	12	n.a.	Very low
Perri 2012 [36]	17	71	6	n.a.	24	n.a.	Low
Kahaleh 2013 [37]	31	80	3	22	n.a.	n.a.	Low
Deviere 2014 [38]	127	80 %	8	10	24	<1	Moderate

Recommendations Based on the Data

Recommendations based upon interpretation of the evidence at hand are summarized in Fig. 26.4.

Therapeutic endoscopy is a reasonable primary approach to the CP related BBS. (Strength of recommendation: Strong; Quality of evidence: Moderate)

Endoscopy can potentially avoid the high reported surgical morbidity. This recommendation is supported by high initial endoscopic success rates (67–100 %). While the durability of endoscopic therapy is inferior to surgery, with long-term success rates of approximately 25 % and some 25–50 % of patients requiring salvage surgery by current strategies, a substantial number of patients will avoid surgery altogether. When analyzed based on intention-to-treat, as per Regimbeau and colleagues, long-term outcomes of surgery are not compromised.

Endoscopic strategy should include balloon cholangioplasty with placement of multiple plastic stents in order to maintain a larger ductal diameter and to avoid premature stent occlusion during therapy. (Strength of recommendation: Strong; Quality of evidence: Moderate)

Fully covered SEMS appear promising based on initial data; comparative effectiveness studies of SEMS versus multiple plastic stents are needed to determine the potential advantages of this technique.

In patients with complications from CP other than biliary tract obstruction requiring surgery (pancreatic duct obstruction with pain, pancreatolithiasis, duodenal obstruction) surgery is a reasonable primary approach. (Strength of recommendation: Strong; Quality of evidence: Low)

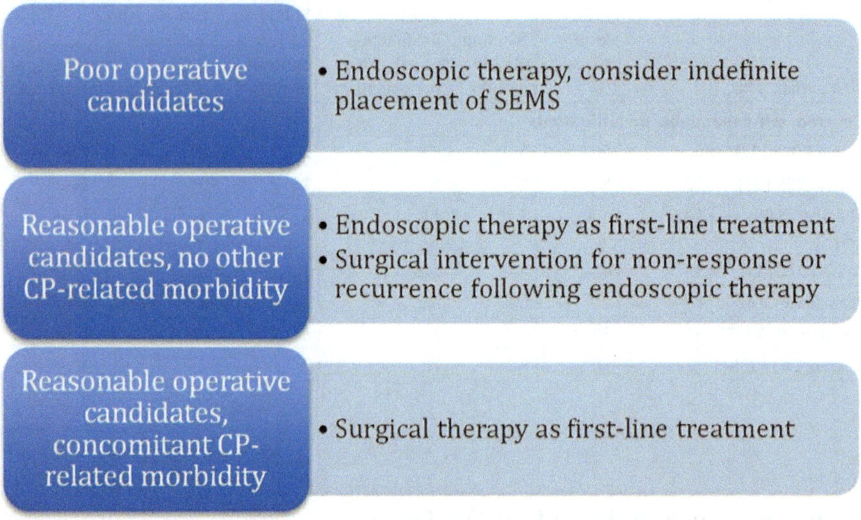
Poor operative candidates
• Endoscopic therapy, consider indefinite placement of SEMS
Reasonable operative candidates, no other CP-related morbidity
• Endoscopic therapy as first-line treatment
• Surgical intervention for non-response or recurrence following endoscopic therapy
Reasonable operative candidates, concomitant CP-related morbidity
• Surgical therapy as first-line treatment

Fig. 26.4 Summary of evidence based recommendations for management of chronic pancreatitis related biliary strictures

Surgery is an effective treatment for CP related BBS. Biliary bypass can be included with pancreatic duct drainage (lateral pancreaticojejunostomy, Frey) with choledochoduodenostomy, Roux-en-Y choledochojejunostomy, or reinsertion of the common bile duct into the pancreatic head resection cavity as described by Izbicki. Generally, choledochoduodenostomy (side-to-side or end-to side) is the most common method of operative biliary bypass for BBS in CP and is safe and durable long term, with minimal morbidity. "Sump syndrome" is an unusual long term complication of CDD and can be avoided by an adequate anastomotic diameter. Roux-en-Y choledochojejunostomy and reinsertion of the CBD into the pancreatic head resection bed are reasonable approaches as well with good outcomes. Laparoscopic biliary bypass is feasible and effective.

Personal View of the Data

Chronic pancreatitis is a heterogenous disease with different clinical and morphological presentations that depend on environmental, genetic, and anatomic factors. There is great geographic variation in the presentation of the disease as exemplified by the calcific chronic pancreatitis of Southern India and the inflammatory head mass reported in studies from Germany [39]. Thus it is hard to classify and directly compare different management strategies for biliary obstruction associated with chronic pancreatitis. Also unanswered is the risk of cholangitis and biliary cirrhosis associated with terminal biliary stenosis. Certainly the patient with cholangitis and multiple medical co-morbidities would be best managed with minimally invasive endoscopic techniques. But what about the asymptomatic patient with mild elevations in serum alkaline phosphatase and bilirubin with common bile duct dilation? What is the natural history of that disorder? Identification of the non-dilatable stricture is difficult and is the crux of the patient selection process. When patients have symptomatic terminal biliary stenosis with fibrosing pancreatitis repeated endoscopic stenting may be needed indefinitely. Choledochoduodenostomy is an attractive long-term solution and may be performed with minimally invasive laparoscopic techniques. However, chronic peripancreatic and peri-duodenal inflammation may make the operation difficult and hazardous. Normal anatomic landmarks may be hidden and simple identification of the inflamed and dilated common bile duct can be a challenge. When duodenal fibrosis is severe, mobilization and anastomosis between a fibrotic duodenum and the bile duct may not be possible. In this situation pre-operatively placed transpapillary biliary stents are useful to protect the anastomosis post-operatively. Alternatively, Roux-en-Y hepaticojejunostomy may be more prudent when the duodenum is unfavorable for anastomosis. Patients who have cavernous transformation of the portal vein associated with CP superior mesenteric and portal vein stenosis can safely undergo CDD though increased operative blood loss is expected, and these patients are frequently directed towards endoscopic therapy. An evidence-based approach to biliary strictures in chronic pancreatitis is problematic and patient selection remains grounded in local experience. As new minimally invasive laparoscopic and endoscopic tools and techniques are developed they can be better tested against traditional open surgical techniques in appropriately classified patient cohorts and evidence will replace experience in clinical practice.

References

1. Regimbeau JM, Fuks D, Bartoli E, Fumery M, Hanes A, et al. A comparative study of surgery and endoscopy for the treatment of bile duct strictures in patients with chronic pancreatitis. Surg Endosc. 2012;26:2902–8.
2. Sanders RL. Indications for and value of choledochoduodenostomy. Ann Surg. 1946;123:847–55.
3. Leppard WM, Shary TM, Adams DB, Morgan KA. Choledochoduodenostomy: is it really so bad? J Gastrointest Surg. 2011;15:754–7.
4. Bosanquet DC, Cole M, Conway KC, Lewis M. Choledochoduodenostomy reevaluated in the endoscopic and laparoscopic era. HepatoGastroenterology. 2012;59:2410–5.
5. Mendes De Almeida A, Dos Santos N, et al. Choledochoduodenostomy in the management of common duct stones or associated pathology- an obsolete method? HPB Surg. 1996;10:27–33.
6. Escudero-Fabre A, Escallon A, et al. Choledochoduodenostomy: analysis of 71 cases followed for 5 to 15 years. Ann Surg. 1991;213:635–42.
7. Blankenstein J, Terpstra O. Early and late results following choledochoduodenostomy and choledochojejunostomy. HPB Surg. 1990;2:151–8.
8. Nealon WH, Urrutia F. Long-term follow-up after bilioenteric anastomosis for benign bile duct stricture. Ann Surg. 1996;6:639–48.

9. Khajanchee YS, Cassera MA, Hammill CW, Swanstrom LL, Hanson PD. Outcomes following laparoscopic choledochoduodenostomy in the management of benign biliary obstruction. J Gastrointest Surg. 2012;16:801–5.
10. Jeyapalan M, Almeida J, et al. Laparoscopic choledochoduodenostomy: review of a 4-year experience with an uncommon problem. Surg Laparosc Endosc Percutaneous Tech. 2002;12:148–53.
11. Howard JM, Zhang Z. Pancreaticoduodenectomy (Whipple resection) in the treatment of chronic pancreatitis. World J Surg. 1990;14:77–82.
12. Frey CF, Suzuki M, Isaji S. Treatment of chronic pancreatitis complicated by obstruction of the common bile duct or duodenum. World J Surg. 1990;14:59–69.
13. Izbicki JR, Bloechle C, Knoefel WT, Wilker DK, Dornschneider G, et al. Complications of adjacent organs in chronic pancreatitis managed by duodenum preserving resection of the head of the pancreas. Br J Surg. 1994;81:1351–5.
14. Izbicki JR, Bloechle C, Broering DC, Broelsch CE. Reinsertion of the distal common bile duct into the resection cavity during duodenum-preserving resection of the head of the pancreas for chronic pancreatitis. Br J Surg. 1997;84:791–2.
15. Cataldegirmen G, Bogoevski D, Mann O, Kaifi JT, Izbicki JR, Yekebas EF. Late morbidity after duodenum-preserving pancreatic head resection with bile duct reinsertion into the resection cavity. Br J Surg. 2008;95:447–52.
16. Rebibo L, Yzet T, Cosse C, Delcenserie R, Bartoli E, Regimbeau JM. Frey procedure for the treatment of chronic pancreatitis associated with common bile duct stricture. Hepatobiliary Pancreat Dis Int. 2013;12:637–44.
17. Davids PH, Rauws EA, Coene PP, Tytgat GN, Huibregtse K. Endoscopic stenting for postoperative biliary strictures. Gastrointest Endosc. 1992;38:12–8.
18. Costamagna G, Pandolfi M, Mutignani M, Spada C, Perri V. Long-term results of endoscopic management of postoperative bile duct strictures with increasing numbers of stents. Gastrointest Endosc. 2001;54:162–8.
19. Costamagna G, Tringali A, Mutignani M, Perri V, Spada C, Pandolfi M, Galasso D. Endotherapy of postoperative biliary strictures with multiple stents: results after more than 10 years of follow-up. Gastrointest Endosc. 2010;72:551–7.
20. Deviere J, Devaere S, Baize M, et al. Endoscopic biliary drainage in chronic pancreatitis. Gastrointest Endosc. 1990;36:96–100.
21. Barthet M, Bernard JP, Duval JL, Affriat C, et al. Biliary stenting in benign biliary stenosis complicating chronic calcifying pancreatitis. Endoscopy. 1994;26:569–72.
22. Smits ME, Rauws EA, van Gulik TM, Gouma DJ, Tytgat GN. Long-term results of endoscopic stenting and surgical drainage for biliary stricture due to chronic pancreatitis. Br J Surg. 1996;83:764–8.
23. Vitale GC, Reed Jr DN, Nguyen CT, et al. Endoscopic treatment of distal bile duct stricture from chronic pancreatitis. Surg Endosc. 2000;14:227–31.
24. Farnbacher MJ, Rabenstein T, Ell C, et al. Is endoscopic drainage of common bile duct stenosis in chronic pancreatitis up to date? Am J Gastroenterol. 2000;95:1466–71.
25. Eickhoff A, Jakobs R, Leonhardt A, et al. Endoscopic stenting for common bile duct stenosis in chronic pancreatitis: results and impact on long-term outcome. Eur J Gastroenterol Hepatol. 2001;13:1161–7.
26. Kahl S, Zimmerman S, Genz I, Glasbrenner B, Pross M, et al. Risk factors for failure of endoscopic stenting in chronic pancreatitis: a prospective follow-up study. Am J Gastroenterol. 2003;98:2448–53.
27. Catalano MF, Linder JD, George S, Alcocer E, Geenen JE. Treatment of symptomatic distal common bile duct stenosis secondary to chronic pancreatitis: comparison of single vs multiple simultaneous stents. Gastrointest Endosc. 2004;60:945–52.
28. Cahen DL, van Berkel A-MM, Oskam D, et al. Long-term results of endoscopic drainage of common bile duct strictures in chronic pancreatitis. Eur J Gastroenterol Hepatol. 2005;17:103–8.

29. Dragonov P, Hoffman B, Marsh W, et al. Long-term outcome in patients with benign biliary strictures treated endoscopically with multiple stents. Gastrointest Endosc. 2002;55:680–6.
30. Pozsar J, Sahin P, Laszlo F, Forro G, Topa L. Medium-term results of endoscopic treatment of common bile duct strictures in chronic calcifying pancreatitis with increasing numbers of stents. J Clin Gastroenterol. 2004;38:118–23.
31. Weber A, Zellner S, Wagenpfeil S, Schneider J, Gerngross C, et al. Long-term follow-up after endoscopic stent therapy for benign biliary strictures. J Clin Gastroenterol. 2014;48:88–93.
32. Cahen D, Rauws EA, Gouma DJ, et al. Removable fully covered self-expandable metal stents to prevent migration in patients with benign biliary strictures: a multicenter, prospective, comparative pilot study. Endoscopy. 2008;40:697–700.
33. Behm B, Brock A, Clarke BW, et al. Partially covered self-expandable metallic stents for benign biliary strictures due to chronic pancreatitis. Endoscopy. 2009;41:547–51.
34. Mahajan A, Ho H, Sauer B, et al. Temporary placement of fully covered self-expandable metal stents in benign biliary strictures: midterm evaluation. Gastrointest Endosc. 2009;70:303–9.
35. Poley JW, Cahen DL, Metselaar HJ, et al. A prospective group sequential study evaluating a new type of fully covered self-expandable metal stent for the treatment of benign biliary strictures. Gastrointest Endosc. 2012;75:783–9.
36. Perri V, Boskoski I, Tringali A, et al. Fully covered self-expandable metal stents in biliary strictures caused by chronic pancreatitis not responding to plastic stenting: a prospective study with 2 years of follow-up. Gastrointest Endosc. 2012;75:1271–8.
37. Kahaleh M, Brijbassie A, Sethi A, et al. Multicenter trial evaluating the use of covered self-expanding metal stents in benign biliary strictures: time to revisit our therapeutic options? J Clin Gastroenterol. 2013;47:695–9.
38. Deviere J, Reddy DN, Puspok A, Ponchon T, Bruno MJ, et al. Successful management of benign biliary strictures with fully covered self-expanding metal stents. Gastroenterol. 2014;147:385–95.
39. Keck T, Marjanovic G, Fernandez-del Castillo C, Makowiec F, Schäfer AO, Rodriguez JR, Razo O, Hopt UT, Warshaw AL. The inflammatory pancreatic head mass: significant differences in the anatomic pathology of German and American patients with chronic pancreatitis determine very different surgical strategies. Ann Surg. 2009;249:105–10.
40. Dumonceau JM, Trinagli A, Blero D, Deviere J, Laugeirs R, Heresbach D, Costamagna, European Society of Gastrointestinal Endoscopy. Biliary stenting: indications, choice of stents and results: European gastrointestinal endoscopy clinical guideline. Endoscopy. 2012;44:277–98.

Chapter 27
Routine or Selective Cholangiography for Elective Laparoscopic Cholecystectomy?

Shane Svoboda and Brian L. Bello

Abstract Laparoscopic cholecystectomy (LC) is one of the most commonly performed surgical procedures today and is considered the standard of care for gallbladder removal. The role of routine versus selective intraoperative cholangiography (IOC) in elective LC to prevent bile duct injury and detect choledocholithiasis remains in dispute. Routine cholangiography may decrease the overall incidence or severity of bile duct injuries. IOC may also play a role in the optimal management of patients with risk of a common duct stone. Controversy arises with routine IOC which may to added operative time, cost, and secondary procedures, suggesting a more selective approach may be more beneficial. Newer techniques such as near-infrared fluorescence cholangiography may be an alternative to traditional IOC.

Keywords Cholangiography • Cholecystectomy • Laparoscopy • Bile duct injury • Fluorescent cholangiography

Introduction

Laparoscopic cholecystectomy (LC) is one of the most commonly performed abdominal procedures in the world. Morbidity associated with LC may be as high as 2–4 % with bile duct injury (BDI) a rare but devastating complication leading to a potential threefold increase in mortality [1]. In the era of laparoscopy, recent studies have demonstrated consistently an increased incidence of bile duct injury of about 0.2–0.6 % [1, 2] compared to that of 0.1–0.3 % for open cholecystectomy [3, 4]. Improving these rates in the technique currently considered standard of care must be addressed.

The use of intraoperative cholangiogram (IOC) during elective LC remains controversial in its role as routine practice for all patients versus selective practice,

S. Svoboda • B.L. Bello (✉)
Department of Surgery, Sinai Hospital of Baltimore,
2435 W Belvedere Avenue, Hoffberger Building Suite 42, Baltimore, MD 21215, USA
e-mail: brianbello@gmail.com

J.M. Millis, J.B. Matthews (eds.), *Difficult Decisions in Hepatobiliary and Pancreatic Surgery*, Difficult Decisions in Surgery: An Evidence-Based Approach, DOI 10.1007/978-3-319-27365-5_27

reserved for those patients with risk for common bile duct stones or difficult anatomy. Differences in training and personal experience have led to varied practices in the use of IOC and remain a matter of surgeon preference. Some surgeons believe that obtaining a "critical view of safety" is sufficient for identification of vital structures while other surgeons see routine IOC as the gold standard for biliary identification and imaging [5, 6]. Selective IOC users believe it changes management in relatively few cases and apply it only in cases where choledocholithiasis is suspected or among patients at high risk for common bile duct injury. Another argument against routine IOC is that cholangiography may be misinterpreted by surgeons over half of the time [7].

This chapter is an evidenced-based review of recent literature focusing on the potential advantages and disadvantages of routine cholangiography compared to selective cholangiography in patients undergoing elective laparoscopic cholecystectomy. Outcomes such as morbidity, secondary procedures, and cost will be specifically examined. We will also address the newer techniques of near-infrared fluorescence cholangiography that may become an alternative to traditional IOC.

Search Strategy

A literature search of English language publications from 2005 to 2014 was used to identify published data on intraoperative cholangiogram using the PICO outline (Table 27.1). Databases searched were PubMed, Medline, Cochrane Evidence Based Medicine, and TRIP database. Terms used in the search were "cholangiogram, routine, selective," "cholangiogram, bile duct injury," "cholangiogram, complications," and "cholangiogram, cost." Randomized controlled studies were reviewed as well as comparative studies with greater than 400 patients. All studies regarding near-infrared cholangiography were reviewed. The data was classified using the GRADE system.

Table 27.1 PICO table for routine versus selective cholangiography for elective laparoscopic cholecystectomy

P (patients)	I (intervention)	C (comparator)	O (outcomes)
Patients undergoing elective laparoscopic cholecystectomy	Routine intraoperative cholangiography	Selective intraoperative cholangiography	Bile duct injury, retained stones, operating time, secondary procedures, false positives, cost

Results

Routine Versus Selective Cholangiography

The role of routine intraoperative cholangiography in laparoscopic cholecystectomy is controversial. When surveyed by the American College of Surgeons, general surgeons had varying opinions. Twenty seven percent identified themselves as "routine users" using IOC in more than 75 % of their cases. "Selective users" tended to be low-volume surgeons with less than 20 LC per year. "Routine users" responded more favorably regarding IOC believing that routine use was overall less costly and more protective of injury [8]. Part of the lack of consensus on this topic among surgeons is the conflicting evidence in the literature.

In the 1990s, there were few randomized, prospective trials conducted comparing routine IOC versus no IOC. Soper and Dunnegan found an increased operative time of 16 min in patients undergoing routine IOC with an increase in total charges by $700 [9]. Nies et al. found no difference in morbidity or mortality between the two groups, and the operations with routine IOC lasted significantly longer (92 vs. 77 min) [10]. Each trial concluded that routine IOC was not justified.

Two more recent randomized controlled trials are summarized in Tables 27.2 and 27.3. Like the two previous trials, Khan et al. in 2011 studied the difference between routine IOC versus no IOC. They studied 190 patients that were at low risk of common duct stones and found a longer operative time (66 vs. 54 min; $p < 0.001$) with no statistical difference in readmission rates and morbidity including retained stones or common bile duct injury. The authors concluded that routine cholangiography was not indicated [11]. In contrast, Amott et al. in 2005 randomized 303 patients to undergo routine or selective IOC. There was no difference in operating time, retained stones or common bile duct injury. However, the authors still changed their practice to performing routine IOC because seven of eight patients who presented with a retained common bile duct stone postoperatively did not undergo IOC. Three of the seven had normal LFTs and a normal ultrasound preoperatively and would have been missed with a selective approach. They also argued an unplanned IOC may lead to a significant increase in operative time versus a routine and planned IOC because the operating room staff would already have the equipment in place [12].

These aforementioned randomized trials were limited by having relatively low numbers at a single center. In fact, due to the low incidence of bile duct injury, the number of patients needed to conduct a randomized, controlled trial with adequate power in order to avoid a type II error would be greater than 30,000 [13].

Despite the lack of randomized trials, it is possible to garner some information from other types of comparative studies. There are several, large prospective registries that examine bile duct injuries in routine IOC versus no IOC. In the Swiss prospective registry, 36.6 % of 31,838 patients underwent IOC which is a similar rate as in the United States. The rate of biliary injuries was 0.3 % in each of the two groups suggesting no effect of IOC on the prevention and detection of biliary

Table 27.2 Routine intraoperative cholangiography versus no intraoperative cholangiography

Author (date)	N (pts)		Bile duct injury (%)		Intraoperative retained stones (%)		Postoperative retained stones (%)		Operating time (min)		Secondary procedures (%)		False positives (%)	Cost ($)	Study type
	IOC	No IOC	IOC	No IOC	IOC	No IOC	IOC	No IOC	IOC	No IOC	IOC	No IOC			
Khan (2011) [11]	91	99	0 (0)	1 (0)[a]	3 (3)	0 (0)[a]	0 (0)	0 (0)[a]	66±2	54±3	NR	NR	0 (0)	NR	RCT level 1B
Giger (2012) [15]	11,642	20,196	40 (0.3)	61 (0.3)[a]	NR	NR	NR	NR	NR	NR	NR	NR	NR	NR	Prospective registry level III
Törnqvist (2012) [15]	51,041		747 (1.5 %), incidence of BDI in IOC group 29 % lower (exact number not reported)		NR	NR	NR	NR	NR	NR	NR	NR	NR	NR	Prospective registry level III

RCT Randomized clinical trial, *NR* not reported
[a]No statistical difference

Table 27.3 Routine intraoperative cholangiography versus selective intraoperative cholangiography

Author (date)	N (pts)		Bile duct injury (%)		Intraoperative retained stones (%)		Postoperative retained stones (%)		Operating time (min)		Secondary procedures (%)		False positives (%)	Cost ($)		Study type
	Routine IOC	Selective IOC	Routine IOC	Selective IOC	Routine IOC	Selective IOC	Routine IOC	Selective IOC	Routine IOC	Selective IOC	Routine IOC	Selective IOC		Routine IOC	Selective IOC	
Amott (2005) [12]	148	155	1 (0.68)	1 (0.64)[a]	12 (8.1)	5 (3.2)[a]	3 (2.0)	5 (3.2)[a]	56	61[a]	12 (8.1 %)	NR	0	NR		RCT level 1B
Nuzzo (2005) [2]	56,591 (Routine IOC done in 10.3 % general surgery units; selective IOC done in 89.7 % general surgery units)		25 (0.32)	210 (0.43)[a]	NR	NR	NR	NR	NR	NR	NR	NR	NR	NR		Retrospective study level III
Ragulin-Coyne (2013) [16]	111,815 (Routine IOC surgeons 10.8 %; Selective IOC surgeons 89.2 %)		(0.25)	(0.26)[a]	NR	NR	NR	NR	NR	NR	(15.8)	(12.7)	NR	10425	9495	Retrospective study level III
Buddingh (2011) [17]	435 (60 % had IOC)	421	11 (2.5); major BDI 0 (0)	15 (3.5)[a]; major BDI 8 (1.9 %)	21 (4.8)	4 (1.0)	NR	NR	110±44	100±47	83 (19.1)	102 (24.2)[a]	NR	NR		Retrospective study level III
Nickkholgh (2006) [18]	1,330	800	0 (0)	2 (0.25)[a]	37 (2.8)	9 (1.1)	NR	NR	NR	NR	NR	NR	0	NR		Retrospective study level III

RCT Randomized clinical trial, *NR* not reported

[a]No statistical difference

injuries [14]. The Swedish prospective registry found 747 bile duct injuries in 51,041 laparoscopic cholecystectomies for a rate of 1.5 %. This relatively high number was likely due to the inclusion of minor bile duct injuries. The incidence of a bile duct injury (BDI) was 29 % lower when IOC was successfully performed or attempted suggesting a possible protective effect [15]. These studies are included Table 27.2. A large, retrospective national survey from Italy examined 56,591 patients in different general surgery units that underwent LC and demonstrated no statistical difference in BDI between routine and selective IOC (0.32 % vs. 0.43 %). However, only 10.3 % of general surgery units surveyed underwent routine IOC much lower than other countries [2]. This study is included in Table 27.3. These sizeable studies are good because of the large numbers but have to be interpreted with caution as the frequency of IOC may be considerably different from other studies and there are very few listed specifics regarding the context of surgery.

Ragulin-Coyne and colleagues queried Nationwide Inpatient Sample data and found 111,815 patients who presented with acute biliary disease who underwent laparoscopic cholecystectomy. They dichotomized surgeons into a routine IOC surgeons and selective IOC surgeons. Their data suggested no significant difference between the rates of biliary injury and the use of routine cholangiography. They found no protective effect of routine IOC with significantly increased cost ($930 more) and slightly higher incidence in morbidity (7.3 vs. 6.8 %; $p=0.04$). Routine IOC was also associated with increased endoscopic retrograde cholangiopancreatography (ERCP) use (15.8 % vs. 12.7 % $p<0.0001$) and higher common bile duct exploration (2.6 % vs. 1.6 %; $p<0.0001$) [16]. This study is summarized in Table 27.3.

A retrospective review by Buddingh et al. examined medical records 3 years prior and following implementation of a routine IOC approach in a university hospital in The Netherlands. Four hundred twenty one patients underwent cholecystectomy with selective IOC prior to the start of the study and this was compared to 435 patients that underwent routine IOC after the study began. In this study, the policy of routine IOC was deliberately not strictly enforced at first. Instead, a period of gradual introduction allowed the surgical team to become more familiar with the technique. Thus, compliance with IOC in the rouine approach was relatively low immediately after introduction. Six percent of the selective IOC group received IOC, and only 60 % of the routine group had IOC both lower than expected limiting this study. They did demonstrate, however, a significant decrease in major BDI in the routine group (0 % versus 1.9 %; $p=0.004$) but no difference in total BDI (major and minor). An increase in intraoperative management of common bile duct stones was also noted (2.8 % vs. 0.7 %; $p=0.023$) [17]. Similarly in Iran, Nickkholgh and colleagues implemented a routine IOC approach and compared 1330 patients that underwent routine IOC versus 800 patients that underwent selective IOC prior to the start of the study. They found an increased rate of retained stones (2.8 % vs. 1.1 %; $p=0.01$) with no significant difference in BDI. These two studies are summarized in Table 27.3.

Literature focused on cost associated with routine intraoperative cholangiography has been sparse. One of the first studies proposed was by Flum et al. in 2003.

They created decision analytic models to calculate costs and benefits of routine IOC. They noted that it would cost approximately $100 more per each case. However, they found that routine IOC would prevent 2.5 deaths for every 10,000 patients at a cost of $390,000 per life saved or $13,900/quality life-year (well below the standard benchmark of <$50,000/quality life-year to be deemed cost-effective). Cost per common bile duct injury avoided ranged from approximately $61,000 to $87,100. These estimates do not consider the high price of litigation costs which many argue that any cost of IOC is worthwhile [13]. Brown et al. designed another decision model to examine patients with symptomatic cholelithiasis with possible common bile duct stones including five different strategies: (1) LC alone, (2) preoperative ERCP followed by LC, (3) LC with IOC ± common bile duct exploration, (4) LC followed by ERCP, (5) and LC with IOC ± postoperative ERCP. Across a common bile duct stone probability range of 4–100 %, LC with IOC ± ERCP was the most cost-effective [19].

Livingston et al. argued against routine IOC when cost and utilization were examined. They reviewed the 2001 Nationwide Inpatient Survey database for IOC utilization and associated charges. IOCs were associated with $706–739 additional charges [20]. This is consistent with the increased cost of $930 of the previously discussed NIS study [16]. Livingston projected a cost of $371,356 to prevent one single bile duct injury by using a routine IOC approach [20].

Near Infrared Fluorescent Cholangiography

Fluorescence cholangiography is a feasible alternative to contrast-dye cholangiography and may have a cost benefit although reduction in bile duct injury has not been proven. A study by Schools and colleagues demonstrated safety and feasibility of near-infrared fluorescence cholangiography (NIRF-C) in patients receiving indocyanine green (ICG) just after induction of anesthesia in 15 patients. Fluorescence imaging was performed with no adverse reactions to the injected ICG with identification of the cystic duct in an average of 23 min [21]. A prospective study that demonstrated the feasibility of NIRF-C was done recently. Eighty two patients underwent elective LC with NIRF-C with successful identification of the cystic duct in 95.1 %, common bile duct in 76.8 % and common hepatic duct in 69.5 %. This was followed by IOC with successful identification of the cystic duct in 72.0 %, common bile duct in 75.6 % and common hepatic duct in 74.3 %. The procedure times were significantly different with NIRF-C and IOC (1.9 min vs. 11.8 min; $p<0.001$). There were no adverse events [22].

A recent study examined cost analysis and effectiveness of fluorescent cholangiography. Identification with fluorescence was successful in 100 % of 43 patients and significantly less costly than IOC ($14.10 vs. $778.43; $p<0.0001$), and was faster than IOC (0.71 vs. 7.15 min; $p<0.0001$) [23]. Prevot and colleagues found in a prospective cohort of 23 patients that identification of the biliary tract was more effective with fluorescence imaging than with IOC after dissection. Analyzability rate was 74 % using indocyanine green, 70 % using IOC with conventional contrast fluid, and 26 % with conventional visual inspection [24].

Recommendations

The literature regarding the routine use of intraoperative cholangiogram is conflicting. Most of the studies are non-experimental comparative data and not Level 1 data. This is due to the fact that bile duct injury occurs rarely and a large multicenter randomized controlled trial is not feasible. Routine IOC is associated with similar rates of bile injury, increased rate of detecting retained stones (though it is unclear if this is clinically significant), longer operative time, increased cost, and low rate of false positives. There is unclear evidence regarding secondary procedures and overall cost-effectiveness. Therefore, the use of routine intraoperative cholangiogram during laparoscopic cholecystectomy should be left to the discretion of the operating surgeon. This is a weak recommendation in light of low-quality data.

There is currently inadequate evidence to suggest replacement of routine IOC with near-infrared fluorescence cholangiography. Additional large volume studies are needed to show protective effect.

A Personal View of the Data

There likely will never be a consensus on the routine versus selective use of intraoperative cholangiogram in elective laparoscopic cholecystectomy. Most recent studies show there is no significant difference in bile duct injury. The more compelling argument is the additional cost of IOC, with a wide variety described in the literature ranging from $77 to $930. The two nationwide analyses reviewed found higher costs ($739–$930) than the values stated in earlier regional studies. In order to ever recommend routine IOC, the cost must be minimal. This is not currently the case.

We eagerly await the results of larger studies of newer techniques such as fluorescence cholangiogram which may facilitate identification of biliary structures with reduced cost and operative time.

Recommendations

1. The safety of laparoscopic cholecystectomy requires correct identification of relevant anatomy (evidence quality low; strong recommendation).
2. The routine use of intraoperative cholangiogram should be used at the discretion of the surgeon (evidence quality low; weak recommendation).

3. Fluorescence cholangiography is a feasible alternative to contrast-dye cholangiography yet larger studies need to be reviewed (evidence quality low; weak recommendation).

References

1. Flum DR, Cheadle A, Prela C, Dellinger EP, Chan L. Bile duct injury during cholecystectomy and survival in Medicare beneficiaries. JAMA. 2003;289(13):1639–44.
2. Nuzzo G, Giuliante F, Giovannini I, Ardito F, D'Acapito F, Vellone M, Murazio M, Capelli G. Bile duct injury during laparoscopic cholecystectomy: results of an Italian national survey on 56 591 cholecystectomies. Arch Surg. 2005;140(10):986–92.
3. Roslyn JJ, Binns GS, Hughes EF, Saunders-Kirkwood K, Zinner MJ, Cates JA. Open cholecystectomy. A contemporary analysis of 42,474 patients. Ann Surg. 1993;218(2):129–37.
4. Strasberg SM, Hertl M, Soper NJ. An analysis of the problem of biliary injury during laparoscopic cholecystectomy. J Am Coll Surg. 1995;180(1):101–25.
5. Avgerinos C, Kelgiorgi D, Touloumis Z, Baltatzi L, Dervenis C. One thousand laparoscopic cholecystectomies in a single surgical unit using the "critical view of safety" technique. J Gastrointest Surg. 2009;13(3):498–503.
6. Sanjay P, Fulke JL, Exon DJ. 'Critical view of safety' as an alternative to routine intraoperative cholangiography during laparoscopic cholecystectomy for acute biliary pathology. J Gastrointest Surg. 2010;14(8):1280–4.
7. Way LW, Stewart L, Gantert W, Liu K, Lee CM, Whang K, Hunter JG. Causes and prevention of laparoscopic bile duct injuries: analysis of 252 cases from a human factors and cognitive psychology perspective. Ann Surg. 2003;237(4):460–9.
8. Massarweh NN, Devlin A, Elrod JA, Symons RG, Flum DR. Surgeon knowledge, behavior, and opinions regarding intraoperative cholangiography. J Am Coll Surg. 2008;207(6):821–30.
9. Soper NJ, Dunnegan DL. Routine versus selective intra-operative cholangiography during laparoscopic cholecystectomy. World J Surg. 1992;16(6):1133–40.
10. Nies C, Bauknecht F, Groth C, Clerici T, Bartsch D, Lange J, Rothmund M. Intraoperative cholangiography as a routine method? A prospective, controlled, randomized study. Chirurg. 1997;68(9):892–7.
11. Khan OA, Balaji S, Branagan G, Bennett DH, Davies N. Randomized clinical trial of routine on-table cholangiography during laparoscopic cholecystectomy. Br J Surg. 2011;98(3):362–7.
12. Amott D, Webb A, Tulloh B. Prospective comparison of routine and selective operative cholangiography. ANZ J Surg. 2005;75(6):378–82.
13. Flum DR, Flowers C, Veenstra DL. A cost-effectiveness analysis of intraoperative cholangiography in the prevention of bile duct injury during laparoscopic cholecystectomy. J Am Coll Surg. 2003;196(3):385–93.
14. Giger U, Ouaissi M, Schmitz SF, Krähenbühl S, Krähenbühl L. Bile duct injury and use of cholangiography during laparoscopic cholecystectomy. Br J Surg. 2011;98(3):391–6.
15. Törnqvist B, Strömberg C, Persson G, Nilsson M. Effect of intended intraoperative cholangiography and early detection of bile duct injury on survival after cholecystectomy: population based cohort study. BMJ. 2012;345:e6457.
16. Ragulin-Coyne E, Witkowski ER, Chau Z, Ng SC, Santry HP, Callery MP, Shah SA, Tseng JF. Is routine intraoperative cholangiogram necessary in the twenty-first century? A national view. J Gastrointest Surg. 2013;17(3):434–42.
17. Buddingh KT, Weersma RK, Savenije RA, van Dam GM, Nieuwenhuijs VB. Lower rate of major bile duct injury and increased intraoperative management of common bile duct stones

after implementation of routine intraoperative cholangiography. J Am Coll Surg. 2011;213(2):267–74.
18. Nickkholgh A, Soltaniyekta S, Kalbasi H. Routine versus selective intraoperative cholangiography during laparoscopic cholecystectomy: a survey of 2,130 patients undergoing laparoscopic cholecystectomy. Surg Endosc. 2006;20(6):868–74.
19. Brown LM, Rogers SJ, Cello JP, Brasel KJ, Inadomi JM. Cost-effective treatment of patients with symptomatic cholelithiasis and possible common bile duct stones. J Am Coll Surg. 2011;212(6):1049–60.
20. Livingston EH, Miller JA, Coan B, Rege RV. Costs and utilization of intraoperative cholangiography. J Gastrointest Surg. 2007;11(9):1162–7.
21. Schols RM, Bouvy ND, Masclee AA, van Dam RM, Dejong CH, Stassen LP. Fluorescence cholangiography during laparoscopic cholecystectomy: a feasibility study on early biliary tract delineation. Surg Endosc. 2013;27(5):1530–6.
22. Osayi SN, Wendling MR, Drosdeck JM, Chaudhry UI, Perry KA, Noria SF, Mikami DJ, Needleman BJ, Muscarella 2nd P, Abdel-Rasoul M, Renton DB, Melvin WS, Hazey JW, Narula VK. Near-infrared fluorescent cholangiography facilitates identification of biliary anatomy during laparoscopic cholecystectomy. Surg Endosc. 2015;29(2):368–752.
23. Dip FD, Asbun D, Rosales-Velderrain A, Lo Menzo E, Simpfendorfer CH, Szomstein S, Rosenthal RJ. Cost analysis and effectiveness comparing the routine use of intraoperative fluorescent cholangiography with fluoroscopic cholangiogram in patients undergoing laparoscopic cholecystectomy. Surg Endosc. 2014;28(6):1838–43.
24. Prevot F, Rebibo L, Cosse C, Browet F, Sabbagh C, Regimbeau JM. Effectiveness of intraoperative cholangiography using indocyanine green (versus contrast fluid) for the correct assessment of extrahepatic bile ducts during day-case laparoscopic cholecystectomy. J Gastrointest Surg. 2014;18(8):1462–8.

Chapter 28
When Is Bile Duct Resection Indicated for Biliary Strictures in Primary Sclerosing Cholangitis?

J. Camilo Barreto and J. Michael Millis

Abstract Primary sclerosing cholangitis (PSC) has a variable clinical course, but often becomes a progressive disease that leads to chronic cholestasis, cirrhosis and liver failure. In addition, PSC is the most common risk factor for cholangiocarcinoma in western countries. The etiology is unclear, and as a result there are no specific medical therapies that change long-term outcomes. Liver transplantation offers the only potentially curative therapy but it is usually reserved for patients with advanced stage or cirrhosis. Earlier stages require alternative invasive treatment modalities to manage symptoms and address dominant strictures, which can be benign or malignant. The distinction between these may be extremely challenging, and has an influence on the treatment options, which include endoscopic dilatation, stenting, or surgery, either biliary bypass or extrahepatic bile duct resection. Endoscopic therapy has less morbidity, but surgical treatment has the advantage of not leaving potentially malignant or dysplastic strictures in place and may be associated with longer survival. When cholangiocarcinoma develops, it tends to appear at an advanced stage and prognosis is poor.

Keywords Primary sclerosing cholangitis • Stricture • Cancer • Endoscopy • Resection • Morbidity

---

J.C. Barreto
Section of General Surgery, University of Chicago Medicine, Chicago, IL, USA

J.M. Millis (✉)
Department of Surgery, University of Chicago Hospitals,
5841 S. Maryland Ave, MC 5027, Chicago, IL 60637, USA
e-mail: mmillis@surgery.bsd.uchicago.edu

J.M. Millis, J.B. Matthews (eds.), *Difficult Decisions in Hepatobiliary and Pancreatic Surgery*, Difficult Decisions in Surgery: An Evidence-Based Approach, DOI 10.1007/978-3-319-27365-5_28

Introduction

Primary sclerosing cholangitis is a chronic disease characterized by multifocal bile duct strictures secondary to idiopathic inflammation and fibrosis of intra and extra-hepatic bile ducts. It is associated in 75 % of patients with concomitant inflammatory bowel disease. PSC has a variable course, and some patients may be asymptomatic, whereas progressive inflammation and obliteration leads to secondary biliary cirrhosis and liver failure in 50 % of cases, with a median survival of 11–18 years [1]. Patients with cirrhosis should be considered for transplant upfront, since their surgical mortality is higher and have poorer survival with non-transplant surgical therapy [2]. The role of transplantation in PSC is well established and out of the scope of this chapter.

For non-cirrhotic patients at earlier stages, treatment options are variable and more controversial. Knowledge of the etiology of PSC is still very limited, likely involving genetic components in a setting of persistent inflammation. Currently, there is no effective targeted therapy, and available medical treatment options (immunosuppressive agents and ursodeoxycholic acid) have limited value and have not proven to halt disease progression. In the absence of specific treatment, a significant aspect in the care of patients with PSC involves managing biliary strictures for symptomatic relief. Dominant strictures happen in 10–20 % of patients [3, 4]. They have been defined in cholangiography as strictures of the common bile duct with a diameter ≤1.5 mm and/or strictures of a hepatic duct ≤1 mm within 2 cm of the hepatic duct bifurcation [5]. Cholangiocarcinoma is a complication occurring in 10–20 % of patients. This should be factored in when deciding what is the best approach for biliary strictures, since at the time of presentation, up to 25 % of strictures are malignant [6]. In previous decades, before the advent of advanced endoscopic interventions and the wider availability of liver transplantation, surgical resection or bypass was the mainstay therapy for dominant strictures. In more recent times, due to its lower complication rate, endoscopic treatment has generally been the first line of treatment, in the form of sphincterotomy followed by stricture dilatation with or without stent placement. The low incidence of PSC makes it difficult to obtain high quality evidence, and there are no randomized trials to identify the best approaches for operative management of strictures.

Search Strategy

A literature search of English language publications was used to identify data on endoscopic and surgical management of dominant biliary strictures, outcomes in terms of complications and survival, as well as risk of cholangiocarcinoma. Data was assessed and processed according to the categories in Table 28.1.

Table 28.1 PICO table for surgery or endoscopic therapy for PSC

P (patients)	I (intervention)	C (comparator group)	O (outcomes measured)
Patients with primary sclerosing cholangitis and dominant stricture	Resection	Endoscopic treatment	Survival
			Cancer risk
			Morbidity

Endoscopic Therapy

Endoscopic therapies have the advantages of lower complication rates, and not altering the biliary anatomy in case patients undergo a liver transplant. Endoscopic dilatation of PSC patients with a dominant stricture can achieve clinical and biochemical response in 80 % of cases [3, 5, 7, 8]. Most patients will require more than one session. Baluyut et al. also showed an increase in survival at 5 years in 63 patients with endoscopic therapy, which primarily consisted of repeated balloon dilatations (83 % vs. 65 % by using the Mayo Survival Model). They concluded that endoscopic attempts to maintain biliary patency are associated with improved survival [8]. Stiehl et al. reported their experience with 106 patients [5], 52 of which developed dominant strictures while also receiving ursodeoxycholic acid. They were managed endoscopically with repeated balloon dilatations, and five patients had a temporary biliary stent. The actuarial survival free of liver transplant at 5 years was 94 %, compared to the Mayo multicenter survival model of 77 %. Another prospective observational study from Germany of 96 patients undergoing endoscopic dilatation showed an actuarial survival free of liver transplant of 68 % at 5 years and 44 % at 10 years when patients had a serum bilirubin greater than 2 mg/dL. With serum bilirubin levels less than 2 mg/dL, the survival was 83 % at 5 years and 56 % at 10 years [9]. A National Institutes of Health panel concluded that balloon dilatation of high grade strictures is beneficial [10].

Stents offer the theoretical advantage of improving patency rates after dilatation. However, some studies have reported an association with increased risk of cholangitis [3, 5, 7]. The difference in stenting protocols and small number of subjects complicate the interpretation of outcomes after stent therapy. A retrospective study [11] compared patients undergoing balloon dilatation alone with a group treated with balloon dilatation plus stenting. Stent placement did not provide additional benefits after dilatation and increased the infectious complication rate.

Biliary Resection and Biliary Bypass

Before liver transplant became a viable option, surgical treatment was the mainstay of treatment for PSC. Non-transplant surgical therapies for patients with PSC are extrahepatic biliary resection or bypass with bilioenteric anastomosis. The disadvantage of the latter is leaving in situ the strictured area at risk of malignant transformation. Resection entails excision of the entire extrahepatic biliary duct including the confluence, since it is frequently involved with a dominant stricture. This is followed by bilateral hepaticojejunostomies and some authors recommend transhepatic stenting for 1 year [12]. Pitt et al. have reported outcomes with different variants of bypass surgery in 22 patients, with an overall survival of 82 % with a median follow-up of 5 years [13]. Johns Hopkins has reported one of the largest experiences with patients undergoing non-transplant surgical therapy. Extrahepatic biliary resection was performed with long term transhepatic stenting. In those patients managed with resection surgical, 50 non-cirrhotic patients had a 5-year survival of 85 % [14]. Operative mortality in cirrhotic patients was 20 %, compared to 2.5 % in non-cirrhotics. The complication rate was 32 %, most commonly from cholangitis. None of the resected patients developed cholangiocarcinoma during a median follow-up of 62 months. Among 35 patients who underwent endoscopic therapy (dilatation with or without stenting), overall 5-year survival was 58 %. Although survival was lower than the 85 % survival achieved with resection, the complication rate associated to endoscopic therapy was lower (14 %, mostly mild pancreatitis). Three patients of 35 (8 %) in the endoscopic group developed cholangiocarcinoma [14]. One of the arguments in favor of endoscopic therapy as first-line treatment quotes that patients who had biliary tract surgery have increased morbidity and mortality should they need liver transplantation [15–18]. In the Johns Hopkins experience, although operative time for liver transplant was shorter in patients with no previous biliary tract surgeries, the estimated blood loss and operative mortality was not statistically different [14]. A more recent report from Johns Hopkins has confirmed the outcomes of extrahepatic bile duct resection including the confluence, with a 5 and 10-year survival of 76 % and 52 % respectively. No patients developed cholangiocarcinoma. Cirrhotic patients had a 10-year survival of only 12 %, compared to 57 % for patients who undergo liver transplant, underscoring that adequate candidate selection is key for good outcomes [19].

The other alternative in surgical therapy is bypass without resection. Pitt et al. reported a survival of 82 % at 5 years with different bypass techniques [13]. Myburgh reported a survival of 100 % in 16 non-cirrhotic patients with a median survival of 6.5 years, managed with hepaticojejunostomy without resection [20]. Another approach involves a choledochojejunostomy with a subcutaneously placed afferent limb, to allow for serial dilatations of the biliary tree [21].

Risk of Malignancy

Patients with PSC have a risk of cholangiocarcinoma of 10–20 % over their lifetime, and PSC is the most common risk factor for its occurrence in Western countries. Half of patients are diagnosed within 1 year of diagnosis of PSC [22]. When it occurs, most tumors develop at the bifurcation (70 % hilar vs. 11 % intrahepatic) [23]. Cholangiocarcinoma tends to be diagnosed at an advanced, unresectable stage.

This is, in part, due to the difficulty in differentiating benign from malignant lesions, and the fact that early strictures are often asymptomatic [24]. Several clinical findings seem to be predictive of malignant transformation, such as rapid clinical and biochemical deterioration, weight loss, marked proximal ductal dilatation [25]. Unfortunately, both screening for the disease and diagnostic confirmation after cancer has appeared can be challenging. Cholangiography alone may not be able to distinguish between benign and malignant strictures. CA 19-9 elevation is non-specific, as there is considerable overlap with elevation secondary to benign strictures. As a consequence, it lacks enough sensitivity and positive predictive values for the diagnosis of cholangiocarcinoma in patients with PSC [2]. In general, endoscopic ultrasound (EUS) guided FNA in suspected cholangiocarcinoma has specificity, sensitivity and positive predictive value of 86, 100 and 100 % respectively [26]. However, these results come from patients without PSC. Tissue-diagnosis is challenging because tumors tend to be highly desmoplastic, with small aggregations of cancer cells in a rich fibrous tissue, and biliary cytology studies are positive in only 30 % of patients. Other modalities, like fluorescent in situ hybridization (FISH) have been used to improve sensitivity, but it still remains low at 34 % [27].

Some reports have suggested that there is an increased risk for cholangiocarcinoma when patients with dominant strictures are treated without resection [14, 28]. In the Johns Hopkins experience, none of the patients that underwent extrahepatic biliary resection later developed cholangiocarcinoma [14], and in contrast, malignancy has been reported in most series of patients treated with endoscopic therapy. In Stiehl et al. series, 3 % were diagnosed with cholangiocarcinoma [5], and 8 % of patients in Baluyut's study developed it [8]. Proponents of endoscopic therapy have argued that the risk of cholangiocarcinoma is still low in their series and that endoscopic therapy is not a risk factor per se for cholangiocarcinoma [8, 29]. However, there is currently a lack of high quality evidence to support either hypothesis. As mentioned before, there are no randomized trials comparing outcomes of endoscopic vs. surgical treatment.

Recommendations

- Liver transplantation provides better survival in cirrhotic patients with PSC (Evidence quality high, strong recommendation).
- Non-cirrhotic patients with PSC and symptomatic, benign-appearing dominant strictures may be treated initially with endoscopic therapy given its lower morbidity, and can be managed with repeated dilatations if needed. (Evidence quality low, weak recommendation)
- Surgical therapy should be performed for non-cirrhotic patients with dominant strictures suspicious for malignancy, equivocal findings on cancer screening, or when endoscopic therapy has failed. (Evidence quality moderate, strong recommendation).

- Extrahepatic bile duct resection should be preferred to biliary bypass in appropriate surgical candidates given the underlying risk of cholangiocarcinoma in unresected bile ducts. (Evidence quality low, weak recommendation)

References

1. Koro NS, Alkaade S. Role of endoscopy in primary sclerosing cholangitis. Curr Gastroenterol Rep. 2003;15:361.
2. Aljiffry M, Renfrew PD, Walsh MJ, Laryea M, Molinari M. Analytical review of diagnosis and treatment strategies for dominant bile duct strictures in patients with primary sclerosing cholangitis. HPB (Oxf). 2011;13:79–90.
3. Van Milligen de Wit AW, Rauws EA, van Bracht J, et al. Endoscopic stent therapy for dominant extrahepatic bile duct strictures in primary sclerosing cholangitis. Gastrointest Endosc. 1996;44:293–9.
4. Olsson RG, Asztely MS. Prognostic value of cholangiography in primary sclerosing cholangitis. Eur J Gastroenterol Hepatol. 1995;7:251–4.
5. Stiehl A, Rudolph G, Kloters-Plachky P, Sauer P, Walker S, et al. Development of dominant bile duct stenoses in patients with primary sclerosing cholangitis treated with ursodeoxycholic acid: outcome after endoscopic treatment. J Hepatol. 2002;36:151–6.
6. Tischendorf JJ, Kruger M, Trautwein C, et al. Cholangioscopic characterization of dominant bile duct stenoses in patients with primary sclerosing cholangitis. Endoscopy. 2006;38:665–9.
7. Ponsloen CY, Lam K, van Milligen de Witt AW, Hulbregtse K, Tytgat GN. Four years experience with short-term stenting in primary sclerosing cholangitis. Am J Gastroenterol. 1999;94:2403–7.
8. Baluyut AR, Sherman S, Lehrman GA, Hoen H, Chalasani N. Impact of endoscopic therapy on the survival of patients with primary sclerosing cholangitis. Gastrointest Endosc. 2001;53:308–12.
9. Gotthardt DN, Rudolph G, Kloters-Plachky P, Kulaksiz H, Stiehl A. Endoscopic dilation of dominant stenoses in primary sclerosing cholangitis: outcome after long-treatment. Gastrointest Endosc. 2010;71:527–34.
10. LaRusso NF, Shneider BL, Black D, et al. Primary sclerosing cholangitis: summary of a workshop. Hepatology. 2006;44:746–64.
11. Kaya M, Petersen BT, Angulo P, et al. Balloon dilation compared to stenting of dominant strictures in primary sclerosing cholangitis. Am J Gastroenterol. 2001;96:1059–66.
12. Domanjko B, Ahrendt SA. Indications for non-transplant surgery in primary sclerosing cholangitis. HPB. 2005;7:292–7.
13. Pitt HA, Thompson HH, Tompkins RK, Longmire WP. Primary sclerosing cholangitis: results of an aggressive surgical approach. Ann Surg. 1982;196:259–68.
14. Ahrendt SA, Pitt HA, Kalloo AN, et al. Primary sclerosing cholangitis. Resect, dilate or transplant? Ann Surg. 1998;227:412–23.
15. Martin FM, Rossi RL, Nugent FW, et al. Surgical aspects of sclerosing cholangitis. Results in 178 patients. Ann Surg. 1990;212:551–6.
16. Ismail T, Angrisani L, Powell JE, et al. Primary sclerosing cholangitis: surgical options, prognostic variables and outcome. Br J Surg. 1991;78:564–7.
17. Farges O, Malassagne B, Sebaugh M, Bismuth H. Primary sclerosing cholangitis: liver transplantation or biliary surgery. Surgery. 1995;117:146–55.
18. Brandsaeter B, Friman S, Broome U, et al. Outcome following liver transplantation for primary sclerosing cholangitis in the Nordic countries. Scand J Gastroenterol. 2003;38:1776–83.

19. Pawlik TM, Olbrecht VA, Pitt HA, et al. Primary sclerosing cholangitis: role of extrahepatic biliary resection. J Am Coll Surg. 2008;206:822–32.
20. Myburgh JA. Surgical biliary drainage in primary sclerosing cholangitis. The role of the Hepp-Couinaud approach. Arch Surg. 1994;129:1057–62.
21. Hutson DG, Russell E, Levi JU, et al. Dilatation of biliary strictures through the afferent limb of a Roux-en-Y choledochojejunostomy in patients with sclerosing cholangitis. World J Surg. 2001;25:1251–3.
22. Bergquist A, Ekbom A, Olsson R, et al. Hepatic and extrahepatic malignancies in primary sclerosing cholangitis. J Hepatol. 2002;36:321–7.
23. Abu-Elmagd KM, Selby R, Iwatsuki S, et al. Cholangiocarcinoma and sclerosing cholangitis: clinical characteristics and effect on survival after transplantation. Transplant Proc. 1993;25:1124–9.
24. Lee JG, Schutz SM, England RE, Leung JW, Cotton PB. Endoscopic therapy of sclerosing cholangitis. Hepatology. 1995;21:661–7.
25. Rosen CB, Nagorney DM, Wiesner RH, Coffey RJ, LaRusso NF. Cholangiocarcinoma complicating primary sclerosing cholangitis. Ann Surg. 1991;213:21–5.
26. Eloubeidi MA, Chen VK, Jhala NC, et al. Endoscopic ultrasound-guided fine needle aspiration biopsy of suspected cholangiocarcinoma. Clin Gastroenterol Hepatol. 2004;2:209–13.
27. Kipp BR, Stadheim LM, Halling SA, et al. A comparison of routine cytology and fluorescence in situ hybridization for the detection of malignant bile duct strictures. Am J Gastroenterol. 2004;99:1675–81.
28. Linder S, Soderlund C. Endoscopic therapy in primary sclerosing cholangitis: outcome of treatment and risk of cancer. Hepatogastroenterology. 2001;48:387–92.
29. Chalasani N, Baluyut A, Ismail A, et al. Cholangiocarcinoma in patients with primary sclerosing cholangitis: a multicenter case-control study. Hepatology. 2000;31:7–11.

Chapter 29
Assessment of Bile Duct Tumors: Endoscopic vs Radiographic

Irving Waxman and Mariano Gonzalez-Haba

Abstract Cholangiocarcinoma (CCA) is the second most common primary liver tumor and it's associated with a poor prognosis. They diagnosis of CCA can be challenging because of its paucicellular nature, anatomic location, and silent clinical character. Cross sectional radiologic studies (MRI/MRCP and multidetector CT scan) are critical for diagnosis and staging CCA but their sensibility is yet improvable and they don't allow tissue acquisition. ERCP has been for years the modality of choice for evaluating and sampling biliary strictures for malignancy. New endoscopic techniques like EUS and cholangioscopy and advances in imaging technologies and cytology processing have the potential of significantly improve the preoperative diagnostic accuracy of this malignancy.

Keywords Cholangiocarcinoma • Diagnosis • Radiologic • MRI/MRCP • CT • Endoscopy • Endoscopic ultrasound • ERCP

Introduction

Cholangiocarcinoma is the second most common primary liver tumor, after hepatocellular carcinoma (HCC), and it can arise anywhere in the biliary tree from the intrahepatic ducts to the distal common bile duct at the ampulla of Vater. On the basis of its location, cholangiocarcinoma can be divided into intrahepatic and extrahepatic tumors. Extrahepatic cholangiocarcinoma can be further subdivided into perihilar (pCCA) and distal extrahepatic cholangiocarcinoma (dCCA). 20 % of all CCA are intrahepatic, according to published series, whereas 50–60 % are perihilar, up to 20 % are distal extrahepatic tumors and 5 % of tumors are multifocal [1]. Given the differences in their frequency, diagnosis and management, in this chapter

I. Waxman (✉) • M. Gonzalez-Haba
Center for Endoscopic Research and Therapeutics (CERT), Center for Care and Discovery, The University of Chicago Medicine and Biological Sciences,
5700 S Maryland Ave. MC 8043, Chicago, IL 60637, USA
e-mail: iwaxman@medicine.bsd.uchicago.edu

J.M. Millis, J.B. Matthews (eds.), *Difficult Decisions in Hepatobiliary and Pancreatic Surgery*, Difficult Decisions in Surgery: An Evidence-Based Approach, DOI 10.1007/978-3-319-27365-5_29

Table 29.1 PICO table for endoscopic versus radiologic diagnosis of bile duct tumors

P (patients)	I (intervention)	C (comparator group)	O (outcomes measured)
Patients with suspected bile duct tumors	Endoscopic diagnosis	Radiologic diagnosis	Yield of preoperative diagnosis
	Endoscopic/radiologic diagnosis	Post-surgical diagnosis	

we will comment separately intrahepatic, perihilar and distal extrahepatic cholangiocarcinomas.

They diagnosis of CCA can be challenging because of its paucicellular nature, anatomic location, and silent clinical character. A multidisciplinary approach that involving radiographic, endoscopic, and biochemical analysis is often required.

Endoscopic retrograde cholangiography (ERC) with brush cytology and intraductal biopsy is the standard approach for diagnosis providing high specificity, but has proven limited diagnostic sensitivity. In this setting, Endoscopic ultrasound (EUS) is increasingly used for CCA diagnosis and staging. Innovative imaging technologies such as Intraductal Ultrasound (IDUS), cholangioscopy or advanced cytologic techniques can improve the diagnostic yield of endoscopic procedures. Patients with primary sclerosis cholangitis (PSC) deserve a special mention in this chapter, as PSC is a major risk factor for developing CCA and its early diagnosis can be particularly challenging.

A literature search of English language publications on PubMed/Medline from 2000 to 2014 was performed to identify published data on endoscopic and radiologic diagnosis on cholangiocarcinoma using the PICO outline (Table 29.1). Terms used in the search were "cholangiocarcinoma" "bile duct tumors" "cholangiocarcinoma AND diagnosis" "endoscopic diagnosis AND cholangiocarcinoma" "radiologic diagnosis AND cholangiocarcinoma" "EUS AND cholangiocarcinoma" "Primary sclerosing cholangitis AND cholangiocarcinoma", "Cholangioscopy AND cholangiocarcinoma" "EUS AND biliary strictures," "Endoscopic diagnosis AND biliary strictures" 22 retrospective studies, 20 prospective studies, 5 guidelines, 3 systematic reviews, and 11 review articles were used. The data was classified using the GRADE system.

Intrahepatic Cholangiocarcinoma (iCCA)

iCCA is often asymptomatic in early stages and can be an incidental finding on cross-sectional imaging performed for other reasons. At more advanced stages, presentation can vary from constitutional syndrome to abdominal pain, jaundice, hepatomegaly, or a palpable abdominal mass. The diagnosis of intrahepatic cholangiocarcinoma is basically radiologic, both MRI and CT scan can provide accurate evaluation of tumor size and detection of satellite lesions. However, CT may be better for assessment of vascular encasement, identification of extrahepatic metastasis and prediction of resectability [2]. Although imaging features of iCCA are often suggestive of the diagnosis, these criteria are insensitive for the diagnosis of iCCA vs HCC in the presence of cirrhosis or from differentiating metastatic adenocarcinoma and iCCA [3]. Pathological diagnosis is currently still required for a definitive diagnosis of iCCA, especially in those patients who are poor candidates for surgical resection [1, 4, 5].

Perihilar Cholangiocarcinoma (pCCA)

Patients with pCCA often present with symptoms of biliary obstruction and less commonly cholangitis. Trans-abdominal ultrasonography can accurately localize the level of obstruction as first approach, but it has a very low yield for detection of strictures or masses [6]. Cross sectional evaluation is critical for detection and evaluation of tumor extent. With the recent technical advances, overall accuracy of CT for determining resectability of CCA is in the range of 60–85 % [2, 6–8]. MRI combined with MRCP is a noninvasive technique is emerging as an excellent tool for evaluating ductal extension and for the preoperative assessment of biliary tract cancers with accuracy up to 95 % [9–11]. However, MRI/ MRCP do not allow any interventions to be performed, such as stent insertion, or tissue acquisition. If at all possible, MRCP should be performed before biliary drainage since evaluation for biliary pathology is more difficult if the biliary tree is collapsed from a preceding biliary drainage [12]. The role of PET scan in the diagnostic algorithm of cholangiocarcinoma is evolving, although its utility for determining resectability of the primary tumor is not superior to MRI/MRCP [13] but it might be a useful tool for identifying occult metastases in patient's a priori surgical candidates.

In an attempt to avoid unnecessary surgeries, staging laparoscopy was widely performed to exclude local metastatic disease in suspected resectable patients; due to improved imaging techniques its role will be probably limited in the upcoming years [14].

Ca 19-9 is an established serum marker for cholangiocarcinoma, although its sensitivity for the diagnosis is limited, in patients without PSC, serum Ca 19-9 values above 100 U/mL have a sensitivity of 53 % and specificity of 75–90 % for the diagnosis of CC [15]. CA 19-9 concentrations >1000 U/mL can predict advanced disease and when elevated at diagnosis can be useful for follow up [16]. Importantly, CA19-9 elevation frequently occurs in PSC and other causes of non-malignant obstructive jaundice, but persistently raised levels of CA19-9 after decompression suggest malignancy.

For years, ERCP has been the modality of choice for evaluating biliary strictures for malignancy. ERCP plays both a diagnostic and therapeutic role in the setting of CCA as it has the power to evaluate the biliary tree and sample it via brush cytology and endoscopic biopsy, but it can also provide means for biliary drainage or ablative therapy, such as PDT or RFA. Brushings for cytology and biopsy samples for histology can confirm the diagnosis of CCA, however, the sensitivity of these tests are limited, ranging from 18 to 60 % [17–19]. This sensitivity can be raised by combining tissue-sampling methods [20–22] and with the addition of newer diagnostic tests, like fluorescence in situ hybridization (FISH) and digital image analysis or flow cytometry [23–25].

In this setting, EUS is becoming and emerging tool for the diagnosis and staging of CCA, [16, 19, 26, 27]. In a prospective evaluation of EUS-FNA on 44 patients with hilar strictures suspicious of HC diagnosed by CT and/or ERCP, but with inconclusive tissue, accuracy, sensitivity, and specificity were 91 %, 89 %, and 100 %, respectively. Furthermore, EUS-FNA changed preplanned surgical approach in 27/44 patients [16]. According to the largest single center recent study, Mohamadnejad et al. reported a sensitivity of EUS-FNA for diagnosing CCA of 73 %, significantly higher in distal than in proximal CCA (81 % vs. 59 %, respectively) [26]. EUS has also shown excellent specificity for malignant biliary strictures but variable results in sensitivity in a recent metaanalysis and prospective studies [28–31]. EUS can also have a great clinical value for the nodal staging in extrahepatic CCA, as locoregional nodal metastasis will preclude liver transplantation and distant nodal involvement can also contraindicate attempting a curative resection. In a study performed by Gleeson et al. on 47 patients with CCA and potential liver transplantation, preoperative EUS-FNA of regional lymph nodes was performed in addition to their standard approach of exploratory laparotomy. EUS identified lymph nodes in all patients and 8/47 patients had positive lymphadenopathy confirmed as malignant by pathologic examination. Based on these results, 17 % of their patients were spared the cost and morbidity of an unnecessary laparotomy. There were no morphologic criteria or echo features to correlate with nodal malignancy. Furthermore, the EUS finding of absent regional lymph-node metastases was confirmed in 20 of 22 by a subsequent exploratory staging laparotomy. Interestingly, seven of these eight patients had PSC [32].

The possibility of tumor seeding during EUS-FNA in patients with suspected extrahepatic CCA is a concern; especially for proximal bile duct lesions. It was reported in a study on 191 patients with locally unresectable enrolled for neoadjuvant chemoradiotherapy followed by LT protocol, a total of 16 underwent transperitoneal FNA biopsy of the primary tumor (13 percutaneous and 3 EUS guided) [33]. It is important to note that percutaneous needle aspiration may carry a greater risk of tumor seeding when compared to EUS-FNA [34]. Although these results have not been reproduced in other studies [35] and until more data are available, tumor seeding during EUS-FNA should be considered before performing a biopsy of a potentially resectable proximal CCA.

Distal Cholangiocarcinoma

Distal biliary strictures frequently present a challenge in terms of diagnosis, which require a multidisciplinary approach. Often carcinomas arising within the area of the major papilla of the duodenum are referred as periampullary carcinomas and include the intrapancreatic distal bile duct, the head and uncinate process of the pancreas and the duodenum. Their origins are often difficult to discern based on clinical settings and results of preoperative imaging, as well as on surgical specimens [36]. CT scan and MRI/MRCP have similar outcomes to those in proximal strictures, although MRI/MRCP can be superior to CT scan on differentiating benign vs malignant strictures [11, 36]. EUS has become the imaging test of choice in patients with distal biliary obstruction, given its relative ease of visualizing and sampling distal bile duct lesions with high sensitivity and accuracy for malignant etiology, which is more frequently associated to pancreatic cancer. In the study of Mohamadnejad, EUS-FNA allowed tissue diagnosis in distal tumors with 81 %, compared to ERCP with brush cytology had only a 27 % sensitivity [26]. Given higher incidence of pancreatic cancer compared with CCA, EUS-FNA should be performed before ERCP in all patients with suspected distal malignant biliary obstruction [37]. Combined EUS and ERCP can be performed in the same procedure with no significant impact on their separate outcomes or complications [38].

EUS might also have an important role in the diagnosis of early stage CCA. In a recent study performed on 142 non icteric patients with an elevated alkaline phosphatase level and biliary dilation, MRCP followed by EUS was highly sensitive (90 %) and specific (98 %) for the diagnosis of extrahepatic bile-duct carcinoma [39].

Primary Sclerosing Cholangitis

Primary sclerosing cholangitis (PSC) is one of the best known risk factor for developing cholangiocarcinoma, with a 10-year cumulative incidence of approximately 7–9 % [40, 41], furthermore, it is estimated that in as many as 50 % of patients with CCA associated with PSC, this one is detected at the time of diagnosis or within the first year. Dominant strictures occurs in 45–58 % of patients during follow up [42–44] and should always raise the suspicion of the presence of a cholangiocarcinoma (CCA). In patients with PSC, the distinction between a benign dominant stricture and CCA can be challenging as because both benign and malignant strictures produce similar cholangiographic findings. Patients with PSC and symptoms such as cholangitis, jaundice, pruritus, right upper quadrant pain or worsening biochemical indices should undergo endoscopic evaluation to rule out dominant strictures and for associated therapy (likely biliary sphincterotomy and balloon dilatation with or without stent placement). Before any attempt at endoscopic therapy, brush cytology and/or endoscopic biopsies should be obtained to help exclude a superimposed malignancy. According to recent meta-analysis, bile duct brushings for diagnosis of CCA in patients with PSC were 43 % and 97 % respectively, with a raise in sensitivity up to 51 % when FISH polysomy was added [45].

In patients with PSC, Ca 19-9 level of 129 units/mL as a cut-off value found a sensitivity, specificity, positive predictive value, and negative predictive value of

78 %, 98 %, 56 % and 99 %, respectively in recent study on 208 [46]. Noteworthy, in another study, more than one-third of patients with this cut-off level of CA 19-9 did not have cholangiocarcinoma after an average of 30 months of follow-up [47]. Cholangioscopy and intraductal US have also been used and are promising technologies for improving the diagnosis of CCA in PSC [48, 49]. Currently there are insufficient data to support any specific screening for CCA in PSC, but most experts suggest an imaging study plus a CA 19-9 at annual intervals [1, 50].

Novel Endoscopic Techniques

Peroral cholangioscopy is a technique for direct endoscopic visualization of the bile ducts, allowing both for targeted tissue sampling and for intraductal interventions. Cholangioscopy and visually targeted biopsies can improve the diagnostic accuracy than standard ERCP [21]. Recent improvements in cholangioscopes with the advent of single operator cholangioscopy system have led to a re-emergence of this technology [51–53]. The use of cholangioscopy with the current available technologies is limited to patients in which other diagnostic tools have been attempted because of potential adverse events and high equipment cost, as was shown in a recent study in which EUS evaluation in patients with difficult biliary stricture prevented the need, cost, and adverse events of cholangioscopy in 60 % of patients [54].

Intraductal ultrasound (IDUS) is based on the use of mini-probes (about 2 mm), which can be passed through standard endoscopes directly into the bile or pancreatic duct. IDUS can overcome EUS limitations in the proximal biliary system and surrounding vascular structures, improving its sensibility when compared to EUS [55–57]. A recent study showed accuracy rates of 92 % of IDUS for the diagnosis of CCA when compared with transpapillary biopsies (74 %) EUS (70 %) or CT scan (79 %) [29].

Confocal laser endomicroscopy (CLE) is novel an imaging technique that provides real-time in vivo microscopic tissue examination during an ongoing endoscopic procedure, it has shown improvement for accuracy in diagnosis of indeterminate pancreaticobiliary strictures in patients with and without PSC [19, 58, 59]. Optical coherence tomography (OCT) uses infrared light reflectance to produce high-resolution cross-sectional tissue images through a probe, and has shown promising results in small studies [60, 61]. These innovative techniques, with the potential of obtaining "true in vivo optical biopsies" are yet limited by their high costs, lack of standardized criteria and insufficient prospective data on clinical outcomes. Multicenter prospective trials are needed to further validate criteria and define the role of this technology compared with conventional tissue sampling techniques in the diagnostic algorithm for indeterminate biliary strictures.

Personal View

Cholangiocarcinoma is associated with a poor prognosis and can often pose a diagnostic challenge, especially in early stages due to difficulties in obtaining an adequate specimen for cytology and the need to rule out benign conditions that can mimic CCA in its early stages. Obtaining a tissue diagnosis is extremely important in certain subgroups of patients such as those who are borderline surgical candidates, PSC patients with dominant strictures or before chemotherapy and radiation therapy in patients non candidate for surgery. Cross sectional imaging like new generation CT scan or especially MRI/MRCP can provide accurate data on resectability and tumor extension but with limited sensibility and no tissue acquisition. ERCP has been for years the first line approach for biliary strictures owing to its significant diagnostic and therapeutic value when there is an additional need for intervention and specimen acquisition power, but biliary brush cytology or forceps biopsies have high specificity with limited sensitivity. These limitations on CCA diagnosis and staging have encouraged development of new technologies. Advances in diagnostic methods like DIA and FISH can have increase the diagnostic yield of brush cytology, but advantages are discrete and limited by price and local availability.

Endoscopic ultrasound (EUS) provides accurate imaging for distinguishing malignancy on indeterminate biliary obstruction, nodal staging for potentially resectable tumors and enables tissue acquisition, however the risk of tumor seeding along the needle tract after FNA has been reported. Despite a lack of prospective data supporting this complication, it should be taken into consideration, especially in patients potentially candidates for liver transplantation, when deciding on a diagnostic approach for cholangiocarcinoma.

The combination of modern cross sectional imaging and endoscopic studies, likely associating ERCP (with advanced cytology sampling) with EUS, and in experienced centers also nouvelle endoscopic techniques (such as cholangioscopy, IDUS or confocal endomicroscopy) when necessary can minimize the proportion of patients requiring diagnostic or staging surgery.

Recommendations

1. For intrahepatic cholangiocarcinoma, cross sectional imaging and tissue acquisition are required for diagnosis and staging. The role of endoscopy is limited in this setting. (Evidence quality high; strong recommendation)
2. Patients with suspected extrahepatic cholangiocarcinoma should have MRI/MRCP and CT scan as initial diagnosis for local and distant staging. (Evidence quality high; strong recommendation)

3. ERCP should be performed when tissue diagnosis and/or when biliary drainage is required. When available, advanced cytology techniques (FISH, DIA) should be added (Evidence quality moderate, strong recommendation)
4. EUS should be considered for nodal staging of extrahepatic cholangiocarcinoma.

   The risk of seeding should be considered before performing FNA in patients potentially candidates for curative surgery or biliary transplantation. (Evidence of quality low, weak recommendation)
5. EUS should be the first endoscopic modality for diagnosis, staging and tissue acquisition on distal biliary obstruction (Evidence of quality moderate, weak recommendation)
6. In indeterminate biliary obstructions, EUS and ultimately advanced endoscopic techniques (cholangioscopy, IDUS, pCLE…) should be attempted prior to surgical approach. (Evidence of quality moderate, weak recommendation)

References

1. Khan SA, et al. Guidelines for the diagnosis and treatment of cholangiocarcinoma: an update. Gut. 2012;61(12):1657–69.
2. Vilgrain V. Staging cholangiocarcinoma by imaging studies. HPB (Oxf). 2008;10(2):106–9.
3. Rimola J, et al. Cholangiocarcinoma in cirrhosis: absence of contrast washout in delayed phases by magnetic resonance imaging avoids misdiagnosis of hepatocellular carcinoma. Hepatology. 2009;50(3):791–8.
4. Bridgewater J, et al. Guidelines for the diagnosis and management of intrahepatic cholangiocarcinoma. J Hepatol. 2014;60(6):1268–89.
5. Marrero JA, Ahn J, Rajender Reddy K. ACG clinical guideline: the diagnosis and management of focal liver lesions. Am J Gastroenterol. 2014;109(9):1328–47; quiz 1348.
6. Aljiffry M, Walsh MJ, Molinari M. Advances in diagnosis, treatment and palliation of cholangiocarcinoma: 1990–2009. World J Gastroenterol. 2009;15(34):4240–62.
7. Lee HY, et al. Preoperative assessment of resectability of hepatic hilar cholangiocarcinoma: combined CT and cholangiography with revised criteria. Radiology. 2006;239(1):113–21.
8. Aloia TA, et al. High-resolution computed tomography accurately predicts resectability in hilar cholangiocarcinoma. Am J Surg. 2007;193(6):702–6.
9. Katabathina VS, et al. Adult bile duct strictures: role of MR imaging and MR cholangiopancreatography in characterization. Radiographics. 2014;34(3):565–86.
10. Kim JY, et al. Contrast-enhanced MRI combined with MR cholangiopancreatography for the evaluation of patients with biliary strictures: differentiation of malignant from benign bile duct strictures. J Magn Reson Imaging. 2007;26(2):304–12.
11. Singh A, et al. Diagnostic accuracy of MRCP as compared to ultrasound/CT in patients with obstructive jaundice. J Clin Diagn Res. 2014;8(3):103–7.
12. Masselli G, Gualdi G. Hilar cholangiocarcinoma: MRI/MRCP in staging and treatment planning. Abdom Imaging. 2008;33(4):444–51.
13. Kim JY, et al. Clinical role of 18F-FDG PET-CT in suspected and potentially operable cholangiocarcinoma: a prospective study compared with conventional imaging. Am J Gastroenterol. 2008;103(5):1145–51.
14. Ruys AT, et al. Staging laparoscopy for hilar cholangiocarcinoma: is it still worthwhile? Ann Surg Oncol. 2011;18(9):2647–53.

15. Patel AH, et al. The utility of CA 19-9 in the diagnoses of cholangiocarcinoma in patients without primary sclerosing cholangitis. Am J Gastroenterol. 2000;95(1):204–7.
16. Fritscher-Ravens A, et al. EUS-guided fine-needle aspiration of suspected hilar cholangiocarcinoma in potentially operable patients with negative brush cytology. Am J Gastroenterol. 2004;99(1):45–51.
17. De Bellis M, et al. Tissue sampling at ERCP in suspected malignant biliary strictures (part 1). Gastrointest Endosc. 2002;56(4):552–61.
18. Fogel EL, et al. Effectiveness of a new long cytology brush in the evaluation of malignant biliary obstruction: a prospective study. Gastrointest Endosc. 2006;63(1):71–7.
19. Rosch T, et al. ERCP or EUS for tissue diagnosis of biliary strictures? A prospective comparative study. Gastrointest Endosc. 2004;60(3):390–6.
20. de Bellis M, et al. Influence of stricture dilation and repeat brushing on the cancer detection rate of brush cytology in the evaluation of malignant biliary obstruction. Gastrointest Endosc. 2003;58(2):176–82.
21. Brugge WR, et al. Techniques for cytologic sampling of pancreatic and bile duct lesions: the Papanicolaou Society of Cytopathology Guidelines. Cytojournal. 2014;11 Suppl 1:2.
22. Curcio G, et al. Intraductal aspiration: a promising new tissue-sampling technique for the diagnosis of suspected malignant biliary strictures. Gastrointest Endosc. 2012;75(4):798–804.
23. Baron TH, et al. A prospective comparison of digital image analysis and routine cytology for the identification of malignancy in biliary tract strictures. Clin Gastroenterol Hepatol. 2004;2(3):214–9.
24. Levy MJ, et al. Prospective evaluation of advanced molecular markers and imaging techniques in patients with indeterminate bile duct strictures. Am J Gastroenterol. 2008;103(5):1263–73.
25. Smoczynski M, et al. Routine brush cytology and fluorescence in situ hybridization for assessment of pancreatobiliary strictures. Gastrointest Endosc. 2012;75(1):65–73.
26. Mohamadnejad M, et al. Role of EUS for preoperative evaluation of cholangiocarcinoma: a large single-center experience. Gastrointest Endosc. 2011;73(1):71–8.
27. Ross WA, et al. Combined EUS with FNA and ERCP for the evaluation of patients with obstructive jaundice from presumed pancreatic malignancy. Gastrointest Endosc. 2008;68(3):461–6.
28. Garrow D, et al. Endoscopic ultrasound: a meta-analysis of test performance in suspected biliary obstruction. Clin Gastroenterol Hepatol. 2007;5(5):616–23.
29. Heinzow HS, et al. Comparative analysis of ERCP, IDUS, EUS and CT in predicting malignant bile duct strictures. World J Gastroenterol. 2014;20(30):10495–503.
30. DeWitt J, et al. EUS-guided FNA of proximal biliary strictures after negative ERCP brush cytology results. Gastrointest Endosc. 2006;64(3):325–33.
31. Byrne MF, et al. Yield of endoscopic ultrasound-guided fine-needle aspiration of bile duct lesions. Endoscopy. 2004;36(8):715–9.
32. Gleeson FC, et al. EUS-guided FNA of regional lymph nodes in patients with unresectable hilar cholangiocarcinoma. Gastrointest Endosc. 2008;67(3):438–43.
33. Heimbach JK, et al. Trans-peritoneal fine needle aspiration biopsy of hilar cholangiocarcinoma is associated with disease dissemination. HPB (Oxford). 2011;13(5):356–60.
34. Micames C, et al. Lower frequency of peritoneal carcinomatosis in patients with pancreatic cancer diagnosed by EUS-guided FNA vs. percutaneous FNA. Gastrointest Endosc. 2003;58(5):690–5.
35. Ikezawa K, et al. Risk of peritoneal carcinomatosis by endoscopic ultrasound-guided fine needle aspiration for pancreatic cancer. J Gastroenterol. 2013;48(8):966–72.
36. Kim JH, et al. Differential diagnosis of periampullary carcinomas at MR imaging. Radiographics. 2002;22(6):1335–52.
37. Weilert F, et al. EUS-FNA is superior to ERCP-based tissue sampling in suspected malignant biliary obstruction: results of a prospective, single-blind, comparative study. Gastrointest Endosc. 2014;80(1):97–104.

38. Aslanian HR, et al. Endoscopic ultrasound and endoscopic retrograde cholangiopancreatography for obstructing pancreas head masses: combined or separate procedures? J Clin Gastroenterol. 2011;45(8):711–3.
39. Sai JK, et al. Early detection of extrahepatic bile-duct carcinomas in the nonicteric stage by using MRCP followed by EUS. Gastrointest Endosc. 2009;70(1):29–36.
40. Chalasani N, et al. Cholangiocarcinoma in patients with primary sclerosing cholangitis: a multicenter case-control study. Hepatology. 2000;31(1):7–11.
41. Burak K, et al. Incidence and risk factors for cholangiocarcinoma in primary sclerosing cholangitis. Am J Gastroenterol. 2004;99(3):523–6.
42. Chapman MH, et al. Cholangiocarcinoma and dominant strictures in patients with primary sclerosing cholangitis: a 25-year single-centre experience. Eur J Gastroenterol Hepatol. 2012;24(9):1051–8.
43. Bjornsson E, et al. Dominant strictures in patients with primary sclerosing cholangitis. Am J Gastroenterol. 2004;99(3):502–8.
44. Stiehl A, et al. Development of dominant bile duct stenoses in patients with primary sclerosing cholangitis treated with ursodeoxycholic acid: outcome after endoscopic treatment. J Hepatol. 2002;36(2):151–6.
45. Navaneethan U, et al. Fluorescence in situ hybridization for diagnosis of cholangiocarcinoma in primary sclerosing cholangitis: a systematic review and meta-analysis. Gastrointest Endosc. 2014;79(6):943–50.e3.
46. Levy C, et al. The value of serum CA 19-9 in predicting cholangiocarcinomas in patients with primary sclerosing cholangitis. Dig Dis Sci. 2005;50(9):1734–40.
47. Sinakos E, et al. Many patients with primary sclerosing cholangitis and increased serum levels of carbohydrate antigen 19-9 do not have cholangiocarcinoma. Clin Gastroenterol Hepatol. 2011;9(5):434–9.e1.
48. Rey JW, et al. Efficacy of SpyGlass(TM)-directed biopsy compared to brush cytology in obtaining adequate tissue for diagnosis in patients with biliary strictures. World J Gastrointest Endosc. 2014;6(4):137–43.
49. Tischendorf JJ, et al. Cholangioscopic characterization of dominant bile duct stenoses in patients with primary sclerosing cholangitis. Endoscopy. 2006;38(7):665–9.
50. EASL. Clinical practice guidelines: management of cholestatic liver diseases. J Hepatol. 2009;51(2):237–67.
51. Keane MG, Marlow NJ, Pereira SP. Novel endoscopic approaches in the diagnosis and management of biliary strictures. F1000Prime Rep. 2013;5:38.
52. Osanai M, et al. Peroral video cholangioscopy to evaluate indeterminate bile duct lesions and preoperative mucosal cancerous extension: a prospective multicenter study. Endoscopy. 2013;45(8):635–42.
53. Ramchandani M, et al. Role of single-operator peroral cholangioscopy in the diagnosis of indeterminate biliary lesions: a single-center, prospective study. Gastrointest Endosc. 2011;74(3):511–9.
54. Nguyen NQ, Schoeman MN, Ruszkiewicz A. Clinical utility of EUS before cholangioscopy in the evaluation of difficult biliary strictures. Gastrointest Endosc. 2013;78(6):868–74.
55. Menzel J, et al. Preoperative diagnosis of bile duct strictures – comparison of intraductal ultrasonography with conventional endosonography. Scand J Gastroenterol. 2000;35(1):77–82.
56. Krishna NB, et al. Intraductal US in evaluation of biliary strictures without a mass lesion on CT scan or magnetic resonance imaging: significance of focal wall thickening and extrinsic compression at the stricture site. Gastrointest Endosc. 2007;66(1):90–6.
57. Stavropoulos S, et al. Intraductal ultrasound for the evaluation of patients with biliary strictures and no abdominal mass on computed tomography. Endoscopy. 2005;37(8):715–21.
58. Heif M, Yen RD, Shah RJ. ERCP with probe-based confocal laser endomicroscopy for the evaluation of dominant biliary stenoses in primary sclerosing cholangitis patients. Dig Dis Sci. 2013;58(7):2068–74.

59. Gabbert C, et al. Advanced techniques for endoscopic biliary imaging: cholangioscopy, endoscopic ultrasonography, confocal, and beyond. Gastrointest Endosc Clin N Am. 2013;23(3):625–46.
60. Arvanitakis M, et al. Intraductal optical coherence tomography during endoscopic retrograde cholangiopancreatography for investigation of biliary strictures. Endoscopy. 2009;41(8):696–701.
61. Kirtane TS, Wagh MS. Endoscopic optical coherence tomography (OCT): advances in gastrointestinal imaging. Gastroenterol Res Pract. 2014;2014:376367.

Chapter 30
Management of Significant Hemobilia: Hepatic Artery Embolization or Stenting?

Mikin V. Patel and Jonathan M. Lorenz

Abstract Hemobilia is a rare but potentially life-threatening cause of upper gastrointestinal bleed. Most common causes include iatrogenic injury and trauma with pseudoaneurysm the most common anomaly identified. Therapeutic options include surgery, arterial embolization, or biliary stenting. Based on the etiology of hemobilia, endoscopic or percutaneous biliary covered stenting can be considered to tamponade the source of hemorrhage. However, in the majority of cases, angiography is required to identify and, ultimately, treat the source of bleeding with arterial embolization. Both arterial embolization and biliary stenting are effective, relatively safe, and cost efficient approaches to treatment of hemobilia which can be used based on the etiology of hemorrhage.

Keywords Hemobilia • Embolization • Biliary stenting

Introduction

Hemobilia is relatively rare and can be difficult to recognize but is an important differential diagnosis for obscure upper gastrointestinal hemorrhage. Hemobilia arises from communication between the biliary tract and vascular structures of the liver, hepatoduodenal ligament, extrahepatic biliary tree, gallbladder, or pancreas. As the pressure differential between the venous system and an obstructed bile tree is relatively low, hemobilia is generally arterial in origin.

Although first described by Francis Glisson in 1654 in a patient who sustained penetrating abdominal trauma during a sword duel, the vast majority of cases today are iatrogenic [1]. A review of 222 reported hemobilia cases from 1996 to 1999 by Green et al. found 147 (66 %) were iatrogenic in etiology with trauma (5 %), most

M.V. Patel • J.M. Lorenz (✉)
Department of Radiology, University of Chicago Medical Center,
5841 S. Maryland Ave. MC2026, Chicago, IL 60037, USA
e-mail: jlorenz@radiology.bsd.uchicago.edu

J.M. Millis, J.B. Matthews (eds.), *Difficult Decisions in Hepatobiliary and Pancreatic Surgery*, Difficult Decisions in Surgery: An Evidence-Based Approach, DOI 10.1007/978-3-319-27365-5_30

commonly motor vehicle accidents, gallstones (5 %), malignancy (6 %), vascular (9 %), and inflammatory etiologies (7 %) comprising the remainder [2]. Rare, isolated cases of hemobilia resulting from ascariasis, amoebiasis, and heterotopic gastric mucosa have also been reported [3–5]. The majority of these reported cases of hemobilia followed percutaneous liver biopsy with an incidence of 0.06–1 %, percutaneous cholangiography with an incidence of 0.7 %, or percutaneous biliary drainage with incidence of 2.2–2.3 % [6–11]. However reports of bleeding as a complication of endoscopic retrograde cholangiopancreatography (ERCP), particularly after sphincterotomy, are also reported with incidence of 2–9 % [12–15].

The cardinal features of hemobilia were described by Quincke in 1871 and included upper gastrointestinal hemorrhage, upper abdominal pain, and jaundice [16]. Based on clinical symptoms, hemobilia can be divided into minor hemobilia, usually treated conservatively, and significant hemobilia, which can be life-threatening. As with any hemorrhage, initial management include resuscitation, achievement of hemodynamic stability, and reversal of coagulopathies. Surgical management of hemobilia focuses on ligation of the bleeding vessel and/or excision of pseudoaneurysm with nonselective embolization of the right or left main hepatic arteries and segmental liver resection as secondary options [2, 17].

As many patients with hemobilia are acutely ill and unable to tolerate surgery, minimally invasive options for therapy are critical for stabilizing patients. Transcatheter arterial embolization (TAE) is considered the interventional treatment of choice; however covered biliary stent placement is a treatment option that can be considered and is seeing increasing use, especially in cases of post-ERCP hemorrhage. This chapter addresses arterial embolization and biliary stenting as potential surgical alternatives for treatment of hemobilia.

Search Strategy

A literature search of English language publications from 1999 to 2014 was used to identity published data on treatment of hemobilia with arterial embolization or biliary stenting using the PICO outline (Table 30.1). Databases searched were PubMed and Embase. Terms used in the search were "hemobilia," "hemobilia/embolization," "hemobilia/stent," "biliary/hemorrhage/embolization," and "biliary/hemorrhage/stent." Articles were excluded if they specifically addressed conservative treatment,

Table 30.1 PICO table for non-surgical treatment options for hemobilia

P (patients)	I (intervention)	C (comparator group)	O (outcomes measured)
Patients with significant hemobilia	Selective hepatic artery embolization	Surgical ligation	Hemobilia requiring surgical intervention, procedure related complication, LOS/return to work
Patients with significant hemobilia	Biliary covered stent placement	Angiographic embolization, surgical ligation	Need for additional intervention, time to stent removal, adverse events

endoscopic treatment other than stenting, or surgical treatment of hemobilia. Thirteen cohort studies, nine case reports, and two reviews were included in our analysis. The data was classified using the GRADE system.

Results

Transcatheter Arterial Embolization

The existing literature regards TAE as the first choice in therapy of significant hemobilia. TAE is used for aneurysms, pseudoaneurysms, arteriovenous malformations, malignancy, and hemangioma both as definitive treatment and as a bridge to surgery for unstable patients. Portal vein thrombosis is a contraindication for TAE as there is a significant risk for infarction. The embolization is performed with gelatin sponge, microcoils, polyvinyl alcohol particles, or cyanoacrylate. Reviews and retrospective studies have shown success rates of TAE to be 75–100 % [2, 17, 18] (Table 30.2). Technical failure occurs due to anomalous vascular anatomy or tortuous vessels. Rebleeding is generally a consequence of collateral vessels. Complications are generally limited to fever, abdominal pain, and elevation of transaminases but also include hepatic or gallbladder necrosis, gallbladder fibrosis, or hepatic abscess.

Most reported cases of hemobilia treated with TAE are either iatrogenic or post-traumatic and, at angiography, pseudoaneurysm is the most common anomaly found irrespective of etiology. Marynissen reported successful treatment of hemobilia with TAE in 12 patients, 6 of which occurred following liver biopsy, but 2 of which followed ERCP with sphincterotomy [19]. Of the remaining patients, 2 had hemobilia following percutaneous biliary drainage, one patient following a radio-frequency ablation, and one patient following cholecystectomy. The angiographic evaluation revealed varying causes of hemobilia, most commonly pseudoaneurysm

Table 30.2 Clinical outcomes for transcatheter arterial embolization in hemobilia

Author (year)	N	Mean age	No cases requiring surgery/failure of TAE	Study type (quality of evidence)
Marynissen (2012)	12	48	0	Retrospective cohort (low)
Murugesan (2014)	12	34	3	Retrospective cohort (low)
Cao (2013)	8	46	0	Retrospective cohort (low)
Moodley (2001)	29	22	0	Retrospective cohort (low)
Srivastava (2006)	32	NR	8	Retrospective cohort (low)
Forlee (2004)	7	27	1	Prospective cohort (low)
Koh (2013)	2	54	1	Retrospective cohort (low)
Rivera-Sanfeliz (2004)	8	53	1	Retrospective cohort (low)
Nicholson (1999)	9	53	0	Retrospective cohort (low)

NR not reported

(n = 6), but also including arteriobiliary and arterioportal fistulae. Angiographic findings of the two cases following ERCP were not specifically identified. Another series of 29 patients successfully treated with TAE, of which 23 had hemobilia related to penetrating or blunt abdominal trauma, found pseudoaneurysm in all patients and associated arterioportal fistulae in 4 patients [20].

Of the largest cohort studies, a series of 32 patients by Srivastava yielded a 75 % success rate of TAE in controlling hemobilia at 1-month followup [21]. Of note, the authors state that microcatheters were not used in this series, only 4-Fr and 5-Fr catheters. A 12 patient series by Murugesan also yielded a 75 % success rate of TAE with three failed embolizations due to inability to isolate the bleeding vessel, incomplete arterial occlusion, and misidentification of the bleeding vessel [22]. However, a number of smaller retrospective series with up to 29 patients report 100 % success of TAE and a comprehensive literature review of cases from 1996 to 1999 reports success of 80–100 % reinforcing an overall high success rate of TAE in controlling significant hemobilia [2, 18, 23–26].

Given the relatively low number of cases of hemobilia reported in the literature and sparse data, it is difficult to estimate the benefit of TAE in terms of the cost of treatment or length of stay reduction. The recovery time from TAE is likely to be considerably less than from surgery and, in a single series of 29 patients, all patients were able to return to work within 2 weeks of embolization [20].

A number of complications of hepatic arterial embolization are reported, the most common of which are fever, abdominal pain, and elevation of transaminases. Post-embolization syndrome, a consequence of ischemic liver damage indicated by transient elevation of liver enzymes is well-recognized and is seen in approximately 20–25 % of cases in most series but was as high as 75 % in a series reported by Cao, although this did resolve with conservative treatment [21, 23, 24]. Major complications related to the embolization procedure are rare but isolated cases were reported in the series reviewed. In one series, a patient who had hemobilia from trauma developed gallbladder necrosis post-embolization which was noted at time of surgery [21]. Additional reported major complications included two separate patients who developed hepatic necrosis, abscess, and sepsis [18, 25]. Overall, however morbidity and mortality is relatively low and hepatic artery embolization is considered the procedure of choice for unstable patients.

Biliary Stenting

As hemobilia typically presents as upper gastrointestinal bleeding, endoscopy is an important diagnostic step in the evaluation of hemobilia to rule out common causes of bleeding such as erosive gastritis, peptic ulcers, esophageal or gastric varices. However, endoscopy is limited in specifically identifying hemobilia because the bleeding is often intermittent and there may be biliary duct obstruction with thrombus preventing direct visualization of blood flowing from the papilla of Vater. Most series which evaluated hemobilia found that endoscopy was able to identify hemobilia in only 24–60 % of cases [19–22]. On the other hand, angiography is typically able to find a vascular anomaly in over 90 % of hemobilia cases [19, 22].

In addition to more commonly seen iatrogenic causes, ERCP with sphincterotomy often results in hemobilia, both immediately and in the delayed setting. This presents a special circumstance because the site of bleeding can typically be visualized endoscopically. First line endoscopic therapy including epinephrine injection, balloon tamponade, or thermal therapy is usually attempted. Typically, if these techniques fail patients require angiographic or surgical treatment. However, the use of covered self-expandable metallic stents (SEMSs) to tamponade the site of bleeding have also been reported.

The largest series of SEMS used to treat hemobilia included 11 patients, 10 of whom presented with delayed post-sphincterotomy, and found successful hemostasis without need for TAE or surgery in all cases [24]. Other series of 6, 5, and 2 patients, most of whom presented with immediate post-sphincterotomy bleeding, also found successful hemostasis in all cases [25–27] (Table 30.3). Theoretical complications include acute cholecystitis or cholangitis induced by obstruction of cystic or other bile ducts, however this complication has not been reported in the literature. Of the larger case series described, spontaneous stent migration was seen in 8 of 22 (36 %) of patients and in one case, rebleeding was seen [24–26]. No stricturing or proximal stent migration was noted. Additional case reports describe the use of endoscopically-placed covered SEMS to successfully treat post-ERCP hemobilia forming a series of four successful cases of hemostasis achieved by endoscopic stenting [28–31].

SEMSs can also be used to treat hemobilia of certain other etiologies such as hepatocellular carcinoma with bile duct invasion [32, 33]. In one of these cases, bleeding could not be stopped with TAE because the patient had undergone multiple prior sessions of transcatheter arterial chemoembolization. Hemobilia can also be treated with percutaneous stenting and can be the preferred option when there is a pre-existing percutaneous biliary drain. Three such reported cases describe successful treatment of portobiliary fistula with percutaneous stent-graft placement [34, 35]. Although isolated, these cases highlight applications in which biliary stent placement in hemobilia when TAE is not feasible or when percutaneous biliary access is already available.

Within the small set of reported cases of hemobilia there is an even smaller subset of cases treated by biliary stent placement. Although cost or length of stay is not directly comparable with TAE or surgery, Shah et al. have suggested that biliary

Table 30.3 Clinical outcomes for biliary covered stenting in hemobilia

Author (year)	N	Mean age	Delayed bleeding	No cases requiring embolization/surgery	Study type (quality of evidence)
Shah (2010)	5	62	2	0	Retrospective cohort (low)
Valats (2013)	6	68	1	0	Prospective cohort (low)
Itoi (2011)	11	76	10	0	Retrospective cohort (low)
Aslinia (2012)	2	42	2	0	Retrospective cohort (low)

SEMS placement for hemobilia is likely a cost-efficient alternative [26]. As ERCP is typically an early step during evaluation of hemobilia, stenting of endoscopically visible sources of bleeding may preclude the need for angiography. However, adequate data to suggest the true rates of success, complications, and cost of stent retrieval are not currently available.

Recommendations

Hemobilia is a relatively rare cause of upper gastrointestinal bleeding with a variety of etiologies and anomalies that can be identified either angiographically or endoscopically. Although there is a distinct lack of high-quality clinical trials or large cohort studies, there are a number of small case series supporting the use of arterial embolization and biliary stenting. The body of evidence supports the use of endoscopic biliary covered stent placement to tamponade the source of bleeding when the anomaly is readily identifiable and accessible such as in the case of post-sphincterotomy bleeding. Additionally, in cases where percutaneous biliary access has already been established, percutaneous biliary stent placement is also an option. However, when there is risk of biliary duct obstruction, arterial embolization may be preferred.

In the majority of reported cases, hemobilia is due to iatrogenic injury from procedure such as liver biopsy or percutaneous biliary drain or from abdominal trauma. In these situations, endoscopy has demonstrated a low yield in identifying the source of hemorrhage. Angiography can identify the vascular anomaly in over 90 % of patients and treatment with TAE is successful in 75–100 % of cases. Reported complications are rare and patient generally recover quickly. Thus, except in cases where the anomaly is easily visualized on endoscopy or accessed percutaneously, we make a weak recommendation that hemobilia be evaluated and treated with angiography and TAE.

A Personal View of the Data

Hemobilia is relatively rare but optimal treatment relies on thorough consideration of the underlying etiology and anomaly. For post-sphincterotomy bleeding, biliary stenting is likely the fastest and most cost efficient option for treatment. Additionally, in the circumstance where the patient has percutaneous biliary access in place and a portobiliary fistula can be identified, biliary stent placement can be a viable option. However, most cases of hemobilia will not be easily amenable to or may be refractory to biliary stenting. Angiography is highly sensitive in identifying the source of bleeding and embolization has a high success rate with relatively rare complications so TAE continues to be the mainstay of treatment. In either case, whether placing a biliary stent for tamponade or embolizing angiographic abnormalities, these interventional options reduce the cost of treatment and time to recovery for patients with hemobilia.

Recommendations

- For the majority of patients with hemobilia, angiography and transcatheter arterial embolization should be the mainstays of evaluation and treatment (evidence quality low; weak recommendation).
- For patients with hemobilia post-endoscopic intervention, we recommend an attempt at biliary covered stent placement at the time of endoscopy (evidence quality low; weak recommendation).
- We recommend considering percutaneous biliary covered stent placement if the patient already has percutaneous biliary access (evidence quality low; weak recommendation).

References

1. Glisson F. Anatomia hepatis. London: O. Pullein; 1654.
2. Green MH, Duell RM, Johnson CD, Jamieson NV. Haemobilia. Br J Surg. 2001;88:773–86.
3. Blumenthal DS. Ascariasis. Cecil textbook of medicine. 18th ed. Philadelphia: WB Saunders; 1988.
4. Koshy A, Khuroo MS, Suri S, Datta DV, Khanna SK. Amoebic liver abscess with hemobilia. Am J Surg. 1979;138:453–5.
5. Adam R, Fabiani B, Bismuth H. Hematobilia resulting from heterotopic stomach in the gallbladder neck. Surgery. 1989;105:564–9.
6. Yoshida J, Donahue PE, Nyhus LM. Hemobilia: review of recent experience with a worldwide problem. Am J Gastroenterol. 1987;82:448–53.
7. Pongchairerks P. Ultrasound-guided liver biopsy: accuracy, safety and sonographic findings. J Med Assoc Thai. 1993;76:597–600.
8. Piccinino F, Sagnelli E, Pasquale G, Giusti G. Complications following percutaneous liver biopsy. A multicenter retrospective study on 68276 biopsies. J Hepatol. 1986;2:165–73.
9. Monden M, Okamura J, Kobayashi N, et al. Hemobilia after percutaneous transhepatic biliary drainage. Arch Surg. 1980;115:161–4.
10. Fidelman N, Bloom AI, Kerlan RK, et al. Hepatic arterial injuries after percutaneous biliary interventions in the era of laparoscopic surgery and liver transplantation: experience with 930 patients. Radiology. 2008;247:880–6.
11. Rivera-Sanfeliz GM, Assar OS, Laberge JM, et al. Incidence of important hemobilia following transhepatic biliary drainage: left-sided versus right-sided approaches. Cardiovasc Intervent Radiol. 2004;27:137–9.
12. Muhldorfer SM, Kekos G, Hahn EG, et al. Complications of therapeutic gastrointestinal endoscopy. Endoscopy. 1992;24:276–83.
13. Masci E, Toti G, Mariani A, et al. Complications of diagnostic and therapeutic ERCP: a prospective multicenter study. Am J Gastroenterol. 2001;96:417–23.
14. Ferreira L, Baron TH. Post-sphincterotomy bleeding: who, what, when, and how. Am J Gastroenterol. 2007;102:2850–8.

15. Wilcox CM, Canakis J, Monkemuller KE, et al. Patterns of bleeding after endoscopic sphincterotomy, the subsequent risk of bleeding, and the role of epinephrine injection. Am J Gastroenterol. 2004;99:244–8.
16. Quinke H. Ein fall von aneurysma der leberarterie. Klin Wochenschr. 1871;8:349–51.
17. Chin MW, Enns R. Hemobilia. Curr Gastroenterol Rep. 2010;12:121–9.
18. Nicholson T, Travis S, Ettles D, et al. Hepatic artery angiography and embolization for hemobilia following laparoscopic cholecystectomy. Cardiovasc Intervent Radiol. 1999;22:20–4.
19. Marynissen T, Maleux G, Heye S, et al. Trancatheter arterial embolization for iatrogenic hemobilia is a safe and effective procedure: case series and review of the literature. Eur J Gastroenterol Hepatol. 2012;24:905–9.
20. Moodley J, Singh B, Lalloo S, et al. Non-operative management of haemobilia. Br J Surg. 2001;88:1073–6.
21. Srivastava DN, Sharma S, Pal S, et al. Transcatheter arterial embolization in the management of hemobilia. Abom Imaging. 2006;31:439–48.
22. Murugesan SD, Sathyanesan J, Lakshmanan A, et al. Massive hemobilia: a diagnostic and therapeutic challenge. World J Surg. 2014;38:1755–62.
23. Cao H, Liu J, Li T, et al. Interventional therapy for the treatment of severe hemobilia after percutaneous transhepatic cholangial drainage: a case series. Int Surg. 2013;98:223–8.
24. Itoi T, Yasuda I, Doi S, et al. Endoscopic hemostasis using covered metallic stent placement for uncontrolled post-endoscopic sphincterotomy bleeding. Endoscopy. 2011;43:369–72.
25. Valats JC, Funakoshi N, Bauret P, et al. Covered self-expandable biliary stents for the treatment of bleeding after ERCP. Gastrointest Endosc. 2013;78(1):183–7.
26. Shah JN, Marson F, Binmoeller KF. Temporary self-expandable metal stent placement for treatment of post-sphincterotomy bleeding. Gastrointest Endosc. 2012;72(6):1274–8.
27. Aslinia F, Hawkins L, Darwin P, et al. Temporary placement of a fully covered metal stent to tamponade bleeding from endoscopic papillary balloon dilation. Gastrointest Endosc. 2012;76(4):911–3.
28. Kawaguchi Y, Ogawa M, Maruno A, et al. A case of successful placement of a fully covered metallic stent for hemobilia secondary to hepatocellular carcinoma with bile duct invasion. Case Rep Oncol. 2012;5:682–6.
29. Layec S, D'Halluin PN, Pagenault M, et al. Massive hemobilia during extraction of a covered self-expandable metal stent in a patient with portal hypertensive biliopathy. Gastrointest Endosc. 2009;70(3):555–6.
30. Song JY, Moon JH, Choi HJ, et al. Massive hemobilia following transpapillary bile duct biopsy treated by using a covered self-expandable metal stent. Endoscopy. 2014;46:E161–2.
31. Bagla P, Erim T, Berzin TM, et al. Massive hemobilia during endoscopic retrograde cholangiopancreatography in a patient with cholangiocarcinoma: a case report. Endoscopy. 2012;44:E1.
32. Goenka MK, Harwani Y, Rai V. Fully covered self-expandable metal biliary stent for hemobilia caused by portal biliopathy. Gastrointest Endosc. 2014;80:1175.
33. Rerknimitr R, Kongkam P, Kullavanijaya P. Treatment of tumor associated hemobilia with a partially covered metallic stent. Endoscopy. 2007;39:E225.
34. Lorenz JM, Zangan SM, Leef JA, et al. Iatrogenic portobiliary fistula treated by stent-graft placement. Cardiovasc Intervent Radiol. 2010;33:421–4.
35. Peynircioglu B, Cwikiel W. Utility of stent-grafts in the treatment of porto-biliary fistula. Cardiovasc Intervent Radiol. 2006;29(6):1156–9.

Chapter 31
The Assessment of Ductal Margin in Curative-Intent Surgery for Perihilar Cholangiocarcinoma

Nobuhisa Akamatsu, Yasuhiko Sugawara, and Norihiro Kokudo

Abstract In the surgical approach for perihilar cholangiocarcinoma, one of the most important aims is to achieve a bile duct margin-negative resection because a negative resection margin is a crucial determinant of prognosis after curative-intent resection. Advances in the knowledge of perihilar anatomy and surgical techniques, including perioperative management, have made an extended hepatectomy with complete resection of the caudate lobe the recommended approach for a promising outcome after curative-intent surgery for perihilar cholangiocarcinoma. Enhanced multidetector-row computed tomography (MDCT) with three-dimensional and multiplanar reconstruction is necessary for both a precise preoperative evaluation of the tumor extent and safe and curative surgical resection, while the gold standard for preoperative assessment of the bile duct margin is cholangiography or MDCT/magnetic resonance cholangiography, depending on the surgeon's preference.

Keywords Ductal margin • Cholangiocarcinoma • Resection • Multidetector-row computed tomography • Tumor extent • Preoperative assessment

Introduction

Perihilar cholangiocarcinoma is a devastating disease, and its surgical resection is technically demanding and highly challenging for hepatobiliary surgeons. Complete surgical resection is the only way to cure this disease, leading many surgeons to adopt an aggressive approach to perihilar cholangiocarcinoma. With advancements in the knowledge and surgical techniques for this disease, curative-intent surgery for perihilar cholangiocarcinoma includes complete extrahepatic bile duct resection,

N. Akamatsu • Y. Sugawara (✉) • N. Kokudo
Hepato-Biliary-Pancreatic Surgery, and Artificial Organ and Transplantation Division, Department of Surgery, Graduate School of Medicine, University of Tokyo, 7-3-1 Hongo, Bunkyo-ku, Tokyo 113-8655, Japan
e-mail: yasusuga-tky@umin.ac.jp

J.M. Millis, J.B. Matthews (eds.), *Difficult Decisions in Hepatobiliary and Pancreatic Surgery*, Difficult Decisions in Surgery: An Evidence-Based Approach, DOI 10.1007/978-3-319-27365-5_31

locoregional lymphadenopathy, and hepatectomy. Although long-term survival after curative-intent surgery for perihilar cholangiocarcinoma has dramatically increased to a 5-year survival rate of more than 30 % along with the evolution of surgical management, the mortality rates and complication rates after this challenging operation remain high, even in high-volume centers (mortality rate is usually under 10 %, but the morbidity rate is up to 70 %) [1].

In this challenging background, surgical management for perihilar cholangiocarcinoma is associated with many controversial 'difficult decisions', including those regarding preoperative biliary drainage; preoperative portal venous embolization; and the extent of surgical resection, such as vascular resection, lymphadenectomy, and hepatectomy [2, 3]. Achieving a bile duct margin-negative resection, however, is one of the most important issues to consider in the surgical approach for perihilar cholangiocarcinoma. Meticulous evaluation of the ductal spread of the tumor is critical.

This chapter addresses the preoperative and intraoperative assessment of the ductal spread of hilar cholangiocarcinoma to achieve a negative margin (R0) in curative-intent aggressive surgery.

Search Strategy

A literature search of English - language publications from 2009 to 2014 (within the last 5 years) was used to identify published data on assessment of the ductal margin in surgery for perihilar cholangiocarcinoma using the PICO outline (Table 31.1). We searched the PubMed, Embase, Science Citation Index/Social sciences Citation Index, and Cochrane Evidence Based Medicine databases. The search terms used were "perihilar cholangiocarcinoma" or "hilar cholangiocarcinoma" AND "surgical treatment" and "diagnosis". Case reports, and studies focusing only on the surgical technique or diagnostic approach, or dealing only with selected cases or specific technique were excluded. Finally, 51 cohort studies and 34 review articles were included in our analysis. No randomized control trials were identified. The data were classified using the GRADE (Grading of Recommendations, Assessment, Development, and Evaluation) system.

Table 31.1 PICO table for assessment of the ductal margin in curative-intent surgery for perihilar cholangiocarcinoma

P (Patients)	I (Intervention)	C (Comparator group)	O (Outcomes measured)
Patients undergoing curative-intent surgery for perihilar cholangiocarcinoma	Curative-intent resection	Preoperative assessment of the tumor extent by cholangiography versus MDCT/MRC	R0 resection rate, 5-year patient survival

Abbreviations: *MDCT* multidetector-row computed tomography, *MRC* magnetic resonance cholangiography

Results

Importance of a Negative Resection Margin for Prognosis After Curative-Intent Surgery for Perihilar Cholangiocarcinoma

In most of the published studies [4–12], a negative resection margin was considered the most important determinant of a better prognosis after curative-intent resection for perihilar cholangiocarcinoma . Median overall survival time was significantly longer after a margin-negative resection than after a margin-positive resection: 24–58 months versus 12–28 months. Accordingly, surgeons have attempted to achieve a negative bile duct margin using various aggressive approaches.

Achieving a Negative Bile Duct Margin: Hepatectomy Versus Bile Duct Resection

Curative-intent surgery for perihilar cholangiocarcinoma has evolved from an extrahepatic bile duct resection to an aggressive approach, including meticulous and challenging hepatectomies. The benchmark study by Tsao and colleagues [13], comparing the Japanese (Nagoya) experience with the USA (Lahey) experience, with a liver resection rate of 89 % vs 16 %, a caudate lobectomy rate of 89 % vs 8 %, and a resectability rate of 79 % vs 25 %, respectively, promoted an aggressive approach for hilar cholangiocarcinoma worldwide. While the mortality rate was higher in Nagoya (8 % vs 4 %), the margin-negative resection and 5-year survival were significantly higher in the Nagoya group (79 % vs 28 %, and 16 % vs 7 %, respectively). Recent convincing evidence indicates that aggressive surgical resection with hepatectomy significantly improves patient survival [4–6, 10, 11, 14]; median overall survival time was 40–47 months in patients with hilar cholangiocarcinoma who underwent liver resection, while it was 15–30 months in those that underwent only bile duct resection. Type of hepatectomy also appears to be associated with margin-negative resection rates and long-term patient survival [15, 16].

Impact of Caudate Lobectomy in Hepatectomy for Hilar Cholangiocarcinoma

Caudate lobectomy in hepatectomy for perihilar cholangiocarcinoma remains controversial [17, 18]. Routine en bloc resection of the caudate lobe was initially advocated by Japanese surgeons based on an anatomic viewpoint [19]. Perihilar cholangiocarcinoma frequently invades the caudate lobe bile duct and the caudate lobe appears to be a common site for locoregional recurrence after curative-intent resection for perihilar cholangiocarcinoma. Further, extended hepatectomy, including caudate lobectomy, increases margin-negative resections. Routine caudate lobectomy for perihilar cholangiocarcinoma is currently accepted in Western institutions [7, 20, 21]. Whether caudate lobectomy improves long-term patient survival, however, is controversial, with some reports [13, 17, 18] of a positive impact on survival and others [7, 10, 21] demonstrating no correlation with patient survival.

Preoperative Assessment of Perihilar Cholangiocarcinoma

Preoperative radiologic evaluation is mandatory for accurate assessment of the tumor extent, which is integral to planning the surgical procedure. Preoperative evaluation of perihilar cholangiocarcinoma in terms of radical resection comprises a multidisciplinary approach with ultrasonography, helical-computed tomography, magnetic resonance imaging (MRI) including MR cholangiography (MRC), direct cholangiography via endoscopic retrograde cholangiography or percutaneous transhepatic biliary drainage, intraductal ultrasonography (IDUS), peroral cholangioscopy, and biopsy [22].

Among these, dynamic multidetector-row computed tomography (MDCT) is now widely used for preoperative evaluation and staging of hilar cholangiocarcinoma, as it provides not only a qualitative diagnosis and indicates the extent of the tumor, but it also shows the relationship between adjacent tissues, such as the hepatic artery, portal vein, and liver parenchyma.

In enhanced MDCT, bile duct cancer is often revealed as a focal thickening of the ductal wall with various enhancement patterns. The accuracy of the differential diagnosis of a malignant lesion from benign stenosis is reported to be over 90 %, with satisfactory accuracy in evaluating major vessel involvement and liver parenchyma invasion. Yet, lymph node metastasis remains difficult to diagnose preoperatively, even with the recent increased resolution of MDCT [23, 24]. Some authors report that MDCT is effective for evaluating longitudinal spread along the bile duct, demonstrating that the efficacy is equivalent to that of evaluation using MRC or direct cholangiography [25, 26]. Additional important information obtained from MDCT and its three-dimensional (3D) and multiplanar reconstruction for surgeons is the precise arterial/portal/venous anatomy around the hepatic hilum and hepatoduodenal ligament in relation to the tumor. MDCT and its 3D images and multiplanar reconstructions are important for preoperative planning and for navigation during the operation [27].

MRI with concurrent MRC provides 3D reconstruction of the biliary tree, and the diagnostic accuracy for evaluating perihilar cholangiocarcinoma is comparable to that of invasive cholangiography via endoscopic retrograde cholangiography or percutaneous transhepatic biliary drainage [28, 29]. MRI also facilitates evaluation of vertical tumor invasion, similar to MDCT. To exclude artifacts of biliary instrumentation and obtain precise images of ductal wall thickening and luminal stenosis/

dilatation, both MDCT and MRC are strongly recommended before decompressing the biliary tree.

Despite the evolution of MDCT and MRC described above, direct cholangiography remains the gold standard for the preoperative evaluation of ductal spread. While there are some drawbacks with the endoscopic or transhepatic approach, these procedures enable bile duct biopsy, IDUS, and choledochoscopy, all of which may enhance preoperative diagnostic accuracy.

Assessment of the Bile Duct Margin and Operative Outcome

To date, there has been no randomized controlled trial or comparative study regarding assessment of the extent of perihilar cholangiocarcinoma. Thus, we collected recent retrospective cohort studies of curative-intent surgery for perihilar cholangiocarcinoma from high-volume centers based on the following inclusion criteria; (1) published within the last 5 years, (2) included over 100 cases, (3) provided the preoperative assessment for ductal spread of the tumor, and (4) provided the R0 rate and 5-year survival rate. Finally, 12 studies comprising 2,343 cases of perihilar cholangiocarcinoma were enrolled in the present review (Table 31.2) [4–6, 10–12, 16, 17, 30–33].

Seven centers used cholangiography as the primary modality for preoperative assessment of the bile duct margin, while five centers used MRC or MDCT as the primary modality for assessing the ductal spread of perihilar cholangiocaricinoma. Intraoperative assessment with frozen sections was routinely performed in four centers. The simultaneous liver resection rate was uniformly high (median 97 %, range 75–100 %), with a median R0 rate of 75 % (range 63–89 %), and a median 5-year survival rate of 33 % (range 29–38 %). These homogeneous results represent the standardization of the surgical approach against perihilar cholangiocarcinoma within the last two decades.

When the cases were divided according to preoperative assessment of the bile duct margin, the R0 rate was 75 % (878/1169) with cholangiography and 77 % (884/1147) with MDCT or MRC, a difference that was not significant. Similarly, collection of intraoperative frozen sections did not significantly affect the R0 rate; with frozen sections, 69 % (554/799), and without frozen sections, 78 % (1208/1544).

Recommendations

In the absence of effective treatment other than surgical resection, curative-intent surgery should be planned for patients with perihilar cholangiocarcinoma. With the evolution of the knowledge of perihilar anatomy and surgical techniques, including perioperative management, extended hepatectomy with complete resection of the

Table 31.2 Studies with a large cohort reporting the results of curative-intent surgery for perihilar Cholangiocarcinoma

Author		Year	Period	Patients, n	Preoperative assessment of the ductal margin	Intraoperative frozen section	Liver resection, %	R0, %	5-year survival rate, %	Study type (quality of evidence)
Chen et al. [30]	Tongji, China	2009	2000–2007	138	Cholangiography	No	100	89	30	Retrospective cohort (low)
Lee et al. [5]	Seoul, Korea	2010	2001–2008	302	Cholangiography	Yes	89	71	33	Retrospective cohort (low)
Shimizu et al. [16]	Chiba Japan	2010	1984–2008	224	Cholangiography	No	100	74	29	Retrospective cohort (low)
Hirano et al. [31]	Hokkaido, Japan	2010	2001–2008	146	Cholangiography	No	94	87	35	Retrospective cohort (low)
Unno et al. [32]	Tohoku, Japan	2010	2001–2008	125	MDCT	Yes	100	63	35	Retrospective cohort (low)
Li et al. [12]	Tianjin, China	2011	1990–2009	215	Cholangiography	Yes	95	66	30	Retrospective cohort (low)
Cho et al. [11]	Seoul, Korea	2012	2000–2009	105	MDCT	No	75	71	34	Retrospective cohort (low)
Matsuo et al. [4]	New York, USA	2012	1991–2008	157	MRC or MDCT	Yes	82	76	32	Retrospective cohort (low)
Cheng et al. [17]	Shanghai, China	2012	2001–2010	171	MRC or MDCT	No	100	78	33	Retrospective cohort (low)
Song et al. [10]	Seoul, Korea	2012	1995–2010	230	MRC or MDCT	No	77	77	33	Retrospective cohort (low)
Nagino et al. [6]	Nagoya, Japan	2013	2001–2010	386	Cholangiography	No	99	78	38	Retrospective cohort (low)
Furusawa et al. [33]	Nagano, Japan	2013	1990–2012	144	Cholangiography	No	99	74	33	Retrospective cohort (low)

Abbreviations: *MDCT* multidetector-row computed tomography, *MRC* magnetic resonance cholangiography caudate lobe is recommended in the absence of clinical restrictions, such as liver dysfunction or apparently insufficient remnant liver. Enhanced MDCT with 3D and multiplanar reconstruction is becoming mandatory both for precise preoperative evaluation of the tumor extent and safe and curative surgical resection of perihilar cholangiocarcinoma. In contrast, direct cholangiography remains the gold standard for preoperative evaluation of the bile duct margin, while the diagnostic accuracy of MDCT or MRC seems comparable to that of direct cholangiography. Given the absence of high quality evidence, the modality for preoperative evaluation of the bile duct margin and surgical planning can be selected based on the surgeon's preference.

A Personal View of the Data

Considering that histopathologic examinations have low sensitivity, non-diagnostic cytology or biopsy results may not rule out cholangiocarcinoma in the presence of appropriate radiologic findings. Further, due to the possibility of procedure-related complications, we do not recommend routine direct cholangiography and biopsy for bile duct margin evaluation in perihilar cholangiocarcinoma. MDCT with 3D and multiplanar reconstruction or MRC can replace these invasive modalities to evaluate tumor extent. In patients with jaundice requiring biliary decompression, direct cholangiography via an inserted tube or IDUS and biopsy at the time of tube insertion facilitates the diagnosis. The benefit of additional resection based on a positive frozen section is controversial [34, 35], and we believe that preoperative surgical planning for an extended resection to achieve a negative margin to the extent possible is much more important. Additional resection of the bile duct may be technically limited. The best modality to gain the maximum diagnostic accuracy, achieve a high R0 resection rate, and improve patient survival remains to be investigated in future prospective studies.

Recommendations

- For patients with perihilar cholangiocarcinoma without distant metastasis, we recommend an extended hepatectomy with complete resection of the caudate lobe in curative-intent surgery.
- Enhanced MDCT with 3D and multiplanar reconstruction is mandatory for both precise preoperative evaluation of tumor extent and safe and curative surgical resection, while the gold standard for evaluation of the bile duct margin can be either cholangiography or MDCT/MRC, depending on the surgeon's preference.
- We recommend that the initial resection be extended as far as possible to achieve a negative margin, rather than performing additional resection based on a positive margin determined from routine intraoperative frozen sections.

References

1. Popescu I, Dumitrascu T. Curative-intent surgery for hilar cholangiocarcinoma: prognostic factors for clinical decision making. Langenbecks Arch Surg. 2014;399:693–705.
2. Nagino M. Perihilar cholangiocarcinoma: a surgeon's viewpoint on current topics. J Gastroenterol. 2012;47:1165–76.
3. Ramos E. Principles of surgical resection in hilar cholangiocarcinoma. World J Gastrointest Oncol. 2013;5:139–46.
4. Matsuo K, Rocha FG, Ito K, D'Angelica MI, Allen PJ, Fong Y, et al. The Blumgart preoperative staging system for hilar cholangiocarcinoma: analysis of resectability and outcomes in 380 patients. J Am Coll Surg. 2012;215:343–55.
5. Lee SG, Song GW, Hwang S, Ha TY, Moon DB, Jung DH, et al. Surgical treatment of hilar cholangiocarcinoma in the new era: the Asan experience. J Hepatobiliary Pancreat Sci. 2010;17:476–89.
6. Nagino M, Ebata T, Yokoyama Y, Igami T, Sugawara G, Takahashi Y, et al. Evolution of surgical treatment for perihilar cholangiocarcinoma: a single-center 34-year review of 574 consecutive resections. Ann Surg. 2013;258:129–40.
7. Nuzzo G, Giuliante F, Ardito F, Giovannini I, Aldrighetti L, Belli G, et al. Improvement in perioperative and long-term outcome after surgical treatment of hilar cholangiocarcinoma: results of an Italian multicenter analysis of 440 patients. Arch Surg. 2012;147:26–34.
8. Ebata T, Kosuge T, Hirano S, Unno M, Yamamoto M, Miyazaki M, et al. Proposal to modify the International Union Against Cancer staging system for perihilar cholangiocarcinomas. Br J Surg. 2014;101:79–88.
9. de Jong MC, Marques H, Clary BM, Bauer TW, Marsh JW, Ribero D, et al. The impact of portal vein resection on outcomes for hilar cholangiocarcinoma: a multi-institutional analysis of 305 cases. Cancer. 2012;118:4737–47.
10. Song SC, Choi DW, Kow AW, Choi SH, Heo JS, Kim WS, et al. Surgical outcomes of 230 resected hilar cholangiocarcinoma in a single centre. ANZ J Surg. 2013;83:268–74.
11. Cho MS, Kim SH, Park SW, Lim JH, Choi GH, Park JS, et al. Surgical outcomes and predicting factors of curative resection in patients with hilar cholangiocarcinoma: 10-year single-institution experience. J Gastrointest Surg. 2012;16:1672–9.
12. Li H, Qin Y, Cui Y, Chen H, Hao X, Li Q. Analysis of the surgical outcome and prognostic factors for hilar cholangiocarcinoma: a Chinese experience. Dig Surg. 2011;28:226–31.
13. Tsao JI, Nimura Y, Kamiya J, Hayakawa N, Kondo S, Nagino M, et al. Management of hilar cholangiocarcinoma: comparison of an American and a Japanese experience. Ann Surg. 2000;232:166–74.
14. Cannon RM, Brock G, Buell JF. Surgical resection for hilar cholangiocarcinoma: experience improves resectability. HPB (Oxf). 2012;14:142–9.
15. Natsume S, Ebata T, Yokoyama Y, Igami T, Sugawara G, Shimoyama Y, et al. Clinical significance of left trisectionectomy for perihilar cholangiocarcinoma: an appraisal and comparison with left hepatectomy. Ann Surg. 2012;255:754–62.
16. Shimizu H, Kimura F, Yoshidome H, Ohtsuka M, Kato A, Yoshitomi H, et al. Aggressive surgical resection for hilar cholangiocarcinoma of the left-side predominance: radicality and safety of left-sided hepatectomy. Ann Surg. 2010;251:281–6.
17. Cheng QB, Yi B, Wang JH, Jiang XQ, Luo XJ, Liu C, et al. Resection with total caudate lobectomy confers survival benefit in hilar cholangiocarcinoma of Bismuth type III and IV. Eur J Surg Oncol. 2012;38:1197–203.
18. Kow AW, Wook CD, Song SC, Kim WS, Kim MJ, Park HJ, et al. Role of caudate lobectomy in type III A and III B hilar cholangiocarcinoma: a 15-year experience in a tertiary institution. World J Surg. 2012;36:1112–21.
19. Nimura Y, Hayakawa N, Kamiya J, Kondo S, Shionoya S. Hepatic segmentectomy with caudate lobe resection for bile duct carcinoma of the hepatic hilus. World J Surg. 1990;14:535–43; discussion 544.

20. Neuhaus P, Thelen A, Jonas S, Puhl G, Denecke T, Veltzke-Schlieker W, et al. Oncological superiority of hilar en bloc resection for the treatment of hilar cholangiocarcinoma. Ann Surg Oncol. 2012;19:1602–8.
21. Dumitrascu T, Chirita D, Ionescu M, Popescu I. Resection for hilar cholangiocarcinoma: analysis of prognostic factors and the impact of systemic inflammation on long-term outcome. J Gastrointest Surg. 2013;17:913–24.
22. Ruys AT, van Beem BE, Engelbrecht MR, Bipat S, Stoker J, Van Gulik TM. Radiological staging in patients with hilar cholangiocarcinoma: a systematic review and meta-analysis. Br J Radiol. 2012;85:1255–62.
23. Akamatsu N, Sugawara Y, Osada H, Okada T, Itoyama S, Komagome M, et al. Diagnostic accuracy of multidetector-row computed tomography for hilar cholangiocarcinoma. J Gastroenterol Hepatol. 2010;25:731–7.
24. Kim HJ, Lee DH, Lim JW, Ko YT. Multidetector computed tomography in the preoperative workup of hilar cholangiocarcinoma. Acta Radiol. 2009;50:845–53.
25. Senda Y, Nishio H, Oda K, Yokoyama Y, Ebata T, Igami T, et al. Value of multidetector row CT in the assessment of longitudinal extension of cholangiocarcinoma: correlation between MDCT and microscopic findings. World J Surg. 2009;33:1459–67.
26. Akamatsu N, Sugawara Y, Osada H, Okada T, Itoyama S, Komagome M, et al. Preoperative evaluation of the longitudinal spread of extrahepatic bile duct cancer using multidetector computed tomography. J Hepatobiliary Pancreat Surg. 2009;16:216–22.
27. Endo I, Matsuyama R, Mori R, Taniguchi K, Kumamoto T, Takeda K, et al. Imaging and surgical planning for perihilar cholangiocarcinoma. J Hepatobiliary Pancreat Sci. 2014;21:525–32.
28. Park MJ, Kim YK, Lim S, Rhim H, Lee WJ. Hilar cholangiocarcinoma: value of adding DW imaging to gadoxetic acid-enhanced MR imaging with MR cholangiopancreatography for preoperative evaluation. Radiology. 2014;270:768–76.
29. Chryssou E, Guthrie JA, Ward J, Robinson PJ. Hilar cholangiocarcinoma: MR correlation with surgical and histological findings. Clin Radiol. 2010;65:781–8.
30. Chen XP, Lau WY, Huang ZY, Zhang ZW, Chen YF, Zhang WG, et al. Extent of liver resection for hilar cholangiocarcinoma. Br J Surg. 2009;96:1167–75.
31. Hirano S, Kondo S, Tanaka E, Shichinohe T, Tsuchikawa T, Kato K, et al. Outcome of surgical treatment of hilar cholangiocarcinoma: a special reference to postoperative morbidity and mortality. J Hepatobiliary Pancreat Sci. 2010;17:455–62.
32. Unno M, Katayose Y, Rikiyama T, Yoshida H, Yamamoto K, Morikawa T, et al. Major hepatectomy for perihilar cholangiocarcinoma. J Hepatobiliary Pancreat Sci. 2010;17:463–9.
33. Furusawa N, Kobayashi A, Yokoyama T, Shimizu A, Motoyama H, Miyagawa S. Surgical treatment of 144 cases of hilar cholangiocarcinoma without liver-related mortality. World J Surg. 2014;38:1164–76.
34. Ribero D, Amisano M, Lo Tesoriere R, Rosso S, Ferrero A, Capussotti L. Additional resection of an intraoperative margin-positive proximal bile duct improves survival in patients with hilar cholangiocarcinoma. Ann Surg. 2011;254:776–81; discussion 781–73.
35. Shingu Y, Ebata T, Nishio H, Igami T, Shimoyama Y, Nagino M. Clinical value of additional resection of a margin-positive proximal bile duct in hilar cholangiocarcinoma. Surgery. 2010;147:49–56.

Chapter 32
Management of Early Post-transplant Portal Vein Thrombosis: Results of Interventional Techniques Versus Surgical

Jonathan M. Lorenz and Mikin V. Patel

Abstract Portal vein thrombosis (PVT) is an uncommon complication of liver transplantation, occurring in less than 4 % of patients. PVT can be immediately life-threatening when it presents with signs and symptoms during the acute stage in the general population or early after liver transplantation. In transplant recipients, most cases present early, which results in a greater risk of loss of the liver graft. Despite substantial morbidity associated with PVT in liver transplant recipients, scant published literature exists to guide clinical management. Limited, small retrospective series address PVT in the general population, but the surgical or endovascular management of PVT in transplant recipients is rarely addressed. Anticoagulation is standard therapy in patients with native livers, but in the setting of early post-transplant PVT, this treatment as a sole option is usually insufficient given the tendency toward clinical progression and graft loss. No consensus exists regarding the appropriate application of surgical or endovascular revascularization, but endovascular therapies may avoid the risks of re-do operations in transplant patients.

Keywords Portal thrombosis • Liver transplant • Thrombolysis • Thrombectomy

Introduction

Portal vein thrombosis (PVT) with or without involvement of the mesenteric vein (portal-mesenteric venous thrombosis: PMVT) is an uncommon complication of liver transplantation [1–4] in the absence of pre-transplant thrombosis or other portal venous pathology. In patients with native livers, up to 75 % of cases of PVT result from an identifiable cause – most commonly hypovolemic and hypercoagulable states, and abdominal infection, inflammation or surgery [5]. Liver transplant

J.M. Lorenz (✉) • M.V. Patel
Department of Radiology, University of Chicago Medical Center,
5841 S. Maryland Ave. MC2026, Chicago, IL 60037, USA
e-mail: jlorenz@radiology.bsd.uchicago.edu

J.M. Millis, J.B. Matthews (eds.), *Difficult Decisions in Hepatobiliary and Pancreatic Surgery*, Difficult Decisions in Surgery: An Evidence-Based Approach, DOI 10.1007/978-3-319-27365-5_32

recipients often have a combination of these factors in addition to an increased risk of mechanical obstruction of the portal vein.

PVT can be immediately life-threatening when it presents with signs and symptoms during the acute stage (<7 days) in the general population or early (<30 days) after liver transplantation. Cases that present in the second to fourth week after thrombosis are considered subacute. Most transplant-related cases occur in this early period [3, 6], which predisposes these patients to a high risk of graft loss. Acute presentation increases the risk of progression to PMVT, which carries a higher risk of bowel infarction, peritonitis, complications of portal hypertension, and death. The need for emergent surgery in such cases adds additional morbidity. Persistence of untreated PVT to the chronic stage may result in portal hypertension and limited options for surgical shunt placement or retransplantation.

Evidence-based evaluation of the risks and outcomes of both surgical and endovascular techniques to manage PVT is made difficult by its low incidence, which has heretofore prevented the publication of prospective comparative trials and limited the publication of large, retrospective series. Surgical or endovascular revascularization may offer a durable solution, but no expert consensus exists regarding the appropriate application of these techniques. Endovascular techniques for PVT remain in the feasibility and pilot stages, but these therapies promise to avoid the risks of re-do operations in select post-surgical patients. Some guidance regarding technical success, clinical success, and complication rates can be gleaned from a review of the few published cases related to transplant patients coupled with published retrospective studies evaluating relevant therapies that have been applied to patients with native livers complicated by PVT.

Search Strategy

A literature search of English language publications from 1980 to 2014 was used to identify published series on the application of surgical or endovascular revascularization for the treatment of PVT and PMVT in liver transplant recipients as well as patients with native livers. The decision to include PVT in non-transplant patients resulted from an exceedingly low number of published cases describing endovascular therapies that are applicable to transplant patients. The PICO outline was used (Table 32.1). Databases searched were PubMed and Embase. Terms used in the

Table 32.1 PICO table for the management of PVT and PVMT

P (Patients)	I (Intervention)	C (Comparator group)	O (Outcomes measured)
Patients with PVT or PMVT	Endovascular revascularization	Surgical revascularization	Restoration of PV patency, resolution of clinical signs and symptoms, recurrence, complications

search were "portal/thrombosis/anticoagulation," "portal/thrombosis/revascularization," "portal/thrombosis/transplant," "portal/thrombosis/thrombolysis," and "portal/thrombosis/thrombectomy." The data was classified using the GRADE system. Seven retrospective cohort studies and one prospective pilot study were included (Table 32.2).

Results

Clinical Relevance of PVT After Liver Transplantation

PVT occurs in less than 4 % [2–4] of liver transplant recipients, but it typically occurs within 30 days of transplantation, resulting in a high risk of graft loss. The relevance of PVT is increasing as transplantation in the setting of pre-transplant PVT has gained support in the published literature [7, 8]. Liver transplantation is performed in patients with pre-existing PVT in 2–26 % of cases, and rethrombosis occurs in 6.2–28.6 % of those patients [9]. Improving surgical options for patients with pre-transplant PVT [10] may result in an increased incidence of post-transplant PVT. Thus, the relevance of the best application of surgical and endovascular therapies is likely to increase. To date, no studies specifically quantify the impact of post-transplant PVT on cost, hospital stay, morbidity and mortality.

Treatment Strategies

The existing published literature regards surgical revascularization as a first-line intervention to salvage the liver graft after early, post-transplant PVT. Since publications addressing treatment options for post-transplant PVT are limited to a few case reports and a short case series, this analysis was expanded to review endovascular treatment options that have been applied to PVT when it occurs in the general population. In such cases, nonsurgical options include anticoagulation alone or in combination with endovascular techniques such as catheter-directed thrombolysis, mechanical thrombectomy, balloon angioplasty, and stent placement – often in combination. The success rates of these therapies in patients with native livers, and their relevance to liver transplant recipients are addressed.

Treatment choices vary with factors such as operator preference, the time interval since major surgery, symptom duration and progression, and the extent of thrombosis. At minimum, the published literature supports the feasibility of endovascular revascularization of acute to subacute PVT not complicated by bowel infarction or peritonitis, and suggests that 30-day mortality rates, complication rates, and long-term patency rates are at least comparable to surgical alternatives.

Table 32.2 Management of PVT or PMVT

Author (year)	N	Mean age	Method	Technical success (%)	Clinical success (%)	Recurrence (%)	Major complications (%)	Study type (quality of evidence)
Jensen (2013) [1]	15	NR	Surgery	60	60	NR	NR	Retrospective cohort (low)
Duffy (2009) [18]	84	21	Variable	Variable	Variable	NR	NR	Retrospective cohort (low)
Hollingshead (2005) [19]	20	37.6	Thrombolysis	75	85	NR	60	Retrospective cohort (low)
Liu (2009) [20]	46	48	Thrombolysis	74	98	9 % at 4 m	0	Retrospective cohort (low)
De Santis (2010) [21]	9	59	Thrombolysis	89	89	NR	0	Prospective pilot (low)
Luo (2013) [22]	18	NR	Mechanical device, thrombolysis, TIPS[a]	100	94.4	28 % at mean 19 m	11	Retrospective cohort (low)
Kim (2005) [23]	11	44.3	Mechanical device, thrombolysis	91	91	0 % at mean 42 m	9.1 %	Retrospective cohort (low)
Cao (2013) [24]	14	61.2	Angioplasty +/– stent	100	100	43 % at mean 16 m	0	Retrospective cohort (low)

[a]*TIPS* transjugular intrahepatic portosystemic shunt

Anticoagulation

Early initiation of anticoagulation has been standard practice for acute PVT for decades, and this approach is endorsed by the American Association for the Study of Liver Diseases (AASLD) guidelines [11]. In patients with native livers, anticoagulation is the most commonly employed sole treatment strategy, and in any patient, anticoagulation limits the risk of clot progression. Senzolo et al. performed a prospective study of 56 cirrhotic patients with PVT in native livers demonstrating that anticoagulation alone achieved a rate of recanalization, either partial or complete, of 63 %, whereas failure to treat with anticoagulation achieved a rate of only 5 % [12]. In addition, with anticoagulation, only 15 % progressed compared to 71 % of patients without anticoagulation. In the general population, anticoagulation to treat PVT has been shown to increase survival and increase symptom-free survival [13, 14], and durable results can be expected as long as patients pass the hurdle of increased morbidity and mortality associated with PVT that presents within 1 month [13].

In patients with native livers, PVT results in late complications in 83.3 % if recanalization is not achieved and in 27.3 % after successful recanalization [15]. At minimum, these results support the use of endovascular techniques for revascularization in cases likely to persist or progress despite anticoagulation. Such cases include liver transplant recipients, cirrhotics, Budd-Chiari patients, and any patient with poor or diminishing liver function. Intrahepatic PVT occurring early after liver transplantation severely limits the application of anticoagulation as a sole treatment option since such cases are associated with biliary stricture formation [16], hepatic infarction [17] and death [18] in published series and case reports. PVT after transplantation causes reduced 5-year survival [6] and a high risk of graft loss, particularly when it presents early [3]. Therefore, early post-transplant PVT is more likely to prompt first-line treatment with invasive revascularization techniques in conjunction with the limited role of anticoagulation as an adjunctive therapy to prevent progression or recurrence. Duffy et al. [18] reported a graft salvage rate of 46 % for 48 patients with post-transplant PVT treated only with anticoagulation, but the interval between transplant and PVT was not specified. In any patient with clinical signs of bowel ischemia, endovascular or surgical management is warranted since mortality rates over 50 % have been described [5, 18].

Surgical Revascularization

Literature supporting surgical over endovascular revascularization for early PVT is limited. Jensen et al. performed a case-control study of pediatric liver transplant recipients. In 15 patients out of 415 recipients, early portal vein thrombosis (occurring in less than 30 days) was noted [1]. Operative restoration of portal flow was achieved in 60 %. The authors noted that patients with early portal vein thrombosis had preserved allograft function and no increase in mortality; they recommended multi-institutional studies. Duffy et al. [18] reported a graft salvage rate of 32 % for

22 patients that underwent surgical revision with thrombectomy for post-transplant PVT, and retransplantation in 20 of 84 cases of post-transplant PVT. Again, for all cases, the interval to PVT was not specified.

Thrombolysis Without Mechanical Methods

Thrombolysis without mechanical thrombectomy has been applied to PVT and PMVT for decades in patients with native livers. Hollingshead et al. retrospectively reviewed 20 acute or subacute cases; thrombolysis alone resulted in partial to complete resolution of thrombus by imaging in 75 %, symptom resolution in 85 %, and a 60 % major complication rate [19]. The route of delivery of thrombolytic agent varied and included cases of catheter-directed venous infusion, mesenteric arterial infusion, or a combination.

Liu et al. retrospectively reviewed 46 patients with acute or subacute PVT or PMVT treated with thrombolysis and reported partial to complete resolution in 74 %, but in this study, no major complications were encountered [20]. For 32 patients (70 %), catheter-directed venous thrombolysis was the sole route of delivery of thrombolytic agent rather than combined mesenteric arterial and venous infusion, a possible explanation for the low complication rate. The majority exhibited both SMV and portal venous thrombosis. Partial or complete clearance of thrombus was observed in 100 %, and the 4-month recurrence rate was only 10 %. This study lends support for the application of venous catheter-directed thrombolysis as a better first-line option than the combination of venous and arterial thrombolytic delivery in the majority of cases. When complete clearance of thrombus fails to establish hepatopetal portomesenteric flow, mesenteric arterial infusion of thrombolytic agents may become an option.

De Santis et al. performed a short prospective pilot study using catheter-directed portal venous thrombolysis to treat PMVT in nine patients with cirrhosis [21]. They achieved partial to complete clearance in eight of nine patients and noted one recurrence. As expected, variceal pressure dropped from 30.7 ± 4.5 mmHg to 21.2 ± 6.6 mmHg ($p = 0.012$).

Mechanical Methods with Thrombolysis

Luo et al. retrospectively reviewed 18 patients that presented with subacute, symptomatic PMVT and were treated with balloon dilatation, sheath-directed thrombus aspiration, and thrombolysis with creation of an intrahepatic portosystemic shunt for access and treatment [22]. Thrombolysis was performed over a mean duration of 65.3 ± 29.5 h. The mean portosystemic gradient dropped from 33.8 ± 4.9 mmHg to 15.4 ± 2.1 mmHg ($p < 0.001$) as a result of treatment. Clinical success rate was 94.4 %. Complications included one death, one patient with mild hepatic encephalopathy, and one patient with hemothorax, the latter two cases managed conservatively.

During a mean follow-up duration of 18.6 ± 17.5 months, five patients experienced symptomatic TIPS malfunction and all others experienced no further recurrence.

While quality data is lacking, mechanical thrombectomy devices promise to improve clot clearance and shorten the interval required for thrombolysis, thereby improving technical success, patency rates, and complication rates in a manner similar to results seen for their application to deep venous thrombosis. Kim et al. performed a small, retrospective cohort study of 11 patients with acute to subacute thrombosis variably involving the portal and superior mesenteric veins [23]. In all patients, the strategy applied was initial therapeutic heparinization followed by percutaneous, transhepatic thrombectomy using an endovascular mechanical device. In 10 of 11 patients, catheter-directed thrombolysis followed via the transhepatic access sheath. Balloon dilatation was used to treat underlying stenoses, and all patients were transitioned from post-procedure heparinization to long-term Warfarin. The authors report immediate restoration of flow in 90.9 % of patients, all of whom experienced rapid symptom relief. One case was complicated by hemothorax requiring a chest tube, and one patient died after unsuccessful restoration of flow. This patient was a poor surgical candidate for whom endovascular recanalization was attempted despite presentation with peritonitis and sepsis. For the remaining nine patients, no recurrent signs or symptoms of PMVT were noted during a mean follow-up period of 42 months ± 22.5. These preliminary results suggest that durable results can be achieved with revascularization followed by long-term anticoagulation.

Mechanical Methods Without Thrombolysis

For patients that require revascularization for acute to subacute PVT or PMVT but for whom thrombolysis may be contraindicated due to factors such as very recent transplantation or ongoing bleeding, some endovascular options may still apply. Cao et al evaluated balloon angioplasty with or without stent placement in 14 patients with PMVT of variable underlying causes and achieved partial to near-complete clearance with brisk hepatopetal flow in all patients and a persistent 50 % residual narrowing in only one patient [24]. Initial clinical success was 93 %. One patient experienced acute rethrombosis in 8 days, and over a mean follow-up period of 16.3 months, rethrombosis occurred in 43 %. Despite the high rethrombosis rate, this small study shows the feasibility of treating some cases of PVT and PMVT without thrombolytic agents.

Recommendations

- Anticoagulation is an option for a sole treatment strategy when subacute PVT or PMVT occurs in patients with native livers, but is rarely an option for early PVT after liver transplantation. Anticoagulation typically augments surgical or endovascular revascularization in liver transplant recipients (evidence quality low, weak recommendation).

- Choice of intervention for revascularization should be made based on local expertise, the timing of symptom progression, the status of the patient as a surgical candidate, and treatment-specific contraindications. Little precedent exists in the published literature for establishing an algorithm for the application of surgical and endovascular therapies for PVT and PMVT, although the success of both options has been established in limited retrospective cohort studies and case reports (evidence quality low, weak recommendation).

A Personal View of the Data

Large, prospective cohort studies that directly address PVT and PMVT in the early period after liver transplantation are unlikely to be forthcoming, given the low incidence of this complication in an already limited cohort of liver transplant recipients. Such studies would require multi-institutional cooperation. As a result, local opinion and expertise tends to trump evidence-based practice when managing this condition. While complication rates vary from 0 to 60 % for endovascular techniques, most morbidity is managed conservatively and tolerated well, especially when compared with the morbidity associated with re-do surgery. At a minimum, in liver transplant patients, PVT threatens graft and patient survival and all therapeutic options should be available in transplant centers.

References

1. Jensen MK, Campbell KM, Alonso MH, et al. Management and long-term consequences of portal vein thrombosis after liver transplantation in children. Liver Transpl. 2013;19(3):315–21.
2. Wozney P, Zajko AB, Bron KM, et al. Vascular complications after liver transplantation: a 5-year experience. Am J Roentgenol. 1986;147(4):657–63.
3. Khalef H. Vascular complications after deceased and living donor liver transplantation: a single-center experience. Transplant Pro. 2010;42:865–70.
4. Buell JF, Funaki B, Cronin DC, et al. Long-term venous complication after full-size and segmental pediatric liver transplantation. Ann Surg. 2002;236(5):658–66.
5. Kumar S. Mesenteric venous thrombosis. N Engl J Med. 2001;345:1683–8.
6. Millis JM, Seaman DS, Piper JB, et al. Portal vein thrombosis and stenosis in pediatric liver transplantation. Transplantation. 1996;62(6):748–54.
7. Hibi T, Nishida S, Levi DM, et al. When and why portal vein thrombosis matters in liver transplantation: a critical audit of 174 cases. Ann Surg. 2014;259(4):760–6.
8. Saidi RF, Jabbour N, Li YF, et al. Liver transplantation in patients with portal vein thrombosis: comparing pre-MELD and MELD era. Int J Organ Transplant Med. 2012;3(3):105–10.
9. Sobhonslidsuk A, Reddy KR. Portal vein thrombosis: a concise review. Am J Gastroenterol. 2002;97:535–41.

10. Paskonis M, et al. Surgical strategies for liver transplantation in the case of portal vein thrombosis – current role of cavoportal hemitransposition and renoportal anastomosis. Clin Transplant. 2006;20(5):551–62.
11. DeLeve LD, Valla DC, Garcia-Tsao G, et al. Vascular disorders of the liver. Hepatology. 2009;49(5):1729–64.
12. Senzolo M, Sartori TM, Rossetto V, et al. Anticoagulation and TIPS for portal vein thrombosis in cirrhosis. Liver Int. 2012;32(6):919–23.
13. Rhee RY, et al. Mesenteric venous thrombosis: still a lethal disease in the 1990s. J Vasc Surg. 1994;20:688–97.
14. Abdu RA, Zakhour BJ, Dallis DJ. Mesenteric venous thrombosis – 1911 to 1984. Surgery. 1987;101:383–8.
15. Hall TC, Garcea G, Metcalfe M, et al. Impact of anticoagulation on outcomes in acute non-cirrhotic and non-malignant portal vein thrombosis: a retrospective observational study. Hepatogastroenterology. 2013;60(122):311–7.
16. Jeng KS, Huang CC, Lin CK, et al. Intrahepatic segmental portal vein thrombosis after living-related donor liver transplantation. Transplant Proc. 2014;46(3):841–4.
17. Gladysz-Polak A, Polak WG, Jazwiec P, et al. Favorable resolution of hepatic infarctions in transplanted liver after portal vein thrombosis treated by surgical thrombectomy: a case report. Transplant Proc. 2006;38(9):3135–7.
18. Duffy JP, Hong JC, Farmer DG, et al. Vascular complications of orthotopic liver transplantation: experience in more than 4200 patients. J Am Coll Surg. 2009;208(5):896–903.
19. Hollingshead M, Burke CT, Mauro MA, et al. Transcatheter thrombolytic therapy for acute mesenteric and portal vein thrombosis. J Vasc Interv Radiol. 2005;16(5):651–61.
20. Liu FY, Wang MQ, Fan QS, et al. Interventional treatment for symptomatic acute-subacute portal and superior mesenteric vein thrombosis. World J Gastroenterol. 2009;15(40):5028–34.
21. De Santis A, Moscatelli R, Catalano C, et al. Systemic thrombolysis of portal vein thrombosis in cirrhotic patients: a pilot study. Dig Liver Dis. 2010;42:451–5.
22. Luo JJ, Yan ZP, Wang JH, et al. Intrahepatic portosystemic shunt assisted by percutaneous transhepatic approach for treatment of portal vein thrombosis. Zhonghua Gan Zang Bing Za Zhi. 2013;21(11):855–9.
23. Kim HS, Patra A, Khan J, et al. Transhepatic catheter-directed thrombectomy and thrombolysis of acute superior mesenteric venous thrombosis. J Vasc Interv Radiol. 2005;16:1685–91.
24. Cao G, Ko GY, Sung KB, et al. Treatment of postoperative main portal vein and superior mesenteric vein thrombosis with balloon angioplasty and/or stent placement. Acta Radiol. 2013;54(5):526–32.

Chapter 33
When Should Patients with Bleeding Esophageal Varices Undergo TIPS Versus Endoscopic Therapy?

John N. Gaetano and K. Gautham Reddy

Abstract Acute variceal bleeding is a serious sequela of cirrhosis and portal hypertension, which carries significant morbidity and mortality. Advances in therapeutic techniques as well as accessibility and overall safety of esophagogastroduodenoscopy (EGD) allowed for endoscopic management to emerge as first line therapy two decades ago, and remain first-line therapy today. Transjugular intrahepatic portosystemic shunt (TIPS) is a critical rescue therapy for those that fail endoscopic management, while rescue TIPS carries significant morbidity and mortality, efforts to identify patients that are likely to fail endoscopy and benefit from early TIPS are ongoing. Surgical portosystemic shunts, particularly distal splenorenal shunt, can be considered for refractory bleeding in ideal patients with minimal comorbidities, where surgeon experience is adequate and TIPS cannot be performed.

Keywords Acute variceal bleeding • Esophageal varices • TIPS • Endoscopic band ligation • Splenorenal shunt

Introduction

Acute hemorrhage of esophageal varices continues to cause significant morbidity and mortality among those with portal hypertension. Primary and secondary prophylaxis, antibiotic and vasoactive drug administration, and improvements in endoscopic therapy have led to a decrease in the rates of hospitalization and decreased rates of mortality over the last two decades [1, 2]. However, the in-hospital mortality of acute variceal bleeding remains strikingly high: up to 32 % in those with

J.N. Gaetano • K.G. Reddy (✉)
Department of Gastroenterology, Section of Gastroenterology, Hepatology and Nutrition, The University of Chicago Medicine and Biological Sciences, 5841 S. Maryland Ave, MC 7120, Chicago, IL 60637, USA
e-mail: greddy@medicine.bsd.uchicago.edu

J.M. Millis, J.B. Matthews (eds.), *Difficult Decisions in Hepatobiliary and Pancreatic Surgery*, Difficult Decisions in Surgery: An Evidence-Based Approach, DOI 10.1007/978-3-319-27365-5_33

Child-Turcotte-Pugh (hereafter referred to as 'Child-Pugh') class C cirrhosis, making the management of acute variceal bleeding a difficult challenge [2].

The backbone of therapy of acute variceal hemorrhage requires prompt attention to airway management, initiation of volume resuscitation, vasoactive therapy, antibiotic prophylaxis, and endoscopic therapy. Endoscopic band ligation, and previously endoscopic sclerotherapy, is the cornerstone of therapy. There remains a need for rescue therapies and alternatives to endoscopy, namely transjugular intrahepatic portosystemic shunt (TIPS) placement, balloon tamponade, and surgical portosystemic shunt formation. Timing and indications of rescue therapies lacks a standardized approach, and is the topic of this chapter.

Search Strategy

A literature search of English language publications from 1990 to present was used to identify published data on surgical shunt, endoscopic therapy and transjugular intrahepatic portosystemic shunt (TIPS) for the management of acute variceal bleeding. Database searched was PubMed. Terms used in the search were "acute variceal hemorrhage/bleeding" AND "endoscopic therapy" OR "TIPS" OR "Surgical portosystemic shunt." The PICO model was used for literature search stratification (Table 33.1).

Results

First Line Therapy

Endoscopic therapy as first-line therapy for acute variceal hemorrhage became consensus in the early 1990s. It was universally accepted in guidelines in 1995 [3], when endoscopic band ligation (EBL) was established as an alternative to endoscopic sclerotherapy (ES). While EBL and ES have almost equal rates of immediate hemostasis (89% and 88 %, respectively), in a meta-analysis of seven randomized trials, ES is associated with higher rates of re-bleeding (31 % vs. 47 %), higher mortality (24 % vs. 32 %), and stricture formation (0 % vs. 11 %) [4]. Furthermore, multiple studies have reported that complications as a result of therapy with EBL are significantly less frequent when compared with ES, 11 % vs. 25 % [5–7].

Table 33.1 Stratification of the literature search using the PICO model

Patients	Acute esophageal variceal hemorrhage
Intervention	Endoscopic band ligation or sclerotherapy
Comparator	TIPS or surgical shunt
Outcomes	Mortality, morbidity

Initial endoscopic therapy fails to control bleeding in 10–20 % of those who present with acute variceal bleeding. Of those that are initially controlled with endoscopic therapy, rebleeding occurs in up to 30 % [8]. Failed therapy is been defined as a failure to control bleeding, if the patient dies, or any one of the following are met: (1) Fresh hematemesis or nasogastric aspiration of ≥100 mL of fresh blood >2 h after the start of a specific therapy, (2) development of hypovolemic shock, or (3) a 3-g hemoglobin drop within any 24 h period if no transfusions are administered. Rebleeding is defined as any bleeding that occurs more than 48 h after the initial admission for variceal hemorrhage, provided there has been at least a 24-h period without bleeding. "Early rebleeding" is defined as rebleeding within 6 weeks of the onset of the initial bleed, while "late rebleeding" is defined as rebleeding after 6 weeks [9].

Rescue Therapies

Patient's at high risk of early rebleeding (within 6 weeks) have the following characteristics: age >60, alcoholic cirrhosis, initial hemoglobin <8, thrombocytopenia, encephalopathy, ascites, bleeding seen at endoscopy, red color signs (red wale signs) on varices, large varices, high hepatic-venous pressure gradient (HVPG), and renal failure. Risk factors associated with late rebleeding include: Liver failure, ascites, hepatocellular carcinoma, active alcohol drinking, and red wale signs [10].

For patients who fail endoscopic therapy or in whom early rebleeding occurs, the next therapeutic option is a critical decision point. In patients with rebleeding following initially successful endoscopic therapy, a second attempt at endoscopic therapy is reasonable, although data is limited in support of this approach [9]. In the event of failure of initial endoscopic therapy or if a second rebleeding event occurs, consensus guidelines from the American Association for the Study of Liver Disease (AASLD), suggest an alternative modality should be considered.

Balloon Tamponade

Balloon tamponade is a temporary measure of achieving hemostasis by direct compression of bleeding varices and should be considered a bridge to a more definitive treatment. Two types of oral-gastric tubes exist, the Sengstaken-Blakemore tube and the Minnesota tube. Both tubes contain a gastric balloon and an esophageal balloon with an aspiration port between the two. The Minnesota tube has an aspiration port proximal to the esophageal balloon as well. The deflated tube is placed with the distal end into the stomach, then, the gastric balloon is inflated and pulled upward until secure at the GE junction. When the gastric balloon alone is insufficient to control bleeding the esophageal balloon is inflated. Esophageal balloon inflation increases the risk of necrosis at the GE junction. The gastric balloon tube should not be inflated for more than 48 h in order to prevent necrosis, and the esophageal balloon should be deflated every 12 h to prevent necrosis. Twenty to thirty percent of patients undergoing balloon tamponade have complications related to tube placement and include aspiration pneumonia, esophageal tears or rupture [11]. One series reported effective control of bleeding with tube placement in 79 % of patients [12], making tamponade an effective means for temporary control of severe hemorrhage while awaiting definitive treatment with TIPS or surgery.

TIPS

Transjugular intrahepatic portosystemic shunt (TIPS) was developed as a minimally invasive shunt, designed to create portosystemic bypass with the primary advantage of avoiding major surgery, while maintaining blood flow to the liver. TIPS is widely considered salvage therapy for the 10–20 % of patients that fail first-line therapy. The first two large series reporting outcomes for TIPS for the management of recurrent variceal bleeding (only 10 % were emergent cases), yielded 92 % success in achieving hemostasis, with overall 1-year survival rates of 75–100 %, 68–86 %, and 49–73 % percent for Child-Pugh A, B, and C, respectively [13, 14].

For patients with acute bleeding refractory to endoscopic therapy, emergent or "salvage" TIPS is also very effective, controlling bleeding in 94 % of patients with low rebleeding rates. However, the 30-day mortality is 30 %, with only half of all patients surviving to 1 year [15]. The high mortality among those requiring rescue therapies likely reflects the severity of liver disease and the underlying degree of portal hypertension in this population. Furthermore, the delay between initial bleed and TIPS placement, number of endoscopic attempts, and need for balloon tamponade correlates with increased mortality when using TIPS as a salvage therapy [11]. In order to decrease the mortality of TIPS, attempts have been made to identify patients most likely to fail endoscopic therapy, and potentially undergo earlier TIPS placement, in order to improve survival. The strongest predictor of negative outcome is a HVPG greater than 20 mmHg, in which patients are 4–5 times more likely to fail medical and endoscopic therapy [16, 17]. HVPG measurement is not routine practice in the setting of acute bleeding in the United States. Risk factors for a HVPG >20 include Child-Pugh C cirrhosis, non-alcohol related cause of cirrhosis, systolic blood pressure at the time of bleeding of less than 100 mmHg, or active bleeding at the time of endoscopy [17, 18].

Early TIPS

Two randomized trials have shown that early TIPS (within 24–72 h of admission) is associated with significant improvement in survival among high-risk patients (Child-Pugh class B and C patients and/or those with hepatic vein-portal gradient (HVPG) >20 mmHg) [12, 19]. The first of these two randomized studies, utilized measurement of hepatic venous pressure gradient within 24 h of admission of acute variceal bleed. All patients received endoscopic sclerotherapy and those with HVPG

>20 were randomized to TIPS or continued medical therapy. Those receiving TIPS had less rebleeding (12 % vs. 50 %), in-hospital mortality (11 % vs. 38 %) and 1-year mortality (31 % vs. 65 %) [19]. Of note, neither control nor treatment group received continuous vasoactive therapy. Furthermore, the decision to place TIPS was determined by HVPG measurement, a tool that is not widely available.

A subsequent randomized trial evaluated early TIPS versus EBL in Child-Pugh B and C patients with acute variceal bleeding. Medical therapy plus EBL had significantly more rebleeding or failure to control bleeding when compared to TIPS (TIPS, 1/32 patients; EBL, 14/31 patients) [12]. ICU stay was shortened in the early TIPS group. The rate of survival at 6 weeks was 97 % in the TIPS group compared with 67 % in the EBL group. No significant differences were reported in serious adverse events, including number or severity of hepatic encephalopathy (TIPS, 25 %; EBL, 39 %). Although not statistically significant, the rate of acute liver failure was 9 % in the TIPS group compared to 3 % in the EBL group [12]. This study was underpowered to show a significant difference in rate of acute liver failure and excluded patients greater than 75 years of age and Child-Pugh score greater than 13 points [12].

Complications of TIPS

Early complications of TIPS are most commonly related to the direct shunting of portal flow into the venous system and include: heart failure (increase venous return/preload), liver failure (ischemia) and hepatic encephalopathy (less toxin clearance). The reported incidence of new onset or worsening hepatic encephalopathy ranges from 13 to 35 % of those undergoing TIPS [20]. In addition, the nature of the procedure itself has risks independent of the effect of shunting. These procedural risks include liver capsular perforation, puncture of the gall bladder or a bile duct, and hepatic artery injury requiring coil embolization or surgery.

Systematic risk stratification for who should undergo TIPS was flawed when the Child-Pugh system was applied as this system was originally designed to determine risk for undergoing surgical portosystemic shunt, and has limitations when applied to TIPS. Most patients requiring emergent TIPS for bleeding are class C, and the system only divides patients into low, intermediate and high risk. Furthermore, the model uses subjective measures such as encephalopathy and ascites, which can be altered by therapy. The creation of the Model for End-stage Liver Disease (MELD) score, which is now universally used for liver transplant listing, was initially designed to predict 3-month mortality in patients undergoing elective TIPS. The MELD score utilizes objective measures of total serum bilirubin, serum creatinine, and prothrombin time to risk stratify patients [21]. The score was later validated to predict 1-month mortality, concluding that patients with a MELD score of >24 undergoing elective TIPS are at higher risk of early death [22].

In the early era of TIPS, bare metal expandable stents were found to be particular vulnerable to stenosis from pseudointimal hyperplasia within the stent, occurring in 30–70 % of patients within 1 year [23], and by 2 years virtually all patient develop some degree of stenosis [24]. The advent of polytetrafluoroethylene (PTFE) covered stents led to a dramatic improvement in stent patency, without an impact of rebleeding, encephalopathy, or survival. The frequency of stenosis declined to 18 % at 1 year, while patency improved from 36 to 76 % at 2 years [25].

There are important contraindications and relative contraindications to TIPS that require consideration (Table 33.2). Absolute contraindications to TIPS are primary prevention of variceal bleeding, congestive heart failure, severe pulmonary hypertension, multiple hepatic cysts, uncontrolled systemic infection or sepsis, and unrelieved biliary obstruction. Relative contraindications include hepatoma if centrally located, obstruction of hepatic veins, portal vein thrombosis, severe coagulopathy (INR >5), platelets <20,000/cm^3, and moderate pulmonary hypertension [26].

Surgical Shunt

For more than half a century, the creation of a surgical portosystemic shunt has been used to bypass the site of increased resistance (cirrhotic liver), thereby decreasing portal venous pressure, and control (and prevent) variceal bleeding. The direct portocaval shunt was prominent in the 1960s–1970s, and while very effective in controlling bleeding, there was significant operative morbidity, induction of liver failure, and worsening of acute and chronic hepatic encephalopathy related to complete redirection of portal blood flow. The distal splenorenal shunt (DSRS) took root in the 1970s–1980s followed by the interposition "C" or "H" graft portocaval shunts in the 1990s and 2000s. These small-diameter portocaval shunts are partial portosystemic shunts that effectively reduce portal pressure while preserving nutrient blood flow to the liver, minimizing postoperative encephalopathy and liver failure. Surgical shunting effectively reduces portal pressure [27] and controls acute bleeding in 99–100 % of patients undergoing surgery [28], however given the poor short term survival among Child-Pugh C patients [27] and considerable morbidity from surgery, the Child-Pugh A patient with minimal comorbidities is the best candidate for this therapy.

In Child-Pugh A and B patients with refractory bleeding, DSRS has been compared to TIPS, which revealed no statistically significant difference in rate of rebleeding (DSRS, 5.5 % and TIPS, 10.5 %,) or survival at 2 years (DSRS, 81 % and TIPS 88 %) or survival at 5 years (DSRS, 62 % and TIPS, 61 %). Half the patients in each group developed hepatic encephalopathy [29].

Table 33.2 Absolute and relative contraindication to transjugular intrahepatic portosystemic shunt (TIPS) placement

Absolute	Relative
Congestive heart failure	Hepatoma, if centrally located
Severe pulmonary hypertension	Moderate pulmonary hypertension
Multiple hepatic cysts	Portal vein thrombosis
Uncontrolled systemic infection or sepsis	Obstruction of hepatic veins
Unrelieved biliary obstruction	Severe coagulopathy (INR >5, platelets <20,000)

Recommendations

It should be reinforced that the backbone of initial therapy for acute bleeding from varices relies upon hemodynamic resuscitation (while avoiding over transfusion), having a low threshold for endotracheal intubation to ensure the patient's airway is protected, and addressing coagulopathies. Prophylactic antibiotics (fluoroquinolone or third generation cephalosporin) as well as vasoactive therapy (octreotide, somatostatin, or terlipressin) must be initiated and maintained for 3–5 days.

After initial resuscitation, airway management, correction of coagulopathy, an EGD should be performed as soon as possible after admission (within 12 h) with appropriate endoscopic therapy if an esophageal variceal bleed is confirmed [9, 26].

In general, those patients who fail endoscopic therapy for variceal bleeding should undergo definitive therapy with either TIPS or a surgical shunt. As noted above, the two procedures are equal in efficacy and appear to have no difference in mortality adverse outcomes, including worsening or new hepatic encephalopathy. The choice of surgical shunt versus percutaneous TIPS should be made based on available expertise and patient preference.

Early TIPS (within 72 h of acute variceal bleeding) appears to be a safe and effective modality to treat acute variceal bleeding in a select patient population in conjunction with medical therapy. The mortality of rescue TIPS (after failure of endoscopic therapy) is associated with a high mortality, which has been attributed, in part, to the delay from the time of initial bleed until TIPS. For this reason, recognition of a patient likely to fail endoscopic and medical therapy should be considered for early TIPS (Fig. 33.1). This recommendation pertains to Child-Pugh class B with active bleeding at the time of initial endoscopy or class C patients, and patients with an HVPG >20. Early-TIPS cannot be recommended in patients with Child-Pugh class A cirrhosis because failure of endoscopic and medical therapy, as well as mortality are low in this patient population. Early TIPS also cannot be recommended in patients with a MELD score >24 given evidence of early mortality after TIPS in these patients [22], as well as patients over the age of 75 or Child-Pugh score over 13 because these patients were excluded from the early-TIPS trial [12].

A Personal View of the Data

Acute variceal bleeding is a serious sequela of cirrhosis and portal hypertension, which still carries significant morbidity and mortality. Advances in therapeutics allowed for endoscopic management to emerge as first line therapy two decades ago. There is ample data demonstrating efficacy of EBL, TIPS, as well as surgical shunting. Given the need for initial endoscopy to prove variceal hemorrhage as the source of GI bleeding, accessibility of endoscopy, as well as limited access to HVPG measurement; TIPS is unlikely to replace EBL as initial therapy in The United States. TIPS remains a crucial rescue therapy for those with refractory bleeding, or

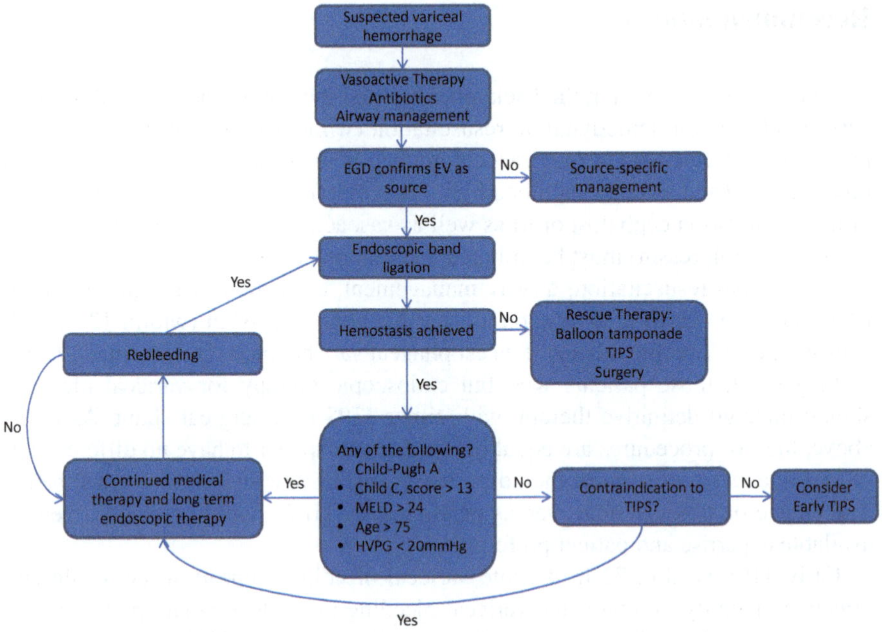

Fig. 33.1 Risk stratified approach to the management of acute variceal bleeding. Abbreviations: *EGD* esophagogastroduodenoscopy, *EV* esophageal varices, *TIPS* transjugular intrahepatic portosystemic shunt, *MELD* Model for End-Stage Liver Disease, *HVPG* hepatic venous pressure gradient

early rebleeding who are considered to have failed an endoscopic approach. Areas of interest for further research within this topic include the role of new pharmacologic therapies with greater effect on HVPG and the role of capsule endoscopy to diagnose acute variceal hemorrhage.

Recommendations

- For patients with suspected acute esophageal variceal hemorrhage, we recommend early (within 12 h) endoscopy as both initial diagnostic and therapeutic procedure. (evidence quality high; strong recommendation)
- In patients with suspected variceal hemorrhage, prompt attention to airway management, volume resuscitation, antimicrobial prophylaxis, and pharmacologic therapy are crucial. (evidence quality high; strong recommendation)
- TIPS is indicated in patients with refractory bleeding, or early rebleeding who are considered to have failed an endoscopic and medical therapy. (Evidence quality moderate, strong recommendation)
- In patients with refractory bleeding, Child A status, with a non-cardiopulmonary contraindication to TIPS (e.g. centrally located hepatoma), distal splenorenal

shunt should be considered if the surgical expertise is available. (Evidence quality moderate, strong recommendation)

- Early TIPS should be considered for bleeding esophageal varices in patients with the following characteristics: Child-Pugh class B with active variceal bleeding at the time of initial endoscopy or class C patients with a Child-Pugh score <14, MELD score <24, and age <75, and with HVPG >20 mmHg in centers where portal gradient measurement is available. (Evidence quality moderate, moderate recommendation)

References

1. Jamal MM, Samarasena JB, Hashemzadeh M, Vega KJ. Declining hospitalization rate of esophageal variceal bleeding in the United States. Clin Gastroenterol Hepatol. 2008;6(6):689–95.
2. Carbonell N, Pauwels A, Serfaty L, Fourdan O, Lévy VG, Poupon R. Improved survival after variceal bleeding in patients with cirrhosis over the past two decades. Hepatology. 2004;40(3):652–9.
3. de Franchis R. Evolving consensus in portal hypertension report of the Baveno IV consensus workshop on methodology of diagnosis and therapy in portal hypertension. J Hepatol. 2005;43(1):167–76.
4. Laine L, Cook D. Endoscopic ligation compared with sclerotherapy for treatment of esophageal variceal bleeding. A meta-analysis. Ann Intern Med. 1995;123(4):280–7.
5. Stiegmann GV, Goff JS, Michaletz-Onody PA, Korula J, Lieberman D, Saeed ZA, Reveille RM, Sun JH, Lowenstein SR. Endoscopic sclerotherapy as compared with endoscopic ligation for bleeding esophageal varices. N Engl J Med. 1992;326(23):1527–32.
6. Lo GH, Lai KH, Cheng JS, Hwu JH, Chang CF, Chen SM, Chiang HT. A prospective, randomized trial of sclerotherapy versus ligation in the management of bleeding esophageal varices. Hepatology. 1995;22(2):466–71.
7. Laine L, el-Newihi M, Migikovsky B, Sloane R, Garcia F. Endoscopic ligation compared with sclerotherapy for the treatment of bleeding esophageal varices. Ann Intern Med. 1993;119(1):1–7.
8. D'amico G, Pagliaro L, Bosch J. The treatment of portal hypertension: a meta-analytic review. Hepatology. 1995;22(1):332–54.
9. de Franchis R, Baveno V Faculty. Revising consensus in portal hypertension: report of the Baveno V consensus workshop on methodology of diagnosis and therapy in portal hypertension. J Hepatol. 2010;53(4):762–8.
10. Habib A, Sanyal AJ. Acute variceal hemorrhage. Gastrointest Endosc Clin N Am. 2007;17(2):223–52.
11. Herrera JL. Management of acute variceal bleeding. Clin Liver Dis. 2014;18(2):347–57.
12. García-Pagán JC, Caca K, Bureau C, Laleman W, Appenrodt B, Luca A, Abraldes JG, Nevens F, Vinel JP, Mössner J, Bosch J. Early use of TIPS in patients with cirrhosis and variceal bleeding. N Engl J Med. 2010;362(25):2370–9.
13. Rossle M, Haag K, Ochs A, Sellinger M, Noldge G, Perarnau J-M, Berger E, Blum U, Gabelmann A, Hauenstein K, Langer M, Gerok W. The transjugular intrahepatic portosystemic stent-shunt procedure for variceal bleeding. N Engl J Med. 1994;330(3):165–71.
14. Laberge JM, Somberg KA, Lake JR, Gordon RL, Kerlan Jr RK, Ascher NL, Roberts JP, Simor MM, Doherty CA, Hahn J, BachettiI P, Ring EJ. Two-year outcome following transjugular intrahepatic portosystemic shunt for variceal bleeding: results in 90 patients. Gastroenterology. 1995;108(4):1143–51.

15. Azoulay D, Castaing D, Majno P, Saliba F, Ichaï P, Smail A, Delvart V, Danaoui M, Samuel D, Bismuth H. Salvage transjugular intrahepatic portosystemic shunt for uncontrolled variceal bleeding in patients with decompensated cirrhosis. J Hepatol. 2001;35(5):590–7.
16. Moitinho E, Escorsell A, Bandi JC, Salmerón JM, García-Pagán JC, Rodés J, Bosch J. Prognostic value of early measurements of portal pressure in acute variceal bleeding. Gastroenterology. 1999;117(3):626–31.
17. Villanueva C, Piqueras M, Aracil C, Gómez C, López-Balaguer JM, Gonzalez B, Gallego A, Torras X, Soriano G, Sáinz S, Benito S, Balanzó J. A randomized controlled trial comparing ligation and sclerotherapy as emergency endoscopic treatment added to somatostatin in acute variceal bleeding. J Hepatol. 2006;45(4):560–7.
18. Vangeli M, Patch D, Burroughs AK. Salvage tips for uncontrolled variceal bleeding. J Hepatol. 2002;37(5):703–4.
19. Monescillo A, Martínez-Lagares F, Ruiz-del-Arbol L, Sierra A, Guevara C, Jiménez E, Marrero JM, Buceta E, Sánchez J, Castellot A, Peñate M, Cruz A, Peña E. Influence of portal hypertension and its early decompression by TIPS placement on the outcome of variceal bleeding. Hepatology. 2004;40(4):793–801.
20. Riggio O, Nardelli S, Moscucci F, Pasquale C, Ridola L, Merli M. Hepatic encephalopathy after transjugular intrahepatic portosystemic shunt. Clin Liver Dis. 2012;16(1):133–46.
21. Malinchoc M, Kamath PS, Gordon FD, Peine CJ, Rank J, ter Borg PCJ. A model to predict poor survival in patients undergoing transjugular intrahepatic portosystemic shunts. Hepatology. 2000;31(4):864–71.
22. Montgomery A, Ferral H, Vasan R, Postoak DW. MELD score as a predictor of early death in patients undergoing elective transjugular intrahepatic portosystemic shunt (TIPS) procedures. Cardiovasc Intervent Radiol. 2005;28(3):307–12.
23. Riggio O, Ridola L, Angeloni S, Cerini F, Pasquale C, Attili AF, Fanelli F, Merli M, Salvatori FM. Clinical efficacy of transjugular intrahepatic portosystemic shunt created with covered stents with different diameters: results of a randomized controlled trial. J Hepatol. 2010;53(2):267–72.
24. Sanyal AJ, Freedman AM, Luketic VA, Purdum PP, Shiffman ML, DeMeo J, Cole PE, Tisnado J. The natural history of portal hypertension after transjugular intrahepatic portosystemic shunts. Gastroenterology. 1997;112(3):889–98.
25. Bureau C, Pagan JCG, Layrargues GP, Metivier S, Bellot P, Perreault P, Otal P, Abraldes J-G, Peron JM, Rousseau H, Bosch J, Vinel JP. Patency of stents covered with polytetrafluoroethylene in patients treated by transjugular intrahepatic portosystemic shunts: long-term results of a randomized multicentre study. Liver Int. 2007;27(6):742–7.
26. Prevention and management of gastroesophageal varices and variceal hemorrhage in cirrhosis – Prevention and Management of Gastro Varices and Hemorrhage.pdf. [Online]. Available: http://www.aasld.org/practiceguidelines/Documents/Bookmarked%20Practice%20 Guidelines/Prevention%20and%20Management%20of%20Gastro%20Varices%20and%20 Hemorrhage.pdf. Accessed: 27 July 2014.
27. Hillebrand DJ, Kojouri K, Cao S, Runyon BA, Ojogho O, Concepcion W. Small-diameter portacaval H-graft shunt: a paradigm shift back to surgical shunting in the management of variceal bleeding in patients with preserved liver function. Liver Transpl. 2000;6(4):459–65.
28. Orloff MJ, Orloff MS, Orloff SL, Rambotti M, Girard B. Three decades of experience with emergency portacaval shunt for acutely bleeding esophageal varices in 400 unselected patients with cirrhosis of the liver. J Am Coll Surg. 1995;180(3):257–72.
29. Henderson JM, Boyer TD, Kutner MH, Galloway JR, Rikkers LF, Jeffers LJ, Abu-Elmagd K, Connor J, DIVERT Study Group. Distal splenorenal shunt versus transjugular intrahepatic portal systematic shunt for variceal bleeding: a randomized trial. Gastroenterology. 2006;130(6):1643–51.

Chapter 34
Management of Symptomatic Portal Hypertension: TIPS vs. Medical Management

Anouar Teriaky and Andrew Aronsohn

Abstract Portal hypertension is a common manifestation of decompensated cirrhosis and can have a profound impact on patient survival and quality of life. Portal hypertension can be managed with medical therapy through use of diuretics or portal pressure lowering agents, however in some cases more invasive procedures such as transjugular intrahepatic portosystemic shunt (TIPS) may be more effective. In this systematic review of the literature, clinical outcomes following medical management and TIPS are compared across various manifestations of portal hypertension. Overall, we found that data favors use of TIPS to prevent recurrent variceal bleeding and recurrent ascites however risk of hepatic encephalopathy is higher than medical management. In addition, in selected patients, TIPS may also improve mortality in those with variceal hemorrhage and refractory ascites. Compared to esophageal varices and ascites, there is limited data supporting use of TIPS vs medical management for conditions such as hepatic hydrothorax, nonesophageal varices and hepatorenal syndrome.

Keywords Portal hypertension • TIPS • Varices • Ascites • Diuretics • Paracentesis • Quality of life

Introduction

Portal hypertension (PH) is a common complication of chronic liver disease [1]. PH can manifest in a variety of forms including gastrointestinal hemorrhage, ascites, hepatic hydrothorax, portopulmonary hypertension, hepatopulmonary syndrome, and hepatorenal syndrome (HRS). It leads to great morbidity and mortality as liver disease further progresses [2]. Most complications of PH are initially managed medically with more invasive measures added when necessary.

A. Teriaky (✉) • A. Aronsohn
Center for Liver Diseases, University of Chicago Medical Center,
5841 S. Maryland Ave, Chicago, IL 60637, USA
e-mail: ateriaky@mail.bsd.uchicago.edu

J.M. Millis, J.B. Matthews (eds.), *Difficult Decisions in Hepatobiliary and Pancreatic Surgery*, Difficult Decisions in Surgery: An Evidence-Based Approach, DOI 10.1007/978-3-319-27365-5_34

Medical management of esophageal varices may involve non-selective beta-blockers or endoscopic variceal ligation (EVL) for primary prophylaxis and variceal hemorrhage is managed with hemodynamic resuscitation, vasoactive agents, antibiotics, and EVL [3]. Rebleeding esophageal varices carry a high mortality [4]. Ascites is initially managed with sodium restriction and diuretics. Refractory ascites can occur in cirrhotic patients that are unresponsive to salt restriction and aggressive diuretic therapy or that develop intolerances to diuretic use [5]. These patients represent 10 % of cirrhotics with ascites [6]. This occurrence predicts poor outcomes with greater than 50 % dying within 1 year without liver transplantation.

Hepatic hydrothorax is managed in a similar fashion to ascites. HRS develops as an end-stage complication of refractory ascites. There are two types with type 1 occurring more rapidly and possessing a higher mortality. Vasoactive agents with albumin have been shown to improve renal function [7]. Portopulmonary hypertension has been managed with vasodilators and hepatopulmonary syndrome with oxygen therapy [8]. Ultimately when PH and its manifestations become severe or refractory, referral to liver transplant centers might provide the greatest survival [9].

Transjugular intrahepatic portosystemic shunt (TIPS) has largely replaced surgical portacaval shunts in decompressing the portal circulation. It has been used for the treatment of severe or refractory complications of PH [5]. TIPS is not without complications and should only be performed when necessary. Complications include transcapsular puncture, intraperitoneal hemorrhage, hepatic infarction, fistulization, hemobilia, hemolysis, encephalopathy, stent infection, stent thrombosis or stenosis, and stent migration [10]. This chapter reviews the evidence for medical management versus TIPS to treat the various manifestations of severe or refractory symptomatic PH.

Search

A literature search on medical management versus TIPS for symptomatic PH (Table 34.1) was conducted on the following databases: Pubmed, Embase, and Cochrane Evidence Based Medicine. English language publications between 1994 and 2014 were reviewed. Terms used in the search query included various combinations of the following terms: transjugular intrahepatic portosystemic shunt, medical management, diuretics, paracentesis, portal hypertension, varices, variceal hemorrhage, ascites, hepatic hydrothorax, portopulmonary hypertension, hepatorenal syndrome, hepatopulmonary syndrome, portal hypertensive gastropathy, control, mortality, morbidity, quality of life, and cost. After reviewing the literature, the

Table 34.1 PICO table for symptomatic portal hypertension management with TIPS

Patients	Intervention	Comparison	Outcomes
Symptomatic patients with portal hypertension	TIPS	Medical management	Control of portal hypertension, morbidity, mortality, and cost

most relevant articles with the highest level of evidence were included. The GRADE system was used to classify data.

Results

Esophageal Varices

Esophageal variceal hemorrhage represents one of the most fatal complications of PH. Patients are generally screened at the time of diagnosis of cirrhosis and regularly thereafter. Primary prophylaxis for esophageal varices is the prevention of first variceal bleed medically with a non-selective beta-blocker or EVL until obliteration. EVL may be considered for large varices, high risk stigmata, and Child Pugh B and C cirrhosis [11]. TIPS is contraindicated for primary prophylaxis of esophageal varices [3].

Acute variceal hemorrhage is a medical emergency and is initially managed with hemodynamic resuscitation, vasoactive drugs, antibiotics, and EVL. Most patients respond to this treatment, but TIPS has been used as rescue therapy when necessary. Controlled studies support the use of early TIPS in esophageal variceal hemorrhage (Table 34.2). Monescillo et al. showed that in patients presenting with a variceal bleed with a hepatic venous pressure gradient greater than 20 mmHg, TIPS within 24 h was superior to endoscopic therapy in reducing treatment failure (12 % vs. 50 % $p=0.0001$) and 1-year mortality (31 % vs. 65 % $p=0.01$) without increasing encephalopathy ($p=31$ % vs. 35 % p = n.s) [12]. A limitation of this study was the use of sclerotherapy instead of EVL, which is the standard of care [3].

Garcia-Pagan et al. showed that in Child-Pugh B and C cirrhotics, early closed stent TIPS combined with medical therapy was superior to medical therapy alone. Medical therapy consisted of vasoactive drugs and endoscopic therapy. The 1-year probability of remaining free of rebleeding was 50 % with the control group and 97 % in the TIPS group ($p<0.001$). The 1-year survival was 61 % in the endoscopic therapy group and 86 % in the combined endoscopic therapy and TIPS group ($p=0.001$). There were no significant differences in adverse events between the two groups [13]. Closed stents have better patency requiring less revisions when compared to open stents and do not increase the risk of encephalopathy [14].

Recurrent variceal hemorrhage is associated with high mortality [4, 15]. Secondary prophylaxis of esophageal varices in patients that have survived an acute variceal bleed can be managed medically with a non-selective beta-blocker and EVL until obliteration [3]. TIPS has also been used in this patient population. When comparing propranolol and isosorbide-5-mononitrate to TIPS, patients who underwent TIPS had lower rebleeding rates and equivalent mortality rates although rates of encephalopathy were higher [16]. However, this is not the standard of care in secondary prophylaxis. Multiple trials including several meta-analyses have compared open stent TIPS to EVL or sclerotherapy with or without beta blockers (Table 34.2) [17–33]. In a recent meta-analysis, Zheng et al., showed that TIPS

Table 34.2 The main outcomes of endoscopic therapy ± pharmacological therapy versus TIPS in the management of variceal hemorrhage

Study (year)	Study type (quality of evidence)	Patients (C vs. T)	Treatment failure (C vs. T)	Hepatic encephalopathy (C vs. T)	Mortality (C vs. T)
Cabrera (1996)	RCT (moderate)	32 vs. 31	52 % vs. 23 %	13 % vs. 33 %	18 % vs. 7 %
			p<0.02	p<0.05	p=n.s
Cello (1997)	RCT (moderate)	25 vs. 24	48 % vs. 13 %	44 % vs 50 %	n.s
			p=0.012	p=0.2	
Jalan (1997)	RCT (strong)	27 vs. 31	52 % vs. 10 %	11 % vs 16 %	n.s
			p<0.0006	p=n.s	
Rossle (1997)	RCT (moderate)	65 vs. 61	52 % vs. 21 %	18 % vs. 36 %	11 % vs. 10 %
			p=0.001	p=0.011	p=n.s
Sanyal (1997)	RCT (moderate)	39 vs. 41	26 % vs. 24 %	13 % vs. 29 %	18 % vs. 29 %
			p=0.2	p=0.01	p=0.02
Sauer (1997)	RCT (moderate)	41 vs. 42	57 % vs. 23 %	13 % vs. 29 %	33 % vs. 31 %
			p=0.0001	p=0.041	p=0.62
Merli (1998)	RCT (moderate)	43 vs. 38	51 % vs. 24 %	26 % vs. 55 %	19 % vs. 24 %
			p=0.11	p=0.006	p=0.50
Garcia-Villarreal (1999)	RCT (moderate)	24 vs. 22	50 % vs. 9 %	25 % vs. 23 %	33 % vs. 15 %
			p<0.001	p=n.s	p<0.05
Narahara (2001)	RCT (moderate)	40 vs. 38	32 % vs. 18 %	15 % vs. 32 %	18 % vs. 29 %
			p>0.05	p<0.05	p=0.35
Pomier-Layrargues (2001)	RCT (strong)	39 vs. 41	66 % vs. 18 %	44 % vs. 47 %	47 % vs. 43 %
			p<0.001	p=n.s	p=n.s
Gulberg (2002)	RCT (moderate)	26 vs. 28	16 % vs. 17 %	4 % vs. 7 %	16 % vs. 8 %
			p=n.s	p=n.s	p=n.s
Sauer (2002)	RCT (strong)	42 vs. 43	30 % vs. 19 %	20 % vs. 40 %	18 % vs. 24 %
			p=0.32	p<0.05	p=n.s
Monescillo (2004)	RCT (moderate)	26 vs. 26	50 % vs. 12 %	35 % vs. 31 %	65 % vs. 31 %
			p=0.0001	p=n.s	p=0.01
Garcia-Pagan (2010)	RCT (strong)	31 vs. 32	50 % vs. 3 %	39 % vs. 25 %	39 % vs. 14 %
			p<0.001	p=n.s	p=0.001

C control group (endoscopic treatment ± pharmacological therapy), *T* treatment groups (TIPS), *RCT* randomized control trial, *n.s* not shown decreased the incidence of recurrent variceal bleeding (odds ratio (OR) = 0.32, 95 % confidence interval (CI) (0.24–0.43), $p < 0.00001$), increased the rate of encephalopathy (OR = 2.21, 95 % CI (1.61–3.03), $p < 0.00001$), decreased deaths due to rebleeding (OR = 0.35, 95 % CI (0.18–0.67), $p = 0.002$) but did not cause an overall mortality benefit (OR = 1.17, 95 % CI (0.85–1.61), $p = 0.33$) [33]. In these studies the range for successful stent placement was 87–100 %, portal pressure gradient decrease was from 10 to 16.2 mmHg, and TIPS dysfunction was from 17 to 89 % [33]. Zheng et al. also separated the studies assessing EVL from sclerotherapy, but this did not change the outcomes [33].

Escorsell et al. compared quality of life in patients that received TIPS to endoscopic therapy for secondary prophylaxis. While there was a small trend towards improvement in quality of life after both interventions, there were no significant differences between the TIPS and endoscopic therapy groups [16]. This might be explained by increased incidence of hepatic encephalopathy in the TIPS group being offset by decreased incidence of variceal bleeding. Two controlled studies compared costs of TIPS to medical management with conflicting results [16, 19]. The cost of TIPS in these studies varied from $11,294 to $21,603. A number of cost-effectiveness analyses on TIPS and medical therapy for secondary prophylaxis have been conducted with varying results in determining the most cost effective procedure [34–36]. This difference can likely be explained by the many variables that will influence the cost such as the number of significant rebleeds, endoscopic technique and sessions required for eradication, variations in institutional procedural costs, the number of TIPS revisions required, complications, and the length of follow up. The cost of TIPS is usually highest in the first year and will decline subsequently if limited interventions are required. Closed stents will likely decrease the cost with fewer revisions required [14].

Ascites

Ascites is initially managed non-invasively with diuretics and dietary changes. Refractory cases may require paracentesis or TIPS. There are six randomized control trials (RCT) (Table 34.3) that have been performed comparing paracentesis ± albumin to TIPS for treatment of refractory ascites [37–42]. All these studies concluded that TIPS was superior to paracentesis for the control of refractory ascites as well as improvement of renal function and hemodynamics. Results were inconsistent when it came to worsening hepatic encephalopathy and a mortality benefit [37–42]. These studies had methodologic variation present that contributed to the differences in results, which included the number of participants, inclusion and exclusion criteria, definitions of refractory ascites, volume of paracentesis, technical skills with TIPS, stents used, and follow up measurements.

Five of these studies were published before 2004 and five meta-analysis between 2005 and 2007 analyzed the same results from these studies [43–47]. There was also great heterogeneity present in the results of these analyses. All analyses agreed

Table 34.3 The main outcomes of studies for refractory ascites comparing medical management (paracentesis ±albumin ± salt restriction ± diuretics) to TIPS

Study (year)	Study type (quality of evidence)	Patients (C vs. T)	Ascites recurrence (C vs. T)	Hepatic encephalopathy (C vs. T)	Mortality (C vs. T)
Lebrec (1996)	RCT (moderate)	12 vs. 13	92 % vs. 77 %	0 % vs. 23 %	40 % vs 71 %
			p=n.s	p=n.s	p=0.03
Rossle (2000)	RCT (strong)	31 vs. 29	76 % vs. 21 %	48 % vs. 58 %	74 % vs. 52 %
			p=0.001	p=n.s	p=n.s
Gines (2002)	RCT (strong)	35 vs. 35	83 % vs. 49 %	66 % vs. 77 %	51 % vs 57 %
			p=0.003	p=0.29	p=0.6
Sanyal (2003)	RCT (strong)	57 vs. 52	84 % vs. 42 %	19 % vs. 38 %	37 % vs. 40 %
			p<0.001	p=0.058	p=0.84
Salerno (2004)	RCT (strong)	33 vs. 33	97 % vs. 39 %	39 % vs. 69 %	61 % vs. 39 %
			p=0.0012	p=n.s	p=0.021
Narahara (2011)	RCT (strong)	30 vs. 30	80 % vs 13 %	17 % vs. 67 %	70 % vs. 57 %
			p<0.001	p<0.001	p=0.422

C control group (medical management), *T* treatment groups (TIPS), *RCT* randomized control trial, *n.s* not shown

that TIPS was significantly superior to paracentesis and albumin in preventing recurrence of ascites. However, hepatic encephalopathy was significantly more common in the TIPS group. Overall there was not a significant mortality difference between the two groups. The quality of the meta-analysis and systematic review varied with a number of limitations.

The study by D'Amico et al. was one of the stronger meta-analysis [45]. They excluded the initial trial by Lebrec as it was identified as an outlier with the lowest successful TIPS placement (77 %), the lowest portal pressure gradient decrease (6 mmHg), the lowest secondary patency rates (46 %), and the only study showing a significantly increased mortality with TIPS placement (40 % vs 71 % p=0.03) [37]. The range of technical success in the four other studies was 89–100 %, reduction in portal pressure gradient was 10.4–14 mmHg, and secondary patency rates were 82–93 %. Surgical shunts were rarely placed if TIPS could not be successfully placed. After excluding this study from their analysis, the pooled odds ratio (OR) for recurrence of ascites with TIPS was 0.14 (CI 0.07–0.27), the OR for hepatic encephalopathy with TIPS was 2.26 (CI 1.35–3.76), and OR for mortality with TIPS was 0.74 (CI 0.40–1.37) [45].

All RCTs had a subset of patients that underwent liver transplantation after TIPS. Salerno et al. performed a meta-analysis on the initial five RCTs using individual patient data from four RCTs evaluating the cumulative effects of transplant-free survival [47]. The actuarial probability of transplant free survival was significantly better in the TIPS groups (p=0.035). The average transplant free survival at 1, 2, and 3 years was 63.1 %, 49.0 %, and 38.1 % for the TIPS group and 52.5 %, 35.2 %, and 28.7 % for the paracentesis group. MELD scores did not alter the mortality difference seen between the TIPS and paracentesis groups. Multivariate analysis identified older age, high bilirubin, low plasma sodium, and treatment allocation as predictors of death [47].

Quality of life for TIPS versus paracentesis was only assessed by Sanyal et al. [40]. The SF-36 questionnaire, consisting of a physical and mental component, was used in both groups before and after the interventions. While the scale score improved significantly amongst both arms after the interventions, there was no significant difference in quality of life between the paracentesis and TIPS group [40, 48]. The lack of a significant change in quality of life may be due to the fact that while ascites may improve with TIPS, hepatic encephalopathy may worsen.

Gines et al. showed that the calculated accumulated cost of TIPS was greater in both the United States and Spain per patient at respectively 103 % and 41 % the cost in the paracentesis and albumin group. In the United States the total cost per patient in the TIPS group was $19,813 and $9,765 for the paracentesis and albumin group [39]. The inflated cost of TIPS was partially due to the open stents requiring multiple revisions [14].

Other Manifestations of Portal Hypertension

Non-esophageal Varices

The evidence for TIPS in controlling other manifestations of PH is limited. First line treatment for gastric variceal bleeding, which can be difficult to control, has involved sclerotherapy with cyanoacrylate [11]. TIPS has been used as salvage therapy. A single RCT by Lo et al showed that TIPS decreased rebleeding from gastric varices compared to cyanoacrylate (11 % vs. 38 % p=0.014) while worsening encephalopathy (26 % vs. 3 % P<0.01) without a difference in mortality or other major complications [49]. Uncontrolled trials showed that transfusion dependent portal hypertensive gastropathy may improve with TIPS while gastric antral vascular ectasia does not [50, 51]. Ectopic varices can occur along the gastrointestinal tract and can bleed. Case studies have shown some benefit with TIPS in reducing bleeding [52, 53].

Hepatic Hydrothorax

Uncontrolled trials have assessed the efficacy of TIPS in hepatic hydrothorax. Singh et al. reviewed eight of these studies, which included 332 patients. The mean improvement in respiratory symptoms and complete and partial response rates to the resolution of the hydrothorax were 74 %, 55.9 % and 24.6 % respectively. The average 30-day mortality, 1-year survival, and incidence of hepatic encephalopathy were 18.6 %, 52.3 %, and 26.7 % respectively [54].

Hepatorenal Syndrome

The efficacy of TIPS to manage patients with HRS type 1 and 2 has been studied in a small number of uncontrolled trials. These studies have identified that renal function, hemodynamics, and ascites can improve in select patients with low MELD and Child-Pugh scores undergoing TIPS, but are not powered to show a survival benefit [55–58].

Other

TIPS had been used in the treatment of Budd-Chiari syndrome. A retrospective study of 221 patients showed that TIPS could be successfully used after failure of medical therapy in appropriately selected patients [59]. Small case studies have looked at the use of TIPS in sinuosoidal obstruction syndrome. While there was an improvement in ascites, most patients still died [60]. Very little literature exists for TIPS in hepatopulmonary syndrome to support its use and portopulmonary hypertension is a contraindication to TIPS [61].

Recommendations

- TIPS is superior to medical management in preventing recurrent variceal bleeding and recurrent ascites while worsening hepatic encephalopathy (evidence quality high; strong recommendation).
- TIPS may improve mortality in well-selected patients with variceal hemorrhage or refractory ascites (evidence quality moderate; recommendation moderate).
- TIPS may have some utility in other manifestations of PH (evidence quality low; recommendation low).

A Personal View of the Data

TIPS has an important role to play in variceal hemorrhage and refractory ascites. It decreases rebleeding and ascites while worsening encephalopathy. It has not consistently shown a mortality benefit, but has displayed a benefit in specific circumstances. However, the technology of TIPS has evolved with closed stents, which have been shown to be superior to open stents with lower rates of occlusion without worsening encephalopathy [14]. Most of the literature has not been done using the closed stent and since this is a newer technology, studies will need to be repeated to see if this changes outcomes. Further studies are also required to study the other manifestations of PH.

References

1. Garcia-Pagan JC, Gracia- Sancho J, Bosch J. Functional aspects on the pathophysiology of portal hypertension in cirrhosis. J Hepatol. 2012;57:458–61.
2. Samonakis DN, Triantos CK, Thalheimer U, Patch DW, Burroughs AK. Management of portal hypertension. Postgrad Med J. 2004;80:634–41.
3. Garcia-Tsao G, Sanyal AJ, Grace ND, Carey W, Practice Guidelines Committee of the American Association for the Study of Liver Disease, Practice Parameters Committee of the American College of Gastroenterology. Prevention and management of gastroesophageal varices and variceal hemorrhage in cirrhosis. Hepatology. 2007;46:922–38.
4. Loffroy R, Estivalet L, Cherblanc V, Favelier S, Pottecher P, Hamza S, et al. Transjugular intrahepatic portosystemic shunt for the management of acute variceal hemorrhage. World J Gastroenterol. 2013;19:6131–43.
5. Boyer TD, Haskal ZJ. AASLD practice guidelines: the role of transjugular intrahepatic portosystemic shunt (TIPS) in the management of portal hypertension. J Vasc Interv Radiol. 2005;16:615–29.
6. Russo MW, Sood A, Jacobson IM, Brown RS. Transjugular intrahepatic portosystemic shunt for refractory ascites: an analysis of the literature on efficacy, morbidity, and mortality. Am J Gastroenterol. 2003;98:2521–7.
7. Rossle M, Gerbes AL. TIPS for the treatment of refractory ascites, hepatorenal syndrome, and hepatic hydrothorax: a critical update. Gut. 2010;59:988–1000.
8. Machicao VI, Balakrishnan M, Fallon MB. Pulmonary complications in chronic liver disease. Hepatology. 2014;59:1627–37.
9. Martin P, DiMartini A, Feng S, Brown R, Fallon M. Evaluation of liver transplantation in adults: 2013 practice guidelines of the American Association for the Study of Liver Diseases and the American Society of Transplantation. Hepatology. 2014;59:1144–65.
10. Boyer TD. Transjugular intrahepatic portosystemic shunt in the management of complications of portal hypertension. Curr Gastroenterol Rep. 2008;10:30–5.
11. Nusrat S, Khan MS, Fazili J, Madhoun MF. Cirrhosis and it's complications: evidence based treatment. World J Gastroenterol. 2014;20:5442–60.
12. Monescillo A, Martinez-Lagares F, Ruiz-del-Arbol L, Sierra A, Guevara C, Jimenez E, et al. Influence of portal hypertension and it's early decompression by TIPS placement on the outcome of variceal bleeding. Hepatology. 2004;40:793–801.
13. Garcia-Pagan JC, Caca K, Bureau C, Laleman W, Appenrodt B, Luca A, et al. Early use of TIPS in patient with cirrhosis and variceal bleeding. N Engl J Med. 2010;362:2370–9.
14. Bureau C, Garcia-Pagan JC, Otal P, Pomier-Layrargues G, Chabbert V, Cortez C, et al. Improved clinical outcome using polytetrafluoroethlene-coated stents for TIPS. Results of a randomized study. Gastroenterology. 2004;126:469–75.
15. Corbett C, Mangat K, Olliff S, Tripathi D. The role of transjugular intrahepatic portosystemic stent-shunt (TIPSS) in the management of variceal hemorrhage. Liver Int. 2012;32:1493–504.
16. Escorsell A, Banares R, Carcia-Pagan JC, Gilabert R, Moitinho E, Piqueras B, et al. TIPS versus drug therapy in preventing variceal rebleeding in advanced cirrhosis: a randomized controlled trial. Hepatology. 2002;35:385–92.

17. Cabrera J, Maynar M, Granados R, Gorriz E, Reyes R, Pulido-Duque JM, et al. Transjugular intrahepatic portosystemic shunt versus sclerotherapy in the elective treatment of variceal hemorrhage. Gastroenterology. 1996;110:832–9.
18. Cello JP, Ring EJ, Olcott EW, Koch J, Gordon R, Sandhu J, et al. Endoscopic sclerotherapy compared with percutaneous transjugular intrahepatic portosystemic shunt after initial sclerotherapy in patients with acute variceal hemorrhage. A randomized, controlled trial. Ann Intern Med. 1997;26:1115–22.
19. Jalan R, Forrest EH, Stanley AJ, Redhead DN, Forbes J, Dillon JF, et al. A randomized trial comparing transjugular intrahepatic portosystemic shunt-shunt with variceal band ligation in the prevention of rebleeding from esophageal varices. Hepatology. 1997;26:1115–22.
20. Rossle M, Deibert P, Haag K, Ochs A, Olschewski M, Siegerstetter V, et al. Randomised trial of tranjugular-intrahepatic-portosystemic shunt versus endoscopy plus propranolol for prevention of variceal bleeding. Lancet. 1997;349:1043–9.
21. Sanyal AJ, Freedman AM, Luketic VA, Purdum PP, Shiffman ML, Cole PE, et al. Transjugular intrahepatic portosystemic shunts compared with endoscopic sclerotherapy for the prevention of recurrent variceal hemorrhage. A randomized controlled trial. Ann Intern Med. 1997;126:849–57.
22. Sauer P, Theilmann L, Stremmel W, Benz C, Richter GM, Stiehl A. Transjugular intrahepatic portosystemic shunt versus sclerotherapy plus propranolol for variceal rebleeding. Gastroenterology. 1997;113:1623–31.
23. Merli M, Salaerno F, Riggio O, de Franchis R, Fiaccadori F, Meddi P, et al. Transjugular intrahepatic portosystemic shunt versus endoscopic sclerotherapy for the prevention of variceal bleeding in cirrhosis: a randomized multicenter trial. Gruppo Italiano Studio TIPS (G.I.S.T). Hepatology. 1998;27:48–53.
24. Garcia-Villarreal L, Martinez-Lagares F, Sierra A, Guevara C, Marrero JM, Jimenez E, et al. Transjugular intrahepatic portosystemic shunt versus endoscopic sclerotherapy for the prevention of variceal rebleeding after recent variceal hemorrhage. Hepatology. 1999;29:27–32.
25. Narahara Y, Kanazawa H, Kawamata H, Tada N, Saitoh H, Matsuzaka S, et al. A randomized clinical trial comparing transjugular intrahepatic portosystemic shunt with endoscopic sclerotherapy in the long-term management of patients with cirrhosis after recent variceal hemorrhage. Hepatol Res. 2001;21:189–98.
26. Pomier-Layrargues G, Villeneuve JP, Deschenes M, Bui B, Perreault P, Fenyves D, et al. Transjugular intrahepatic portosystemic shunt (TIPS) versus endoscopic variceal ligation in the prevention of variceal rebleeding in patients with cirrhosis: a randomized trial. Gut. 2001;48:390–6.
27. Gulberg V, Schepke M, Geigenberger G, Holl J, Brensing KA, Waggershauser T, et al. Transjugular intrahepatic portosystemic shunting is not superior to endoscopic variceal band ligation for prevention of variceal rebleeding in cirrhotic patients: a randomized, controlled trial. Scand J Gastroenterol. 2002;37:338–43.
28. Sauer P, Hansmann J, Richter GM, Stremmel W, Stiehl A. Endoscopic variceal ligation plus propranolol vs. transjugular intrahepatic portosystemic stent shunt: a long-term randomized trial. Endoscopy. 2002;34:690–7.
29. Luca A, D'Amico G, La Galla R, Midiri M, Morabito A, Pagliaro L. TIPS for prevention of recurrent bleeding in patients with cirrhosis: meta-analysis of randomized clinical trials. Radiology. 1999;212:411–21.
30. Papatheodoridis GV, Goulis J, Leandro G, Patch D, Burroughs AK. Transjugular intrahepatic portosystemic shunt compared with endoscopic treatment for prevention of variceal rebleeding: a meta-analysis. Hepatology. 1999;30:612–22.
31. Burroughs AK, Vangeli M. Transjugular intrahepatic portosystemic shunt versus endoscopic therapy: randomized trials for secondary prophylaxis of variceal bleeding: an updated meta-analysis. Scan J Gastroenterol. 2002;37:249–52.
32. Khan S, Tudur SC, Williamson P, Sutton R. Portosystemic shunts versus endoscopic therapy for variceal rebleeding in patients with cirrhosis. Cochrane Database Syst Rev. 2006;18:CD000553.

33. Zheng M, Chen Y, Bai J, Zeng Q, You J, Jin R, et al. Transjugular intrahepatic portosystemic shunt versus endoscopic therapy in the secondary prophylaxis of variceal rebleeding in cirrhotic patients. J Clin Gastroenterol. 2008;42:507–16.
34. Russo MW, Zacks SL, Sandler RS, Brown RS. Cost-effectiveness analysis of transjugular intrahepatic portosystemic shunt (TIPS) versus endoscopic therapy for the prevention of recurrent esophageal variceal bleeding. Hepatology. 2000;31:358–63.
35. Rubenstein JH, Eisen GM, Inadomi JM. A cost-utility analysis of secondary prophylaxis for variceal hemorrhage. Am J Gastroenterol. 2004;99:1274–88.
36. Harman DJ, McCorry RB, Jacob RP, Lim TR, O'Neill R, Ryder SD, et al. Economic modeling of early transjugular intrahepatic portosystemic shunt insertion for acute variceal hemorrhage. Eur J Gastroenterol Hepatol. 2013;25:201–7.
37. Lebrec D, Giuily N, Hadengue A, Vilgrain V, Moreau R, Poynard T, et al. Transjugular intrahepatic portosystemic shunts: comparison with paracentesis in patients with cirrhosis and refractory ascites: a randomized control trial. J Hepatol. 1996;25:135–44.
38. Rossle M, Ochs A, Gulberg V, Siegerstetter V, Holl J, Deibert P, et al. A comparison of paracentesis and transjugular intrahepatic portosystemic shunting in patients with ascites. N Engl J Med. 2000;342:1701–7.
39. Gines P, Uriz J, Calahorra B, Garcia-Tsao G, Kamath PS, Del Arbol LR, et al. Transjugular intrahepatic portosystemic shunting versus paracentesis plus albumin for refractory ascites in cirrhosis. Gastroenterology. 2002;123:1839–47.
40. Sanyal AJ, Genning C, Reddy KR, Wong F, Kowdley KV, Benner K, et al. The North American study for the treatment of refractory ascites. Gastroenterology. 2003;124:634–41.
41. Salerno F, Merli M, Riggio O, Cazzaniga M, Valeriano V, Pozzi M, et al. Randomized controlled study of TIPS versus paracentesis plus albumin in cirrhosis with severe ascites. Hepatology. 2004;40:629–35.
42. Narahara Y, Kanazawa H, Fukuda T, Matsushita Y, Harimoto H, Kidokoro H, et al. Transjugular intrahepatic portosystemic shunt versus paracentesis plus albumin in patients with refractory ascites who have good hepatic and renal function: a prospective randomized trial. J Gastroenterol. 2011;46:78–85.
43. Deltenre P, Mathurin P, Dharancy S, Moreau R, Bulois P, Henrion J, et al. Transjugular intrahepatic portosystemic shun in refractory ascites: a meta-analysis. Liver Int. 2005;25:349–56.
44. Albillos A, Banares R, Gonzalez M, Catalina MV, Molinero LM. A meta-analysis of 9. transjugular intrahepatic portosystemic shunt versus paracentesis for refractory ascites. J Hepatol. 2005;43:990–6.
45. D'Amico G, Luca A, Morabito A, Miraglia R, D'Amico M. Uncovered transjugular intrahepatic portosystemic shunt for refractory ascites: a meta- analysis. Gastroenterology. 2005;129:1282–93.
46. Saab S, Nieto JM, Lewis SK, Runyon BA. TIPS versus paracentesis for cirrhotic patients with refractory ascites. Cochrane Database Syst Rev. 2006; (4):CD004889.
47. Salerno F, Camma C, Enea M, Rossle M, Wong F. Transjugular intrahepatic portosystemic shunt for refractory ascites: a meta-analysis of individual patient data. Gastroenterology. 2007;133:825–34.
48. Campbell MS, Brensinger CM, Sanyal AJ, Gennings C, Wong F, Kowdley KV, et al. Quality of life in refractory ascites: transjugular intrahepatic poral-systemic shunting versus medical therapy. Hepatology. 2005;42:635–40.
49. Lo GH, Lian HL, Chen WC, Chen MH, Lai KH, Hsu PI, et al. A prospective, randomized controlled trial of transjugular intrahepatic portosystemic shunt versus cyanoacrylate injection in the prevention of gastric variceal bleeding. Endoscopy. 2007;39:679–85.
50. Spahr L, Villeneuve JP, Dufresne MP, Tasse D, Bui B, Willems B, et al. Gastric antral vascular ectasia in cirrhotic patients: absence of relation with portal hypertension. Gut. 1999;44:739–42.
51. Kamath PS, Lacerda M, Ahlquist DA, McKusick MA, Andrews JC, Nagorney DA. Gastric mucosal responses to intrahepatic portosystemic shunting in patients with cirrhosis. Gastroenterology. 2000;118:905–11.

52. Vangeli M, Patch D, Terreni N, Tibballs J, Watkinson A, Davies N, Burroughs AK. Bleeding ectopic varices – treatment with transjugular intrahepatic porto-systemic shunt (TIPS) and embolisation. J Hepatol. 2004;41:560–6.
53. Vidal V, Joly L, Perreault P, Bouchard L, Lafortune M, Pomier-Layrargues G. Usefulness of transjugular intrahepatic portosystemic shunt in the management of bleeding ectopic varices in cirrhotic patients. Cardiovasc Intervent Radiol. 2006;29:216–9.
54. Singh A, Bajwa A, Shujaat A. Evidence-based review of the management of hepatic hydrothorax. Respiration. 2013;86:155–73.
55. Guevara M, Gines P, Bandi JC, Gilabert R, Sort P, Jimenez W, et al. Transjugular intrahepatic portosystemic shunt in hepatorenal syndrome: effects on renal function and vasoactive systems. Hepatology. 1998;28:416–22.
56. Brensing KA, Textor J, Peerz J, Scheidermaier P, Raab P, Strunk H, et al. Long term outcome after transjugular intrahepatic portosystemic stent-shunt in non-transplant cirrhotics with hepatorenal syndrome: a phase 2 study. Gut. 2000;47:288–95.
57. Testino G, Ferro C, Sumberaz A, Messa P, Morelli N, Gaudagni B, et al. Type-2 hepatorenal syndrome and refractory ascites: role of transjugular intrahepatic portosystemic stent-shunt in eighteen patients with advanced cirrhosis awaiting orthotopic liver transplantation. Hepatogastroenterology. 2003;50:1753–5.
58. Wong F, Pantea L, Sniderman K. Midodrine, octreotide, albumin, and TIPS in selected patients with cirrhosis and type 1 hepatorenal syndrome. Hepatology. 2004;40:55–64.
59. Garcia-Pagan JC, Heydtmann M, Raffa S, Plessier A, Murad S, Fabris F, Vizzini G, Gonzales Abraldes J, Olliff S, Nicolini A. TIPS for Budd-Chiari syndrome: long-term results and prognostics factors in 124 patients. Gastroenterology. 2008;135:808–15.
60. Azoulay D, Castaing D, Lemoine A, Hargreaves GM, Bismuth H. Transjugular intrahepatic portosystemic shunt (TIPS) for severe veno-occlusive disease of the liver following bone marrow transplantation. Bone Marrow Transplant. 2000;25:987–92.
61. Paramesh AS, Husain SZ, Shneider B, Guller J, Tokat I, Gondolesi GE, et al. Improvement in hepatopulmonary syndrome after transjugular intrahepatic portosystemic shunt: case report and review of the literature. Pediatr Transplant. 2003;7:157–62.

Chapter 35
Should All Hepatic Arteriovenous Fistulas Be Embolized?

Darren van Beek and Brian Funaki

Abstract Hepatic arteriovenous fistulae (AVF) are rare but increasingly encountered clinical entities. Due to their poorly understood natural history and multiple underlying etiologies, treatment currently represents a clinical quandary. There are no definitive studies regarding management, but rather, only small published case series. A better understanding of the underlying mechanisms of AVF formation, factors affecting clinical significance, and knowledge of the risks and benefits of treatment can help guide physicians in their management of this complex clinical dilemma.

Keywords Arteriovenous fistula • Arterioportal fistula • Embolization • Hepatic transplant

Introduction

A hepatic arteriovenous fistula (AVF) is a rare clinical entity that has been increasingly diagnosed in recent decades. As the natural history and management options are unclear, it poses a diagnostic dilemma for clinicians.

Part of the confusion regarding a hepatic AVF arises from the fact that it is a catch-all term for multiple pathophysiologic entities arising from numerous underlying causes. Anatomically, this group can be divided into intrahepatic and extrahepatic shunts. Much of the early literature on the topic focused on extrahepatic shunts between the visceral arterial and portal venous systems. A review published in 1987 showed 30 cases of fistulas between the arterial and portal venous systems, of which only 3 were intrahepatic [1, 2]. Some authors have speculated that this early reported

D. van Beek • B. Funaki (✉)
Department of Radiology, Section of Vascular and Interventional Radiology, University of Chicago Medical Center, 5841 S. Maryland Avenue MC 2026, Room Q-219, Chicago, IL 60637, USA
e-mail: bfunaki@radiology.bsd.uchicago.edu

J.M. Millis, J.B. Matthews (eds.), *Difficult Decisions in Hepatobiliary and Pancreatic Surgery*, Difficult Decisions in Surgery: An Evidence-Based Approach, DOI 10.1007/978-3-319-27365-5_35

preponderance of extrahepatic AVFs was related to their more sensational clinical presentations and dramatic, typically traumatic, etiologies [3].

In the last 30 years, intrahepatic AVFs have been found to represent the vast majority of arterioportal fistulae. This book chapter will focus exclusively on intrahepatic AVFs as the underlying mechanisms and clinical management differ from their extrahepatic counterparts. Intrahepatic AVFs are also more clinically pertinent, as they are much more likely to be encountered by clinicians.

Intrahepatic AVFs may be congenital, post-traumatic, or malignant in etiology. Like extrahepatic AVFs, arteriovenous shunting related to intrahepatic tumors is a unique clinical entity with additional management complexities. The physiology of malignant shunting also tends to be more multifocal in nature and there are additional available treatment options including chemotherapy, chemoembolization, and ablation. For these reasons, malignant intrahepatic AVFs are beyond the scope of this book chapter.

Search Strategy

A literature search of English language publications from 1994 to 2014 was used to identify published data on hepatic AVFs using the PICO outline (Table 35.1). Databases searched were PubMed, Embase, and Cochrane Evidence Based Medicine. Terms used in the search were "hepatic arteriovenous fistula", "hepatic arterioportal fistula", "hepatic arteriovenous fistula management", "hepatic arteriovenous fistula treatment", "hepatic arteriovenous fistula embolization", "hepatic arterioportal fistula management", "hepatic arterioportal fistula treatment", "hepatic arterioportal fistula embolization", "hepatic arteriovenous malformation management", "hepatic arteriovenous malformation treatment", and "hepatic arteriovenous malformation embolization." Articles specifically addressing AVFs in the setting of malignancy or exclusively reviewing extrahepatic AVFs were excluded. The results yielded 82 case series/reports, 4 additional case reports containing systematic reviews of the literature, and 6 review articles. No prospective clinical trials or guidelines statements were found. Additional articles published prior to 1994 that are cited in the more modern literature are referenced only for historical background.

Table 35.1 PICO table for perioperative arrhythmia prophylaxis for lung resection

P (Patients)	I (Intervention)	C (Comparator group)	O (Outcomes measured)
Patients with intrahepatic arteriovenous fistulae occurring outside the setting of malignancy or HHT	Embolization	Surgical management or observation	Rate of symptom reduction, complications, conversion to surgical management

Results

After applying the aforementioned exclusion criteria, a total of 134 unique cases of intrahepatic AVFs were identified. The majority of these are presented in small reports detailing one or two patients with a handful of authors presenting series of 5–7 patients [4–8]. Analysis of the treatments and outcomes presented in the literature is complicated by the wide variety of approaches (percutaneous versus trans-arterial embolization), choice of embolic agent (coils, detachable balloons, liquid embolics, thrombin impregnated gelatin, occlusion devices, and a combination of any of the above), and patient population (ages 1 month to 83 years). Some general trends, however, can be gleaned from the data. In the 134 patients, 125 underwent attempted embolization while 9 were followed clinically. Of the 125 undergoing embolization, 106 (85 %) achieved complete resolution or clinically significant improvement in their presenting symptoms after embolization alone. Of the remaining 19, 1 died of fulminant liver failure while the other 18 underwent surgical management with either partial hepatectomy or transplant. Multiple embolization procedures were performed in 25 (20 %) of the patients, 17 of which achieved clinical improvement without surgical intervention.

Prevalence and Clinical Importance

The prevalence of hepatic AVFs is unknown. This is largely due to the fact that the majority are asymptomatic, and therefore the condition is presumed to be dramatically underreported [2, 9, 10]. Several case series have examined the prevalence of AVFs in liver transplant recipients undergoing hepatic angiograms. The prevalence was found to be between 0 and 5.4 % [3, 11–13]. This figure, however, is expected to be much higher compared to the general population as these transplanted livers have typically undergone many more percutaneous interventions that directly increase the risk of AVF. Saad et al. showed that while 5.4 % of patients had angiographically detectable AVFs, only 0.2 % of patients were symptomatic. This underscores both how underreported and potentially how benign these AVFs may be.

Risk Factors

One of the primary reasons for the increasing incidence of hepatic AVFs is the well-established link between AVFs and percutaneous hepatic procedures [9, 10]. As the number of these percutaneous interventions has increased, so too has the number of hepatic AVFs. Iatrogenic causes are now responsible for greater than 50 % of AVFs [10, 14]. Percutaneous biliary drain placement and percutaneous cholangiography can both lead to AVF formation, however, percutaneous liver biopsy is the most common cause of iatrogenic AVF due to its commonality. Various case series have reported AVFs occurring after 0.008–5 % of liver biopsies [9, 15]. While a wide range, this is likely related to the length of follow-up time between biopsy and imaging investigation. As described below, many biopsy-induced AVFs resolve quickly and spontaneously.

Detection and Evaluation

Asymptomatic AVFs may be detected incidentally in patients undergoing hepatic angiography, ultrasound, or CT angiography for other indications. Symptoms from AVFs typically relate to portal hypertension, which may occur in larger shunts that cause arterialization of the portal venous system. Ascites and varix formation, with or without associated gastrointestinal hemorrhage, are the most common presentations. Hemobilia secondary to erosion into the biliary tree, heart failure, and mesenteric ischemia due to high volume shunting away from the visceral arterial system are less common presenting symptoms. In contrast to other causes of portal hypertension such as cirrhosis, AVFs may also be accompanied by an abdominal bruit detectable on physical exam.

As with other vascular conditions involving the liver, ultrasound is the main diagnostic modality used to evaluate AVFs [16]. While angiography remains the gold standard, it is also more expensive and invasive and therefore typically reserved for cases in which embolization is planned. In a short series evaluating orthotopic liver transplant patients with known AVFs, it was shown that ultrasound detected all hemodynamically significant AVFs which the authors defined as opacification of the main portal vein or a first order branch in the early arterial phase [2]. Various authors have also examined the utility of CT angiography in the evaluation of AVFs. Nguyen et al. proposed a "double barrel sign," which showed early opacification of a portal venous branch running parallel to a feeding hepatic artery [17]. This "double barrel sign" had a sensitivity of 64 % and a specificity of 100 % for the identification of AVFs in the 33 patients studied.

In addition to detecting AVFs, ultrasound can provide information regarding their hemodynamic significance. Vascular manifestations include decreased resistive indices in the involved hepatic artery relative to the contralateral side, along with increased resistance and eventual reversal of flow in the portal vein. Again, no prospective studies have been conducted to determine cut-off values at which intervention is warranted.

Natural History

The natural history of hepatic AVFs remains poorly elucidated. Detection of AVFs may occur years after the inciting event that created the fistula. There are numerous case reports of AVFs first manifesting clinical symptoms 15–52 years after a known traumatic event or hepatic intervention [18–22]. Because of this delay, a detailed clinical history is required in any patient presenting with a hepatic AVF. These cases of delayed presentation also indicate that, in at least a portion of cases, previously asymptomatic AVFs progress to become clinically significant. Unfortunately, with the majority of AVFs being asymptomatic and the absence of prospective longitudinal studies, the percentage of AVFs which enlarge over long periods remains unclear.

Several smaller studies have evaluated the short-term natural history of AVFs after percutaneous liver biopsy (PLB). As described above, the rate of biopsy-induced AVFs has been reported to be up to 5 %. In patients undergoing angiography immediately after PLB, hemorrhage, pseudoaneurysms, and AVFs are relatively common. AVFs represent 37 % of vascular injuries immediately after biopsy [23]. Of these vascular injuries, however, AVFs are most likely to persist. By 1 week after biopsy, AVFs account for 86 % of residual vascular abnormalities and at 1 month after biopsy only AVFs will persist [9, 23].

Despite being the most persistent of the intervention-related vascular injuries, the majority of AVFs resolve spontaneously and only a minority progress [9, 10]. By 1 week post-biopsy, only 10 % of initially detectable AVFs remain [24]. While there are no definitive criteria to determine which AVFs will persist, observational evidence suggests that peripherally-located AVFs are more likely to resolve spontaneously [25]. Size also appears important as smaller AVFs tend to resolve spontaneously [26]. This has led many authors to advocate for observation, typically with serial ultrasound, as the primary management of small, asymptomatic AVFs. Even if an AVF persists under observation, it may not require intervention, as there are reports of several asymptomatic AVFs spontaneously closing months and even years after initial diagnosis [27].

Treatment Indications and Outcomes

Treatment of hepatic AVFs was previously the exclusive domain of surgical interventions including hepatic artery ligation, fistula division and repair, hepatic segmentectomy, or liver transplant. In current clinical practice, endovascular intervention with embolization has become the mainstay of treatment [10, 13, 28]. Coil embolization is most common, but the effective use of liquid embolic, sclerosing, and thrombotic agents have all been reported. In addition, specialized closure devices, i.e. Amplatzer plugs, can be used for large diameter fistulae [26].

No indications have been established for the treatment of asymptomatic AVFs [29]. As discussed previously, it is reasonable to believe that the vast majority of hepatic AVFs are asymptomatic and undiagnosed. However, it has also been shown that a percentage of these eventually progress to become symptomatic. For this reason, regular observation of known fistulae appears prudent in order to identify hemodynamic progression prior to the manifestation of high-morbidity clinical entities such as variceal bleeding and liver failure.

Once AVFs are symptomatic, intervention is warranted [6]. The technical aspects of embolization are beyond the scope of this chapter, but it is worth noting that the goal of treatment is not necessarily complete occlusion of the shunt, but rather improvement in the hemodynamic derangement. It is not uncommon that after embolization of the main fistula, the change in hemodynamics may reveal smaller adjacent fistulae. Before proceeding with further embolization, physicians must carefully consider the increased risk of complications associated with more extensive embolization and weigh these against the expected clinical significance of smaller fistulae.

Special considerations must also be made with regard to the management of AVFs occurring in transplanted livers. Within liver grafts, there is a higher risk of hepatic artery thrombosis occurring during super-selective embolization as well as more devastating consequences. Despite this, one prominent author on the subject has advocated for earlier treatment of AVFs in transplanted livers citing the increased risk of embolization complications if the lesion is allowed to grow [2, 4].

An additional special situation not included in this literature review, but worthy of brief discussion, is the management of hepatic arteriovenous malformations in hereditary hemorrhage telangiectasia (HHT). Early attempts to embolize these lesions were associated with unacceptably high morbidity and mortality [30]. Based on this, current treatment guidelines recommend that embolization be reserved only for symptomatic patients that have failed medical management [31, 32].

Recommendations

Hepatic AVFs represent a collection of diverse and complex clinical entities. The relatively limited volume of observational research and a complete lack of systematic, prospective studies limit recommendations regarding management. Limited evidence based on small case series suggests that asymptomatic and hemodynamically insignificant hepatic AVFs merit observation with serial ultrasound exams until either resolution or progression to hemodynamic significance. Yearly observation is reasonable in incidentally detected lesions. AVFs noted acutely as a consequence of an associated hepatic intervention or trauma merit more frequent initial observation before spacing out to annual examinations.

Available evidence suggests that once AVFs become symptomatic or display altered portal venous hemodynamics, immediate endovascular intervention is warranted. Limited evidence suggests that earlier intervention should be considered in the setting of liver transplants or other patients in whom it is reasonable to expect worse outcomes if the lesion progresses.

Recommendations

- Not all hepatic arteriovenous fistula should be embolized.
- Once diagnosed, asymptomatic hepatic AVFs merit surveillance with ultrasound until resolution or progression to hemodynamic significance.

- Symptomatic or hemodynamically significant AVFs merit prompt treatment with embolization.
- Earlier intervention can be considered in the setting of liver transplants or other patients in whom it is reasonable to expect worse outcomes if the lesion progresses.

References

1. Strodel WE, et al. Presentation and perioperative management of arterioportal fistulas. Arch Surg. 1987;122(5):563–71.
2. Saad WE, et al. Endoluminal management of arterioportal fistulae in liver transplant recipients: a single-center experience. Vasc Endovascular Surg. 2006;40(6):451–9.
3. Saad W, et al. Prevalence, presentation, and endovascular management of hemodynamically or clinically significant arterio-portal fistulae in living and cadaveric donor liver transplant recipients. Clin Transplant. 2012;26(4):532–8.
4. Saad WE. Management of nonocclusive hepatic artery complications after liver transplantation. Tech Vasc Interv Radiol. 2007;10(3):221–32.
5. Falkenstein K, et al. Arterial-venous fistulas following pediatric liver transplant case studies. Pediatr Transplant. 2007;11(6):683–8.
6. Kumar A, et al. Hepatic arteriovenous fistulae: role of interventional radiology. Dig Dis Sci. 2012;57(10):2703–12.
7. Tasar M, et al. Intrahepatic arterioportal fistula and its treatment with detachable balloon and transcatheter embolization with coils and microspheres. Clin Imaging. 2005;29(5):325–30.
8. Vauthey JN, et al. The arterioportal fistula syndrome: clinicopathologic features, diagnosis, and therapy. Gastroenterology. 1997;113(4):1390–401.
9. Okuda K, et al. Frequency of intrahepatic arteriovenous fistula as a sequela to percutaneous needle puncture of the liver. Gastroenterology. 1978;74(6):1204–7.
10. Jabbour N, et al. Arterioportal fistula following liver biopsy. Three cases occurring in liver transplant recipients. Dig Dis Sci. 1995;40(5):1041–4.
11. Zajko AB, et al. Angiography of liver transplantation patients. Radiology. 1985;157(2):305–11.
12. Wozney P, et al. Vascular complications after liver transplantation: a 5-year experience. AJR Am J Roentgenol. 1986;147(4):657–63.
13. Karatzas T, et al. Vascular complications, treatment, and outcome following orthotopic liver transplantation. Transplant Proc. 1997;29(7):2853–5.
14. Kakati BR, et al. Hepatic arterioportal fistula presenting as gastric variceal hemorrhage. J Gastrointestin Liver Dis. 2014;23(2):211–4.
15. Van Thiel DH, et al. Liver biopsy. Its safety and complications as seen at a liver transplant center. Transplantation. 1993;55(5):1087–90.
16. Itri JN, Heller MT, Tublin ME. Hepatic transplantation: postoperative complications. Abdom Imaging. 2013;38(6):1300–33.
17. Nguyen CT, et al. MDCT diagnosis of post-traumatic hepatic arterio-portal fistulas. Emerg Radiol. 2013;20(3):225–32.
18. Blecher GA, Bohmer R. Hepatoportal fistula in an 83-year-old male, presenting with hematemesis 52 years after blunt trauma. Surg Laparosc Endosc Percutan Tech. 2013;23(2):e84–6.
19. Nojiri K, Sugimoto K, Shiraki K. Ascites caused by arterioportal fistula 15 years after liver biopsy. Clin Gastroenterol Hepatol. 2011;9(4):e31–2.
20. Guha IN, et al. Case report of an arterioportal fistula, presenting with accelerated decompensation and sepsis, twenty-six years after initial liver biopsy. Hepatol Res. 2005;32(4):252–5.

21. Pohle T, Fischbach R, Domschke W. Arterioportal fistula: a rare cause of portal hypertension and abdominal pain. Scand J Gastroenterol. 2001;36(11):1227–9.
22. Kayser S, et al. Rapidly progressive portal hypertension 23 years after post-traumatic arterioportal fistula of the liver. Am J Gastroenterol. 1996;91(7):1442–6.
23. Hellekant C. Vascular complications following needle puncture of the liver. Clinical angiography. Acta Radiol Diagn (Stockh). 1976;17(2):209–22.
24. Quiroga S, et al. Complications of orthotopic liver transplantation: spectrum of findings with helical CT. Radiographics. 2001;21(5):1085–102.
25. Guzman EA, McCahill LE, Rogers FB. Arterioportal fistulas: introduction of a novel classification with therapeutic implications. J Gastrointest Surg. 2006;10(4):543–50.
26. Ward TJ, Marin ML, Lookstein RA. Embolization of a giant arterioportal fistula requiring multiple Amplatzer vascular plugs. J Vasc Surg. 2015;62(6):1636–9.
27. Horiike N, et al. Spontaneous closure of intrahepatic portovenous shunt in a noncirrhotic patient with recurrent encephalopathy. Dig Dis Sci. 2003;48(3):551–5.
28. Chavan A, et al. Transcatheter coil occlusion of an intrahepatic arterioportal fistula in a transplanted liver. Bildgebung. 1993;60(4):215–8.
29. Kittaka H, Akimoto H, Tashiro K. A case report of spontaneous closure of a posttraumatic arterioportal fistula. Case Rep Emerg Med. 2013;2013:623704.
30. Chavan A, et al. Hepatic artery embolization for treatment of patients with hereditary hemorrhagic telangiectasia and symptomatic hepatic vascular malformations. Eur Radiol. 2004;14(11):2079–85.
31. Buscarini E, et al. Liver involvement in hereditary hemorrhagic telangiectasia: consensus recommendations. Liver Int. 2006;26(9):1040–6.
32. Faughnan ME, et al. International guidelines for the diagnosis and management of hereditary haemorrhagic telangiectasia. J Med Genet. 2011;48(2):73–87.

Chapter 36
Early or Delayed Cholecystectomy in Acute Gallstone Pancreatitis

Darren S. Bryan and Mustafa Hussain

Abstract

Introduction
Acute biliary pancreatitis is one of the most common gastrointestinal illnesses necessitating inpatient hospital admission. With an increasing incidence of gallstone disease, in the setting of a changing healthcare landscape, surgical indications must be carefully examined. The principles of management, including common duct clearance, bowel rest, and interval cholecystectomy to avoid recurrent disease have not changed, however with the refinement of minimally invasive techniques, timing of intervention deserves re-examination. We seek to make evidence based recommendations on the timing of cholecystectomy following acute biliary pancreatitis.

Methods
OVID Medline, EMBASE, and Cochrane Review databases were queried in systematic fashion for English language articles published after 1994 using "Cholecystectomy, laparoscopic" and "Pancreatitis". To be included, studies must state a laparoscopic success rate, morbidity, and mortality. Studies not classifying severity of pancreatitis (or mixing mild and severe patients), those with fewer than ten patients, and those not identifying time until laparoscopic cholecystectomy were excluded. Identified articles were examined for relevance.

Results
Four hundred sixty-two unique publications were identified. Nine met inclusion criteria and were subsequently included in analysis. Eight were retrospective studies. One prospective randomized trial was identified and included.

D.S. Bryan • M. Hussain (✉)
Department of Surgery, Biological Sciences Division, The University of Chicago, 5841 S Maryland Ave, Chicago, IL 60637, USA
e-mail: hussainm@uchicago.edu

J.M. Millis, J.B. Matthews (eds.), *Difficult Decisions in Hepatobiliary and Pancreatic Surgery*, Difficult Decisions in Surgery: An Evidence-Based Approach, DOI 10.1007/978-3-319-27365-5_36

Conclusions
Management recommendations are made based on severity of pancreatitis. For patients with mild, stable pancreatitis, we make a strong recommendation for laparoscopic cholecystectomy at the earliest convenience. In patients with severe pancreatitis, there is insufficient evidence to make a recommendation for an appropriate interval for laparoscopic cholecystectomy, however patients should be considered for endoscopic sphincterotomy as a bridging procedure.

Keywords Early cholecystectomy • Delayed cholecystectomy • Laparoscopic cholecystectomy • Gallstone pancreatitis • Biliary pancreatitis

Introduction

In the modern era, acute pancreatitis is one of the most common upper gastrointestinal illnesses requiring inpatient hospital admission. While many etiologies exist, gallstone pancreatitis remains the most frequent inciting factor in the western world [1, 2]. Transient gallstone impaction within the common channel of the biliary tree is hypothesized to lead to intraparenchymal trypsin activation. The subsequent enzymatic cascade, resulting in intra- and potentially extra-pancreatic inflammation leads to the clinical constellation of symptoms constituting acute pancreatitis [3]. While a multitude of grading systems have been utilized, the 2012 working group revision of the Atlanta criteria defines the disease process of pancreatitis as it is known today. Extent of acute disease is classified as either interstitial/edematous, or as necrotizing according to the gross appearance of the gland and peri-pancreatic tissue on cross sectional imaging. Severity ranges greatly along a continuum, from patients with mild abdominal pain and lab abnormalities, to patients with life threatening hemodynamic instability. Classifications are divided into mild, moderately severe, and severe, according to a group of physiological parameters defined by the working group [4].

Treatment for gallstone pancreatitis has changed considerably over the past three decades with the advent of minimally invasive surgical technique and endoscopy. Basic tenets of care include: resuscitation, bowel rest, common bile duct clearance (if necessary) via common duct exploration or endoscopic retrograde cholangiopancreatography (ERCP) with endoscopic sphincterotomy (ES), and eventual cholecystectomy to avoid recurrent pancreatitis.

Cholecystectomy in the setting of acute, active pancreatitis has long been considered an endeavor fraught with morbidity [5]. Delaying cholecystectomy in patients with acute onset of both mild and severe pancreatitis became standard practice during the era of open cholecystectomy and was carried over with the advent of laparoscopy. The timing of cholecystectomy however, has remained a subject of debate within the literature [3, 6–9].

Recognizing the disease spectrum that constitutes acute pancreatitis, we look to make evidence based recommendations for timing of laparoscopic cholecystectomy

Table 36.1 PICO table for patients with acute gallstone pancreatitis

P (Patients)	I (Intervention)	C (Comparator group)	O (Outcomes measured)
Patients with acute gallstone pancreatitis	Early laparoscopic cholecystectomy	Delayed laparoscopic cholecystectomy	Morbidity (surgical or recurrent biliary pathology), mortality, LOS

following acute gallstone pancreatitis, stratified by severity of pancreatitis (Table 36.1).

Search Strategy

The OVID Medline, EMBASE, and Cochrane Review databases were queried for MESH terms "Cholecystectomy, laparoscopic" with Boolean operator AND "Pancreatitis". Results were reviewed for relevancy. Laparoscopic cholecystectomy was widely adopted in the early 1990s, and in 1993 the United States National Institutes of Health released a consensus statement declaring laparoscopic cholecystectomy as the standard of care in the treatment of acute cholecystitis [10]. Articles prior to 1995 were excluded in an attempt to limit confounding morbidity stemming from technical failures early in the life of laparoscopic surgery. Search results were limited to English language articles. Studies were included which evaluated patients undergoing laparoscopic cholecystectomy following gallstone pancreatitis. Certain outcome measures were considered to be essential for study inclusion (laparoscopic success rate, morbidity, and mortality). Studies were excluded if: (1) no time period from symptom onset or hospital admission to cholecystectomy was noted, (2) fewer than ten patients were evaluated, (3) pancreatitis severity was not noted, or (4) if results mixed patients with various severities of pancreatitis. Four hundred sixty-two unique publications were identified. Of these, nine met inclusion criteria and were subsequently included in analysis. Eight were retrospective studies. One prospective randomized trial was identified and included.

Results

Patients with Interstitial, Edematous, or Mild Gallstone Pancreatitis

The aim of early cholecystectomy for acute gallstone pancreatitis is to minimize the risk of recurrent biliary events [8]. However, patients with pancreatitis who are early in the course of their disease have long been considered to be at increased risk for perioperative morbidity secondary to increased difficulty of dissection [9]. A multitude of retrospective observational studies and one randomized controlled trial exist which evaluate early versus delayed cholecystectomy in patients with mild pancreatitis (Table 36.2).

Tang and colleagues were among the first to publish their experiences in 1995, retrospectively examining outcomes and incidence of surgical morbidity in patients operated on within 1 week of symptom onset [11]. Patients were categorized according to severity of pancreatitis using Ranson's criteria [12], and underwent either early (<1 week since symptom onset) or delayed (>1 week since symptom onset) laparoscopic cholecystectomy. All operations were performed during the index admission, at least 48 h after biochemical and clinical resolution of pancreatitis. Among patients categorized as "mild" pancreatitics (<3 Ranson criteria), there was no significant difference in surgical morbidity, conversion to open operation, mortality, or post operative length of stay between groups undergoing early and delayed laparoscopic cholecystectomy. Patients who underwent early cholecystectomy were noted to have a significantly shorter overall hospitalization. Since Teng's seminal paper, numerous retrospective reviews have arrived at similar results, advocating same-admission laparoscopic cholecystectomy for stable patients with resolved mild, or interstitial/edematous pancreatitis.

Some have advocated for earlier laparoscopic cholecystectomy in carefully selected patients. Taylor and colleagues reported on a group of retrospectively examined patients who presented with mild gallstone pancreatitis and were operated on either after complete normalization of the physical exam and serum amylase, or after physical examination and serum amylase had begun to trend towards normalization [13]. Patients in the early cholecystectomy group were operated on an average of 1.8 days after presentation and were found to have a significantly shorter overall hospitalization than those who were postponed for complete resolution of pancreatitis. Additionally, no benefit was found when postponing intervention until complete resolution of pancreatitis.

To date, one randomized controlled trial has addressing the timing of laparoscopic cholecystectomy in patients with acute biliary pancreatitis. In 2012, Aboulian and colleagues reported on 50 patients that presented with mild gallstone pancreatitis, defined by fewer than three Ranson criteria, who were randomized to either early laparoscopic cholecystectomy within the first 48 h of admission, or to cholecystectomy after symptom and laboratory resolution of pancreatitis [14]. Patients received intervention as long as post admission serum amylase values documented stable pancreatitis. The early surgery group was operated on at a mean of 35 h compared to 77.8 h in the control group. Overall hospital stay was significantly shorter in the early operative group (3.8 vs. 5.8 days, $P=0.0016$). No patients were readmitted, had post-operative complications, or required conversion to open operation. At interim analysis (50 of 100 total patients), the study was terminated due to the significant decrease in total hospitalization without increased morbidity among the early operation group. As with previous retrospective, non-randomized studies, results indicate that cholecystectomy can be safely performed in patients with mild pancreatitis soon after admission, and that delaying operation until full symptomatic and biochemical resolution is unnecessary and adds to hospital stay.

Table 36.2 Clinical outcomes in patients with interstitial edematous/mild ABP with early versus delayed cholecystectomy

Author (year)	N	Time until operation (d)	Success (laparoscopic completion)	LOS (d)	Morbidity	Mortality	Pancreatitis severity grading	Study type (quality of evidence)
Tang (1995) [11]	122	<7 (early)	114/122 (93 %)	7.8 (early)	0	0	Ranson <3	Retrospective cohort (low)
		>7 (late)		14 (late)				
Uhl (1999) [18]	35	10	30/35 (86 %)	5	1/30 (3 %)	0	CT	Prospective observational (low)
Taylor (2004) [13]	46	1.8 (early)	26/26 (100 %)	3.5 (early)	3/26 (11 %)	0	Ranson <3	Retrospective observational (low)
		2.3 (late)	18/20 (90 %)	4.7 (late)	2/20 (10 %)			
Griniatsos (2005) [27]	44	7–14 (early)	20/20 (100 %)	2 (post-op)	1/20 (5 %)	0	Glasgow <3	Retrospective cohort (low)
		60 (late)	24/24 (100 %)	2 (post-op)	1/24 (4 %)			
Rosing (2007) [28]	220	<2 (early)	40/41 (98 %)	4	1/20 (5 %)	0	Ranson <3	Prospective cohort (medium)
		5 (late)	177/177 (100 %)	7 (post-op)	1/41 (2.4 %)			
Aboulian (2010) [14]	49	1.8 (early)	25/25 (100 %)	3.5	0/25	0	Ranson <3	Randomized controlled trial (high)
		3.2 (late)	24/24 (100 %)	5.8	0/24			
Falor (2012) [29]	303	<2 (early)	114/117 (97 %)	3	5/117 (4.2 %)	0	Ranson <3	Retrospective cohort (low)
		>2 (late)	172/186 (93 %)	6	9/186 (4.8 %)			
Mador (2014) [25]	80	3.3	43/45 (96 %)	8.8	4/45 (9 %)	0	Ranson <3	Retrospective observational (low)
		141	32/35 (91 %)	10	5/35 (15 %)			

Patients with Severe or Necrotizing Pancreatitis

As with patients with more mild disease, those with severe or necrotizing gallstone pancreatitis should undergo clearance of the common duct and cholecystectomy after disease stabilization [15]. With 10–20 % of patients with gallstone pancreatitis developing necrotizing pancreatitis and systemic organ failure, timing of surgical intervention differs from those with less severe disease [16, 17]. Few studies exist evaluating the timing of laparoscopic cholecystectomy in patients with severe or necrotizing pancreatitis. Three were identified and included for review (Table 36.3). In the classic paper by Kelly and Wagner published in 1988, patients with acute gallstone pancreatitis were randomized to early (<48 h) or delayed (>48 h) open cholecystectomy [5]. Those with severe acute pancreatitis (greater than 3 Ranson criteria) randomized to the early surgery group were found to have significantly higher rates of morbidity and mortality. Numerous other retrospective studies were published in the 1970s and 1980s detailing the dangers associated with open cholecystectomy in those with acute, active, severe pancreatitis.

These findings were translated to the laparoscopic era with Tang's paper in 1995 [11]. A subset of patients with severe gallstone pancreatitis (>3 Ranson's criteria) underwent early (<1 week) or delayed laparoscopic cholecystectomy. Those in the early surgery group had a significantly increased overall length of hospital stay.

In 1999 Uhl and colleagues published a retrospective report on 60 patients with acute biliary pancreatitis [18]. All received cross sectional imaging (contrast enhanced CT scanning) and were categorized as having necrotizing pancreatitis or acute interstitial pancreatitis. Of the 21 with necrotizing disease, 13 underwent laparoscopic cholecystectomy an average of 14 days after symptom onset. Five of thirteen (38 %) required conversion to an open operation. The remainder underwent open cholecystectomy at the time of necrosectomy. Extent of necrosis demonstrated on CT was shown to correlate with the development of infected pancreatic necrosis. The authors recommend postponing laparoscopic cholecystectomy for at least 7 days in the case of necrotizing pancreatitis, and for at least 3 weeks in patients with extended pancreatic necrosis involving more than 50 % of the gland due to an increased risk for late development of pancreatic necrosis.

The Role for Endoscopic Sphincterotomy

It remains clear that both open and laparoscopic intervention in patients with severe and necrotizing pancreatitis is morbid. Delaying cholecystectomy after discharge in patients with resolved pancreatitis is similarly risky and has been recognized to be associated with a significant risk of recurrent biliary events, occurring in 30–50 % of patients within the first 2 months [16, 19]. As recurrent acute pancreatitis in patients with prior severe or necrotizing disease can prove fatal, endoscopic sphincterotomy performed during initial admission has been proposed as a bridging procedure to interval cholecystectomy.

Table 36.3 Clinical outcomes in patients with necrotizing/moderately severe to severe ABP with early versus delayed cholecystectomy

Author (year)	N	Time until operation (days)	Success	LOS (days)	Morbidity	Mortality	Pancreatitis severity grading	Study type (quality of evidence)
Tang (1995) [11]	9 (early)	4.2 (early)	3/9 (33 %)	9.8	1/9 (11 %)	0/9	Ranson >3	Retrospective cohort (low)
	11 (late)	9.8 (late)	9/11 (82 %)	11.9	0/11 (0 %)	0/11		
Uhl (1999) [18]	13	14	8/13 (62 %)	6	2/8 (25 %)	0/8	CT	Prospective observational (low)
Heider (2005) [16]	30	102	25/27 (93 %)	3	2/27 (3 %)	0	CT	Retrospective observational (low)

Several studies have addressed the utility of ES in patients with acute gallstone pancreatitis. Those who undergo ES prior to discharge are less likely to have recurrent episodes of pancreatitis, however are not spared from all biliary complications secondary to gallstones [6, 20]. In looking at patients with interstitial edematous pancreatitis with fluid collections, as well as patients with necrotizing pancreatitis, Heider and colleagues found that 23 % of those who had received endoscopic sphincterotomy were readmitted after discharge, but prior to eventual cholecystectomy [16]. While multiple patients experienced biliary symptomatology (cholangitis, pain, nausea/emesis, and infected peri-pancreatic fluid collections), there were no noted episodes of recurrent pancreatitis.

Some have advocated endoscopic retrograde cholangiopancreatography and endoscopic sphincterotomy for all patients with acute gallstone pancreatitis. A Cochrane review in 2012 examined the role for early ERCP, defined as conservative medical management with the addition of ERCP within the first 72 h of admission [21]. A total of 7 trials and 757 patients were included in the review. The early ERCP strategy, when applied broadly to all presenting patients, was not found to reduce morbidity or mortality when compared to normal conservative management. The potential benefit of decreased local complications (i.e. fluid collections) and systemic complications was identified when the strategy was applied to subgroups of patients with suspected cholangitis or suspected persistent choledocholithiasis.

Cost Implications

The incidence of both gallstone disease and pancreatitis in the United States and the western world are increasing, which has been hypothesized to be secondary to increasing trends in obesity [2, 22, 23]. An estimated 700,000 cholecystectomies are performed annually at a cost of $6.5 billion [24]. With changing healthcare landscapes and payor structures, it is important to acknowledge the impact of management decisions on total cost of care.

A significant cost is associated with recurrent biliary symptomatology. The risk of recurrent symptoms and readmissions is not negligible, and must be considered in patients with resolved pancreatitis awaiting interval cholecystectomy. Recurrent pancreatitis has been reported to occur with a frequency of roughly 10 %, and overall biliary complication rates have been reported to be as high as 60 % in patients waiting 20 weeks for cholecystectomy [8, 25].

The patients most likely to experience cost savings secondary to early cholecystectomy are those with mild biliary pancreatitis [16]. A recently published UK study considered treatment costs associated with laparoscopic cholecystectomy performed at various intervals. Total cost of care for patients undergoing definitive operation within the first 3 days of symptom onset was compared with cost of care for patients undergoing subsequent admission (interval) cholecystectomy. Early intervention was found to yield a cost savings of nearly 27 % [26].

Recommendations

Management of patients with acute gallstone pancreatitis can be stratified according to severity. Those with mild biliary pancreatitis, without systemic complications or organ failure, are appropriate for evaluation for early laparoscopic cholecystectomy. To date, multiple retrospective and observational studies have compared early and delayed surgery in patients with mild gallstone pancreatitis, however there is a paucity of prospective evidence, with a single randomized trial in the literature. Based on the available data, we make a recommendation for laparoscopic cholecystectomy within the first 2 days of admission, provided the patient has shown clinical stability. Among patients with mild disease, further delay appears to add to total cost of care and length of stay.

In patients with severe, or necrotizing pancreatitis, there is inadequate evidence to recommend an appropriate interval for laparoscopic cholecystectomy following resolution of the acute disease.

A Personal View of the Data

Therapy for gallstone pancreatitis includes patient resuscitation, clearance of the common bile duct (if necessary), and cholecystectomy to remove the nidus for future attacks. Pancreatitis represents a spectrum of disease and severity varies greatly, and multiple severity grading systems exist. Ranson's criteria, though outdated, are the most frequently used in the literature to risk stratify patients with gallstone pancreatitis. Among those with mild disease (commonly defined as <3 Ranson's criteria), which has been shown to be stable by physical examination and laboratory values, laparoscopic cholecystectomy should be pursued, regardless of the time since symptom onset. Patients with suspected choledocholithiasis should undergo ERCP and ES. Those with severe or necrotizing pancreatitis should be initially resuscitated and stabilized. When performed after stabilization and prior to hospital discharge, ERCP and ES can provide an important bridge to eventual laparoscopic cholecystectomy.

Recommendations

- Patients with mild gallstone pancreatitis that is stable in severity should undergo laparoscopic cholecystectomy at earliest convenience, provided they are of acceptable surgical risk (evidence quality moderate; strong recommendation).
- Patients with severe or necrotizing gallstone pancreatitis should undergo interval cholecystectomy with endoscopic ERCP and ES utilized as a bridging procedure, if necessary (evidence quality low; weak recommendation).

References

1. Swaroop VS, Chari ST, Clain JE. Severe acute pancreatitis. JAMA. 2004;291:2865–8.
2. Spanier BW, Dijkgraaf MG, Bruno MJ. Epidemiology, aetiology and outcome of acute and chronic pancreatitis: an update. Best Pract Res Clin Gastroenterol. 2008;22(1):45–63.
3. Banks PA, Freeman ML, Practice Parameters Committee of the American College of Gastroenterology. Practice guidelines in acute pancreatitis. Am J Gastroenterol. 2006;101(10):2379–400.
4. Banks PA, et al. Classification of acute pancreatitis – 2012: revision of the Atlanta classification and definitions by international consensus. Gut. 2013;62(1):102–11.
5. Kelly TR, Wagner DS. Gallstone pancreatitis: a prospective randomized trial of the timing of surgery. Surgery. 1988;104:600–4.
6. Wilson CT, de Moya MA. Cholecystectomy for acute gallstone pancreatitis: early vs delayed approach. Scand J Surg. 2010;99(2):81–5.
7. Working Party of the British Society of Gastroenterology, Association of Surgeons of Great Britain and Ireland, Pancreatic Society of Great Britain and Ireland, Association of Upper GI Surgeons of Great Britain and Ireland. UK guidelines for the management of acute pancreatitis. Gut. 2005;54 Suppl 3:iii1–9.
8. Bakker OJ. Timing of cholecystectomy after mild biliary pancreatitis. Br J Surg. 2011;98(10):1446–54.
9. Tate JJ, Lau WY, Li AK. Laparoscopic cholecystectomy for biliary pancreatitis. Br J Surg. 1994;81(5):720–2.
10. NIH Consensus conference. Gallstones and laparoscopic cholecystectomy. JAMA. 1993;269(8):1018–24.
11. Tang E, et al. Timing of laparoscopic surgery in gallstone pancreatitis. Arch Surg. 1995;130(5):496–9.
12. Ranson JHC, Rifkind KM, Roses DF. Prognostic signs and the role of operative management in acute pancreatitis. Surg Gynecol Obstet. 1974;139:69–74.
13. Taylor E, Wong C. The optimal timing of laparoscopic cholecystectomy in mild gallstone pancreatitis. Am Surg. 2004;70(11):971–5.
14. Aboulian A, et al. Early cholecystectomy safely decreases hospital stay in patients with mild gallstone pancreatitis: a randomized prospective study. Ann Surg. 2010;251(4):615–9.
15. Schirmer B. Timing of and indications for biliary tract surgery in acute necrotizing pancreatitis. J Gastrointest Surg. 2001;5(3):229–31.
16. Heider TR, et al. Endoscopic sphincterotomy permits interval laparoscopic cholecystectomy in patients with moderately severe gallstone pancreatitis. J Gastrointest Surg. 2006;10(1):1–5.
17. Beger HG, et al. Natural course of acute pancreatitis. World J Surg. 1997;21(2):130–5.
18. Uhl W, et al. Acute gallstone pancreatitis: timing of laparoscopic cholecystectomy in mild and severe disease. Surg Endosc. 1999;13(11):1070–6.
19. Steinberg W, Tenner S. Acute pancreatitis. N Engl J Med. 1994;330(17):1198–210.
20. Ito K, Ito H, Whang EE. Timing of cholecystectomy for biliary pancreatitis: do the data support current guidelines? J Gastrointest Surg. 2008;12(12):2164–70.
21. Tse F, Yuan Y. Early routine endoscopic retrograde cholangiopancreatography strategy versus early conservative management strategy in acute gallstone pancreatitis. Cochrane Database Syst Rev. 2012;5:CD009779.
22. Fagenholz PJ, et al. Increasing United States hospital admissions for acute pancreatitis, 1988–2003. Ann Epidemiol. 2007;17(7):491–7.

23. Mokdad AH, et al. The spread of the obesity epidemic in the United States, 1991–1998. JAMA. 1999;282(16):1519–22.
24. Shaffer EA. Gallstone disease: epidemiology of gallbladder stone disease. Best Pract Res Clin Gastroenterol. 2006;20(6):981–96.
25. Mador BD, Panton ON, Hameed SM. Early versus delayed cholecystectomy following endoscopic sphincterotomy for mild biliary pancreatitis. Surg Endosc. 2014;28(12):3337–42.
26. Morris S, et al. Cost-effectiveness of early laparoscopic cholecystectomy for mild acute gallstone pancreatitis. Br J Surg. 2014;101(7):828–35.
27. Griniatsos J, Karvounis E, Isla A. Early versus delayed single-stage laparoscopic eradication for both gallstones and common bile duct stones in mild acute biliary pancreatitis. Am Surg. 2005;71(8):682–6.
28. Rosing DK, et al. Early cholecystectomy for mild to moderate gallstone pancreatitis shortens hospital stay. J Am Coll Surg. 2007;205(6):762–6.
29. Falor AE, et al. Early laparoscopic cholecystectomy for mild gallstone pancreatitis: time for a paradigm shift. Arch Surg. 2012;147(11):1031–5.

Chapter 37
Nutritional Support in Acute Necrotizing Pancreatitis

Andreas Mykoniatis

Abstract Enteral nutrition (EN) is now considered the standard of care for patients with severe acute pancreatitis and patients with pancreatic necrosis. Several randomized controlled trials and meta-analyses have shown that the administration of EN nutrition reduces complications and mortality of patients with severe pancreatitis including patients with pancreatic necrosis compared to parenteral nutrition (PN). PN had been the standard of care for many decades, based on the concept of "pancreatic rest". Avoidance of alimentary stimulation of pancreatic exocrine secretion was assumed to limit or prevent ongoing pancreatic inflammation. Current practice guidelines recommend the use of enteral nutrition for feeding patients with acute pancreatitis, including those with pancreatic necrosis. Accumulating evidence suggests that the use of the gut through EN may promote the maintenance of gut barrier and immune functions. Provision of luminal nutrition via the gastric approach appears to be equally tolerated as the enteral route and may be more cost effective. However, larger randomized controlled trials and other studies focused on optimization of nutritional support during the acute and convalescent phases of necrotizing pancreatitis are needed. Pharmaconutriton or the use of defined elemental formulae has not yet been shown to be beneficial. The use of PN should be limited to patients that cannot tolerate EN.

Keywords Acute pancreatitis • Pancreatic necrosis • Enteral nutrition • Parenteral nutrition • Enteral feedings • Parenteral feedings • Severe pancreatitis

---

A. Mykoniatis (✉)
Department of Medicine, The University of Chicago Medicine,
5841 S. Maryland Ave. Rm. M408, MC4076, Chicago, IL 60637, USA
e-mail: amykonia@medicine.bsd.uchicago.edu

J.M. Millis, J.B. Matthews (eds.), *Difficult Decisions in Hepatobiliary and Pancreatic Surgery*, Difficult Decisions in Surgery: An Evidence-Based Approach, DOI 10.1007/978-3-319-27365-5_37

Introduction

Patients with severe acute pancreatitis are defined as those with ≥3 Ranson criteria; APACHE II score of ≥8; and a CRP level of ≥150 mg/dl [1]. The Atlanta classification [2] determines the severity of acute pancreatitis by the presence of organ failure, systemic failure, or other prognostic indicators (i.e.:≥3 Ranson criteria or APACHE II ≥8). The revised Atlanta classification includes the use of morphologic CECT (Contrast-enhanced computed tomography) criteria to diagnose acute necrotizing pancreatitis by the presence of necrosis and evidence of infection.

The exact pathophysiology [3] of acute pancreatitis (AP) is not clear, but it is thought to be caused by the abnormal activation of pancreatic proenzymes that results in autodiegestion of the pancreas. In theory, "pancreatic rest" might help decrease pancreatic exocrine secretion and thereby retard disease progression. It is now known that several other factors are involved in the progression of pancreatitis that involve the integrity of the intestinal mucosa [4].

In about 15–20 % of patients, the disease progresses to severe illness with a prolonged disease course; multiple organ failure; and sepsis. The overall mortality of AP is about 5 % and can reach up to 20–30 % in patients with severe AP and infected necrosis [5, 6]. Parenteral nutrition was regarded as the standard nutritional management for many decades based on the theory of pancreatic rest [7]. Optimal management now includes resuscitation with IV fluids, pain management, and early enteral nutrition. Several pieces of evidence have shown that early enteral nutrition is superior to PN. Enteral nutrition (EN) preserves mucosal integrity and reduces the risk of infections. In comparison to PN, EN seems to be equally tolerated and is more cost effective. This chapter will address and grade the evidence for the use of enteral nutrition in patients with severe acute pancreatitis and pancreatic necrosis. It will also evaluate the existing evidence for the use of gastric vs. jejunal tube feeding (TF); early vs. late nutrition; and the use of polymeric vs. elemental formula and probiotics in the setting of severe acute pancreatitis and pancreatic necrosis.

Search Strategy

In order to evaluate the use of enteral nutrition, a literature search of English language publications from 2000 to 2013 was used to identify published data on acute pancreatitis and nutrition using the PICO outline (Tables 37.1 and 37.2). Databases searched were PubMed, Web of Sciences, Cochrane library, and Embase Database. Terms used in the search were "acute pancreatitis," "pancreatic necrosis", "enteral nutrition/parenteral nutrition", or "enteral feeding/parenteral feedings". Eight randomized controlled trials were included in the analyses that evaluated the use of EN vs. PN. Four randomized controlled trials that studied the use of NG vs. NJ tube feeds in patients with acute pancreatitis were included. The data was classified using the GRADE system.

Table 37.1 PICO table for enteral nutrition vs. parenteral nutrition in acute pancreatitis

P (Patients)	I (Intervention)	C (Comparator group)	O (Outcomes measured)
Patients with severe acute pancreatitis	Enteral	Parenteral nutrition	Mortality, organ failure, pancreatic infection

Table 37.2 PICO table for G tube vs. J tube in acute pancreatitis

P (Patients)	I (Intervention)	C (Comparator group)	O (Outcomes measured)
Patients with acute pancreatitis	Gastric	Jejunal	Incidence of infection

Results

Feeding in Severe Acute Pancreatitis and Pancreatic Necrosis-EN vs. PN

The data supporting the use of EN are based on more than eight prospective randomized controlled trials. In particular, comparison of PN to EN in patients with severe acute pancreatitis has been addressed by these trials [8–15] (Table 37.3); and the results were analyzed in several meta-analyses [16–18].

In the most recent randomized study by Wu et al. [14], 107 patients were enrolled between 2003 and 2007. Fifty-four patients were fed with PN and 53 patients were fed with EN. Those individuals with pancreatic necrosis determined by CT scan and confirmed by a C-reactive protein (CRP) level (greater than 19.5 mg/dL, 48 h after the onset of the disease), were included in this study. Eighty percent of the patients developed organ failure in the PN group vs. 21 % ($P<0.05$) in the EN group. Similarly, 80 % and 22 % ($P<0.05$) in the PN and EN groups respectively underwent surgical intervention. Seventy-two percent of the PN patients ($P<0.05$) and 23 % of the EN patients developed pancreatic septic necrosis. The mortality rate in the PN and EN groups was 43 % and 11 % respectively.

In a meta-analysis by Petrov et al. [18] published in 2008, the aim was to evaluate PN and EN with regards to infectious complication and mortality. Five randomized controlled trials compared parenteral to enteral nutrition in patients with predicted severe acute pancreatitis. EN reduced the risk of infectious complications (relative risk, 0.47; 95 % CI, 0.28–0.77; $P<0.001$); pancreatic infections (0.48; 0.26–0.91; $P=0.02$); and mortality (0.32; 0.11–0.98; $P=0.03$).

According to the international consensus guideline committee [19] that published their guidelines in 2012, there was almost uniform agreement on the following items. Patients with mild to moderate disease should be treated with IV fluids and nil per os (NPO) with gradual advancement of their diet. The need for EN or PN therapy should be considered in mild to moderate disease when the patient has been NPO for 5–7 days. In severe disease, EN should be started early with a small

Table 37.3 Clinical outcomes of EN vs. PN

Author (year)	EN N[a]	PN N[a]	Results	Study type (quality of evidence)
Kalfarent-zos et al. (1997)	18	20	Lower pancreatic infection and sepsis rate in EN	Prospective (high)
Gupta (2003)	8	9	Non-significant lower pancreatic infection rate in EN	Prospective (high)
Louie (2005)	10	18	Non-significant lower pancreatic infection rate in EN	Prospective (high)
Eckerwall (2006)	23	25	Significant higher pancreatic infection rate in EN	Prospective (high)
Petrov (2007)	35	34	Significant lower pancreatic infection and mortality rate in EN	Prospective (high)
Casas (2007)	11	11	Non-significant lower pancreatic infection rate and length of stay	Prospective (high)
Doley (2008)	25	25	Non-significant pancreatic infection and mortality rate	Prospective (high)
Wu (2010)	53	54	Significant lower pancreatic necrosis rate in EN	Prospective (high)

[a]N: number of patients

peptide-based medium-chain triglyceride (MCT) oil formula into the stomach or small intestine. EN can be continued despite the presence of complications such as fistula, ascites, or pseudocyst. PN should be initiated if EN is contraindicated or not well tolerated. The guidelines conclude that EN is the evidence based standard of care for patients with severe acute pancreatitis and pancreatic necrosis.

Route of Enteral Feeding in Acute Pancreatitis-NG vs. NJ

The administration of nasogastric (NG) tube feeding does not require specialized invasive procedures. However, it is thought to increase the risk of aspiration resulting in prolonged hospitalization. Conversely, the provision of nasojejunal (NJ) tube feeds usually requires the insertion of a NJ tube that requires endoscopic or radiological guidance for insertion, procedures that may delay the initiation of feeding.

The effect of NG vs. NJ tube feeds has been investigated in four randomized clinical studies (Table 37.4) [20–23]. These studies included patients with severe acute pancreatitis (SAP) and pancreatic necrosis. There were no significant differences in clinical outcomes or in tolerance.

In the most recent randomized controlled study published by Singh et al. in 2012 [22], 78 patients were randomized to feeding by either the NG or the NJ route. This was a non-inferiority study. Thirty-six of the patients had necrotizing pancreatitis. Early enteral feeding through NG was not inferior to NJ in patients with SAP. The presence of infectious complications in the NG and NJ groups was 23.1 % and 35.9 % ($P<0.05$) respectively. The infectious complications were within the

Table 37.4 Clinical outcomes of NG vs. NJ tube feedings

Author (year)	NG N*	NJ N*	Results	Study type (quality of evidence)
Eatock (2000)	20	18	Non-significant differences in outcome and tolerance	Cohort (low)
Eatock (2005)	9	8	Non-significant difference in pancreatic infection rate and tolerance	Prospective (low due to flaws)
Kumar (2006)	15	16	Non-significant difference in outcome measure and tolerance	Prospective (low due to flaws)
Singh (2012)	39	39	Infectious complication within the inferiority limit and similar tolerance	Prospective (low due to flaws)

* = number of patients

non-inferiority limit. All other complications such as pain in refeeding intestinal permeability and endotoxemia were comparable in both groups.

In the meta-analysis published by Petrov [24], four studies [20–25] investigated the use of NG tube feedings, and a total of 92 patients with predicted severe acute pancreatitis were included. Eleven of those patients (16.9 %) had severe necrotizing pancreatitis. There was no statistically significant difference in the mortality rate (RR=0.77; 95 % CI: 0.37–1.62; P=0.50) between the patients fed via NG vs. NJ. Likewise, there was no difference in the feeding tolerance in the two groups (RR=1.09; 95 % CI: 0.46–2.59; P=0.84).

A meta-analysis published by Zhang et al. [26] in June 2013 included many studies in nutrition in the ICU setting and showed that jejunal feeding can deliver a higher proportion of the estimated energy requirement compared to gastric feeding. However, mortality (OR, 1.05; 95 % CI, 0.77–1.44); new-onset pneumonia (OR, 0.77; 95 % CI, 0.53–1.13); and aspiration (OR, 1.20; 95 % CI, 0.64–2.25) were not improved in the NJ tube feed group.

The concept of NG vs. NJ tube feeds needs to be further investigated in a large randomized trial that is adequately powered. As stated by Petrov et al. [27], this will require the enrollment of 440 patients to demonstrate a 10 % absolute risk reduction in feeding intolerance. Such a study is technically difficult requiring multicenter involvement. Current randomized studies each have flaws that were discussed by Petrov [28]. For example, the study by Eatock [21] used a duodenal and not jejunal tube. In the study by Kumar [23] and Singh [22], there was a delay in initiating the TF.

The practical preference of using NJ rather than NG feeds in patients with necrotizing pancreatitis is related to the clinical observation that necrotizing pancreatitis patients commonly develop gastric ileus [29]. Therefore, they are at an increased risk for non-tolerance to NG tube feeds. In addition, the use of NJ tube feeds is intuitively more consistent with the concept of pancreatic rest which is an area of ongoing investigation. However, hard data showing the advantage of NJ over NG routes has not yet been established.

The anatomic level below which pancreatic stimulation is prevented is another area that requires further investigation. There was a loss of pancreatic stimulatory effect from 20 to 120 cm post ligament of Treitz as stated by O'Keefe et al. [30]. A study by Kumar et al. [23] that aimed to investigate the stimulatory effects of feeding by inserting NJ tubes 60 cm beyond the ligament of Treitz was inconclusive due to inadequate statistical power.

There is a weak recommendation for NJ tube feed placement in patients with severe acute pancreatitis and pancreatic necrosis because of possible gastric ileus resulting in inadequate nutrition. The optimal length of the feeding tube insertion below the ligament of Treitz has to be further investigated.

Type of TF

There are multiple tube feeding products available. These can be divided into three large groups. These groups include the elemental or semielemental; polymeric; and immunomodulating products (i.e., glutamine, omega-3 fatty acids, antioxidants, or probiotics) [31].

The use of an elemental or semielemental formulation during the treatment of severe acute pancreatitis was thought to be advantageous because it was absorbed easier resulting in better tolerance. On the other hand, polymeric formulations are less expensive. In a meta-analyses published by Petrov et al. [32], the different feeding products were compared with respect to their feeding tolerance. The following endpoints were evaluated: temporary reduction or cessation of feeding; infectious complications; and in-hospital mortality. The study reviewed 20 randomized controlled trials and included a total of 1070 patients with acute pancreatitis. Eight-hundred twenty-five of the patients had severe acute pancreatitis. In the study, it was shown that the use of an elemental formulation did not result in a statistically significant difference in the risk of infectious complications and death. Polymeric and elemental formulations were equally tolerated.

The use of probiotics was studied in a multicenter randomized double blind controlled trial entitled PROPATRIA [33]. In this study, 298 patients with predicted severe acute pancreatitis were randomized to receive either a multispecies probiotic preparation or placebo for 28 days. The primary endpoints were infectious complications (infected pancreatic necrosis, bacteremia, pneumonia, urosepsis, or infected ascites) during admission and at 90-day follow-up. Infectious complications occurred in 30 % of patients in the probiotics group and 28 % in the placebo group. Sixteen percent of patients in the probiotics group died, compared with 6 % in the placebo group. In addition, nine patients in the probiotics group developed bowel ischemia compared with none in the placebo group. The PROPATRIA study was preceded by two lower powered studies by Olah et al. [34, 35] that showed decreased rates of infected necrosis; hospital stay; SIRS; and organ failure in patients with acute pancreatitis using lactobacillus. Because of the conflicting results of these studies, and the surprising yet unexplained increase in death and intestinal ischemia in the PROPATRIA study, the use probiotic prophylaxis in patients with severe acute pancreatitis remains highly controversial and in need of further investigation.

Timing of Feeding Initiation- Early vs. Late

The role of very early (in the first 24 h) EN in patients with severe acute pancreatitis has yet to be adequately investigated in randomized trials. The initiation of TF in the first 24–48 h after admission is the current practice of timing enteral nutrition support.

Initiation of very early enteral nutrition in patients with severe pancreatitis is thought to prevent mucosal barrier dysfunction; bacterial overgrowth; and bacterial translocation. This concept was examined in a meta-analysis by Bakker [36] that included eight trials. In the subgroups of patients with predicted severe acute pancreatitis and pancreatic necrosis, results were consistently better if EN was started within 24 h. However, these results were not statistically significant. Therefore, the current guideline is to start the enteral nutrition in the first 24–48 h which is considered early by American Society of Enteral and Parenteral Nutrition standards [37].

Numerous meta-analyses have examined the use of early enteral nutrition in severe acute pancreatitis. In a meta-analysis by Li et al. [38], early enteral nutrition within 48 h in severe acute pancreatitis showed protection against infectious complications. There was another meta-analysis by Petrov et al. in 2008 [32] that aimed to analyze the timing of enteral nutrition. This study showed a significant risk reduction of multiple organ failure; pancreatic infectious complications; hyperglycemia; and length of hospitalization if EN was started within the first 48 h. The limiting factor of this study was the lack of a standard definition for early vs. late enteral nutrition, which varied from 24 to 72 h after admission. Taken together, the available evidence base suggests that EN can be safely initiated within the first 24–48 h after resuscitation.

Another approach used to nourish patients with acute necrotizing pancreatitis is early volume oral feeds containing 248–330 kcal/day given to patients within the first 72 h. A retrospective study published in 2014 by Pupelis et al. [39], examined 10 years of data. In this study, there was a statistically significant improvement in CRP level, the need for surgical intervention, and ICU stay. The concept of early oral nutrition in necrotizing pancreatitis should be further investigated in a prospective randomized study.

Future Directions

Several advances have been made in defining the role of nutritional support in the treatment of severe acute necrotizing pancreatitis [40]. One of the most important changes is the early initiation of proper enteral nutrition. The use of PN to achieve pancreatic rest is no longer recommended. The appropriate site of tube insertion for patients with severe acute pancreatitis and pancreatic necrosis needs to be further elucidated.

The use of antioxidants for patients with acute pancreatitis should be evaluated further in a large scale study since there are studies that have shown that glutamine or other antioxidants [41] can be beneficial in the ICU setting.

Recommendations

In severe acute pancreatitis and pancreatic necrosis, enteral feeds are recommended (evidence quality high: strong recommendation).

If there is normal gut function and tolerance, NG tube feeds can be attempted (quality moderate: weak recommendation).

If there is gut dysfunction, NJ tube should be inserted (evidence quality moderate: weak recommendation).

EN should be initiated within 24–48 h after admission (evidence quality high: strong recommendation).

A Personal View of the Data

In most of tertiary medical centers, feeding in patients with acute necrotizing pancreatitis usually starts after completion of the initial resuscitation process. The administration of feeding stimulates the gut and preserves gut function [27]. Prolongation of intestinal dysfunction increases pancreatic infection rate and mortality [42].

There is a clear role for the use of PN in the management of severe acute pancreatitis when EN is not able to achieve hutritional goals [43] or when the route is compromised [44] such as in the presence of ileus, enteric fistula, pancreatic pseudocyst, ascites, or other severe complications. Nutrition in necrotizing pancreatitis is an important medical decision that can influence the progression of the disease and reduce complication rates. Further studies are needed to address the optimal anatomic level used for nutrition, the use of immunonutrition, and the prophylactic administration of probiotics.

References

1. Wilson C, Heads A, Shenkin A, et al. C-reactive protein, antiproteases and complement factors as objective markers of severity in acute pancreatitis. Br J Surg. 1989;76(2):177–81.
2. Bradley EL. A clinically based classification system for acute pancreatitis. Summary of the International Symposium on Acute Pancreatitis, Atlanta, Ga, September 11 through 13, 1992. Arch Surg. 1993;128(5):586–90.
3. Pandol SJ, Saluja AK, Imrie CW, et al. Acute pancreatitis: bench to the bedside. Gastroenterology. 2007;132(3):1127–51.

4. Powell JJ, Murchison JT, Fearon KC, et al. Randomized controlled trial of the effect of early enteral nutrition on markers of the inflammatory response in predicted severe acute pancreatitis. Br J Surg. 2000;87(10):1375–81.
5. Pavlidis P, Crichton S, Lemmich Smith J, et al. Improved outcome of severe acute pancreatitis in the intensive care unit. Crit Care Res Pract. 2013;2013:897107.
6. Banks PA, Freeman ML. Practice guidelines in acute pancreatitis. Am J Gastroenterol. 2006;101(10):2379–400.
7. McClave SA. Nutrition support in acute pancreatitis. Gastroenterol Clin North Am. 2007;36(1):65–74, vi.
8. Kalfarentzos F, Kehagias J, Mead N, et al. Enteral nutrition is superior to parenteral nutrition in severe acute pancreatitis: results of a randomized prospective trial. Br J Surg. 1997;84(12):1665–9.
9. Gupta R, Patel K, Calder PC, et al. A randomised clinical trial to assess the effect of total enteral and total parenteral nutritional support on metabolic, inflammatory and oxidative markers in patients with predicted severe acute pancreatitis (APACHE II > or =6). Pancreatology. 2003;3(5):406–13.
10. Louie BE, Noseworthy T, Hailey D, et al. 2004 MacLean-Mueller prize enteral or parenteral nutrition for severe pancreatitis: a randomized controlled trial and health technology assessment. Can J Surg. 2005;48(4):298–306.
11. Eckerwall G, Olin H, Andersson B, et al. Fluid resuscitation and nutritional support during severe acute pancreatitis in the past: what have we learned and how can we do better? Clin Nutr. 2006;25(3):497–504.
12. Casas M, Mora J, Fort E, et al. Total enteral nutrition vs. total parenteral nutrition in patients with severe acute pancreatitis. Rev Esp Enferm Dig. 2007;99(5):264–9.
13. Doley RP, Yadav TD, Wig JD, et al. Enteral nutrition in severe acute pancreatitis. JOP. 2009;10(2):157–62.
14. Wu X-MM, Ji K-QQ, Wang H-YY, et al. Total enteral nutrition in prevention of pancreatic necrotic infection in severe acute pancreatitis. Pancreas. 2010;39(2):248–51.
15. Petrov MS, Kukosh MV, Emelyanov NV. A randomized controlled trial of enteral versus parenteral feeding in patients with predicted severe acute pancreatitis shows a significant reduction in mortality and in infected pancreatic complications with total enteral nutrition. Dig Surg. 2006;23(5–6):336–44; discussion 344–5.
16. Marik PE, Zaloga GP. Meta-analysis of parenteral nutrition versus enteral nutrition in patients with acute pancreatitis. BMJ. 2004;328(7453):1407.
17. McClave SA, Chang W-KK, Dhaliwal R, et al. Nutrition support in acute pancreatitis: a systematic review of the literature. JPEN J Parenter Enter Nutr. 2006;30(2):143–56.
18. Petrov MS, van Santvoort HC, Besselink MG, et al. Enteral nutrition and the risk of mortality and infectious complications in patients with severe acute pancreatitis: a meta-analysis of randomized trials. Arch Surg. 2008;143(11):1111–7.
19. Mirtallo JM, Forbes A, McClave SA, et al. International consensus guidelines for nutrition therapy in pancreatitis. JPEN J Parenter Enter Nutr. 2012;36(3):284–91.
20. Eatock FC, Brombacher GD, Steven A, et al. Nasogastric feeding in severe acute pancreatitis may be practical and safe. Int J Pancreatol. 2000;28(1):23–9.
21. Eatock FC, Chong P, Menezes N, et al. A randomized study of early nasogastric versus nasojejunal feeding in severe acute pancreatitis. Am J Gastroenterol. 2005;100(2):432–9.
22. Singh N, Sharma B, Sharma M, et al. Evaluation of early enteral feeding through nasogastric and nasojejunal tube in severe acute pancreatitis: a noninferiority randomized controlled trial. Pancreas. 2012;41(1):153–9.
23. Kumar A, Singh N, Prakash S, et al. Early enteral nutrition in severe acute pancreatitis: a prospective randomized controlled trial comparing nasojejunal and nasogastric routes. J Clin Gastroenterol. 2006;40(5):431–4.

24. Petrov MS, Correia MI, Windsor JA. Nasogastric tube feeding in predicted severe acute pancreatitis. A systematic review of the literature to determine safety and tolerance. JOP. 2008;9(4):440–8.
25. Eckerwall GE, Axelsson JB, Andersson RG. Early nasogastric feeding in predicted severe acute pancreatitis: a clinical, randomized study. Ann Surg. 2006;244(6):959–65; discussion 965–7.
26. Zhang Z, Xu X, Ding J, et al. Comparison of postpyloric tube feeding and gastric tube feeding in intensive care unit patients: a meta-analysis. Nutr Clin Pract. 2013;28(3):371–80.
27. Petrov MS. Gastric feeding and "gut rousing" in acute pancreatitis. Nutr Clin Pract. 2014;29(3):287–90.
28. Petrov M. Nutrition, inflammation, and acute pancreatitis. ISRN Inflamm. 2013;2013:341410.
29. O'Keefe S, Rolniak S, Raina A, et al. Enteral feeding patients with gastric outlet obstruction. Nutr Clin Pract. 2012;27(1):76–81.
30. O'Keefe SJ, McClave SA. Feeding the injured pancreas. Gastroenterology. 2005;129(3):1129–30.
31. Silk DB. Formulation of enteral diets. Nutrition. 1999;15(7–8):626–32.
32. Petrov MS, Loveday BP, Pylypchuk RD, et al. Systematic review and meta-analysis of enteral nutrition formulations in acute pancreatitis. Br J Surg. 2009;96(11):1243–52.
33. Besselink MG, van Santvoort HC, Buskens E, et al. Probiotic prophylaxis in predicted severe acute pancreatitis: a randomised, double-blind, placebo-controlled trial. Lancet. 2008;371(9613):651–9.
34. Olah A, Belagyi T, Issekutz A, et al. Randomized clinical trial of specific lactobacillus and fibre supplement to early enteral nutrition in patients with acute pancreatitis. Br J Surg. 2002;89:1103–7.
35. Oláh A, Belágyi T, Pótó L, et al. Synbiotic control of inflammation and infection in severe acute pancreatitis: a prospective, randomized, double blind study. Hepatogastroenterology. 2007;54(74):590–4.
36. Bakker OJ, van Brunschot S, Farre A, et al. Timing of enteral nutrition in acute pancreatitis: meta-analysis of individuals using a single-arm of randomised trials. Pancreatology. 2014;14:340–6.
37. Kreymann KG, Berger MM, Deutz NE, et al. ESPEN guidelines on enteral nutrition: intensive care. Clin Nutr. 2006;25(2):210–23.
38. Li J-YY, Yu T, Chen G-CC, et al. Enteral nutrition within 48 hours of admission improves clinical outcomes of acute pancreatitis by reducing complications: a meta-analysis. PLoS One. 2013;8(6):e64926.
39. Pupelis G, Plaudis H, Zeiza K, et al. Oral feeding in necrotizing pancreatitis. Acta Chir Belg. 2014;114(1):34–9.
40. McClave SA. Drivers of oxidative stress in acute pancreatitis: the role of nutrition therapy. JPEN J Parenter Enter Nutr. 2012;36(1):24–35.
41. Petrov MS, Pylypchuk RD, Uchugina AF. A systematic review on the timing of artificial nutrition in acute pancreatitis. Br J Nutr. 2009;101(6):787–93.
42. Sun J-KK, Li W-QQ, Ni H-BB, et al. Modified gastrointestinal failure score for patients with severe acute pancreatitis. Surg Today. 2013;43(5):506–13.
43. Gianotti L, Meier R, Lobo D, et al. ESPEN guidelines on parenteral nutrition: pancreas. Clin Nutr. 2009;28(4):428–35.
44. Schneider A, Boyle A, McCluckie A, et al. Acute severe pancreatitis and multiple organ failure: total parenteral nutrition is still required in a proportion of patients. Br J Surg. 2000;87(3):362–73.

Chapter 38
Management of Symptomatic Pancreatic Pseudocyst

Benjamin D. Ferguson and Vivek N. Prachand

Abstract Management options for pancreatic pseudocyst are numerous and include endoscopic and surgical approaches. Much debate exists regarding which of these approaches is superior and when each is most appropriate. While endoscopy offers less post-procedural pain, shorter length of stay, and fewer complications, laparoscopic surgical approaches are more suitable for pseudocysts whose locations or other characteristics present significant technical challenge or are otherwise unamenable to endoscopic drainage. Endoscopic management should be attempted when technically feasible, and a laparoscopic approach should be employed when endoscopic drainage would be technically difficult or in symptom recurrence following initial endoscopic management.

Keywords Pancreatic pseudocyst • Laparoscopy • Endoscopy • Cystgastrostomy

Introduction

Pancreatic pseudocysts are collections of pancreatic fluid and necrotic tissue surrounded by a non-epithelial perimeter persisting for greater than 6 weeks and arising following pancreatitis or trauma. Although usually asymptomatic, pseudocysts can cause symptoms by mass effect (abdominal or back pain, obstructive symptoms, or jaundice), infection, or hemorrhage. Though spontaneous resolution is typical, serious complications, such as rupture, infection, bleeding, or obstruction, can occur. Management options can be broadly classified as surgical or endoscopic. Within the surgical domain, laparoscopy has emerged as a safe and effective method for management of pancreatic pseudocysts and typically is associated with less postoperative pain, shorter length of stay, and non-inferior success rates compared to open surgical management. Endoscopic approaches offer even less pain,

B.D. Ferguson • V.N. Prachand (✉)
Department of Surgery, University of Chicago Medical Center,
5841 S Maryland Ave, Chicago, IL 60637, USA
e-mail: vprachan@surgery.bsd.uchicago.edu

J.M. Millis, J.B. Matthews (eds.), *Difficult Decisions in Hepatobiliary and Pancreatic Surgery*, Difficult Decisions in Surgery: An Evidence-Based Approach, DOI 10.1007/978-3-319-27365-5_38

procedural invasiveness, and hospital length of stay, but may require more than one treatment to achieve pseudocyst resolution. As a result, there is significant controversy and uncertainty regarding optimal management of pancreatic pseudocyst.

Several laparoscopic surgical techniques have been described. The most common among these include pseudocystgastrostomy via anterior (intraluminal) or posterior (extraluminal) approaches, pseudocystduodenostomy, and Roux-en-Y pseudocystjejeunostomy. Likewise, several endoscopic options have been described, including the use of ultrasound or fluoroscopic guidance for pseudocyst localization, plastic vs. metal stent use, single vs. multiple stent placement, and concomitant ERCP to identify need for and facilitate pancreatic duct (PD) stent placement. For the purpose of this review, studies involving any combination of these techniques have been considered collectively as either laparoscopic or endoscopic management techniques, respectively.

Search Strategy

A Medline search was performed in PubMed using the following search strings based on PICO elements (Table 38.1): "pancreatic AND pseudocyst AND (laparoscopic OR laparoscopy OR endoscopic OR endoscopy)". The search was limited to studies on human subjects written in the English language since 2000. All results were read and reviewed, and irrelevant results were excluded from the analysis. Single-case reports, systematic and other reviews, and editorials and commentaries were also excluded.

Results

There is a paucity of prospective clinical trials comparing surgical and endoscopic management of pancreatic pseudocysts. No studies have directly compared laparoscopic management to endoscopy, and there is substantial heterogeneity in the techniques and adjuncts used in the series that are available. Furthermore, numerous series include both pseudocysts and necrotic fluid collections, further complicating the interpretation of their outcomes given the reduced efficacy of endoscopic

Table 38.1 PICO table for management of symptomatic pancreatic pseudocyst

P (Patients)	I (Intervention)	C (Comparator group)	O (Outcomes measured)
Patients with symptomatic pancreatic pseudocyst undergoing curative management	Laparoscopic operative management	Endoscopic management	Resolution of symptoms, complications, recurrence, need for additional or more invasive management

management of walled-off necrotic fluid collections. Finally, much of the literature represents experience of a single surgeon or endoscopist or within a single institution, limiting their generalizability and comparative usefulness.

Surgical Versus Endoscopic Management

In a prospective randomized clinical trial involving 40 patients at a single institution with symptomatic pancreatic pseudocysts, Varadarajulu et al. compared open surgical and endoscopic management. Twenty patients underwent either ultrasound- and fluoroscopic-guided cystgastrostomy with stoma balloon dilation and placement of two plastic stents immediately followed by ERCP and PD stent placement if PD leak was identified or open surgical cystgastrostomy by a single surgeon via an upper midline laparotomy and an anterior (intraluminal) gastric approach using an endovascular stapler to create a 6-cm communication. Successful treatment was noted in 95 % (19/20) of patients undergoing endoscopic management and in 100 % (20/20) of patients undergoing surgical management, although one surgical patient developed a recurrent pseudocyst with ongoing alcohol use. There were no complications in the endoscopy group, while one wound infection and one upper GI bleed occurred in the surgical group, the latter of which required endoscopic cauterization at the anastomosis. Another patient had a surgical feeding tube placed for persistent intolerance of oral intake, and another developed a pancreatic duct stricture at the tail requiring distal pancreatectomy after attempted stent placement via ERCP. Overall, there were no significant differences between arms in success rates, complications, or need for further interventions with or without crossover. However, hospital length of stay was significantly shorter in the endoscopic group (2 days versus 6 days), and overall treatment cost per patient was significantly lower in the endoscopic group. The utility of the study was limited by its small sample size and its inclusion of data generated by only one surgeon and two endoscopists at a single institution [1].

Melman et al. performed a retrospective review of a series of 83 patients who had undergone endoscopic, laparoscopic, or open cystgastrostomy over the prior 8 years at a single institution. Primary success, defined as resolution of symptoms or pseudocysts following the initial intervention, was more common in patients with laparoscopic and open surgical management compared to endoscopic management (87.5 %, 81.2 %, and 51.1 %, respectively; $p<0.01$). However, overall success, defined as resolution of symptoms or pseudocysts at last patient follow-up regardless of number of attempts of or techniques for intervention, was not significantly different between laparoscopic, open, and endoscopic groups (93.8 %, 90.9 %, and 84.6 %, respectively; $p>0.05$). One patient in the laparoscopic group had recurrent symptomatic pseudocyst and underwent successful endoscopic management. One patient in the open group had recurrent pancreatitis and underwent necrosectomy, and another who had a residual pseudocyst was managed with percutaneous drainage. In the endoscopic group, 13 initial failures were managed via open surgical management, and 3 had percutaneous drainage. Six initial failures were successfully managed with repeat endoscopic procedures; the overall success rate among endoscopic patients who did not require subsequent surgical or percutaneous procedures was 64.4 % (29/45). Surgical complications in the laparoscopic group were encountered in 25 % (4/16) of patients and included two upper gastrointestinal hemorrhages, one of which required endoscopic management. Among open surgical patients, complications occurred in 22.7 % (5/22) and included one patient who developed a wound infection, two patients with incisional hernias, and one patient who developed multi-system organ failure and prolonged respiratory failure requiring tracheostomy. Complications in the endoscopic group occurred in 15.6 % (7/45) of patients and included three patients who needed urgent laparotomy for unspecified reasons, two with gastric perforation, one with cystgastrostomy unable to be managed endoscopically, and one with upper gastrointestinal hemorrhage who was managed conservatively. The complication rates did not differ significantly between groups ($p=0.6448$). However, crossover rates from endoscopic to any surgical management and from laparoscopic or open surgical to endoscopic management for either treatment failure or management of complications was significantly higher in the initial endoscopic group (15.6 % versus 2.6 %, $p=0.0475$). Interpretation of these results is made complicated by the inclusion of debris-containing fluid collections (suggestive of walled-off necrosis, which has lower rate of successful endoscopic treatment) and the lack of clarification as to the conduct of interventions (i.e. PD stent placement) when PD leak was identified. This study was further limited by inclusion of patients within a single institution and bias associated with non-randomized patient groups [2].

Nealon et al. retrospectively reviewed 79 patients over a 10-year period at a single institution who developed complications after initial endoscopic and/or percutaneous management of pancreatic pseudocysts and compared outcomes and characteristics of this cohort with those of 100 consecutive patients who underwent initial open operative management. Additionally, pancreatic ductal anatomy and the relationship of the pseudocyst to the rest of the pancreas were assessed and classified in all patients using ERCP or MRCP. There were no statistical differences in disease severity, pseudocyst size or location, or anatomic relationship of the pseudocyst to the main pancreatic duct between patients undergoing initial endoscopic and/or percutaneous management versus operative management. Treatment failure was noted in 83.5 % (66/79) patients undergoing endoscopic and/or percutaneous management; all 66 patients required subsequent open operative management. Of these, two-thirds were noted to have pancreatic duct disruption and had not had PD stent placement prior to referral for operative management. Sepsis eventually occurred in 91.1 % (72/79) of patients with initial endoscopic and/or percutaneous management. The most common operative technique in patients with initial failed therapy was open cystjejunostomy (47/66, 71.2 %). There were no mortalities or need for reoperation among this group. While the rate of patients requiring ICU admission, ICU admissions per patient, episodes of sepsis, complications related to bleeding or renal failure, need for mechanical ventilation, and persistent pancreatic fistula were significantly lower among patients with initial operative management compared to those with initial endoscopic and/or percutaneous management ($p<0.05$), these results must be interpreted with caution as the non-operatively managed patients included in this study only included those who were initially unsuccessful or developed complications, and included percutaneous drainage as a treatment modality, which is not currently accepted as a definitive treatment modality. Finally, details regarding the specific non-operative approaches used are not provided [3].

Laparoscopic Management

We identified six retrospective reports of case series primarily involving laparoscopic management of pancreatic pseudocysts. Overall, treatment success was noted in 83–100 % of patients, with complications occurring in 0–27 %. The recurrence rates were 0–20 %, and 0–20 % of patients required operative or other procedural management following the initial operative therapy.

In the largest case series by Palanivelu et al., which included 106 patients who underwent laparoscopic management, the treatment success rate was 100 %. Complications occurred in 6.6 % of patients, and recurrence was noted in 0.9 %, while the need for further surgical or other management was noted in 1.9 %. Laparoscopic cystgastrostomy was the most common procedure, accounting for 83.4 % of the cases in this series [4].

No other case series involving primarily laparoscopic patients included more than 17 patients, limiting the significance of their conclusions. However, a summary of the findings from these smaller studies is presented in Table 38.2.

Endoscopic Management

We identified 11 retrospective reports of case series primarily involving endoscopic management of pancreatic pseudocysts. Overall, treatment success was noted in 75–100 % of patients, with complications occurring in 0–26 %. The recurrence rates were 0–16 %, and 0–28 % of patients required additional operative management following the initial endoscopic therapy.

The largest case series involving primarily endoscopic management was reported by Weckman et al. Among 165 patients who underwent endoscopic therapy and completed follow-up, treatment success (i.e. those with no or only mild pancreatic symptoms) was noted in 75.2 %. The 170 patients examined in this study underwent a total of 380 endoscopic procedures; complications occurred in 10.0 % of these. Recurrence was noted in 5.6 % of patients, and 13.9 % of patients initially managed endoscopically subsequently underwent a surgical procedure in their course of treatment [10].

In another series, Varadarajulu et al. compiled outcomes of patients treated for pancreatic pseudocysts, abscesses, or necrosis. In 154 patients undergoing endo-

Table 38.2 Studies involving laparoscopic management of pancreatic pseudocyst

Study	n	Male	Male %	Resolution	Resolution %	Complications	Complications %	Recurrence	Recurrence %	Further surgery required	Further surgery %	Follow up	Notes
Dávila-Cervantes (2004)	10	6	60.0 %	9	90.0 %	2	20.0 %	0	0.0 %	2	20.0 %	22 months	Study compared open vs laparoscopic procedures; among 10, 4 RY cyst-J, 4 extraluminal cyst-G, 2 intraluminal cyst-G; 2 required further procedures (1 endoscopic cyst-D, 1 open surgery); lap less morbidity, less pain, shorter LOS
Hauters (2004)	17	9	52.9 %	16	94.1 %	2	11.8 %	0	0.0 %	2	11.8 %	12 months	Complications: 1 open conversion followed by retrocolic abscess requiring perc drainage, 1 with residual infection secondary to gastrotomy closure requiring endoscopic stent
Hindmarsh (2005)	15	5	33.3 %	10	83.3 %	4	26.7 %	2	20.0 %	2	13.3 %	37 months	12 of 15 underwent lap operation; 3 conversions to open; recurrences were prior to discharge and managed by open cyst-G; (1 also underwent subsequent open panc/splenic for path with serous cystadenoca)

Barragan (2005)	8	1	12.5 %	8	100.0 %	0	0.0 %	1	12.5 %	1	12.5 %	NR	All secondary to gallstone pancreatitis s/p lap chole; 4 anterior (intraluminal), 4 posterior (extraluminal); posterior deemed superior due to no gastrotomy closure and better visualization of cyst
Palanivelu (2007)	108	76	70.4 %	106[a]	100.0 %	7[a]	6.6 %	1	0.9 %	2	1.9 %	54 months	[a]among 106 who underwent initial laparoscopic drainge
Oida (2009)	7	7	100.0 %	7	100.0 %	0	0.0 %	0	0.0 %	0	0.0 %	65 months	

References for table in order: [4–9]

[a]Refers to the columns "complication" and "resolution" in the same row to deliniate specific subsets of the study

scopic management for pancreatic pseudocysts or abscesses, successful treatment was achieved in 93.5 %. Complications and recurrence were noted in 5.2 % and 5.0 %, respectively, of patients undergoing endoscopic therapy for pseudocyst, abscess, or necrosis. Operative management was required in 13.3 % of treated patients [11].

These and several smaller studies, none including more than 60 patients, are summarized in Table 38.3.

Recommendations Based on the Data

1. For patients with favorable size and location of pseudocyst (with respect to the stomach and/or duodenum) and favorable pancreatic duct anatomy, endoscopic management is recommended (evidence quality moderate, moderate recommendation).
2. Evaluation of pancreatic ductal anatomy for identification of associated pancreatic duct disruption or stricture and the presence of communication between the duct and pseudocyst should be performed. If disruption or stricture is identified, particularly in the setting of communication with the pseudocyst, placement of a pancreatic duct stent to bridge the disruption/stricture may increase the likelihood of successful endoscopic management (evidence quality moderate, moderate recommendation).
3. If "disconnected duct" syndrome is identified, laparoscopic drainage may be preferable to endoscopic management as the latter may require pseudocyst stent placement of indeterminate length with attendant increased risks of stent migration and associated complications (evidence quality weak, recommendation weak).
4. For patients in whom endoscopic pseudocyst drainage would be technically challenging or has already been attempted with procedural failure or symptom recurrence related to unanticipated presence of necrotic debris, surgical management is recommended (evidence quality moderate, moderate recommendation).
5. Laparoscopic approaches should be attempted during surgical drainage procedures when technically feasible and commensurate with the proficiency of the surgeon (evidence quality moderate, moderate recommendation).

A Personal View of the Data

Numerous minimally invasive techniques exist in the management of pancreatic pseudocyst. Definitive algorithms are lacking due to inconsistent application of appropriate pancreatic fluid collection terminology (2013 revised Atlanta classification) and variability of local expertise in both endoscopic and laparoscopic techniques. Endoscopic management appears to result in shorter length of stay and fewer complications, though at the cost of more frequent interventions. Laparoscopic

Table 38.3 Studies involving endoscopic management of pancreatic pseudocyst

Study	n	Male	Male %	Resolution	Resolution %	Complications	Complications %	Recurrence	Recurrence %	Surgery required	Surgery %	Follow up	Notes
Sharma (2002)	38	25	65.8 %	37	97.4 %	5	13.2 %	6	16.2 %	2	5.3 %	44 months	Usefulness of ERCP for stenting or stone removal; selection of only patients with bulging/communicating pseudocysts; 50 % of recurrences symptomatic
Baron (2002)	95	54	56.8 %	82	86.3 %	17	17.9 %	9	11.0 %	7	7.4 %	766 days	Divided into acute/chronic pseudocyst + pancreatic necrosis groups; surgery crossover figure combined amonth groups; endoscopic drainage most favorable for chronic pseudocysts >4 weeks
Will (2006)	13	NR	NR	11	84.6 %	1	7.7 %	0	0.0 %	0	0.0 %	NR	Study also included patient groups treated by percutaneous transgastric drainage and by EUS-guided cystagastrostomy with necrosectomy; success, recurrence, and complication rates similar among groups
Kahalek (2006)	99	76	76.8 %	93[a]	93.9 %	19	19.2 %	NR	NR	2	2.0 %	13.9 months	Included patients undergoing EUS-guided or conventional transmural drainage; success and complication rates were similar between groups, [a]at 1 month follow-up; resolution rates at 13.9 months were 84 % (27/32, EUS) and 91 % (41/45, CTD)

(continued)

Table 38.3 (continued)

Study	n	Male	Male %	Resolution	Resolution %	Complications	Complications %	Recurrence	Recurrence %	Surgery required	Surgery %	Follow up	Notes
Weckman (2006)	170	125	73.5 %	124[a]	75.2 %	38[b]	10.0 %	8	5.6 %	23	13.9 %	34 months	[a]124 of 165 patients with full follow-up and with no or only mild pancreatic symptoms; [b]among 380 total endoscopic procedures
Varadarajulu (2008)	20	18	62.1 %	27	93.1 %	2	6.9 %	0	0.0 %	2	6.9 %	142 days	
Sharma (2008)	9	6	66.7 %	9	100.0 %	0	0.0 %	0	0.0 %	0	0.0 %	5.7 years	Pediatric population
Park (2009)	60	47	78.3 %	50	83.3 %	5	8.3 %	4	8.5 %	4[a]	6.7 %	26 months	[a]Surgical or percutaneous management
Varadarajulu (2011)	154[a]	88	57.1 %	144	93.5 %	8	5.2 %	9[b]	5.0 %	28[c]	13.3 %	367 days[a]	[a]Among only study patients with pancreatic pseudocyst or abscess, [b]among all study patients with successful treatment, [c]among all study patients treated
Will (2011)	113	76	67.3 %	110	97.3 %	19	16.8 %	17	15.5 %	13	11.5 %	21 months	
Seewald (2012)	80	49	61.3 %	67	83.8 %	21	26.3 %	9	13.4 %	22	27.5 %	31 months	

References for table in order: [10–20]

[a]Refers to the columns in the same row to deliniate specific subsets of the study

[b]Refers to the columns in the same row to deliniate specific subsets of the study

[c]Refers to the columns in the same row to deliniate specific subsets of the study

[d]Refers to the columns in the same row to deliniate specific subsets of the study

management as first-line therapy may be more successful in resolution of symptoms and reducing the need for additional procedural intervention, though length of stay is longer and complications can be more serious. The first important clinical clarification is whether the pancreatic fluid collection (PFC), typically seen initially on computerized tomography (CT) imaging, represents a pseudocyst or walled-off pancreatic necrosis. The presence of solid debris may reduce the efficacy and increase the risk of adverse outcomes of standard endoscopic pseudocystgastrostomy and may favor the use of a laparoscopic approach given the more thorough concomitant debridement that can be performed. Because computerized tomography (CT) cannot reliably identify the presence of solid (necrotic) debris within a PFC, EUS or MRI/MRCP can be invaluable during the formulation of the treatment plan. These modalities also offer an opportunity to differentiate the PFC from features consistent with pancreatic cystic neoplasm. The second important anatomic clarification required in the formulation of a treatment plan is assessment of the PD anatomy and its relationship to the pseudocyst, with appropriate PD stent placement to enhance the likelihood of success with endoscopic pseudocystgastrostomy. Alternatively, if "disconnected duct" with a viable pancreatic tail remnant is identified, laparoscopic drainage or even distal pancreatic resection may be more appropriate.

Given the complexity and range of the available treatment modalities and the relative infrequency and clinical heterogeneity of patients presenting with pancreatic pseudocysts, a multidisciplinary approach to treatment plan formulation involving surgeons, endoscopists, and other interventionalists should be an integral part of the management of patients with pancreatic pseudocyst. On the whole, given the presence of appropriate local expertise and anatomic features, endoscopic approach should be given strong consideration as first-line treatment, but may require several interventions before resolution is complete. Laparoscopic management may be a more definitive approach, particularly in the setting of disconnected duct syndrome, but is associated with greater morbidity, and requires that the patient be able to undergo general anesthesia.

References

1. Varadarajulu S, Bang JY, Sutton BS, Trevino JM, Christein JD, Wilcox CM. Equal efficacy of endoscopic and surgical cystogastrostomy for pancreatic pseudocyst drainage in a randomized trial. Gastroenterology. 2013;145(3):583–90.
2. Melman L, Azar R, Beddow K, Brunt LM, Halpin VJ, Eagon JC, Frisella MM, Edmundowicz S, Jonnalagadda S, Matthews BD. Primary and overall success rates for clinical outcomes after laparoscopic, endoscopic, and open pancreatic cystgastrostomy for pancreatic pseudocysts. Surg Endosc. 2009;23(2):267–71.
3. Nealon WH, Walser E. Surgical management of complications associated with percutaneous and/or endoscopic management of pseudocyst of the pancreas. Ann Surg. 2005;241(6):948–57.
4. Palanivelu C, Senthilkumar K, Madhankumar MV, Rajan PS, Shetty AR, Jani K, Rangarajan M, Maheshkumaar GS. Management of pancreatic pseudocyst in the era of laparoscopic surgery – experience from a tertiary centre. Surg Endosc. 2007;21(12):2262–7.

5. Dávila-Cervantes A, Gómez F, Chan C, Bezaury P, Robles-Díaz G, Uscanga LF, Herrera MF. Laparoscopic drainage of pancreatic pseudocysts. Surg Endosc. 2004;18(10):1420–6.
6. Hauters P, Weerts J, Navez B, Champault G, Peillon C, Totte E, Barthelemy R, Siriser F. Laparoscopic treatment of pancreatic pseudocysts. Surg Endosc. 2004;18(11):1645–8.
7. Hindmarsh A, Lewis MPN, Rhodes M. Stapled laparoscopic cystgastrostomy: a series with 15 cases. Surg Endosc. 2005;19(1):143–7.
8. Barragan B, Love L, Wachtel M, Griswold JA, Frezza EE. A comparison of anterior and posterior approaches for the surgical treatment of pancreatic pseudocyst using laparoscopic cystogastrostomy. J Laparoendosc Adv Surg Tech A. 2005;15(6):596–600.
9. Oida T, Mimatsu K, Kawasaki A, Kano H, Kuboi Y, Aramaki O, Amano S. Long-term outcome of laparoscopic cystogastrostomy performed using a posterior approach with a stapling device. Dig Surg. 2009;26(2):110–4.
10. Weckman L, Kylänpää M-L, Puolakkainen P, Halttunen J. Endoscopic treatment of pancreatic pseudocysts. Surg Endosc. 2006;20(4):603–7.
11. Varadarajulu S, Bang JY, Phadnis MA, Christein JD, Wilcox CM. Endoscopic transmural drainage of peripancreatic fluid collections: outcomes and predictors of treatment success in 211 consecutive patients. J Gastrointest Surg. 2011;15(11):2080–8.
12. Sharma SS, Bhargawa N, Govil A. Endoscopic management of pancreatic pseudocyst: a long-term follow-up. Endoscopy. 2002;34(3):203–7.
13. Baron TH, Harewood GC, Morgan DE, Yates MR. Outcome differences after endoscopic drainage of pancreatic necrosis, acute pancreatic pseudocysts, and chronic pancreatic pseudocysts. Gastrointest Endosc. 2002;56(1):7–17.
14. Will U, Wegener C, Graf K-I, Wanzar I, Manger T, Meyer F. Differential treatment and early outcome in the interventional endoscopic management of pancreatic pseudocysts in 27 patients. World J Gastroenterol. 2006;12(26):4175–8.
15. Kahaleh M, Shami VM, Conaway MR, Tokar J, Rockoff T, La Rue De SA, de Lange E, Bassignani M, Gay S, Adams RB, Yeaton P. Endoscopic ultrasound drainage of pancreatic pseudocyst: a prospective comparison with conventional endoscopic drainage. Endoscopy. 2006;38(4):355–9.
16. Varadarajulu S, Christein JD, Tamhane A, Drelichman ER, Wilcox CM. Prospective randomized trial comparing EUS and EGD for transmural drainage of pancreatic pseudocysts (with videos). Gastrointest Endosc. 2008;68(6):1102–11.
17. Sharma SS, Maharshi S. Endoscopic management of pancreatic pseudocyst in children-a long-term follow-up. J Pediatr Surg. 2008;43(9):1636–9.
18. Park DH, Lee SS, Moon S-H, Choi SY, Jung SW, Seo DW, Lee SK, Kim M-H. Endoscopic ultrasound-guided versus conventional transmural drainage for pancreatic pseudocysts: a prospective randomized trial. Endoscopy. 2009;41(10):842–8.
19. Will U, Wanzar C, Gerlach R, Meyer F. Interventional ultrasound-guided procedures in pancreatic pseudocysts, abscesses and infected necroses – treatment algorithm in a large single-center study. Ultraschall Med. 2011;32(2):176–83.
20. Seewald S, Ang TL, Richter H, Teng KYK, Zhong Y, Groth S, Omar S, Soehendra N. Long-term results after endoscopic drainage and necrosectomy of symptomatic pancreatic fluid collections. Dig Endosc. 2012;24(1):36–41.

Chapter 39
Antibiotic Prophylaxis for Acute Necrotizing Pancreatitis

Brodie Parent and E. Patchen Dellinger

Abstract In patients with severe acute pancreatitis complicated by pancreatic parenchymal necrosis, one of the feared complications is infected pancreatic necrosis and/or infected peripancreatic tissue. Because of this concern many patients with severe pancreatitis have been treated with prophylactic antibiotics in an attempt to prevent this complication, and one early open label trial in 1993 appeared to show benefit for this approach. Since that time multiple additional studies have been carried out, and review of these trials fails to demonstrate any reduction in infectious complications or the need for operative intervention when prophylactic antibiotics are used. An analysis of trials comparing prophylactic antibiotics with placebo shows that the highest quality studies (rigorous blinding, placebo protocols, inclusion only of severe disease, detailed patient flow descriptions) uniformly fail to show benefit for prophylaxis.

Patients with severe acute pancreatitis or necrotizing pancreatitis should not receive prophylactic antibiotics, but they should be carefully observed in order to facilitate early diagnosis and specific treatment if infection occurs. This is facilitated by fine needle, CT-guided aspiration of suspicious areas. This is an accurate and safe mechanism for determining the presence of infection and identifying the responsible organisms.

Keywords Severe acute pancreatitis • Necrotizing pancreatitis • Infected pancreatic necrosis • Prophylactic antibiotics • Septic complications • Operative intervention • Fine needle aspiration • Clinical trials

---

B. Parent • E.P. Dellinger (✉)
Department of General Surgery, University of Washington,
Room BB 428, 1959 N.E. Pacific Street, 356410, Seattle, Washington 98195-6410, USA
e-mail: bparent@u.washington.edu; patch@u.washington.edu

J.M. Millis, J.B. Matthews (eds.), *Difficult Decisions in Hepatobiliary and Pancreatic Surgery*, Difficult Decisions in Surgery: An Evidence-Based Approach, DOI 10.1007/978-3-319-27365-5_39

Introduction

Acute pancreatitis has a wide range of clinical severity, potential complications and outcomes. Approximately 80 % of patients have mild disease with a relatively quick recovery. Mild pancreatitis patients do not require antibiotic treatment and generally discharge from the hospital within 1 week. However, 15–20 % of patients develop severe acute pancreatitis (SAP) and necrosis of peri-pancreatic tissue or of the parenchyma itself [1–3]. Those patients with necrosis of >30 % of the gland demonstrated by contrast enhanced CT scan are at high risk of developing infected necrosis; overall, 15–35 % of patients with SAP develop infected pancreatic necrosis, typically in the second to fourth week of hospitalization [1, 2, 4, 5]. If the necrosis becomes infected, this increases systemic complications, raises rates of multiple organ failure, and increases the overall SAP mortality rate from 10 % to 30–40 % [2, 6, 7]. Organisms from the gastrointestinal tract are the most common causative agents and include *Escherichia coli*, *Pseudomonas aeruginosa*, Clostridium species, Bacteroides species, enterococci, Klebsiella species, Proteus species and Enterobacter species [2, 5, 7, 8]. Gram positive, drug-resistant and fungal organisms are also becoming more common [1, 9–11].

Making the diagnosis of infected pancreatic necrosis can be difficult. Patients with SAP and pancreatic necrosis almost always present with an impressive systemic inflammatory response syndrome (SIRS) with tachypnea, tachycardia, fever and leukocytosis. This initial clinical presentation is similar to one resulting from an underlying infection (sepsis), regardless of whether sterile necrosis or infected necrosis is present. Although this goes against the intuition of the treating physician, clinical parameters in SAP patients do not reliably distinguish between infected versus sterile necrosis [12–14].

In the face of clinical uncertainty and the potential for high mortality with infected necrosis, treating clinicians have often initiated early broad-spectrum antimicrobial prophylaxis for patients with SAP. The rationale is clear: one can surmise that prophylactic antibiotics in these critically-ill patients would reduce the incidence of infected necrosis and improve patient morbidity and mortality. Myriad trials and meta-analyses spanning the past four decades have attempted to show this anticipated benefit, but the published data have led to mixed and sometimes directly contradictory conclusions.

Our aim in this chapter is to determine if antibiotic prophylaxis benefits patients with severe acute pancreatitis (SAP). We will address the apparent impact of antibiotic prophylaxis on the incidence of infected necrosis, septic complications, length of stay, need for operative intervention, mortality and emerging antibiotic resistance.

Search Strategy

Using the PICO format (Table 39.1), a literature search using the PubMed database was performed to survey available published data on acute pancreatitis and antibiotic prophylaxis. Results were limited to English-language publications, human

Table 39.1 'PICO' literature search strategy for antibiotic prophylaxis in severe acute pancreatitis

P (Patients)	I (Intervention)	C (Comparator group)	O (Outcomes measured)
Patients with severe acute pancreatitis (inclusive of those with pancreatic and peri-pancreatic necrosis)	Antibiotic prophylaxis	No prophylaxis/placebo	Incidence of infected necrosis, septic complications, mortality, need for operative intervention, length of stay, antibiotic resistance

studies only, with publication range from 1993 to August 2014. Exceptions were made for publications prior to 1993 if they were widely referenced studies. Search terms were as follows: "antibiotic prophylaxis," "antibiotics," "antibacterial agent," "antifungal agent," "antibiotic resistance," AND ("acute necrotizing pancreatitis" OR "acute pancreatitis" OR "necrotizing pancreatitis" OR "severe acute pancreatitis").

We performed a validation of our search strategy using the bibliographies from several recent review articles and meta-analyses [1, 3, 15, 16]. A search of published literature from 1993 to 2009 was performed using the terms: "antibiotics," "antibiotic prophylaxis" AND ("acute pancreatitis" OR "necrotizing pancreatitis"). This strategy returned all but 3 of 43 relevant studies in the reference list by Wittau et al., all but 3 of 40 in Howard et al., all but 2 of 28 in Jiang et al., and all but 1 of 45 relevant references cited by De Waele et al. These unique references were included in our review.

Studies were excluded if they were case reports only or if they were studies devoted primarily to surgical decision making/surgical technique. Studies were also excluded if they primarily addressed regional arterial infusion of antibiotics or selective gastrointestinal decontamination.

Results

Early Studies: Prophylaxis and Decreased Infected Necrosis

Two randomized trials in 1975 by Howes et al. [17] and Finch et al. [18] (Tables 39.2 and 39.3) first assessed the efficacy of prophylactic ampicillin in acute pancreatitis. Both papers conclude that there was no difference in clinical outcomes between groups who received prophylaxis versus no prophylaxis. However, these initial studies have several limitations. Both included very mild cases of pancreatitis in their study populations, which introduced considerable heterogeneity in the study groups. Moreover, the rate of pancreatic necrosis and subsequent pancreatic infections was so low in the study groups that both papers were underpowered to detect a difference in treatments (high probability of a type II error).

In 1993, Pederzoli et al. [19] completed a randomized multicenter trial which compared imipenem prophylaxis versus no antibiotic treatment in acute pancreatitis

Table 39.2 Characteristics of studies on antibiotic prophylaxis in severe acute pancreatitis, with grading of evidence

Author (year)	Inclusion criteria	n	Study type	Quality of evidence (GRADE)
Finch (1975)	AP, amylase >160	58	RCT	Low
Howes (1975)	AP, amylase >160	95	RCT	Low
Pederzoli (1993)	SAP, PN	74	RCT	Low
Sainio (1995)	SAP, PN, CRP >120	60	RCT	Low
Declenserie (1996)	AP, ≥2 fluid collections on CT	23	RCT	Low
Bassi (1998)[a]	SAP, PN >50 %, CRP >100	60	RT	Low
Nordback (2001)[b]	AP, PN, CRP >150	58	RCT	Low
Manes (2003)[a]	SAP, PN, CRP >120	176	RT	Low
Isenmann (2004)	SAP, PN, CRP >150	114	DB-PC-RCT	High
Manes (2006)[b]	AP	59	RCT	Low
Dellinger (2007)	SAP, PN >30 %, CRP >120 or Balthazar E, MOD score >2	100	DB-PC-RCT	High
Rokke (2007)	SAP, CRP >120 at 24 h or CRP >200 at 48 h	73	RCT	Low
Garcia-Barrasa (2009)	SAP, PN	41	DB-PC-RCT	Moderate
Xue (2009)	SAP, PN >30 %	56	RCT	Low
Ignatavicius (2012)	SAP, CRP >120	210	NRPC	Low

AP acute pancreatitis, *CRP* C-reactive protein, *DB-PC-RCT* double-blind, placebo-controlled, randomized controlled trial, *MOD* multiple organ dysfunction, *NRPC* non-randomized prospective cohort; *PN* pancreatic necrosis (visualized on computed tomography scan), *RCT* randomized controlled trial, *RT* randomized trial, *SAP* severe acute pancreatitis

[a]Control groups in both these studies received imipenem, making comparison to other studies difficult. These studies' controls were compared to groups who received different antibiotics

[b]Control groups in both these studies were also given the designated intervention arm antibiotics later in the study, making comparisons to the other studies difficult. These two studies primarily evaluated antibiotics given early (intervention) vs late (control)

(n = 74). The authors reported an impressive 18 % decrease in the incidence of pancreatic sepsis with the use of prophylactic antibiotics. However, they were unable to show a difference in ultimate clinical endpoints like organ failure rates, operative rates, or mortality. Moreover, this study had several methodological flaws, most significant of which is the lack of any blinding. Lack of blinding is particularly problematic for pancreatitis studies because of historically ambiguous criteria for diagnosing patients with infection vs sepsis vs SIRS (as previously discussed). In addition, un-blinded studies may create a tendency to initiate more off-protocol antibiotics in control patients, leading to crossover between study arms [20]. Other methodological limitations in this study include the lack of a placebo, a heterogeneous study sample (varying severity pancreatitis patients were included), unbalanced study arms, and lack of any comments on patient recruitment/study flow.

Subsequent trials published in the 1990s concluded that pancreatic infections were reduced with prophylactic antimicrobials, but these studies were similarly limited methodologically. Limitations included heterogeneous severity of pancreatitis in study groups, lack of blinding, lack of placebo, low samples sizes (underpowered analyses), and frequent changes in antibiotic regimens in both intervention and control arms. Moreover, although many of these studies showed decreased pancreatic infections and systemic infections with prophylaxis, they failed to show any difference in observed mortality or the need for operations [21–28] (Tables 39.2 and 39.3). Notable exceptions include studies by Sainio et al. [22] and Nordback, et al. [23], who respectively noted a significant mortality benefit and a reduced operative rate in prophylaxis groups. However, both of these studies chose unique methods for defining pancreatic infection, and one study used only clinical parameters to define pancreatic infection (which we have previously described as inherently inaccurate). Finally, it is noteworthy that none of the aforementioned studies documented detailed methods of nutrition for sample populations. The use of enteral nutrition in pancreatitis studies is a highly significant potential confounding factor, given its demonstrated significant benefits for patients with SAP in terms of decreased systemic infections, need for operations, multiple organ failure and death [2, 6, 29, 30].

Recent Randomized Trials: Prophylaxis Reconsidered

Three more recent double-blinded placebo-controlled, randomized controlled trials (DBPCRCT) avoided several of the aforementioned methodological limitations and represent the highest quality evidence yet published. In the first double-blinded study in 2004, Isenmann et al. [31] (Tables 39.2 and 39.3) enrolled 114 pts with SAP and randomized them into two groups (metronidazole and ciprofloxacin versus placebo). No significant differences were noted in mortality, need for operations, length of stay or infected necrosis. Subgroup analysis of those with confirmed pancreatic necrosis >30 % (those deemed at higher risk of pancreatic infection) also showed no differences between groups. Notably, 46 % in placebo group required conversion to open antibiotic treatment due to systemic and septic complications, compared with just 28 % of patients in the intervention group. The next DBPCRCT was performed in 2007 by Dellinger et al. [5] and included 100 patients who had necrotizing SAP. Patients received either meropenem or placebo, and after 42 days follow-up, groups showed similar rates of mortality, infection and need for operative intervention. The authors concluded that the data do not support early prophylactic antibiotics in SAP. Finally, in 2009, Garcia-Barrasa et al. [32] performed a DBPCRCT in 41 patients diagnosed with SAP who had a CT scan showing evidence of pancreatic necrosis. No significant differences between groups were found for infected pancreatic necrosis, mortality, systemic complications, need for operations or length of stay. Of note, due to limitations inherent to this study's design (described below), the authors stated that no conclusions could be drawn regarding efficacy of prophylactic antibiotics in SAP.

These three DBPCRCTs have methodological strengths that are worth reviewing, but they also contain several limitations. Notable strengths of these studies

Table 39.3 Studies on antibiotic prophylaxis in severe acute pancreatitis, with comparison of clinical outcomes

Author (year)	Infected necrosis			Septic/systemic complications[a]			Mortality		
	Intervention	Control	p-value	Intervention	Control	p-value	Intervention	Control	p-value
Finch (1975)	na	na	na	19 %	18 %	na	3 %	0 %	na
Howes (1975)	4 %	2 %	na	10 %	13 %	na	0 %	0 %	na
Pederzoli (1993)	12 %	30 %	0.01	15 %	49 %	<0.01	3 %	4 %	na
Sainio (1995)	15 %	20 %	na	50 %	90 %	0.01	2 %	12 %	0.03
Declenserie (1996)	0 %	30 %	0.03	58 %	0 %	0.03	9 %	25 %	NS
Bassi (1998)[b]	34 %	10 %	0.03	44 %	20 %	0.06	24 %	10 %	0.18
Nordback (2001)[c]	8 %	42 %	0.03	20 %	30 %	NS	8 %	15 %	NS
Manes (2003)[b]	11 %	14 %	na	22 %	24 %	na	14 %	11 %	na
Isenmann (2004)	12 %	9 %	0.58	28 %	46 %	na	5 %	7 %	na
Manes (2006)[c]	13 %	31 %	0.10	17 %	45 %	<0.05	10 %	10 %	NS
Dellinger (2007)	23 %	15 %	0.39	32 %	48 %	<0.2	20 %	18 %	0.97
Rokke (2007)	8 %	19 %	0.01	14 %	43 %	0.04	8 %	11 %	NS
Garcia-Barrasa (2009)	36 %	42 %	0.70	27 %	42 %	0.30	18 %	11 %	0.60
Xue (2009)	28 %	27 %	NS	62 %	55 %	NS	10 %	15 %	NS
Ignatavicius (2012)	9 %	7 %	0.79	13 %	11 %	0.83	13 %	20 %	0.19

ICU intensive care unit, *LOS* length of stay, *NA* not available, *NS* not significant, *RO* resistant organisms

[a]Septic/systemic complications include incidence rates of nosocomial infections, newly developed SIRS or sepsis

[b]Control groups in both these studies received imipenem, making comparison to other studies difficult. These studies' controls were compared to groups who received different antibiotics

Need for operation			Mean ICU/hospital LOS (days)			Antibiotic resistance		
Intervention	Control	p-value	Intervention	Control	p-value	Intervention	Control	p-value
3 %	0 %	na	na, 10.4	na, 11.3	na	na	na	na
4 %	2 %	na	na, 9	na, 12	NS	na	na	na
12 %	11 %	na	na	na	na	na	na	na
12 %	23 %	0.01	33, 12	43, 23	0.24, 0.06	na	na	na
0 %	25 %	na	na, 22	na, 27.8	NS	na	na	na
na	na	na	na, 31	na, 29	na	na	na	na
8 %	36 %	NS	8, 20	8,20	na	na	na	na
17 %	18 %	na	na, 24	na, 23	na	na	na	na
17 %	11 %	na	8,21	6,18	na	18 RO	6RO	<.001
12 %	38 %	<0.05	na,18.5	na,29.6	<0.01	4 RO	3RO	na
26 %	20 %	0.47	na	na	na	7 RO	3 RO	na
8 %	8 %	NS	na, 18	na, 22	NS	na	na	na
50 %	42 %	0.61	17,21	18,19	0.82, 0.79	2 RO	1 RO	na
30 %	35 %	NS	na,28	na, 21	NS	36 % fungal	14 % fungal	$p<0.05$
8 %	20 %	0.02	2,14	3,11	0.14, 0.24	8 RO	5 RO	0.52

[c]Control groups in both these studies were also given the designated intervention arm antibiotics later in the study, making comparisons to the other studies difficult. These two studies primarily evaluated antibiotics given early (intervention) vs late (control)

include rigorous blinding and placebo protocols, homogeneity of patients (designed to include only *severe* disease), and detailed patient flow descriptions. Moreover, the 2007 DBPCRCT is one of the first studies that ensured standardized nutrition protocols between study groups, thus controlling for this significant source of bias. One limitation inherent to all three studies is small sample size, which diminishes the power to detect a small magnitude effect. Moreover, the conclusions from these studies must be interpreted with caution because all study protocols allowed substantial heterogeneity in both the time of initiation (range: 3–10 days) and duration of therapy among patients (range 6–21 days). Finally, large proportions (up to half) of patients in control and intervention arms received non-protocol antibiotics for other clinical indications.[1] Taken together, the limitations of these three DBPCRCTs have the potential to bias results toward acceptance of a null hypothesis (type II error). That is, all these described limitations would more likely diminish the effect seen from prophylactic antibiotics and make it more likely to conclude that no significant difference exists between groups.

A Review of Disparate Results

The meta-analyses, reviews, editorials and observational studies published on this topic are too numerous to review individually [6, 15, 20, 33–48], but some trends are worth noting. Results from the meta-analyses on this topic must be interpreted with caution because of the myriad differences between available trials. Any comparison among the previously described trials is limited because of variety in: (a) sampled severities of pancreatitis, (b) definitions for pancreatic infections, (c) outcomes evaluated, (d) thresholds for operative intervention, and (e) antibiotics administered. The majority of these meta-analyses found a significant difference in pancreatic infections for those patients who received antibiotic prophylaxis, but found no differences in mortality, LOS or the need for operations. In contrast, some meta-analyses *did* show significant differences in mortality, LOS and operative interventions, but these authors failed to include data from relevant DBPCRCTs published after 2004 [36, 41, 43, 45, 47, 48]. Those meta-analyses that included data from DBPCRCTs published after 2004 showed that prior perceived differences in outcomes failed to achieve significance [15, 16, 46].

Some meta-analyses have used unique approaches and explanations to highlight trends in the available data on antibiotic prophylaxis for SAP. One meta-analysis by De Vries et al. [20] reviewed six randomized controlled trials addressing antibiotic prophylaxis in SAP and noted a significant inverse relationship between their methodological quality and the reported effect of antibiotic prophylaxis on mortality. In

[1] However, Dellinger et al. [5] note that the vast majority of 'off-protocol' antibiotics given in this trial occurred three or more weeks after randomization. This permits evaluation of the efficacy of *early* antibiotic prophylaxis and does not diminish the validity of their conclusions. This is strengthened by evidence that bacterial seeding of pancreatic and peri-pancreatic necrosis often occurs as early as the first 1–2 weeks of hospitalization [13].

other words, studies that were assessed as methodologically rigorous tended to report negligible differences in mortality with the use of prophylaxis. Moreover, after grading for quality, and including studies only with a standardized score >5, the meta-analysis revealed that there was no difference found in infection of pancreatic necrosis or mortality. A subsequent meta-analysis by Wittau et al. in 2010 [15] independently confirmed this correlation between study quality and reported outcomes. The authors concluded that prophylaxis had no associated reduction in mortality, infected necrosis, systemic complications or the need for operations. Moreover, the authors found a "borderline significant" pooled relative risk for infected necrosis (RR = 0.78, [95 % CI 0.60–1.02]) but note that this is a surrogate outcome, and that the "real effects" seen by the patient (mortality or need for an operation) are not close to achieving significant differences. Finally, a meta-analysis from 2012 [16] pooled results from studies prior to the year 2000 and demonstrated a relative risk reduction for mortality (RR 0.31, [95 % CI, 0.12–0.79], $p = 0.01$). This difference was not present when results were pooled for studies after the year 2000 (RR 1.01, 95 % CI 0.65–1.56 p 0.98). Interestingly, the authors note a high potential for publication bias prior to the year 2000 based on the asymmetric results of a funnel plot analysis. The combination of this publication bias and un-blinded study designs prior to 2000 created an environment which would be more likely to produce studies showing a significant effect with prophylactic antibiotics in SAP.

Antimicrobial Resistance and Atypical Organisms

Published studies of moderate quality are available regarding antimicrobial resistance patterns in relation to antibiotics and SAP; overall trends indicate that exposure to broad-spectrum prophylaxis is associated with atypical and resistant organisms. A study in 2002 by Howard et al. [9] compared operative cultures taken from SAP patients before (1977–1992) and after (1993–2001) institution of routine prophylactic antibiotics at a single institution. There was a significant change in bacteriology between groups from gram negative organisms to predominantly gram positive organisms (52 % gram positive organisms in recent samples versus 23 % in older samples). The organisms most frequently cultured in antibiotic-treated patients were *S. aureus*, *S. epidermidis* and Corynebacterium. Of note, there were no differences in B-lactam resistance noted between groups. A subsequent case series of 46 patients with SAP and infected necrosis found that approximately 52 % of the patients developed infection with resistant organisms [10]. Those who developed resistant organisms were treated with antibiotics, on average, for 9 days longer than those without resistant organisms ($p < 0.05$). The authors note that patients with resistant organisms required longer ICU stays, and tended to have higher mortality (37 % vs 23 %, $p = 0.28$). Other studies have confirmed that the prevalence of antibiotic resistant microorganisms is increasing in patients with SAP and exposure to antibiotic prophylaxis [5, 11, 27, 28, 31, 32, 49, 50]. Classic pathophysiologic teaching on infected pancreatic necrosis cultures has attributed the predominant growth of gram negative species to a prior translocation event from the gastrointestinal tract [2, 4, 6]. However, in the new antibiotic era, increased growth of gram positive flora and fungal organisms may indicate that sources of infection are changing. Some authors speculate that these atypical and resistant organisms may emanate from central lines, catheters, and endotracheal tubes [9, 11]. This was corroborated by a retrospective study which found that patients who had any bacteremia episode while under treatment for SAP with pancreatic necrosis had an increased risk of infected necrosis (65 % vs 37 %) [4].

Available data suggest that SAP patients who have a longer exposure to broad spectrum antibiotics are also at a higher risk of infections with Candida species. In one retrospective study of 92 patients, the authors found that patients with fungal infections were on antibiotics for a mean of 19 days versus 6.4 days in patients without fungal infections ($p = 0.0001$) [51]. This trend was independently confirmed by a case series of 46 patients in 2004 [10], a prospective study of 50 SAP patients in 2009 [52], and a randomized trial in 2009 [28]. A more recent nonrandomized prospective cohort study of 210 SAP patients [50] found that candida species from pancreatic cultures were significantly more frequent in the patients who received prophylactic antibiotics versus those who did not (10.7 % vs 3.8 %, p 0.04). The mortality rate for SAP patients with Candida has been reported at 65 % versus about 20 % in non-Candida patients [4, 51]. Some studies have found less impressive differences in mortality but still note that SAP patients who develop fungal infections suffer more in-hospital morbidity and have longer hospital and ICU stays [10, 50, 53, 54].

Nevertheless, the reviewed studies on atypical and resistant organisms constitute moderate to low-quality evidence. Much of the published data is un-blinded, non-randomized, and considers two different time periods. Moreover, some considered studies [50] had control groups where large proportions of patients actually received prophylaxis while intervention groups had large proportions of patients who actually did not receive prophylaxis, making the labels 'control' and 'intervention' less meaningful. Finally, much of the available data on resistance patterns comes from larger studies which assessed this only as a secondary outcome. There is a need for larger epidemiological studies focused specifically on atypical and resistant organisms in patients with SAP who receive antibiotic prophylaxis.

A detailed review of the evidence for antifungal prophylaxis in SAP is beyond the scope of this chapter. In brief, there is insufficient evidence to recommend routine antifungal prophylaxis for all patients with SAP, but there is evidence of a survival benefit in high risk subsets of critically-ill surgical patients [1, 7, 39, 52, 55]. More research is needed to determine if patients with SAP fall within these subsets of patients that could benefit from anti-fungal prophylaxis.

Evidence-Based Protocol for "On-Demand" Antibiotics

The use of prophylactic antibiotics remains suspect, but "on-demand" antibiotics [31] should be initiated in clear cases of infection. If patients with SAP continue to deteriorate or fail to improve after the first or second week of hospitalization, obtaining a CT with or without fine needle aspiration (FNA) of pancreatic tissue is warranted. If the CT shows retroperitoneal air inside pancreatic fluid collections, this is pathognomonic for infection. If the diagnosis remains ambiguous, FNA should be obtained [56, 57]. FNA results can help tailor antibiotic therapy and identify drug-resistant organisms as well. If a positive CT or FNA is obtained, antibiotics should be initiated and source control should be obtained via a "step-up approach" (percutaneous drainage, followed by surgical or endoscopic debridement if necessary) [1–3, 31, 58]. While awaiting full speciation on culture, empiric antibiotics should be initiated and should cover enteric organisms. Standard empiric regimens include carbapenems or quinolones plus metronidazole [1, 39]. Since infected necrosis rarely presents before 10 days, clinical worsening during this time period is typically the result of SIRS evolution rather than infected necrosis. Therefore, it is generally safe to wait up to 10 days to perform a diagnostic FNA [4, 8]. FNA of pancreatic necrosis is relatively sensitive and specific and is reported overall at 88 % and 90 % respectively. After the first week, the FNA sensitivity increases to 97 % and specificity increases to 100 % [1, 8, 56, 59, 60]. Some patients fail to improve after several weeks despite a negative culture results on FNA. In this case, repeat FNA or even empiric drainage/debridement may be warranted [7, 8, 61].

Summary and Recommendations

In summary, we performed a literature review to survey published data on antibiotic prophylaxis in patients with SAP (inclusive of those with pancreatic and peripancreatic necrosis). The relevant outcomes reviewed included the incidence of infected necrosis, septic complications, mortality, need for operative interventions, length of stay, and antibiotic resistance. Search results revealed a myriad of studies with diverse results and conclusions.

Early studies reported decreased pancreatic and systemic infections with prophylaxis, but largely failed to show corresponding differences in ultimate outcomes like operative rates, length of stay or mortality. Early studies constitute low-quality evidence (Table 39.2) because they were limited by publication bias, lack of blinding, lack of placebo, limited recruitment/study flow descriptions, high cross-over from control to intervention arms, and small sample sizes (underpowered). Moreover, early studies were limited by heterogeneity of disease severity and heterogeneity in nutrition methods. As a result of these limitations, no recommendations can be made based on these data.

Later DBPCRCTs constitute high-quality evidence (Table 39.2). These studies failed to show any significant differences between prophylaxis and placebo groups; rates of pancreatic infections, operations, mortality and length of stay were similar. While these studies did show trends toward decreased systemic infections in patients who received prophylaxis, they showed no significant differences in ultimate clinical outcomes for those treated "on-demand" [31] with antibiotics as soon as nosocomial infections arose. On the basis of these studies, we strongly recommend against using antibiotics to prevent infection in patients with SAP or in patients who develop sterile pancreatic necrosis. Antibiotics should only be used for patients with already proven pancreatic or systemic infections. However, even these high quality studies are limited by small sample sizes (under-powered analyses), variation in initiation/duration of antibiotics, and frequent use of additional 'off-protocol' antibiotics in both placebo and control groups. The net effect of these limitations may diminish small magnitude effects from prophylaxis and may result in failure to appreciate subtle but real differences (a type II error).

As previously discussed, it is largely impossible to differentiate sterile from infected pancreatic necrosis on the basis of clinical signs alone. Additional tools like CT and FNA are needed to help obtain a definitive diagnosis. Available moderate-quality evidence suggests that FNA is a sensitive and specific tool. Observational studies and randomized trials have noted that infected necrosis is extremely rare prior to day 7–10 of hospitalization. Therefore, we strongly recommend investigation with a CT with or without an FNA in any patient with pancreatic or peri-pancreatic necrosis if clinical deterioration or failure to improve occurs beyond 7–10 days of hospitalization. Treatment with empiric antibiotics should occur only if positive FNA cultures are obtained. Nevertheless, a negative FNA should be interpreted with caution in a patient who fails to improve and should not be used to definitively rule-out infected necrosis.

Available published data on prophylaxis and antimicrobial resistance/atypical organisms is of moderate to low quality. Many of these studies were observational in nature, but some evidence was from larger randomized trials. These studies have shown that drug-resistant organisms are frequent in patients with SAP and that the prevalence of resistant bacteria and fungi is associated with both exposure and *duration* of exposure to broad-spectrum antibiotics. It is unclear whether infections with resistant and/or atypical organisms lead to increased mortality, but fungal infections have been associated with increased morbidity and longer length of hospital stay. On the basis of these data, we recommend caution in all decisions to initiate antibiotics and limitation of the treatment duration whenever possible (weak recommendation).

A Personal View of the Data

Despite mounting evidence against the use of prophylactic antibiotics in SAP, a recent survey of intensivists and surgeons indicates that routine prophylaxis is an ongoing and common practice [62]. If the data are becoming more convincing, what can we infer from this generalized reluctance to adopt evidence-based practices? Certainly the cacophony of contradictory results and conclusions in the literature contributes to this slow uptake. Perhaps more importantly, as an individual clinician taking care of a critically-ill deteriorating patient, making the diagnosis of infected pancreatic necrosis is difficult and decisions must often be made quickly. In this context, antibiotic prophylaxis may be employed to allay the fears and anxieties of the clinician rather than to treat the patient. Prescribing prophylactic antibiotics 'buys time' while the patient stabilizes and while diagnostic workup occurs.

We caution against this practice and encourage a more rigorous application of evidence-based practice. Despite aforementioned limitations in the current evidence, we must balance the proven risks of antimicrobial resistance against the (at best) nominal potential and unproven benefits of prophylactic antibiotics. Moreover, we are a priori suspect regarding the use of antibiotics to prevent an infection of any necrotic tissue. Dead tissue lacks adequate perfusion and therefore lacks an adequate conduit for any antibiotic; studies of antibiotic penetration and tissue concentrations in *living* pancreatic tissue may not be applicable to this topic. Finally, the risk of infection in pancreatitis starts at the onset of inflammation and persists over several weeks. Generally accepted teaching dictates that infectious risks which persist over long periods of time do not benefit from antibiotic prophylaxis (for example, prophylaxis has been found ineffective for foley catheters, endotracheal tubes, central lines, burns, etc…).

Further studies to clarify this subject are needed, but improvements beyond currently published literature will prove challenging. Obtaining early access to patients for enrollment continues to be difficult due to frequent transfers from outside hospitals. Moreover, defining strict inclusion criteria often mandates obtaining a CT scan, but necrosis of pancreatic parenchyma often is not adequately depicted on CT until an interval of 2–3 days past initial presentation [27]. This further limits timeliness of enrollment. Finally, given the high prevalence of systemic (nonpancreatic) infections in these patients, studies on patients with SAP will likely always require frequent initiation of non-protocol, open-label antibiotics.

Future DBPCRCTs could be structured to evaluate specifically early versus late administration of prophylactic antibiotics and would offer methodological improvements beyond currently published studies on this topic [23, 27]. In any future studies, efforts must be focused on creating larger samples so that adequately powered analyses can occur. As it currently stands, the proven risks of antibiotic prophylaxis in SAP outweigh the potential nominal benefits, and available evidence indicates that the use of prophylaxis is not warranted.

Recommendations

1. We recommend against using antibiotics to prevent infection in patients with severe acute pancreatitis and in patients who develop sterile pancreatic necrosis. Antibiotics should only be used for patients with already proven pancreatic or systemic infections. (High-quality evidence, strong recommendation).
2. We recommend investigation with a CT +/– FNA in any patient with pancreatic or peri-pancreatic necrosis if clinical deterioration or failed improvement occurs beyond 7–10 days of hospitalization. Treatment with empiric antibiotics should

occur only if positive FNA cultures are obtained (moderate-quality evidence, strong recommendation).

3. If patients with severe acute pancreatitis have a confirmed infection, we recommend judicious initiation and limited duration of antibiotic treatment when possible to decrease the development of drug-resistant organisms (moderate-low quality evidence, weak recommendation).

References

1. Howard TJ. The role of antimicrobial therapy in severe acute pancreatitis. Surg Clin N Am. 2013;93(3):585–93. PubMed Epub 2013/05/02. eng.
2. da Costa DW, Boerma D, van Santvoort HC, Horvath KD, Werner J, Carter CR, et al. Staged multidisciplinary step-up management for necrotizing pancreatitis. Br J Surg. 2014;101(1):e65–79. PubMed.
3. De Waele JJ. Acute pancreatitis. Curr Opin Crit Care. 2014;20(2):189–95. PubMed.
4. Besselink MG, van Santvoort HC, Boermeester MA, Nieuwenhuijs VB, van Goor H, Dejong CH, et al. Timing and impact of infections in acute pancreatitis. Br J Surg. 2009;96(3):267–73. PubMed.
5. Dellinger EP, Tellado JM, Soto NE, Ashley SW, Barie PS, Dugernier T, et al. Early antibiotic treatment for severe acute necrotizing pancreatitis: a randomized, double-blind, placebo-controlled study. Ann Surg. 2007;245(5):674–83. PubMed Pubmed Central PMCID: PMC1877078, Epub 2007/04/26. eng.
6. Bakker OJ, Issa Y, van Santvoort HC, Besselink MG, Schepers NJ, Bruno MJ, et al. Treatment options for acute pancreatitis. Nat Rev Gastroenterol Hepatol. 2014;11(8):462–9. PubMed.
7. Tenner S, Baillie J, DeWitt J, Vege SS, American College of G. American College of Gastroenterology guideline: management of acute pancreatitis. Am J Gastroenterol. 2013;108(9):1400–15; 16. PubMed.
8. Hasibeder WR, Torgersen C, Rieger M, Dunser M. Critical care of the patient with acute pancreatitis. Anaesth Intensive Care. 2009;37(2):190–206. PubMed Epub 2009/04/30. eng.
9. Howard TJ, Temple MB. Prophylactic antibiotics alter the bacteriology of infected necrosis in severe acute pancreatitis. J Am Coll Surg. 2002;195(6):759–67. PubMed Epub 2002/12/24. eng.
10. De Waele JJ, Vogelaers D, Hoste E, Blot S, Colardyn F. Emergence of antibiotic resistance in infected pancreatic necrosis. Arch Surg (Chicago, Ill : 1960). 2004;139(12):1371–5. PubMed Epub 2004/12/22. eng.
11. Behrman SW, Bahr MH, Dickson PV, Zarzaur BL. The microbiology of secondary and postoperative pancreatic infections: implications for antimicrobial management. Arch Surg. 2011;146(5):613–9. PubMed Epub 2011/05/18. eng.
12. Block S, Buchler M, Bittner R, Beger HG. Sepsis indicators in acute pancreatitis. Pancreas. 1987;2(5):499–505. PubMed Epub 1987/01/01. eng.
13. Beger HG, Bittner R, Block S, Buchler M. Bacterial contamination of pancreatic necrosis. A prospective clinical study. Gastroenterology. 1986;91(2):433–8. PubMed Epub 1986/08/01. eng.
14. Gerzof SG, Banks PA, Robbins AH, Johnson WC, Spechler SJ, Wetzner SM, et al. Early diagnosis of pancreatic infection by computed tomography-guided aspiration. Gastroenterology. 1987;93(6):1315–20. PubMed Epub 1987/12/01. eng.
15. Wittau M, Mayer B, Scheele J, Henne-Bruns D, Dellinger EP, Isenmann R. Systematic review and meta-analysis of antibiotic prophylaxis in severe acute pancreatitis. Scand J Gastroenterol. 2011;46(3):261–70. PubMed Epub 2010/11/12. eng.

16. Jiang K, Huang W, Yang XN, Xia Q. Present and future of prophylactic antibiotics for severe acute pancreatitis. World J Gastroenterol. 2012;18(3):279–84. PubMed Pubmed Central PMCID: PMC3261546, Epub 2012/02/02. eng.
17. Howes R, Zuidema GD, Cameron JL. Evaluation of prophylactic antibiotics in acute pancreatitis. J Surg Res. 1975;18(2):197–200. PubMed Epub 1975/02/01. eng.
18. Finch WT, Sawyers JL, Schenker S. A prospective study to determine the efficacy of antibiotics in acute pancreatitis. Ann Surg. 1976;183(6):667–71.
19. Pederzoli P, Bassi C, Vesentini S, Campedelli A. A randomized multicenter clinical trial of antibiotic prophylaxis of septic complications in acute necrotizing pancreatitis with imipenem. Surg Gynecol Obstet. 1993;176(5):480–3. PubMed Epub 1993/05/01. cng.
20. de Vries AC, Besselink MG, Buskens E, Ridwan BU, Schipper M, van Erpecum KJ, et al. Randomized controlled trials of antibiotic prophylaxis in severe acute pancreatitis: relationship between methodological quality and outcome. Pancreatology. 2007;7(5–6):531–8. PubMed.
21. Rokke O, Harbitz TB, Liljedal J, Pettersen T, Fetvedt T, Heen LO, et al. Early treatment of severe pancreatitis with imipenem: a prospective randomized clinical trial. Scand J Gastroenterol. 2007;42(6):771–6. PubMed.
22. Sainio V, Kemppainen E, Puolakkainen P, Taavitsainen M, Kivisaari L, Valtonen V, et al. Early antibiotic treatment in acute necrotising pancreatitis. Lancet. 1995;346(8976):663–7. PubMed Epub 1995/09/09. eng.
23. Nordback I, Sand J, Saaristo R, Paajanen H. Early treatment with antibiotics reduces the need for surgery in acute necrotizing pancreatitis – a single-center randomized study. J Gastrointest Surg. 2001;5(2):113–8; discussion 8–20. PubMed Epub 2001/05/02. eng.
24. Delcenserie R, Yzet T, Ducroix JP. Prophylactic antibiotics in treatment of severe acute alcoholic pancreatitis. Pancreas. 1996;13(2):198–201. PubMed Epub 1996/08/01. eng.
25. Bassi C, Falconi M, Talamini G, Uomo G, Papaccio G, Dervenis C, et al. Controlled clinical trial of pefloxacin versus imipenem in severe acute pancreatitis. Gastroenterology. 1998;115(6):1513–7. PubMed Epub 1998/12/03. eng.
26. Manes G, Rabitti PG, Menchise A, Riccio E, Balzano A, Uomo G. Prophylaxis with meropenem of septic complications in acute pancreatitis: a randomized, controlled trial versus imipenem. Pancreas. 2003;27(4):e79–83. PubMed Epub 2003/10/25. eng.
27. Manes G, Uomo I, Menchise A, Rabitti PG, Ferrara EC, Uomo G. Timing of antibiotic prophylaxis in acute pancreatitis: a controlled randomized study with meropenem. Am J Gastroenterol. 2006;101(6):1348–53. PubMed.
28. Xue P, Deng LH, Zhang ZD, Yang XN, Wan MH, Song B, et al. Effect of antibiotic prophylaxis on acute necrotizing pancreatitis: results of a randomized controlled trial. J Gastroenterol Hepatol. 2009;24(5):736–42. PubMed Epub 2009/02/18. eng.
29. Cao Y, Xu Y, Lu T, Gao F, Mo Z. Meta-analysis of enteral nutrition versus total parenteral nutrition in patients with severe acute pancreatitis. Ann Nutr Metab. 2008;53(3–4):268–75. PubMed Epub 2009/01/13. eng.
30. Al-Omran M, Albalawi ZH, Tashkandi MF, Al-Ansary LA. Enteral versus parenteral nutrition for acute pancreatitis. Cochrane Database Syst Rev. 2010;(1):CD002837. PubMed Epub 2010/01/22. eng.
31. Isenmann R, Rünzi M, Kron M, Kahl S, Kraus D, Jung N, et al. Prophylactic antibiotic treatment in patients with predicted severe acute pancreatitis: a placebo-controlled, double-blind trial1 ☆. Gastroenterology. 2004;126(4):997–1004.
32. Garcia-Barrasa A, Borobia FG, Pallares R, Jorba R, Poves I, Busquets J, et al. A double-blind, placebo-controlled trial of ciprofloxacin prophylaxis in patients with acute necrotizing pancreatitis. J Gastrointest Surg. 2009;13(4):768–74. PubMed.
33. Bai Y, Gao J, Zou DW, Li ZS. Prophylactic antibiotics cannot reduce infected pancreatic necrosis and mortality in acute necrotizing pancreatitis: evidence from a meta-analysis of randomized controlled trials. Am J Gastroenterol. 2008;103(1):104–10. PubMed Epub 2007/10/11. eng.

34. Jafri NS, Mahid SS, Idstein SR, Hornung CA, Galandiuk S. Antibiotic prophylaxis is not protective in severe acute pancreatitis: a systematic review and meta-analysis. Am J Surg. 2009;197(6):806–13. PubMed Epub 2009/02/17. eng.
35. Mazaki T, Ishii Y, Takayama T. Meta-analysis of prophylactic antibiotic use in acute necrotizing pancreatitis. Br J Surg. 2006;93(6):674–84. PubMed Epub 2006/05/17. eng.
36. Sharma VK, Howden CW. Prophylactic antibiotic administration reduces sepsis and mortality in acute necrotizing pancreatitis: a meta-analysis. Pancreas. 2001;22(1):28–31. PubMed Epub 2001/01/04. eng.
37. Heinrich S, Schafer M, Rousson V, Clavien PA. Evidence-based treatment of acute pancreatitis: a look at established paradigms. Ann Surg. 2006;243(2):154–68. PubMed Pubmed Central PMCID: PMC1448904, Epub 2006/01/25. eng.
38. De Waele JJ. A role for prophylactic antibiotics in necrotizing pancreatitis? Why we may never know the answer. Crit Care. 2008;12(6):195. PubMed Pubmed Central PMCID: PMC2646304. Epub 2008/12/19. eng.
39. De Waele JJ. Rational use of antimicrobials in patients with severe acute pancreatitis. Semin Respir Crit Care Med. 2011;32(2):174–80. PubMed Epub 2011/04/21. eng.
40. Beger HG, Rau B, Isenmann R, Schwarz M, Gansauge F, Poch B. Antibiotic prophylaxis in severe acute pancreatitis. Pancreatology. 2005;5(1):10–9. PubMed Epub 2005/03/19. eng.
41. Dambrauskas Z, Gulbinas A, Pundzius J, Barauskas G. Meta-analysis of prophylactic parenteral antibiotic use in acute necrotizing pancreatitis. Medicina (Kaunas). 2007;43(4):291–300. PubMed Epub 2007/05/09. eng.
42. Tellado JM. Prevention of infection following severe acute pancreatitis. Curr Opin Crit Care. 2007;13(4):416–20. PubMed Epub 2007/06/30. eng.
43. Xu T, Cai Q. Prophylactic antibiotic treatment in acute necrotizing pancreatitis: results from a meta-analysis. Scand J Gastroenterol. 2008;43(10):1249–58. PubMed Epub 2008/07/09. eng.
44. Yao L, Huang X, Li Y, Shi R, Zhang G. Prophylactic antibiotics reduce pancreatic necrosis in acute necrotizing pancreatitis: a meta-analysis of randomized trials. Dig Surg. 2010;27(6):442–9. PubMed Epub 2010/11/13. eng.
45. Villatoro E, Bassi C, Larvin M. Antibiotic therapy for prophylaxis against infection of pancreatic necrosis in acute pancreatitis. Cochrane Database Syst Rev. 2006;(4):CD002941. PubMed Epub 2006/10/21. eng.
46. Villatoro E, Mulla M, Larvin M. Antibiotic therapy for prophylaxis against infection of pancreatic necrosis in acute pancreatitis. Cochrane Database Syst Rev. 2010;(5):CD002941. PubMed Epub 2010/05/14. eng.
47. Golub R, Siddiqi F, Pohl D. Role of antibiotics in acute pancreatitis: a meta-analysis. J Gastrointest Surg. 1998;2(6):496–503. PubMed Epub 1999/08/24. eng.
48. Zhou YM, Xue ZL, Li YM, Zhu YQ, Cao N. Antibiotic prophylaxia in patients with severe acute pancreatitis. Hepatobiliary Pancreat Dis Int. 2005;4(1):23–7. PubMed Epub 2005/02/26. eng.
49. Israil AM, Palade R, Chifiriuc MC, Vasile D, Grigoriu M, Voiculescu D, et al. Spectrum, antibiotic susceptibility and virulence factors of bacterial infections complicating severe acute pancreatitis. Chirurgia (Bucur). 2011;106(6):743–52. PubMed Epub 2012/02/09. eng.
50. Ignatavicius P, Vitkauskiene A, Pundzius J, Dambrauskas Z, Barauskas G. Effects of prophylactic antibiotics in acute pancreatitis. HPB (Oxf). 2012;14(6):396–402. PubMed Pubmed Central PMCID: PMC3384864, Epub 2012/05/10. eng.
51. Isenmann R, Schwarz M, Rau B, Trautmann M, Schober W, Beger HG. Characteristics of infection with Candida species in patients with necrotizing pancreatitis. World J Surg. 2002;26(3):372–6. PubMed Epub 2002/02/28. eng.
52. Kochhar R, Ahammed SK, Chakrabarti A, Ray P, Sinha SK, Dutta U, et al. Prevalence and outcome of fungal infection in patients with severe acute pancreatitis. J Gastroenterol Hepatol. 2009;24(5):743–7. PubMed Epub 2009/02/18. eng.

53. Vege SS, Gardner TB, Chari ST, Baron TH, Clain JE, Pearson RK, et al. Outcomes of intra-abdominal fungal vs. bacterial infections in severe acute pancreatitis. Am J Gastroenterol. 2009;104(8):2065–70. PubMed Epub 2009/06/06. eng.
54. Trikudanathan G, Navaneethan U, Vege SS. Intra-abdominal fungal infections complicating acute pancreatitis: a review. Am J Gastroenterol. 2011;106(7):1188–92. PubMed.
55. He YM, Lv XS, Ai ZL, Liu ZS, Qian Q, Sun Q, et al. Prevention and therapy of fungal infection in severe acute pancreatitis: a prospective clinical study. World J Gastroenterol. 2003;9(11):2619–21. PubMed Epub 2003/11/08. eng.
56. Buchler MW, Gloor B, Muller CA, Friess H, Seiler CA, Uhl W. Acute necrotizing pancreatitis: treatment strategy according to the status of infection. Ann Surg. 2000;232(5):619–26. PubMed Pubmed Central PMCID: PMC1421214, Epub 2000/11/07. eng.
57. van Baal MC, Bollen TL, Bakker OJ, van Goor H, Boermeester MA, Dejong CH, et al. The role of routine fine-needle aspiration in the diagnosis of infected necrotizing pancreatitis. Surgery. 2014;155(3):442–8. PubMed Epub 2013/11/30. eng.
58. van Santvoort HC, Besselink MG, Bakker OJ, Hofker HS, Boermeester MA, Dejong CH, et al. A step-up approach or open necrosectomy for necrotizing pancreatitis. N Engl J Med. 2010;362(16):1491–502. PubMed Epub 2010/04/23. eng.
59. Schoenberg MH, Rau B, Beger HG. New approaches in surgical management of severe acute pancreatitis. Digestion. 1999;60 Suppl 1:22–6. PubMed Epub 1999/02/23. eng.
60. Ashley SW, Perez A, Pierce EA, Brooks DC, Moore Jr FD, Whang EE, et al. Necrotizing pancreatitis: contemporary analysis of 99 consecutive cases. Ann Surg. 2001;234(4):572–9. PubMed Pubmed Central PMCID: PMC1422080, discussion 9–80. Epub 2001/09/27. eng.
61. Rodriguez JR, Razo AO, Targarona J, Thayer SP, Rattner DW, Warshaw AL, et al. Debridement and closed packing for sterile or infected necrotizing pancreatitis: insights into indications and outcomes in 167 patients. Ann Surg. 2008;247(2):294–9. PubMed Pubmed Central PMCID: 3806106.
62. De Waele JJ, Rello J, Anzueto A, Moreno R, Lipman J, Sakr Y, et al. Infections and use of antibiotics in patients admitted for severe acute pancreatitis: data from the EPIC II study. Surg Infect. 2014;15(4):394–8. PubMed Epub 2014/05/14. eng.

Chapter 40
Endoscopic or Minimally Invasive Debridement of Walled-Off Pancreatic Necrosis?

Ajaypal Singh and Andres Gelrud

Abstract Acute necrotizing pancreatitis comprises 10–15 % of acute pancreatitis cases but is associated with significant mortality of around 15 % that further increases up to 30 % if the necrotic tissue becomes infected. Historically, open surgical debridement has been the most common intervention but over the last two decades various minimally invasive modalities have been developed including percutaneous, endoscopic, laparoscopic, retroperitoneal debridement or combinations of the above. Due to constantly evolving nature of minimally invasive techniques and lack of consensus definition of the collections in the past, there is a lack of prospective data comparing the different interventions. Our understanding of the pancreatic fluid collections has improved and a standardized classification of pancreatic and peripancreatic fluid collections was recently proposed in the form of revised Atlanta Classification in 2012. Now conclusive evidence exists that minimally invasive techniques are associated with lower morbidity and mortality compared to open surgical debridement. Amongst the minimally invasive techniques, endoscopic debridement is associated with lower morbidity compared to laparoscopic or retroperitoneal approaches though mortality benefit is not clear and long-term outcomes data is lacking. Step up approach allows for more aggressive interventions only in patients failing conservative therapy or percutaneous drainage and hence can prevent aggressive and morbidity associated debridement procedures in a fraction of symptomatic walled-off necrosis patients.

Keywords Walled-off necrosis • Pancreatic necrosis • Necrosectomy • Minimally invasive necrosectomy • Endoscopic necrosectomy • Retroperitoneal necrosectomy

A. Singh • A. Gelrud (✉)
Center for Endoscopic Research and Therapeutics, Department of Medicine, University of Chicago, 5700S. Maryland Avenue, MC 8043, Chicago, IL 60637, USA
e-mail: agelrud@uchicago.edu

J.M. Millis, J.B. Matthews (eds.), *Difficult Decisions in Hepatobiliary and Pancreatic Surgery*, Difficult Decisions in Surgery: An Evidence-Based Approach, DOI 10.1007/978-3-319-27365-5_40

Introduction

Acute pancreatitis is a leading cause of hospitalization for gastrointestinal disorders with approximately 275,000 admissions in 2009 and more than 2 billion US dollars in annual health care costs [1, 2]. The overall mortality amongst patients with acute pancreatitis is around 5 % but 10–15 % of the patients can develop necrotizing pancreatitis with mortality rates as high as 15 % [3] and even higher when multi organ failure and/or infection is present. This necrosis can develop over days after the onset of pain and hence can be missed on imaging done very early in the disease course [4, 5]. The revised Atlanta classification of pancreatic and peripancreatic fluid collections was published in 2012 and categorizes these collections based on presence or absence of solid material within and well defined capsule surrounding these collections [6]. The four types of fluid collections associated with acute pancreatitis are acute fluid collection (AFC), pancreatic pseudocyst (PP), acute necrotic collection (ANC) and walled-off necrosis (WON). AFCs develop early in acute interstitial edematous pancreatitis, do not contain any solid debris, are homogenous on contrast enhanced imaging, do not have well developed capsule and usually resolve without any intervention. If these persist beyond 4 weeks, they develop a well-demarcated capsule and are known as pseudocysts that also do not contain any solid material. Acute necrotic collection, usually seen during the first 4 weeks in necrotizing pancreatitis, contains both fluid and necrotic components and is without a well-demarcated wall. These can develop a well-defined encapsulation after 4 weeks and are known as walled-off necrosis. Infection can occur in approximately 40–70 % of necrotizing pancreatitis patients and dramatically increases the mortality from 15 % for sterile necrosis to 40 % in infected necrosis [7]. It is usually difficult to differentiate between AFC and ANC during the first week or two of acute pancreatitis since both can appear homogenous with fluid consistency on contrast imaging and hence imaging should be delayed for the first 2 weeks after admission if clinically feasible.

Majority of acute collections resolve within a few weeks while less than 10 % of these persist beyond 4 weeks, develop a well demarcated capsule and evolve in to either PP or WON. In a recent study, it was shown that 41 % patients with ANCs had spontaneous resolution while 49 % evolved in to WON [8]. Up to one third of patients with WON develop infection. It is of utmost importance to carefully select patients who require intervention for pancreatic fluid collections. Only symptomatic patients due to infection, obstruction of adjacent viscera (gastric outlet obstruction, pancreatobiliary obstruction), abdominal pain and less frequently rupture or bleeding require intervention. There has been a rapid increase in the availability of minimally invasive debridement techniques over the last couple of decades and there is marked variability in each technique based on local expertise. This is compounded by lack of high quality prospective, randomized studies comparing the different modalities; hence no standard guidelines exist for management of walled-off necrosis.

Search Strategy

A literature search of publications in English language from 1995 to 2014 was performed to identify studies reporting outcomes of various debridement methods for walled-off necrosis using the PICO outline (Table 40.1). Since the term walled-off necrosis was widely adopted after the revised Atlanta Classification of 2012, we used the previously used term "pancreatic necrosis" for our literature search. The databases that were searched include PubMed, Google Scholar, Embase, Cochrane library and SUMSearch. The search terms included necrotizing pancreatitis, infected pancreatic necrosis, pancreatic necrosis, walled-off necrosis AND debridement or necrosectomy or minimally invasive necrosectomy or laparoscopic necrosectomy/debridement or retroperitoneal necrosectomy/debridement or endoscopic necrosectomy/debridement. Only studies that reported definite outcomes (morbidity, mortality and complications) were included. The selected articles included 20 retrospective studies, 3 randomized controlled trials, 3 prospective cohort studies, 4 systematic reviews and meta-analyses and 2 guideline papers.

Management of Symptomatic Walled-Off Necrosis (WON)

Successful management of walled-off necrosis requires a multi-disciplinary approach with involvement of gastroenterologists, radiologists, pancreato-biliary surgeons, nutritionists and critical care specialists. Optimal nutrition and if present, management of sepsis and organ failure are of paramount significance.

Indication of Drainage

It is important to realize that asymptomatic collections do not need to be drained irrespective of the size and location. Intervention is usually needed in patients with suspected or documented infection in the collection, persistent organ failure in the absence of infection, obstruction of viscera, persistent symptoms (pain, nausea/vomiting, early satiety) and disconnected duct syndrome (since these are less likely to resolve without intervention). There is no role for endoscopic drainage of acute collections and if possible surgical intervention should be avoided in the first 4

Table 40.1 PICO table for management of walled-off necrosis

P (Patients)	I (Intervention)	C (Comparator group)	O (Outcomes measured)
Patients with walled-off necrosis after necrotizing pancreatitis	Endoscopic debridement	Minimally invasive debridement (transperitoneal or retroperitoneal)	Resolution of collection
			Incidence of fistula formation, repeat intervention, organ failure and mortality

weeks since a direct correlation exists between success of endoscopic intervention and degree of encapsulation [9] and early intervention is associated with poor outcomes [10].

Over the last few years, few studies have reported that even selected patients with infected WON who are clinically stable, can be managed without debridement with supportive care, antibiotics and percutaneous drainage [11–13]. Prior to advent of endoscopic drainage, symptomatic WON was traditionally managed by surgical debridement, which usually required multiple sessions and had significant morbidity including organ failure, external fistulas, and incisional hernias. Endoscopic necrosectomy must be avoided till a well-defined capsule has developed and success of debridement has been shown to be directly associated with the degree of encapsulation [14, 15]. Besselink et al. [16] showed that mortality after surgical necrosectomy in patients with necrotizing pancreatitis (more than 80 % with infected necrosis) decreased significantly with increasing the time interval from initial admission (8 % vs. 45 % vs. 75 % for more than 30 days, 15–29 days and 1–14 days respectively; $p<0.001$).

Which Modality to Choose

The Diminishing Role of Open Necrosectomy

Open necrosectomy with wide drainage and placement of abdominal drains for lavage was the most common approach for patients with infected pancreatic necrosis. This usually required repeat interventions and was associated with significant morbidity 34–95 % and mortality ranging from 11 to 50 % [17–22]. The re-intervention rates in high volume series from Europe and the United States have been high 30–70 %. A study from Fernandez del Castillo et al. in which 167 patients with suspected pancreatic necrosis underwent single step debridement and abdominal closure were noted to develop post operative pancreatic fistulas in 41 %, enteric fistulas in 15 %, endocrine pancreatic insufficiency in 16 % and exocrine insufficiency in 20 % patients. Post-operative Intensive care unit stay was needed in 57 % patients [18]. Even though there is no prospective comparison between open and laparoscopic necrosectomy, Tan et al. retrospectively reviewed their data of 76 patients with severe acute necrotizing pancreatitis who underwent either open or laparoscopic necrosectomy and showed that laparoscopic group was associated with significantly lower complications (including pancreatic fistulae, infections) and length of hospitalization. There was however no difference in overall mortality in the two groups [23]. Bakker et al. compared surgical necrosectomy with endoscopic transgastric necrosectomy in a randomized controlled trial (ten patients in each group) [24]. They showed that patients undergoing endoscopic necrosectomy had lower systemic inflammatory response as measured by IL-6 levels ($p=0.004$) and also lower composite clinical end point of major complications including new onset organ failure, pancreatic/enterocutaneous fistula, intra-abdominal bleeding or death (20 % vs. 80 %, risk difference 0.60, 95 % CI 0.16–0.80, $p = 0.03$).

A meta-analysis of comparative studies (one randomized and three clinical controlled trials) published by Cirocchi et al. compared open necrosectomy (ON) with minimally invasive necrosectomy (MIN) in patients with infected pancreatic necrosis (total of 336 patients, 215 with MIN and 121 with ON) [25]. MIN included laparoscopic transperitoneal, retroperitoneal as well as endoscopic procedures. They showed that MIN was associated with significantly lower incidence of multi-organ failure (OR 0.16, 95 % CI 0.06–0.39, $p < 0.001$), surgical reintervention (OR 0.16, 95 % CI, 0.00–3.07, $p = 0.19$), incisional hernias (OR 0.23, 95 % CI 0.06–0.90, $p = 0.03$), new onset diabetes (OR 0.32, 95 % CI 0.12–0.88, $p = 0.03$) and need for pancreatic enzymes (OR 0.005, 95 % CI 0.04–0.57, $p = 0.005$) compared to open necrosectomy. There was also trend towards lower mortality, intra-abdominal bleeding, pancreatic fistula and entero-cutaneous fistulae formation after MIN but these did not achieve statistical significance. Significant heterogeneity amongst the included studies was a major limitation of this analysis.

Minimally Invasive Necrosectomy (MIN)

Even though there is data to show the MIN is associated with better outcomes compared to open surgical necrosectomy, there is wide variation in the technique for MIN depending on the route and instrumentation used. These techniques include laparoscopic necrosectomy (trans or intraperitoneal), retroperitoneal necrosectomy (video assisted retroperitoneal debridement or sinus tract endoscopy with debridement) and percutaneous approach. The instruments used for these can include laparoscopes, flexible endoscopes and nephroscopes. Hence the published data for MIN is severely limited by lack of randomized trials, small numbers of patients and marked heterogeneity in the techniques.

Laparoscopic Necrosectomy

Laparoscopic necrosectomy was first described by Gagner et al. in 1996 [26]. In the first published series of laparoscopic intraperitoneal necrosectomy in 2000, Zhu et al. performed laparoscopic debridement in ten patients followed by large volume peritoneal lavage for 7–14 days [27]. Interestingly all surgeries were done within 24–72 h after disease onset and they reported 30-day mortality of 30 % without any other major complications (pancreatic fistula, abscess or bleeding). Another retrospective series was published from China by Zhou et al. in 2003 in which laparoscopic debridement was done in patients with early as well as later stage of severe acute pancreatitis with 92 % resolution of collections at 6 months following 2–7 weeks of drainage [28]. Parekh for the first time in 2006, published a retrospective series of 19 patients with persistently symptomatic or infected pancreatic necrosis who underwent hand assisted laparoscopic debridement [29]. All procedures were done at least 3 weeks after onset of symptoms (median 65 days). One patient required conversion to open surgery while two others required open surgery during follow-up and there were two deaths. Pancreatic fistulae developed in 11 out of 14 patients treated primarily with laparoscopic intervention.

Repeat surgery is needed in up to 20 % of patients and external drainage is needed in majority of the patients undergoing laparoscopic debridement (range 9 days–7 weeks based on studies in Table 40.2) [27–29]. There is also high incidence of pancreatic fistula formation though lower than that associated with open debridement. Laparoscopic cholecystectomy can be done at the same time as laprascopic necrosectomy. In a systematic review of minimally invasive necrosectomy, Babu et al. [30] showed that 11 % patients required laparotomy and mortality was 7 % though the six studies included in the review were all retrospective, had a total of 46 patients and involved significant variation in patient selection (timing of intervention, previous interventions and indication for intervention) and operative technique. With the advent of retroperitoneal and endoscopic debridement techniques, laparoscopic transperitoneal debridement is being used less frequently these days.

Retroperitoneal Necrosectomy

Alverdy et al. described the technique of laparoscopic intracavitary debridement after percutaneous drain placement in two patients with WON in 2000 for the first time [31]. This was followed by a case series of ten patients with confirmed infected pancreatic necrosis who underwent retroperitoneal necrosectomy as the primary modality for debridement [32]. A median of two explorations was needed with a median inpatient stay of 42 days. One patient required conversion to open laparotomy due to bleeding from injury to splenic vessels and a total of two patients died post procedure.

Castellanos et al. [33] performed translumbar retroperitoneal debridement in 15 patients with mortality of 27 % and complications in 40 % (6/15) patients (one pancreatic fistula, one duodenal, one colonic perforation, two pseudocysts and one lumbotomy eventeration). Only one patient required pancreatic enzyme and insulin replacement during follow up. Numerous smaller, retrospective case series have confirmed the use of retroperitoneal debridement for infected WON [32, 34, 35]. The major studies that investigated role of retroperitoneal necrosectomy for WON are listed in Table 40.3.

Hovarth et al. for the first time reported prospective data of a step up approach in a multicenter trial involving 40 patients with infected pancreatic necrosis. All patients initially underwent percutaneous drains and if more than 75 % of necrosis persistent after 10–14 days, more invasive (VARD or open necrosectomy) were performed. Thirty-one (77 %) patients had less than 75 % decrease in necrosis and 25 out of these underwent VARD. VARD was successful in 60 % patients while remaining had conversion to open surgery.

Table 40.2 Outcomes of laparoscopic transperitoneal debridement for

Author/year	N	Infected necrosis n (%)	Time to surgery after disease onset (days)	Success n (%)	Re-intervention n (%)	Morbidity/ complications, n (%)	Mortality n (%)
Gagner 1996 [26]	8	NA	NA	6 (75)	38 %	NA	0
Zhu 2001 [27]	10	0	1–3	7 (70)	NA	NA	10 %
Zhou 2003 [28]	13	4 (31)	NA	12 (92)	0	NA	15 %
Parekh 2006 [29]	19	9 (47)	NA	16 (84)	11 %	21 %	11 %
Bucher 2008 [46]	8	8 (100)	31 (13–59)	8 (100)	25 %	0	0
Tan 2012 [23]	25	25 (100)	30 (13–46)	NA	4 %	48.3 %	4 %

Table 40.3 Review of studies of retroperitoneal necrosectomy

Author/year	N	Infected necrosis n (%)	Time to surgery after disease onset (ds)	Success n (%)	Necrosectomy Sessions per patient	Need for laparotomy, n (%)	Morbidity/ complications n (%)	Mortality (%)
Gambiez 1998 [47]	20	13 (65)	18 (13–26)	75 %	5±4	NA	60 %	10 %
Carter 2000 [32]	10	10 (100)	40 (13–187)	80 %	2.4 (1–4)	1 (7 %)	28 %	20 %
Castellanos 2002 [33]	15	15 (100)	NA	73 %	1	0	40 %	27 %
Connor 2005 [34]	47	38 (41)	28 (3–161)	75 %	3 (1–5)	12 (26 %)	92 %	19 %
Cheung 2005 [35]	8	4 (50)	3–22 weeks	62.5 %	NA	3 (37.5 %)	50 %	12.5 %
Horvath 2010 [48]	25	25 (100)	80 (33–208)	60 %	1 (1–2)	10 (40 %)	42 %	4 %
Raraty 2010 [49]	137	88 (64)	32 (1–181)	84 %	3 (1–9)	19 (14 %)	55 %	19 %
Bakker 2012 [24]	10	9 (90)	59 (29–69)	60 %	1 (1–2)	4 (40 %)	80	40 %
Baush 2012 [50]	14	13 (93)	39 (15–184)	57 %	NA	3 (21 %)	57 %	21 %
Castellanos 2013 [36]	32	32 (100)	19 (11–28)	NA	3 (1–10)	NA	9.3 %	15.6 %
Zhao 2014 [51]	17	17 (100 %)	29 (14–45)	NA	2	2 (12 %)	9 (53 %)	0

In a systematic review of nine reports on retroperitoneal necrosectomy [30], 141 patients were evaluated. There was significant heterogeneity in the technique and inclusion criteria, but the overall mortality for retroperitoneal debridement was 16 % and 13 % patients required laparotomy. The complication rate was 41 % and majority of the patients required more than one debridement session. Castellanos et al. [36] updated their prospectively collected data of retroperitoneal necrosectomy by describing 32 patients who underwent the procedure for confirmed infected pancreatic necrosis. A median of three debridement sessions was performed, with a reported mortality of 15.6 % and morbidity of 9.3 %. There was clinical complete resolution of symptoms in 27/32 patients after a median follow up of 84 months. It is important to note that they did not use the step up approach or percutaneous catheter drainage prior to retroperitoneal debridement. Most of the studies for VARD have used catheter drainage for lavage of the necrotic cavity for many days though no consensus on the optimal drainage exists.

Percutaneous Drainage

Percutaneous approach involves placement of percutaneous drains in to the collections under ultrasound or CT guidance followed by frequent flushing of the cavity. The three main advantages of percutaneous drainage are that the drain tract can be used in future for further necrosectomy (either video assisted or endoscopic), the complications and mortality associated with percutaneous drainage are low and percutaneous drainage can be performed in critically ill patients early in the course of disease when a well defined capsule is not present. But since no debridement is done initially, the success rate is not very high and more invasive interventions are usually needed, particularly in large cavities or if infection is present). Even though the data is mainly retrospective and from small sized studies, approximately 44 % patients can avoid further invasive interventions after percutaneous drainage of pancreatic necrosis [37]. In a systematic review, Baal et al. evaluated percutaneous catheter drainage (PCD) as the primary intervention for management of pancreatic necrosis [38]. They found that no additional surgical intervention was needed in 55.7 % of the patients and mortality in the PCD group was 15.4 %.

Endoscopic Necrosectomy

Over the last decade endoscopic necrosectomy has emerged as the most common debridement intervention for walled-off necrosis due to improvements in technology, endoscopist expertise and use of carbon dioxide for insufflation. Multiple non-randomized studies have shown the efficacy of endoscopic transmural necrosectomy in managing walled-off necrosis. Baron et al. for the first time in 1996 published a case series of 11 patients who had cystgastrostomy and nasocystic irrigation for walled off necrosis. Trans-luminal direct endoscopic necrosectomy was first reported in 2000 [39]. Since then multiple studies have shown efficacy of transgastric access into the retroperitoneum and debridement of necrotic tissue followed by placement of stents to allow for subsequent drainage [24, 40, 41].

EUS guidance should be used when puncturing the gastric wall if a definite bulge is not seen endoscopically or if gastric varices are present [42]. EUS also helps assess the degree of necrotic debris inside the cavity. Once the cavity is punctured, it is followed by balloon dilatation and placement of plastic or metal stents. This allows for access to the retroperitoneum for debridement, which can be done using various tools including forceps, snares, baskets, nets as well as vigorous irrigation. The data about placement of nasocystic drains and use of hydrogen peroxide is still not conclusive. Repeat debridement can be done using the cystgastrostomy tract.

A multi-center study from the United States involved 104 patients with symptomatic WON who underwent direct endoscopic necrosectomy with successful resolution in 91 % patients after a mean period of 4.1 months and a median of three procedures [9]. Peri-procedural complications occurred in 14/103 patients and included significant bleeding requiring blood transfusion and 2 deaths. In the first randomized trial comparing endoscopic transgastric necrosectomy with surgical necrosectomy (ten patients in each group, PENGUIN trial: the Pancreatitis Endoscopic Transgastric vs Primary Necrosectomy in Patients with Infected Necrosis), Bakker et al. showed that endoscopic necrosectomy reduced proinflammatory response and was associated with markedly decreased incidence of major complications or death (20 % vs. 80 %) [24]. The endoscopic approach involved transgastric puncture, balloon dilation, followed by retroperitoneal drainage and necrosectomy while surgical approach consisted of video-assisted retroperitoneal debridement (VARD) or laparoscopic if VARD was not feasible. Patients who underwent endoscopic transgastric necrosectomy had lower post procedure IL-6 levels ($p=0.004$), lower incidence of new onset multiple organ failure (0 % vs 50 %; $p=0.03$), lesser pancreatic fistulas (10 % vs 70 %, $p=0.02$) and a non-significant trend towards lower mortality (10 % vs. 40 %; $p=0.3$). The data about long-term outcomes of endoscopic transluminal necrosectomy is still limited but promising. Seifert et al. showed an 84 % clinical success rate with 26 % complication rate and 7.5 % mortality in 93 patients undergoing endoscopic necrosectomy after a mean follow-up interval of 43 months. The mean number of endoscopic procedures required was six and only 4 % patients required surgical interventions while 16 % had recurreht pancreatitis episodes [40]. The studies that reported outcomes for endoscopic debridement of WON are listed in Table 40.4. It is important to note that most of these studies are non-randomized, retrospective, observational studies. The overall success of endoscopic debridement in these studies ranges from 69 % to 100 % with a mortality of 0–15 %. The number of debridement sessions reported range from 1.4 to 6 though one study reported up to 15 debridement sessions.

Table 40.4 Review of studies with endoscopic debridement

Author/year	N	Infected necrosis n (%)	Time to surgery after disease onset (days)	Success n (%)	Necrosectomy Sessions per patient	Need for surgery, n (%)	Morbidity/ complications n (%)	Mortality n (%)
Seifert 2000 [39]	3	1 (33)	14–64	100 %	NA	0	NA	0
Seewald 2005 [52]	13	13 (100 %)	NA	77 %	1 (1–4)	4 (31 %)	30 %	0
Charnley 2006 [53]	13	11 (85 %)	27	100 %	4 (1–10)	2 (15 %)	NA	15 %
Papachristou 2007 [41]	53	26 (49 %)	49 (20–300)	81 %	3 (1–12)	12 (23 %)	49 %	6 %
Voermans 2007 [54]	25	19 (76 %)	84 (21–385)	93 %	2 (1–4)	2 (8 %)	40 %	0
Hocke 2008 [55]	30	30 (100 %)	NA	97 %	2.7 (1–16)	3 (10 %)	10 %	7 %
Escourrou 2008 [56]	13	13 (100 %)	28 (21–32)	100 %	1.8 (1–3)	0	46 %	0 %
Seifert 2009 [40]	93	50 (54 %)	43	84 %	6	14 (15 %)	26 %	8 %
Ross 2010 [57]	15	9 (60 %)	29 (4–207)	100 %	1.4	0	13 %	0 %
Gardner 2011 [9]	104	40 (39 %)	63	91 %	3 (1–14)	1 (1 %)	14 %	2 %
Bakker 2012 [24]	10	19 (100 %)	59 (29–69)	100 %	3 (2–6)	2 (20 %)	20 %	10 %
Smoczynski 2014 [58]	112	NA	16.3 weeks (3–78 weeks)	93 %	2.7 (1–6)	7 (6.25 %)	26 %	1.8 %

Step-Up Approach

A step-up approach that aims at control of infection source rather than complete removal of infected necrosis has been proposed. In the PANTER trial (minimally invasive step up approach vs. maximal necrosectomy in patients with acute necrotizing pancreatitis), Van Sanvoort et al. randomized patients with necrotizing pancreatitis and confirmed or suspected infection in the necrosis to either primary open necrosectomy or a step-up approach [13]. The step-up approach involved either percutaneous or endoscopic drainage followed by VARD if no improvement. They showed that primary end point of death or major complications was seen in 40 % patients with minimally invasive step up compared to 69 % patients who underwent primary open necrosectomy (RR = 0.57, 95 % CI 0.38–0.87, $p = 0.006$). A very important outcome of the study was that up to 40 % of patients with infected necrosis could be managed by drainage along thus obviating the need for debridement. The limitations of this study included not using laparoscopic necrosectomy instead of open necrosectomy in patients undergoing surgery and endoscopic necrosectomy was not performed in majority of the patients (only 5 % of the patients in the step up group underwent endoscopic necrosectomy).

More prospective trials comparing percutaneous drainage, VARD, endoscopic necrosectomy and hybrid techniques (combination of drainage techniques) are needed. In a recently published retrospective, observational study of 100 patients with symptomatic walled-off necrosis, Bang et al. [43] showed that adoption of a step-up approach for WON based on collection size, location and response to intervention led to improved treatment success compared with the conventional endoscopic management (91 % vs. 60 %, $p < 0.001$). Management based on step-up algorithm was the only predictor of treatment success on multivariate logistic regression analysis (OR 6.51, 95 % CI 2.19–19.37 $p = 0.001$). But conflicting data exists as well. Kumar et al. compared step up approach with direct endoscopic necrosectomy in a recently published matched cohort study (12 patients with infected WON in each group) [44]. They showed that direct endoscopic necrosectomy led to higher rates of clinical success (11/12 vs 3/12), decreased need for surgical intervention, lesser new antibiotics use, respiratory failure, endocrine insufficiency, shorter length of stay and lower health care utilization. To compare the outcomes between endoscopic step up and surgical step up approaches, the results of ongoing randomized controlled, superiority multicenter trial from the Netherlands (the TENSION trial) will be important [45].

Conclusion/Recommendations

- Open surgical debridement of walled-off necrosis is associated with higher morbidity and mortality compared to minimally invasive necrosectomy approaches and should be avoided unless absolutely necessary (evidence quality high; strong recommendation)

- Step-up approach starting with percutaneous drainage and followed by endoscopic or retroperitoneal debridement if percutaneous drainage fails should be adopted (evidence quality high; strong recommendation)
- If accessible endoscopically, endoscopic debridement should be preferred over retroperitoneal debridement (evidence quality moderate; weak recommendation)

A Personal View of the Data

Multi disciplinary approach is imperative. Debridement should be avoided in the early stages of necrotizing pancreatitis if possible. Around 15–20 % of WON with infection can be managed conservatively with antibiotics, though very close monitoring for any change in clinical status is very important. If absolutely necessary, percutaneous catheter drainage should be used in early stages, in 20–25 % of patients this approach will be curative. If no improvement despite antibiotics and catheter drainage, minimally invasive debridement should be considered. The choice is determined by local expertise and location of the WON. For endoscopically accessible WON collections, transmural approach should be preferred. It is associated with decreased systemic inflammatory response and is also without external fistulae or drains and still allows repeat debridement sessions to be performed. VARD should be considered if no improvement despite endoscopic necrosectomy and percutaneous drainage or if the collection is not accessible endoscopically or to large. Laparoscopic transperitoneal debridement followed by open necrosectomy should be reserved if none of the above interventions lead to clinical improvement or if the necrosis is extensive and cannot be fully debrided by endoscopic or retroperitoneal approaches.

References

1. Peery AF, Dellon ES, Lund J, et al. Burden of gastrointestinal disease in the United States: 2012 update. Gastroenterology. 2012;143:1179–87.e1–3.
2. Fagenholz PJ, Fernandez-del Castillo C, Harris NS, et al. Direct medical costs of acute pancreatitis hospitalizations in the United States. Pancreas. 2007;35:302–7.
3. van Santvoort HC, Bakker OJ, Bollen TL, et al. A conservative and minimally invasive approach to necrotizing pancreatitis improves outcome. Gastroenterology. 2011;141:1254–63.
4. Bollen TL, Singh VK, Maurer R, et al. A comparative evaluation of radiologic and clinical scoring systems in the early prediction of severity in acute pancreatitis. Am J Gastroenterol. 2011;107:612–9.
5. Spanier BWM, Nio Y, van der Hulst RWM, et al. Practice and yield of early CT scan in acute pancreatitis: a Dutch Observational Multicenter Study. Pancreatology. 2010;10:222–8.
6. Banks PA, Bollen TL, Dervenis C, et al. Classification of acute pancreatitis – 2012: revision of the Atlanta classification and definitions by international consensus. Gut. 2013;62:102–11.

7. Trikudanathan G, Attam R, Arain MA, et al. Endoscopic interventions for necrotizing pancreatitis. Am J Gastroenterol. 2014;109:969–81.
8. Sarathi Patra P, Das K, Bhattacharyya A, et al. Natural resolution or intervention for fluid collections in acute severe pancreatitis. Br J Surg. 2014;101:1721–8.
9. Gardner TB, Coelho-Prabhu N, Gordon SR, et al. Direct endoscopic necrosectomy for the treatment of walled-off pancreatic necrosis: results from a multicenter U.S. series. Gastrointest Endosc. 2011;73:718–26.
10. Takahashi N, Papachristou GI, Schmit GD, et al. CT findings of walled-off pancreatic necrosis (WOPN): differentiation from pseudocyst and prediction of outcome after endoscopic therapy. Eur Radiol. 2008;18:2522–9.
11. Garg PK, Sharma M, Madan K, et al. Primary conservative treatment results in mortality comparable to surgery in patients with infected pancreatic necrosis. Clin Gastroenterol Hepatol. 2010;8:1089–94.
12. Mouli VP, Sreenivas V, Garg PK. Efficacy of conservative treatment, without necrosectomy, for infected pancreatic necrosis: a systematic review and meta-analysis. Gastroenterology. 2013;144:333–40.e2.
13. van Santvoort HC, Besselink MG, Bakker OJ, et al. A step-up approach or open necrosectomy for necrotizing pancreatitis. N Engl J Med. 2010;362:1491–502.
14. Mier J, León EL-D, Castillo A, et al. Early versus late necrosectomy in severe necrotizing pancreatitis. Am J Surg. 1997;173:71–5.
15. Wittau M, Scheele J, Gölz I, et al. Changing role of surgery in necrotizing pancreatitis: a single-center experience. Hepatogastroenterology. 2010;57:1300–4.
16. Besselink MGH, Verwer TJ, Schoenmaeckers EJP, et al. Timing of surgical intervention in necrotizing pancreatitis. Arch Surg. 2007;142:1194–201.
17. Besselink MG, de Bruijn MT, Rutten JP, et al. Surgical intervention in patients with necrotizing pancreatitis. Br J Surg. 2006;93:593–9.
18. Rodriguez JR, Razo AO, Targarona J, et al. Debridement and closed packing for sterile or infected necrotizing pancreatitis. Ann Surg. 2008;247:294–9.
19. Babu BI, Sheen AJ, Lee SH, et al. Open pancreatic necrosectomy in the multidisciplinary management of postinflammatory necrosis. Ann Surg. 2010;251:783–6.
20. Tsiotos, Luque-De Leon, Sarr. Long-term outcome of necrotizing pancreatitis treated by necrosectomy. Br J Surg. 1998;85:1650–3.
21. Howard TJ, Patel JB, Zyromski N, et al. Declining morbidity and mortality rates in the surgical management of pancreatic necrosis. J Gastrointest Surg. 2007;11:43–9.
22. Parikh PY, Pitt HA, Kilbane M, et al. Pancreatic necrosectomy: North American mortality is much lower than expected. J Am Coll Surg. 2009;209:712–9.
23. Tan J, Tan H, Hu B, et al. Short-term outcomes from a multicenter retrospective study in China comparing laparoscopic and open surgery for the treatment of infected pancreatic necrosis. J Laparoendosc Adv Surg Tech A. 2012;22:27–33.
24. Bakker OJ, van Santvoort HC, van Brunschot S, et al. Endoscopic transgastric vs surgical necrosectomy for infected necrotizing pancreatitis: a randomized trial. JAMA. 2012;307:1053–61.
25. Cirocchi R, Trastulli S, Desiderio J, et al. Minimally invasive necrosectomy versus conventional surgery in the treatment of infected pancreatic necrosis: a systematic review and a meta-analysis of comparative studies. Surg Laparosc Endosc Percutan Tech. 2013;23:8–20.
26. Gagner M. Laparoscopic treatment of acute necrotizing pancreatitis. Semin Laparosc Surg. 1996;3:21–8.
27. Zhu JF, Fan XH, Zhang XH. Laparoscopic treatment of severe acute pancreatitis. Surg Endosc. 2001;15:146–8.
28. Zhou Z-G, Zheng Y-C, Shu Y, et al. Laparoscopic management of severe acute pancreatitis. Pancreas. 2003;27:e46–50.
29. Parekh D. Laparoscopic-assisted pancreatic necrosectomy: a New surgical option for treatment of severe necrotizing pancreatitis. Arch Surg. 2006;141:895–903.

30. Babu BI, Siriwardena AK. Current status of minimally invasive necrosectomy for post-inflammatory pancreatic necrosis. HPB (Oxf). 2009;11:96–102.
31. Alverdy J, Vargish T, Desai T, et al. Laparoscopic intracavitary debridement of peripancreatic necrosis: preliminary report and description of the technique. Surgery. 2000;127:112–4.
32. Carter CR, McKay CJ, Imrie CW. Percutaneous necrosectomy and sinus tract endoscopy in the management of infected pancreatic necrosis: an initial experience. Ann Surg. 2000;232:175–80.
33. Castellanos G, Pinero A, Serrano A, et al. Infected pancreatic necrosis: translumbar approach and management with retroperitoneoscopy. Arch Surg. 2002;137:1060–3.
34. Connor S, Raraty MGT, Howes N, et al. Surgery in the treatment of acute pancreatitis minimal access pancreatic necrosectomy. Scand J Surg. 2005;94:135–42.
35. Cheung M-T, Ho CN-S, Siu K-W, et al. Percutaneous drainage and necrosectomy in the management of pancreatic necrosis. ANZ J Surg. 2005;75:204–7.
36. Castellanos G, Piñero A, Doig LA, et al. Management of infected pancreatic necrosis using retroperitoneal necrosectomy with flexible endoscope: 10 years of experience. Surg Endosc. 2013;27:443–53.
37. Bello B, Matthews JB. Minimally invasive treatment of pancreatic necrosis. World J Gastroenterol. 2012;18:6829–35.
38. Van Baal MC, van Santvoort HC, Bollen TL, et al. Systematic review of percutaneous catheter drainage as primary treatment for necrotizing pancreatitis. Br J Surg. 2011;98:18–27.
39. Seifert H, Wehrmann T, Schmitt T, et al. Retroperitoneal endoscopic debridement for infected peripancreatic necrosis. Lancet. 2000;356:653–5.
40. Seifert H, Biermer M, Schmitt W, et al. Transluminal endoscopic necrosectomy after acute pancreatitis: a multicentre study with long-term follow-up (the GEPARD Study). Gut. 2009;58:1260–6.
41. Papachristou GI, Takahashi N, Chahal P, et al. Peroral endoscopic drainage/debridement of walled-off pancreatic necrosis. Ann Surg. 2007;245:943–51.
42. Freeman ML, Werner J, van Santvoort HC, et al. Interventions for necrotizing pancreatitis: summary of a multidisciplinary consensus conference. In: Vol 41. 2012:1176–1194.
43. Bang JY, Holt BA, Hawes RH, et al. Outcomes after implementing a tailored endoscopic step-up approach to walled-off necrosis in acute pancreatitis. Br J Surg. 2014;101:1729–38.
44. Kumar N, Conwell DL, Thompson CC. Direct endoscopic necrosectomy versus step-up approach for walled-off pancreatic necrosis: comparison of clinical outcome and health care utilization. Pancreas. 2014;43:1334–9.
45. van Brunschot S, van Grinsven J, Voermans RP, et al. Transluminal endoscopic step-up approach versus minimally invasive surgical step-up approach in patients with infected necrotising pancreatitis (TENSION trial): design and rationale of a randomised controlled multicenter trial [ISRCTN09186711]. BMC Gastroenterol. 2013;13:161.
46. Bucher P, Pugin F, Morel P. Minimally invasive necrosectomy for infected necrotizing pancreatitis. Pancreas. 2008;36:113–9.
47. Gambiez LP, Denimal FA, Porte HL, et al. Retroperitoneal approach and endoscopic management of peripancreatic necrosis collections. Arch Surg. 1998;133:66–72.
48. Horvath K, Freeny P, Escallon J. Safety and efficacy of video-assisted retroperitoneal debridement for infected pancreatic collections: a multicenter, prospective, single-arm phase 2 study. Arch Surg. 2010;145:817–25.
49. Raraty MGT, Halloran CM, Dodd S, et al. Minimal access retroperitoneal pancreatic necrosectomy. Ann Surg. 2010;251:787–93.
50. Bausch D, Wellner U, Kahl S, et al. Minimally invasive operations for acute necrotizing pancreatitis: comparison of minimally invasive retroperitoneal necrosectomy with endoscopic transgastric necrosectomy. Surgery. 2012;152:S128–34.
51. Zhao G, Hu M, Liu R, et al. Retroperitoneoscopic anatomical necrosectomy: a modified single-stage video-assisted retroperitoneal approach for treatment of infected necrotizing pancreatitis. Surg Innov. 2014;22(4):360–5.

52. Seewald S, GROTH S, Omar S, et al. Aggressive endoscopic therapy for pancreatic necrosis and pancreatic abscess: a new safe and effective treatment algorithm (videos). Gastrointest Endosc. 2005;62:92–100.
53. Charnley R, Lochan R, Gray H, et al. Endoscopic necrosectomy as primary therapy in the management of infected pancreatic necrosis. Endoscopy. 2006;38:925–8.
54. Voermans RP, Veldkamp MC, Rauws EA, et al. Endoscopic transmural debridement of symptomatic organized pancreatic necrosis (with videos). Gastrointest Endosc. 2007;66:909–16.
55. Hocke M, Will U, Gottschalk P, et al. Transgastral retroperitoneal endoscopy in septic patients with pancreatic necrosis or infected pancreatic pseudocysts. Z Gastroenterol. 2008;46:1363–8.
56. Escourrou J, Shehab H, Buscail L, et al. Peroral transgastric/transduodenal necrosectomy: success in the treatment of infected pancreatic necrosis. Ann Surg. 2008;248:1074–80.
57. Ross A, Gluck M, Irani S, et al. Combined endoscopic and percutaneous drainage of organized pancreatic necrosis. Gastrointest Endosc. 2010;71:79–84.
58. Smoczyński M, Marek I, Dubowik M, et al. Endoscopic drainage/debridement of walled-off pancreatic necrosis. Pancreatology. 2014;14:137–42.

Chapter 41
Surgical Debridement in Necrotizing Pancreatitis

Baddr Shakhsheer and John Alverdy

Abstract Pancreatic necrosis is a feared complication following acute pancreatitis, carrying a 10–20 % mortality. When surgical intervention is indicated, open necrosectomy remains the gold standard approach. Recent evidence demonstrating the advantage of delaying or even avoiding surgical intervention altogether has changed treatment paradigms and has opened the door for minimally invasive techniques. This chapter discusses open versus minimally invasive necrosectomy with respect to morbidity and outcome.

Keywords Complicated pancreatitis • Pancreatic necrosis • Necrosectomy

Introduction

Approximately 10–25 % of patients diagnosed with acute pancreatitis go on to develop pancreatic necrosis, an often devastating complication that carries a 10–20 % mortality rate [1]. Recommendations to intervene surgically in the management of pancreatic necrosis have varied over the last several decades so significantly that previous experience may be no longer applicable in the current era of high resolution imagining, newer antibiotics, and minimally invasive techniques. The indications for surgery to treat pancreatic necrosis have historically been based on the surgeon's clinical perception of the severity of disease and the rate of clinical deterioration. The tradition of aggressive surgical debridement of the pancreas to treat a rapidly evolving progression from pancreatitis to necrosis has waned significantly in the face of emerging evidence that "less is more" when treating this highly morbid condition. In the last decade with the advent of guidelines from the International Association of Pancreatology and other consensus working groups, evidence has emerged that pancreatic necrosis itself, independent of its clinical manifestations and anastomotic

B. Shakhsheer (✉) • J. Alverdy
Department of Surgery, Pritzker School of Medicine, University of Chicago,
5841 S Maryland Ave, MC 6040, Chicago, IL 60637, USA
e-mail: baddr.shakhsheer@uchospitals.edu

J.M. Millis, J.B. Matthews (eds.), *Difficult Decisions in Hepatobiliary and Pancreatic Surgery*, Difficult Decisions in Surgery: An Evidence-Based Approach, DOI 10.1007/978-3-319-27365-5_41

extent, is no longer an absolute indication for surgery [2]. Rather surgery has become the default position when source control cannot be achieved non- surgically and when the progression from necrosis to infected necrosis leads to clinical deterioration, abscess formation, bacteremia, and non- resolving organ dysfunction [3].

Today most centers perform a step-up approach that avoids invasive surgery in favor of early non-operative management with source control of infected pancreatic necrosis achieved by either percutaneous or minimally invasive (i.e. endoluminal or laparoscopic) drainage. Despite the many advances in care for the patient with necrotizing pancreatitis, surgery is often indicated. The purpose of this chapter is to compare minimally invasive necrosectomy to open necrosectomy, when indicated for necrotizing pancreatitis, on key outcome variables including morbidity, development of multi-organ failure (MOF), fistula formation, diabetes, recovery times, and mortality. We will make this comparison in the current era of high resolution CT imaging of the pancreas, the availability of modern intensive care medicine, improved anesthesia, application of broader, more powerful and highly penetrating antibiotics and advances in surgical techniques such as the damage control laparotomy, wound vacuum devices, and reconstructive surgery.

Search Strategy

A literature search was performed of publications in English-language from 200 to the current using the PICO outline (Table 41.1). Databases utilized for the search include PubMed, Google Scholar, and Embase. Searches were constructed from combinations of the following terms: "pancreatic necrosis," "necrosectomy," "pancreatic debridement," "multisystem organ failure," "new-onset diabetes," "retroperitoneal debridement," "step up," and "minimally invasive." The GRADE system was used for evaluation of the data.

Results

Open Procedure

At the present time, it is fair to state that open pancreatic debridement to treat necrotizing pancreatitis in its acute phase, absent a compelling suspicion for infected pancreatic necrosis, is ill-advised and rarely practiced at high volume tertiary care

Table 41.1 PICO outline

P (Patients)	I (Intervention)	C (Comparator)	O (Outcomes)
Patients with pancreatic necrosis	Minimally invasive necrosectomy	Open necrosectomy	Mortality, multisystem organ failure, new-onset diabetes mellitus

centers. Abandonment of open pancreatic debridement has been based on exceedingly high morbidity and mortality rates with no established effect on improved outcome. A single-institution study by Ashley et al. in 2001 evaluated 99 consecutive patients with necrotizing pancreatitis, employing a non-operative management strategy followed by delayed intervention [4]. Mortality was approximately 10 % and in all cases, were related to multisystem organ failure. In 2007, Howard et al. published an observational series of 102 patients undergoing laparotomy for surgical debridement of pancreatic necrosis at a single institution over two time periods: 1993–2001 vs 2002–2005 [5]. Patients in the latter group were treated in accordance with the International Association of Pancreatology guidelines which mandated use of fine needle aspiration or CT evidence of infection as indicators for surgery and avoiding operating on patients within 14 days of the onset of disease unless otherwise indicated. The earlier treatment group (1993–2001) did not differ significantly from the latter group in terms of severity of illness. The latter group showed a decreased operative morbidity (89 % vs 72 %, $p=0.03$), length of stay, and overall mortality (18 % vs 4 %, $p=0.03$). There were no differences in culture result patterns between the two groups and the average time from acute presentation to surgical debridement were the same. What then made up for the dramatic decrease in mortality over the two time periods? There are likely highly conspicuous differences in management between these two groups that perhaps were not accounted for in the description of the study. For example, were the anesthetics, pain management or surgical debridement approaches different? Were the indications for surgery identical in both groups? Despite no differences in culture results, did patient in the latter group receive broader antibiotics with better pancreatic tissue penetration? Were the antibiotics delivered with greater attention to their pharmacodynamics and pharmacokinetics by pharmacy services in the latter period? The most important finding in this study was difference in mortality of 18–4 % and a decrease length of stay of 20 %. Pancreatic fistula rates were high in both groups (49 vs 60 %). Diabetes incidence was not reported. Despite the lack of detail available in this study to account for the improved mortality rates, today among surgeons dealing with pancreatitis, there is a general sense that the morbidity and mortality of open surgery to treat necrotizing pancreatitis has decreased significantly perhaps owing to more strict adherence to the indications for surgery, improved imaging, better anesthesia and pain management, better antibiotics and their pharmacologic application and the availability of newer surgical techniques such as the damage control laparotomy and the wound vac. There are few observational trials in the last few years that can substantiate today that fistula formation, number of procedures (take backs) required, extent of pancreatic debridement, incidence of diabetes development, and multiple organ failure incidence are decreased overall following open surgery. The reason for this is twofold: open surgery is performed less often and less repeatedly for a given patient and the patient populations are extremely heterogeneous making most comparisons problematic. Experienced surgeons are quick to accept that each patient with severe necrotizing pancreatitis represents his or her own unique odyssey. Patients today, compared to several decades previously, can be safely managed with an open abdomen. Yet distinct from years past, the open abdomen is now generally closed within days using newer biologic materials, some of which are reported to resist infection. Today there is a sense however that with repeated imaging, delaying surgery, and use of percutaneous drainage, open surgery enjoys a much lower mortality than in previous years. Regarding morbidity however, this is a much more complicated issue. For example, fistula formation is not necessarily lowered by the use of percutaneous drainage [6, 7]. Diabetes development following open necrosectomy is as much function of the amount of pancreatic parenchyma lost by necrosis and infection as it is by surgical debridement. Similarly, the incidence of multiple organ failure is as much a function of the virulence of the pancreatitis as it is the virulence of bacteria that infect the pancreas and the bacterial that colonize the gut and drive systemic inflammation [8, 9]. In the aggregate these complications remain significant following severe necrotizing pancreatitis and are not necessarily a function of the surgery itself. It may be prudent therefore, in the absence of reliable data, to conclude that there is no evidence that these complications, in the aggregate, have decreased as a result of modern care, but rather, they just have become less lethal.

Endoscopic Drainage

Peroral endoscopic techniques via transgastric or transduodenal incisions and drain placement can achieve debridement in select patients [10]. There are several important advantages of this technique that are obvious relative to the complications of fistula formation, diabetes mellitus development, multiple organ failure, and time to recovery. Entering the pancreatic necroma through the gastric wall minimizes the tissue injury and trauma of an open procedure. In addition the technique does not traverse otherwise sterile tissue planes and thus the potential for bacteremia and disseminated infection are theoretically less. Also, the technique creates an internal fistula thus avoiding the possibility of an external one. Perhaps its greatest advantage is that it can be repeatedly performed with low morbidity thus lessening the often compelling need to excise as much pancreatic parenchyma as possible in a single sitting. This may result in less pancreatic parenchyma excised over the entire course of the disease with the potential to decrease the overall incidence of diabetes. Whether this approach strikes the balance of adequate source control of infection while at the same time better preserving islet cell function remains to be proven. Certainly it has the potential to do so. Theoretically, the open connection between the stomach and the pancreatic necroma cavity may allow for digestive enzymes to more gradually debride tissues and preserve the native pancreas. As an example, Papachristou et al. showed in a retrospective review of 53 patients that this method could be successful in both sterile and infected pancreatic necrosis [11]. However 40 % of the patients in the series needed concurrent percutaneous drainage and 23 % went on to need operative intervention. Predictors of need for open intervention included patients with pre-existent diabetes mellitus and larger areas of necrosis extending into anatomic areas difficult to access endoscopically, including the paracolic gutters. A meta-analysis of four studies yielded a 69 % success rate with a 2 % mortality for endoscopic drainage [12]. Obviously patient selection is critical and there is the general sense that less critically ill patient are the best candidates for this procedure, perhaps explaining the overall improved outcomes [13].

Laparoscopic Procedures

Laparoscopic pancreatic debridement to treat infected necrosis has involved two general approaches: transperitoneal laparoscopic debridement and video-assisted retroperitoneal debridement (VARD) [14]. Both procedures have the advantage of avoiding a major laparotomy incision and exploration, one of the major causes of the morbidity of open pancreatic debridement. Also theoretically, multiple repeated procedures may be attempted with the laparoscopic approach thus providing a similar advantage to endoscopy of lessening the need to radically debride all necrotic tissue in a single sitting. Without a large abdominal laparotomy wound, theoretically fistula formation and bleeding should be lessened. In addition, for the same reasons stated above with endoscopy, the incidence of diabetes development has the potential to be decreased using less aggressive and repeated laparoscopy.

Transperitoneal laparoscopy today is rarely performed owing to the more popular approach of direct access to the necroma cavity first percutaneously via interventional radiology and then laparoscopically using the radiologically placed catheter as a guide (VARD) [15]. The conventional approach today is a "step up" approach starting with percutaneous drainage and antibiotics moving to necrosectomy via laparoscopic approaches. Transperitoneal approaches, nonetheless, have been described with excellent outcomes. Parekh et al.'s series of 19 patients underwent hand-assisted laparoscopic necrosectomy, 18 of whom were able to have the procedure laparoscopically, 14 of whom had prior percutaneous drainage by interventional radiology. These patients had a 79 % rate of external pancreatic fistulization, but all but one closed spontaneously [16]. In another series, a transperitoneal approach was used with no mortality and excellent outcomes [17]. However both series included a small number of patients and the patient populations consisted of those self-selecting who would tolerate the procedure. The incidence of diabetes, fistula formation, and multiple organ failure of transperitoneal necrosectomy relative to other procedures is unknown as one cannot compare this approach to the others given the variability in clinical presentations, the variable timing of the procedures along the course of necrotizing pancreatitis and the use of adjunctive procedures that often follow when residual infected necromas are present.

VARD utilizes a retroperitoneal drainage catheter as a tract for insufflation and retroperitoneal debridement [18]. This approach seeks to minimize the morbidity of other techniques by avoidance of contamination of unaffected anatomic spaces, namely the peritoneum. By debriding only the retroperitoneal, the intact peritoneum acts as a natural barrier to reduce the systemic immune response. In 2008, a meta-analysis of VARD reported a 64 % success rate with a 14 % mortality [12].

In 2010, van Santvoort et al. published the results of the Dutch Pancreatitis Study Group's PANTER study (PAncreatitis, Necrosectomy versus sTEp up appRoach), a multicenter trial randomizing 88 patients to primary open necrosectomy versus a "step up approach," utilizing percutaneous drainage followed by minimally invasive retroperitoneal drainage, if necessary [19]. Of the 43 patients in the "step up" arm, 35 % were treated with percutaneous drainage alone. When compared to the open necrosectomy cohort, patients in the "step up" arm had less multi-system organ failure (12 % vs 40 %, $p=0.002$) and less new onset diabetes mellitus (16 % vs 38 %, $p=0.002$). Though mortality was unchanged in this study, it was not designed nor powered for that outcome to be measured. Currently there is an ongoing trial by the Dutch cooperative group using the step up approach trial comparing endoscopic debridement to minimally invasive (laparoscopic) debridement. Common endpoints such as fistula formation, diabetes development and multiple organ failure will be determined. The idea here is, based on the principles outlined above, that endoscopic debridement will result in less fistula formation and less diabetes development [20].

Recommendations Based on the Data

The management of necrotizing pancreatitis remains a major challenge to reduce morbidity and mortality, contain costs, and minimize long term disabilities. Current trends suggest that necrosectomy should be delayed as long as is safely possible with the idea in mind of percutaneously draining the necroma when it is suspected to be infected and the patient is not improving (evidence quality moderate, weak recommendation). Initially this is attempted percutaneously and then, if needed, via minimally invasive approaches if repeat imaging and the clinical course indicate that adequate source control has not been achieved. The decision to proceed with endoscopic, minimally invasive (laparoscopic/VARD) versus open surgery will depend on clinical circumstances. Open surgery should be reserved for those situations where neither endoscopy nor laparoscopy is feasible or when the extent or severity of the disease mandates open exploration (evidence quality moderate, weak recommendation). This latter situation may involve rapidly evolving severe sepsis, hemodynamic instability or widespread intraperitoneal disease. The PANTER trial presents the best evidence in favor of a minimally-invasive treatment paradigm, showing decreased morbidity without any change in mortality (evidence quality moderate, weak recommendation).

1. Necrosectomy should be delayed as long as is safely possible, temporizing by percutaneous drainage when it is suspected to be infected and the patient is not improving (evidence quality moderate, weak recommendation)
2. Open necrosectomy should be reserved for those situations where neither endoscopy nor laparoscopy is feasible or when the extent or severity of the disease mandates open exploration (evidence quality moderate, weak recommendation).

3. A minimally-invasive treatment paradigm shows decreased morbidity without any change in mortality (evidence quality moderate, weak recommendation).

A Personal View of the Data

The management of necrotizing pancreatitis remains a clinical challenge. The indications for surgery continue to evolve along a continuum of delayed intervention, multiple imaging, percutaneous drainage and then operative intervention based on a clinical suspicion of infected necrosis and inadequate source control. A patient who is stable, ambulatory, and presents with pain and pancreatic necrosis on axial imaging differs significantly from a septic patient with multisystem organ failure. Each patient is unique and may require various procedures either as the primary intervention or as the default procedure when the primary approach fails. As such, the "step-up" approach advocated by the Dutch Pancreatitis Study Group represents, to date, the best paradigm for management of these patients. Patients are often treated "a la carte" and carefully monitored for clinical improvement and image-based evidence that source control is proceeding along steady course of completion. Deployment of either endoscopic or open surgery is then decided upon based on several factors including the patients' anatomy, extent of necroma, technical expertise, and the evolving course of the physiologic response to the inflammation and infection. A major advancement has been the widespread belief by experienced clinicians in the field that surgery need not be implicitly considered urgent when infection is suspected or identified and that a given surgical approach need not be considered to be the single operative intervention. Clinicians should be aware of the multi-pronged approaches across disciplines that are available and deploy them in a rational and customized way based on the patient presentation and course.

References

1. Whitcomb DC. Clinical practice. Acute pancreatitis. N Engl J Med. 2006;354(20):2142–50.
2. Uhl W, Warshaw A, Imrie C, Bassi C, McKay CJ, Lankisch PG, Carter R, Di Magno E, Banks PA, Whitcomb DC, Dervenis C, Ulrich CD, Satake K, Ghaneh P, Hartwig W, Werner J, McEntee G, Neoptolemos JP, Büchler MW, International Association of Pancreatology. IAP guidelines for the surgical management of acute pancreatitis. Pancreatology. 2002;2(6):565–73.
3. Büchler MW, Gloor B, Müller CA, Friess H, Seiler CA, Uhl W. Acute necrotizing pancreatitis: treatment strategy according to the status of infection. Ann Surg. 2000;232(5):619–26.
4. Ashley SW, Perez A, Pierce EA, Brooks DC, Moore Jr FD, Whang EE, Banks PA, Zinner MJ. Necrotizing pancreatitis: contemporary analysis of 99 consecutive cases. Ann Surg. 2001;234(4):572–9; discussion 579–80.
5. Howard TJ, Patel JB, Zyromski N, Sandrasegaran K, Yu J, Nakeeb A, Pitt HA, Lillemoe KD. Declining morbidity and mortality rates in the surgical management of pancreatic necrosis. J Gastrointest Surg. 2007;11(1):43–9.

6. Freeny PC, Hauptmann E, Althaus SJ, Traverso LW, Sinanan M. Percutaneous CT-guided catheter drainage of infected acute necrotizing pancreatitis: techniques and results. AJR Am J Roentgenol. 1998;170(4):969–75.
7. Sikora SS, Khare R, Srikanth G, Kumar A, Saxena R, Kapoor VK. External pancreatic fistula as a sequel to management of acute severe necrotizing pancreatitis. Dig Surg. 2005;22(6):446–51; discussion 452.
8. Li Q, Wang C, Tang C, He Q, Li N, Li J. Bacteremia in patients with acute pancreatitis as revealed by 16S ribosomal RNA gene-based techniques. Crit Care Med. 2013;41(8):1938–50.
9. Hanna EM, Hamp TJ, McKillop IH, Bahrani-Mougeot F, Martinie JB, Horton JM, Sindram D, Gharaibeh RZ, Fodor AA, Iannitti DA. Comparison of culture and molecular techniques for microbial community characterization in infected necrotizing pancreatitis. J Surg Res. 2014;191(2):362–9.
10. Charnley RM, Lochan R, Gray H, O'Sullivan CB, Scott J, Oppong KE. Endoscopic necrosectomy as primary therapy in the management of infected pancreatic necrosis. Endoscopy. 2006;38:925–8.
11. Papachristou GI, Takahashi N, Chahal P, Sarr MG, Baron TH. Peroral endoscopic drainage/debridement of walled-off pancreatic necrosis. Ann Surg. 2007;245(6):943–51.
12. Bradley 3rd EL, Howard TJ, van Sonnenberg E, Fotoohi M. Intervention in necrotizing pancreatitis: an evidence-based review of surgical and percutaneous alternatives. J Gastrointest Surg. 2008;12(4):634–9.
13. Navaneethan U, Vege SS, Chari ST, Baron TH. Minimally invasive techniques in pancreatic necrosis. Pancreas. 2009;38(8):867–75.
14. Wysocki AP, McKay CJ, Carter CR. Infected pancreatic necrosis: minimizing the cut. ANZ J Surg. 2010;80(1-2):58–70.
15. Alverdy J, Vargish T, Desai T, Frawley B, Rosen B. Laparoscopic intracavitary debridement of peripancreatic necrosis: preliminary report and description of the technique. Surgery. 2000;127(1):112–4.
16. Parekh D. Laparoscopic-assisted pancreatic necrosectomy: a new surgical option for treatment of severe necrotizing pancreatitis. Arch Surg. 2006;141(9):895–902; discussion 902–3.
17. Wani SV, Patankar RV, Mathur SK. Minimally invasive approach to pancreatic necrosectomy. J Laparoendosc Adv Surg Tech A. 2011;21(2):131–6.
18. Horvath KD, Kao LS, Wherry KL, Pellegrini CA, Sinanan MN. A technique for laparoscopic-assisted percutaneous drainage of infected pancreatic necrosis and pancreatic abscess. Surg Endosc. 2001;15(10):1221–5.
19. van Santvoort HC, Besselink MG, Bakker OJ, Hofker HS, Boermeester MA, Dejong CH, van Goor H, Schaapherder AF, van Eijck CH, Bollen TL, van Ramshorst B, Nieuwenhuijs VB, Timmer R, Laméris JS, Kruyt PM, Manusama ER, van der Harst E, van der Schelling GP, Karsten T, Hesselink EJ, van Laarhoven CJ, Rosman C, Bosscha K, de Wit RJ, Houdijk AP, van Leeuwen MS, Buskens E, Gooszen HG, Dutch Pancreatitis Study Group. A step-up approach or open necrosectomy for necrotizing pancreatitis. N Engl J Med. 2010;362(16):1491–502.
20. van Brunschot S, van Grinsven J, Voermans RP, Bakker OJ, Besselink MG, Boermeester MA, Bollen TL, Bosscha K, Bouwense SA, Bruno MJ, Cappendijk VC, Consten EC, Dejong CH, Dijkgraaf MG, van Eijck CH, Erkelens GW, van Goor H, Hadithi M, Haveman JW, Hofker SH, Jansen JJ, Laméris JS, van Lienden KP, Manusama ER, Meijssen MA, Mulder CJ, Nieuwenhuis VB, Poley JW, de Ridder RJ, Rosman C, Schaapherder AF, Scheepers JJ, Schoon EJ, Seerden T, Spanier BW, Straathof JW, Timmer R, Venneman NG, Vleggaar FP, Witteman BJ, Gooszen HG, van Santvoort HC, Fockens P, Dutch Pancreatitis Study Group. Transluminal endoscopic step-up approach versus minimally invasive surgical step-up approach in patients with infected necrotising pancreatitis (TENSION trial): design and rationale of a randomised controlled multicenter trial [ISRCTN09186711]. BMC Gastroenterol. 2013;13:161.

Chapter 42
Surgery or Endotherapy for Large Duct Chronic Pancreatitis

Jason B. Liu and Marshall S. Baker

Abstract For chronic pancreatitics who have a glandular morphology characterized by a dilated main pancreatic duct, pain is thought to be due to ductal hypertension and glandular/capsular stretch. Decompression of the pancreatic duct by either endoscopic transampullary stenting or surgical drainage is the principle method of treating symptoms in these patients. Surgical intervention is commonly thought to carry increased risk of perioperative morbidity, thus current practice involves an intervention sequence starting with endoscopic stenting and falling back to surgery in cases of recalcitrant pain. There is, however, little evidence to argue that an "endoscopy first" approach is better than early surgical intervention. Few studies prospectively examine outcomes of endoscopy compared to surgery in terms of pain relief, morbidity and mortality, number of repeated interventions, and preservation of pancreatic function. The evidence that is available suggests surgical management of large duct chronic pancreatitis results in better long term outcomes when compared to endoscopic therapy without incurring prohibitive risk of significant perioperative morbidity. In our view, surgical drainage of the pancreas should be considered as a primary method of managing patients with chronic pancreatitis and a dilated main pancreatic duct.

Keywords Chronic pancreatitis • Endoscopy • Surgery • Outcomes • Large duct

J.B. Liu
Department of Surgery, University of Chicago, Pritzker School of Medicine, 5841 S. Maryland Ave. Rm O-217 MC6040, Chicago, IL 60637, USA
e-mail: jason.liu@uchospitals.edu

M.S. Baker (✉)
Department of Surgery, Division of Surgical Oncology, University of Chicago, Pritzker School of Medicine, 5841 S. Maryland Ave. Rm O-217 MC6040, Chicago, IL 60637, USA

NorthShore University Health System, 2650 Ridge Ave. Walgreen Bldg., 2nd floor, Evanston, IL 60201, USA
e-mail: mbaker3@northshore.org

J.M. Millis, J.B. Matthews (eds.), *Difficult Decisions in Hepatobiliary and Pancreatic Surgery*, Difficult Decisions in Surgery: An Evidence-Based Approach, DOI 10.1007/978-3-319-27365-5_42

Introduction

Pain is the symptom leading to treatment in patients with chronic pancreatitis. For some patients, obstruction of the main pancreatic duct by stones or by progressive fibrosis in the pancreatic head results in a marked dilation of the main pancreatic duct. Ductal and parenchymal hypertension and capsular stretch are purported to be the major etiologic factors of pain in these patients. In later stages of the disease, the pain may be neuropathic in nature, driven by nerve injury from repeated bouts of retroperitoneal inflammation.

Endoscopic or surgical decompression of the pancreatic duct is the mainstay of therapy for chronic pancreatitics with dilation of the main pancreatic duct. Both methods aim to alleviate pain by promoting adequate drainage of the pancreas thereby relieving ductal and parenchymal hypertension. To date, there is no clear consensus as to which modality is superior in relieving pain and improving quality of life, or as to when to use one approach over the other. In general, current practice involves a conservative "step up" approach in which patients are first managed medically with diet modification (e.g. alcohol abstinence, low fat diet, enzyme supplementation), then endoscopically with transampullary stenting, and are lastly referred to consider surgery when other modes of therapy fail to alleviate or control pain. There is little evidence to suggest that this is the most efficacious way to manage these patients. Longitudinal studies show that of all patients with chronic pancreatitis, up to 75 % will require surgical management at some point during the course of their disease [1, 2]. Prospective studies evaluating endoscopic methods in isolation find these methods to be safe, technically successful and achieve long-term pain relief. Similar claims are made for surgical therapies when examining resection, decompression and hybrid resection-drainage procedures in isolation [2–9].

This chapter attempts to answer the question which mode of therapy, early endoscopic or surgical intervention for patients with large duct chronic pancreatitis, is best by means of an evaluation of the literature focused on studies that offer comparisons between endoscopic and surgical approaches.

Search Strategy

A literature search was performed to identify relevant studies comparing the outcomes of endoscopic and operative interventions in the treatment of large duct chronic pancreatitis. A PICO approach was constructed for the search (Table 42.1). English language publications between August 1, 2000 and August 1, 2014 involving adult patients aged 18 years or older were queried from the following databases: PubMed, Science Citation Index/SCI-Expanded, and Cochrane Evidence Based Medicine. A combination of the following terms in their various forms were used to complete the search: "chronic pancreatitis," "surgery," "endoscopy," "extracorporeal shockwave lithotripsy," "drainage," "decompression," "outcomes," "pain,"

Table 42.1 PICO table for management of large duct chronic pancreatitis

P (Patients)	I (Intervention)	C (Comparator)	O (Outcomes)
Patients with large duct chronic pancreatitis	Surgery	Endoscopy	Pain relief, morbidity/mortality, need for repeated interventions, progression to endocrine/exocrine insufficiency

"Izbicki pain score," "pancreatectomy," "resection," "endocrine function," and "exocrine function." Articles were excluded if they examined either surgical therapies alone or endoscopic therapies alone. One paper was exempt from the publication date limitation due to its relevance to the discussion and was included. In all, three randomized controlled trials, six cohort studies, three review articles, two systematic reviews, and one study protocol were evaluated. The data was classified using the GRADE system. A summary of discussed data is provided in Table 42.2.

Results

Pain Relief

In general, comparative studies have demonstrated that both endoscopic and surgical methods of pancreatic duct drainage provide effective improvement in patients' symptoms with most studies demonstrating an advantage to surgical intervention with regard to both initial rates of improvement in symptoms and durability of the response.

The North American Pancreatitis Study 2 (NAPS2) was a prospective, 20-center case-control study of 1000 recurrent acute pancreatitis and chronic pancreatitis patients in the United States in which standardized questionnaires were used to capture information on the use and effectiveness of medical, endoscopic, and surgical therapies. Gland morphology was not considered in this study. The authors analyzed their cohort of patients who only had chronic pancreatitis with regard to the frequency of endoscopic and surgical therapies, and their subjective effectiveness [5]. Of the 515 patients studied, 185 (35.9 %) underwent endoscopic pancreatic duct stenting with reported effectiveness in 87 (47 %) patients. Fifty-one (9.9 %) patients underwent a surgical drainage procedure, which was effective in 36 (70.6 %) patients. Overall, endotherapy was considered effective in 42.8 % of patients compared to 68.5 % in patients treated with either surgical drainage or resection ($p<0.0001$). Surgical procedures, however, were performed less frequently than endoscopic procedures (32.8 % vs. 60.8 %, $p<0.0001$). Studying their group of patients that participated in NAPS2, Clarke et al. reported that endoscopically managed patients achieved clinical success in 51 % of patients [6]. Of those who failed endotherapy and subsequently underwent surgery, 50 % had successful outcomes. The NAPS2 did not record the specific symptom being treated with each procedure,

Table 42.2 Summary of clinical outcomes comparing surgery and endoscopy in the treatment of large duct chronic pancreatitis

Author	Year	N	Follow up (months)	Pain relief[b]			Morbidity			Mortality			Repeated intervention[d]			Endocrine insufficiency[f]			Exocrine insufficiency[f]			Quality of evidence (grade)
				Endoscopy	Surgery	*p*	Endoscopy	Surgery	*p*	Endoscopy	Surgery	*p*	Endoscopy	Surgery	*p*	Endoscopy	Surgery	*p*	Endoscopy	Surgery	*p*	
Clarke	2012	146	96	51 %	50 %	NR	12 %	NR	NR	0 %	NR	NR	–	–	–	–	–	–	–	–	–	Very low
Cahen	2007	39	24	32 %	75 %	0.007	58 %	35 %	0.15	5 %	0 %	0.49	8 (1–21)	3 (1–9)	<0.001	17 %	5 %	0.48	33 %	5 %	0.05	Moderate
Cahen	2011	31	79	38 %	80 %	0.042	–	–	–	–	–	–	2 (0–43)	0 (0–20)	0.51	44 %	20 %	0.32	38 %	13 %	0.13	Moderate
Dite	2003	72	60	15 %	33.8 %	0.002	8 %	8 %	NR	0 %	0 %	NR	6 (4–9)	1 (1–3)	NR	34.2 %	38.8 %	NR	28.6 %	47.2 %	0.003	Low
Glass	2014	515	72	38.8 %	69.6 %	<0.0001	–	–	–	–	–	–	–	–	–	–	–	–	39.8 %	67.2 %	0.0008	Very low
Hirota[c]	2011	68	40	0.21	0.16	NS	–	–	–	–	–	–	–	–	–	–	–	–	–	–	–	Low
Hong	2011	62	60	47 %	77 %	0.04	7 %	14 %	0.66	0 %	3 %	1	2 (1–4)	1 (1–2)	<0.001	65 %	87 %	0.16[g]	54 %	29 %	0.17	Low
Rutter	2010	292	58	–	–	–	32 %	32 %	NA	0 %	5 %	NA	2.1	0.43	<0.001[e]	–	–	–	–	–	–	Low
				Non-Op												*Non-Op*			*Non-Op*			
Nealon[a]	1993	32	47	13 %	94 %	<0.001	–	–	–	–	–	–	–	–	–	15 %	83 %	0.001	7 %	79 %	<0.001	Low

NR not reported, *NS* not significant, *Non-Op*: non-operative management
[a]Secondary analysis from [9]
[b]Percentage of partial and complete pain relief
[c]Incidence of acute pancreatitis per person-year
[d]Median (range)
[e]Comparison between means
[f]New onset endocrine or exocrine insufficiency unless otherwise specified
[g]Preservation of independent endocrine function

and effectiveness was reported as the interpretation of the treating physician. There was little effort to control for disease morphology – to limit the study to patients with diffuse dilation of the main pancreatic duct and no pancreatic head mass. There was also a relatively limited effort to use standardized methods to assess pain in these studies.

A smaller retrospective study of 62 patients with chronic pancreatitis and main pancreatic duct dilation treated with either endoscopic intervention or surgical drainage calculated the Izbicki pain scores before and after intervention [7]. They demonstrated a significant difference in complete or partial pain relief over a 5-year follow up period in those who underwent surgery (77 % vs 47 %, $p = 0.04$).

Very few prospective randomized studies have compared the outcomes of medical and surgical management of chronic pancreatitis patients with regard to pain. The earliest study reported by Nealon and Thompson was done at a time when endoscopic procedures had not been fully developed [8]. This study randomized 17 patients with mild/moderate pancreatitis and non-debilitating abdominal pain to either non-operative (medical, non-endoscopic intervention) or operative management with a mean follow up period of 39 months. One quarter of patients in the non-operative group remained with mild/moderate pancreatitis while the others progressed to more severe symptoms. Seventy-eight percent of patients in the operated group remained with mild/moderate pancreatitis at the end of follow up. Unfortunately, no objective measures of pain were used in this study. Substantial pain relief was reported in 16/17 (94 %) patients in the surgical group compared to only 2/15 (13 %) patients in the non-operative group [9]. At a time in which endoscopic decompression was not readily available, the investigators concluded that surgical ductal decompression delayed the progression of chronic pancreatitis.

In 2003, Dite et al. published a pseudo-randomized (i.e. 1:1 alternating patient allocation) prospective study of 72 patients embedded in a cohort of 140 patients [10]. All patients had failed medical management for at least 3 years. Endoscopy did not utilize extracorporeal shock wave lithotripsy, and surgery entailed both drainage and resection procedures. At 5-year follow up, complete pain relief as assessed by the Melzack score was achieved in a greater number of patients who underwent surgery compared to endotherapy (34 % vs. 15 %, $p = 0.002$).

The most well done prospective randomized trial was carried out by Cahen et al. and published in the *New England Journal of Medicine* in 2007 [11]. For this study, the authors randomized 39 patients with advanced chronic pancreatitis and proximal obstruction of the pancreatic duct without pancreatic head enlargement to multimodal endoscopic therapy or operative decompression. The primary end point was the average Izbicki pain score during a median of 24 (range 6–24) months of follow up. Patients who underwent surgery reported an Izbicki pain score significantly lower than those who underwent endotherapy (mean difference 24, 95 % confidence interval [CI], 11–36, $p < 0.001$). Moreover, after surgical drainage, pain relief was present by 6 weeks postoperatively and persisted during the follow up period. Complete or partial pain relief was achieved in 32 % of patients in the endoscopy group and 75 % of patients in the surgery group ($p = 0.007$). The study was prematurely terminated on the basis of a significant difference in outcome favoring the surgical group. After 79 months of follow up, 31 of the 39 patients were re-evaluated [12]. The Izbicki pain score difference in favor of the surgical group was no longer significant (39 vs. 22, $p=0.12$). However, the secondary outcome measure of either partial or complete pain relief was still significantly higher in the surgically treated group (80 % vs. 38 %, $p=0.042$).

A more recently published Cochrane review pooled the data from these two randomized studies [9]. Of the 111 patients, surgery achieved a higher proportion of patients with pain relief compared to endoscopy (RR 1.62, 95 % CI, 1.22–2.15). The proportion of patients with complete pain relief was higher in the surgical group (RR 2.45, 95 % CI, 1.18–5.09), but there was no difference in the proportion of patients with partial pain relief.

Morbidity and Mortality

Proponents of endoscopic management of chronic pancreatitis cite high morbidity and mortality in those undergoing surgical intervention as the primary reason for pursuing endoscopy prior to or in place of surgery. Both comparative studies and longitudinal examinations of endoscopic and surgical drainage in isolation generally support the contention that the absolute risk of peri-procedure morbidity is higher in the surgically treated patients. But, there is no clear indication from the existing literature that the increased morbidity is prohibitive or that it justifies an “endoscopy first” or “endoscopy alone” approach to these patients.

In their cohort of endoscopically managed patients, Clarke et al. reported an overall complication rate of 12 % of which 59 % were hospitalizations for post-procedure monitoring [6]. There were no deaths. In a retrospective study of 292 patients with chronic pancreatitis of any morphology, Rutter et al. reported an equivalent complication rate of 32 % between patients treated by endoscopy and by surgery [13]. Infectious complications were more common in patients managed surgically (14.1 % vs. 0.7 %, $p<0.001$), while acute on chronic pancreatitis and formation of pseudocyst were more often seen in patients after endoscopic treatment (14.7 % vs. 5.1 % and 14.7 % vs. 10.1 %, respectively). Hong et al. noted a trend toward increased rates of complication following surgical management, but that trend did not achieve statistical significance (14 % vs. 7 %, $p=0.66$) [7].

Similarly, Dite et al. reported 8 % morbidity and no mortality in both their endoscopic and surgical groups when they combined their randomized and non-randomized groups [10]. Cahen et al. also demonstrated no significant difference in morbidity and mortality between the endoscopic and surgical groups (58 % vs. 35 %, $p=0.15$ and 5 % vs. 0 %, $p=0.49$, respectively) [11].

None of these studies formally grade the complications that happen following either endoscopic or surgical interventions. Given this, we have a very limited understanding of the true burden that these procedures bring to patients.

Repeated Interventions, Hospitalizations, and Costs

The need for repeated interventions, prolonged hospitalization, and increased costs have been identified as potential disadvantages to endoscopic therapy. Rutter et al. reported patients with an initial surgical intervention had the fewest consecutive interventions compared with endotherapy [13]. Of the 99 surgically treated patients, 13 (13 %) required a second intervention, and 9 (9 %) required up to four interventions. Of the 150 endoscopically managed patients, 47 (31 %) patients needed a second intervention and 63 (42 %) patients received up to 12 interventions. Patients with an initial surgical intervention had the lowest number of subsequent interventions compared with patients who had an initial endoscopic intervention (mean number, 0.43 vs. 2.1, $p<0.001$). Furthermore, the intervention-free interval was significantly longer after initial surgical treatment compared with endotherapy (mean months, 18.8 vs. 4.8, $p<0.001$). Patients treated endoscopically spent a significantly greater number of days hospitalized compared to those who underwent surgery (mean days, 25.3 vs. 34.4, $p<0.001$). However, the single mean admission time in patients with surgical treatment was longer than those who received endoscopic therapy (mean days, 20 vs. 10.7, $p<0.001$).

A small retrospective study of 65 patients with chronic pancreatitis and main pancreatic duct dilation treated with either endoscopic or surgical drainage done by Hirota et al. reported no difference between groups in the number of total hospitalized days per year (29.3 vs. 18.6, $p=0.055$) over an average follow up period of 40 months [14]. However, the number of hospitalizations per year was significantly more frequent in those treated endoscopically compared to those managed surgically (1.6 vs. 0.67, $p<0.001$). They did not report the indications for repeated hospitalizations. Hong et al. were able to demonstrate similar results [7]. They reported a significantly greater number of interventions in the endoscopy group compared to the surgery group (median number of procedures, 2 vs. 1, $p<0.001$). Although patients undergoing endotherapy had a shorter initial hospital stay (mean days, 12 vs. 28, $p<0.001$), they had a significantly greater number of readmissions at 5-year follow up compared to the surgical group (median, 2 vs. 0, $p<0.001$).

Interestingly, when Hirota et al. stratified their endoscopy group into patients that required endoscopic therapy for shorter than or longer than 1 year, they noted that patients who required endoscopic therapy for longer than 1 year had significantly greater annual hospitalized days (41.3 vs. 18.6, $p=0.0016$), more frequent annual hospitalizations (2.5 vs. 0.67, $p<0.0001$), and incurred greater annual costs ($20,300 vs. $10,200, $p=0.0027$) [14]. They concluded endoscopic therapy should not persist past 1 year of therapy before considering surgery.

Dite et al. reported an average of six endoscopic interventions per patient (range 4–9) compared to one surgical intervention per patient (range 1–3) [10]. When including the initial endoscopic or surgical intervention, Cahen et al. reported more overall diagnostic and therapeutic interventions in the group treated with endotherapy compared to the group treated with surgery (median, 8 vs 3, $p<0.001$) [11]. This trend continued to hold true at their long-term analysis (median, 12 vs. 4, $p=0.001$) [12]. There was no difference in median hospital length of stay (13 vs. 11, p=0.33), rate of readmission (2 vs. 0, p=0.194), or costs ($31,048 vs. $25,042, p=0.29). Nine (47 %) patients treated initially with endoscopy underwent surgical intervention at the time of the long-term analysis.

Endocrine and Exocrine Insufficiency

Disease progression results in exocrine and endocrine insufficiency. Both endoscopic and surgical modalities have been shown to delay the progression of pancreatic insufficiency. Some studies have demonstrated an advantage to surgery compared to endoscopy in terms of the time to exocrine insufficiency. Others have shown no advantage.

In the NAPS2 cohort, Glass et al. reported perceived improvement in exocrine insufficiency in patients treated with surgery compared to endoscopy (93 % vs. 55 % over 5 years of follow up, p=0.0008) [5]. However, Hong et al. demonstrated no significant difference in either endocrine or exocrine preservation or deterioration at 12-month or 60-month follow up (Table 42.2) [7].

As mentioned earlier, Nealon and Thompson evaluated the outcomes of pancreatic function in patients undergoing operative management compared to medical management [8]. Their grade of disease was based wholly upon endocrine and exocrine function. New onset endocrine and exocrine pancreatic insufficiency were respectively observed in 2/13 (15 %) patients and 1/15 (7 %) in the surgery group compared to 10/12 (83 %) patients and 11/14 (79 %) patients in the non-operative group [4]. They did not report the time to diagnosis of new insufficiency during their follow up period.

Dite et al. examined body weight changes and new onset diabetes mellitus during their 5-year follow up period [10]. Patients who underwent surgery gained significantly more body weight compared to those who underwent endotherapy (47.2 % vs 28.6 %, p=0.003). There was no difference in new onset diabetes mellitus between groups. Cahen et al. reported preservation of exocrine function in patients who underwent surgery, but no difference in new onset endocrine insufficiency between groups [11]. A pooled analysis also demonstrated no significant difference in endocrine insufficiency between surgical and endoscopic management (RR 0.98, CI 0.55–1.76). Long-term analysis by Cahen et al. trended towards a greater loss of pancreatic exocrine and endocrine function in the endoscopy group but this was not significant [12].

Timing of Intervention

Few studies have adequately compared surgical to endoscopic therapy head-to-head with the intent to identify appropriate timing of intervention. Most patients with chronic pancreatitis present for intervention late in the course of the disease and are a heterogeneous group in terms of glandular morphology. Nealon and Thompson were the first to demonstrate early surgical intervention in patients with mild to moderate disease had better pain control and sustained pancreatic function relative to best medical management [8]. A more recent study by Ahmed Ali identified surgery within 3 years of the onset of symptoms, fewer than five previous endoscopic treatments, and the absence of preoperative opioid use as independent factors associated with achievement of greater postoperative pain relief [15]. The two currently available randomized studies by Dite et al. and Cahen et al. seem to show improved results from surgery but also identify a benefit in select patients treated with endoscopy alone. From the available data we can surmise that surgical intervention early in the disease course might mitigate disease progression, reduce pain durably, and slow deterioration of pancreatic function. There is, however, probably a cohort of patients that would benefit permanently from one or two transampullary stenting procedures. Unfortunately no consensus as to the sequence or the timing of endoscopy and surgery presently exists. The Dutch Pancreatitis Study Group is currently recruiting patients for the ESCAPE trial (Early Surgery versus Optimal Current Step-Up Practice for Chronic Pancreatitis trial; ISRCTN 45877994), which will help to answer the question of whether early surgical intervention improves pain control and pancreatic function compared to the current "step up" approach [4].

Recommendations

Quality evidence includes only patients with severe late-stage chronic pancreatitis. This is a heterogeneous population of patients with variable glandular morphology, degrees of fibrosis and calcification, and narcotic addiction. The available studies are themselves also variable in terms of the way pain assessments are made, and the types of endoscopic and surgical interventions evaluated. Nevertheless, most investigations would support the contention that endoscopic drainage offers less durable symptom relief in patients with advanced chronic pancreatitis and a dilated main duct compared to surgical management (evidence quality moderate). Patients managed endoscopically require more repeated interventions than patients who undergo early surgical intervention. This translates to more hospitalization days and to greater costs. There appears to be no difference in the morbidity and mortality between each method (evidence quality low). There is no long-term difference in the preservation of endocrine and exocrine function (evidence quality low). Our recommendation is to consider surgical decompression for dilated duct chronic pancreatitis early in the course of its management.

A Personal View of the Data

The pain associated with chronic pancreatitis is debilitating. For patients with a diffuse dilation of the main pancreatic duct, surgical and endoscopic decompression can offer significant improvement in symptoms and allow patients to return to high quality of life. Endoscopy is rarely a durable solution, meaning patients treated endoscopically will almost always require multiple subsequent interventions to manage the progression of disease. In the end, repeated bouts of pancreatitis are the only known risk factor for intractable, untreatable pain syndromes and endoscopy would seem more likely than early surgical intervention to allow for repeated bouts of pancreatitis to occur. Undoubtedly, there is a small population of chronic pancreatitics who will have durable relief of pain with a limited number of endoscopic interventions. In our opinion, it is reasonable to pursue endotherapy once or twice. This will serve to confirm a benefit to drainage but not contribute risk of permanent neuropathy. For patients who only have temporary or limited relief with endotherapy, surgical drainage should be promptly pursued.

Recommendations

- For patients with chronic pancreatitis, pain and ductal dilation, we recommend no more than two attempts at endoscopic management prior to consideration of surgical decompression to alleviate pain and slow the progression of disease (evidence quality moderate; weak recommendation).
- Available evidence is too limited to allow a statement concerning the morbidity and mortality of endoscopy versus surgery in the treatment of large duct chronic pancreatitis.
- Available evidence is too limited to allow a statement concerning the preservation of pancreatic function for patients who are managed endoscopically or surgically in the treatment of large duct chronic pancreatitis.

References

1. D'Haese JG, Ceyham GO, Demir IE, et al. Treatment options in painful chronic pancreatitis: a systematic review. HPB (Oxf). 2014;16:512–21.
2. Issa Y, van Santvoort HC, van Goor H, et al. Surgical and endoscopic treatment of pain in chronic pancreatitis: a multidisciplinary update. Dig Surg. 2013;30:35–50.
3. Issa Y, Bruno MJ, Bakker OJ, et al. Treatment options for chronic pancreatitis. Nat Rev Gastroenterol Hepatol. 2014;11:556–64. doi:10.1038/nrgastro.2014.74.
4. Ali Ahmed UA, Issa Y, Bruno M, et al. Early surgery versus optimal current step-up practice for chronic pancreatitis (ESCAPE): design and rational of a randomized trial. BMC Gastroenterol. 2013;13:49.
5. Glass LM, Whitcomb DC, Yadav D, et al. Spectrum of use and effectiveness of endoscopic and surgical therapies for chronic pancreatitis in the United States. Pancreas. 2014;43:539–43.
6. Clarke B, Silvka A, Tomizawa Y, et al. Endoscopic therapy is effect for patients with chronic pancreatitis. Clin Gastroenterol Hepatol. 2012;10:795–802.
7. Hong J, Wang J, Keleman AM, et al. Endoscopic versus surgical treatment of downstream pancreatic duct stones in chronic pancreatitis. Am Surg. 2011;77(11):1531–8.
8. Nealon WH, Thomson JC. Progressive loss of pancreatic function in chronic pancreatitis is delayed by main pancreatic duct decompression. A longitudinal prospective analysis of the modified Puestow procedure. Ann Surg. 1993;217:458–66.

9. Ali Ahmed UA, Pahlplatz JM, Nealon WH, et al. Endoscopic or surgical intervention for painful obstructive chronic pancreatitis (review). Cochrane Libr. 2012;(1):CD007884. doi:10.1002/14651858.CD007884.pub2.
10. Dite P, Ruzicka M, Zboril V, Novotny I. A prospective, randomized trial comparing endoscopic and surgical therapy for chronic pancreatitis. Endoscopy. 2003;35(7):553–8.
11. Cahen DL, Gouma DJ, Nio Y, et al. Endoscopic versus surgical drainage of the pancreatic duct in chronic pancreatitis. N Eng J Med. 2007;356(7):676–84.
12. Cahen DL, Gouma DJ, Laramee P, et al. Long-term outcomes of endoscopic vs surgical drainage of the pancreatic duct in patients with chronic pancreatitis. Gastroenterology. 2011;141:1690–5.
13. Rutter K, Ferlitsch A, Sautner T, et al. Hospitalization, frequency of interventions and quality of life after endoscopic, surgical, or conservative treatment in patients with chronic pancreatitis. World J Surg. 2010;34:2642–7.
14. Hirota M, Asakura T, Kanno A, et al. Long-period pancreatic stenting for painful chronic calcified pancreatitis required high medical costs and frequent hospitalizations compared with surgery. Pancreas. 2011;40:946–50.
15. Ahmed Ali UA, Nieuwenhuijs VB, van Eijck CH, et al. Clinical outcome in relation to timing of surgery in chronic pancreatitis: a nomogram to predict pain relief. Arch Surg. 2012;147:825–32.

Chapter 43
Pancreatic Head Resection for Painful Chronic Pancreatitis

Minh B. Luu and Daniel J. Deziel

Abstract This chapter compares the outcomes of operations for chronic painful pancreatitis performed with or without duodenal preservation. The results of published, randomized clinical trials and systematic reviews are examined with regard to quality of evidence and strength of recommendations. Both pancreaticoduodenectomy and duodenal preserving resection of the head of the pancreas can provide pain relief for the majority of patients with chronic pancreatitis who undergo these operations. Current evidence is not adequate to clearly establish the superiority of either of these approaches, or of any specific variation of duodenal preserving resection, in terms of pain relief, peri-operative morbidity, post-operative pancreatic function or quality of life. Delayed gastric emptying may be more frequent following pancreaticoduodenectomy. The functional benefits of duodenum preserving resections that were noted in some early reports are absent at longer term follow up.

Keywords Chronic pancreatitis • Duodenal preserving pancreaticoduodenectomy • Beger procedure • Frey procedure • Quality of evidence

Introduction

Pancreatic head enlargement occurs in approximately 30–50 % of patients with chronic pancreatitis (CP) [1, 2]. These inflammatory masses are considered responsible for the development of chronic pain and may be associated with obstruction of the common bile duct or duodenum as well as portal vein thrombosis. Resection of the pancreatic head is indicated in patients with CP and intractable pain, but the most beneficial method of resection remains controversial. Resection by pancreaticoduodenectomy (PD) with or without pylorus preservation yields initial pain relief in a large proportion of patients. However, long-term follow-up has demonstrated

M.B. Luu • D.J. Deziel (✉)
Department General Surgery, Rush University Medical Center,
1653 West Congress Parkway, 785 Jelke, Chicago, IL 60612, USA
e-mail: Minh_B_Luu@rush.edu; Daniel_J_Deziel@rush.edu

J.M. Millis, J.B. Matthews (eds.), *Difficult Decisions in Hepatobiliary and Pancreatic Surgery*, Difficult Decisions in Surgery: An Evidence-Based Approach, DOI 10.1007/978-3-319-27365-5_43

high rates of insulin dependent diabetes and gastrointestinal complaints and diminished quality of life (QoL) [3, 4]. The importance of duodenal preservation for insulin homeostasis has been demonstrated in several studies [5–7]. Rationalizing that PD is overtreatment of CP, Beger [8] developed a duodenum-preserving pancreatic head resection (DPPHR) to minimize the rates of postoperative pancreatic insufficiency and gastrointestinal symptoms. Frey and colleagues subsequently introduced a modification of DPPHR involving less pancreatic dissection over the portal vein and a simplified reconstruction [9]. Several other modifications of DPPHR have also been described [10, 11].

This chapter uses the PICO format (Table 43.1) to compare PD to DPPHR for the treatment of patients with CP. The PD intervention group includes procedures performed either with or without gastric and pyloric preservation. The comparator group includes any version of the DPPHR operation reported. Outcomes measured were pain relief, perioperative morbidity, pancreatic endocrine and exocrine function and QoL.

Search Strategy

A search of English language publications from 1994 to 2014 on the surgical treatment for chronic pancreatitis was conducted. Databases searched were Medline (via PubMed and Ovid), Scopus, Cochrane Database of Systematic Reviews, Database of Abstracts of Reviews of Effectiveness (DARE) and Embase. Controlled vocabulary were used in Medline (MeSH) and Embase (Embase). Terms used in the search were "pancreatitis," AND "Frey" or "Beger". In Medline, 3116 articles related to surgery/pancreatitis contained 128 articles relating to Beger or Frey procedures. Of the 128 articles, 50 were in English pertaining to adult patients. In Embase, 44,308 articles relating to pancreatitis, were cross referenced with the 1086 related to Beger or Frey procedures, resulting in 42 articles. Of these 42 articles, 12 were of adult patient populations. Duplicate articles identified in the Medline and Embase searches were excluded. Reference lists from selected articles were hand searched for additional relevant citations. Retrospective or non-randomized observational studies were excluded. Four prospective randomized clinical trials (RCT) with their subsequent follow-up reports and three meta-analyses were analyzed. A fifth RCT, available only in the German language, was subsequently identified and included.

Table 43.1 PICO table for pancreatic head resection to treat chronic pancreatitis

P (Patients)	I (Intervention)	C (Comparator group)	O (Outcomes measured)
Patients with pain from chronic pancreatitis undergoing pancreatic head resection	Pancreaticoduodenectomy (Whipple with or without pylorus preservation)	Duodeno-preserving pancreatic head resection (Frey, Beger)	Pain relief, perioperative morbidity, pancreatic function, quality of life

The quality of evidence from the included studies and strength of recommendations were determined using the GRADE approach.

Results

Randomized Clinical Trials

Five original prospective randomized trials were identified, grouped with their subsequent follow-up reports and listed in Table 43.2. The first listed randomized trial, by Buchler et al. [12] in 1995, consisted of 20 patients who underwent a pylorus preserving (pp) PD and 20 patients who underwent DPPHR (Beger). They reported no perioperative mortality and the postoperative morbidity rates (15 % versus 20 %) were similar in both groups. Outcomes were initially reported after 6 months of follow-up. Pain was assessed by a visual analog scale. A standard meal stimulation test was performed measuring blood glucose, insulin and glucagon to assess pancreatic endocrine function. Additionally, preoperative and postoperative pancreolauryl serum test and an oral glucose load were performed to verify pancreatic endocrine and exocrine functions. Patients who underwent DPPHR had less pain, greater weight gain, better glucose tolerance and higher insulin secretion capacity. The long-term outcome of Buchler's study was reported by Muller et al. [10] in 2008 with a median follow-up of 7 and 14 years. Fourteen (70 %) patients who underwent PD and 15 (75 %) patients who underwent DPPHR from the original study were available to be assessed. No differences were noted in pain relief, pancreatic exocrine or endocrine function. QoL was evaluated with the European Organization for Research and Treatment of Cancer's (EORTC) Quality of Life Questionnaire-30 (QLQ-30). Although the ppPD group reported significantly worse appetite compared to the DPPHR patients, all other QoL parameters were similar. They concluded that the early advantages of the DPPHR reported by Buchler were no longer present at the later follow-up intervals. The study population was balanced with proper follow up reporting and adequate definition of outcome parameters. The sample size calculation, allocation concealment, blinding of outcome assessment and intention to treat (ITT) analysis were not described. The quality of evidence is moderate according to the GRADE system.

The second listed randomized trial, by Klempa et al. [13] in 1995, consisted of 21 patients who underwent PD and 22 patients who underwent DPPHR (Beger). There was no mortality in the PD group and one postoperative death (4.5 %) in the DPPHR group. Postoperative morbidity rates were similar for both groups although median length of stay was significantly longer in the PD group (21.7 vs. 16.5 days). The follow-up range was done in intervals following surgery (range 6–24 months and 36–60 months). Complete pain relief, based on a questionnaire, was reported in 60 % of patients who underwent PD and 70 % of patients who underwent DPPHR ($p<0.05$). New onset diabetes mellitus was higher in the PD group (38 %) com-

Table 43.2 Outcomes of prospective randomized trials comparing PD versus DPPHR

Study #	Author (year)	Patients PD/ DPPHR	Median follow-up months	Postop morbidity type, significance	Pain relief % pain free, significance	Pancreatic endocrine function	Pancreatic exocrine function	Quality of life	Study type (quality of evidence)
1	Buchler et al. (1995)	20/20 ppPD/ Beger 14/15	6	NS	40/75	PD < DPPHR	NS	NA	PRT (moderate)
	Muller et al. (2008)		84, 168	NS	(p<0.05) NS	NS	NS	NS	
2	Klempa et al. (1995)	21/22 PD/Beger	Range 36–60	LOS less in DPPHR	60/70 NS	NS	PD < DPPHR	NA	PRT (low)
3	Izbicki et al. (1998)	30/31 ppPD/Frey	24	DGE less in DPPHR	87/90, NS	NS	NS	PD < DPPHR	PRT (moderate)
	Strate et al. (2008)	24/23	84	NA	NS	NS	NS	NS	
	Bachman et al. (2013)	14/21	180	NA	NS	NS	NS	NS	
4	Farkas et al. (2006)	20/20 ppPD/Frey	12	DGE and PC less in DPPHR	90/85, NS	NS	NS	NA	PRT (low)
5	Keck et al. (2012)	45/47 ppPD/ Beger and Frey	66	NS	67/67, NS	NS	NS	NS	PRT (moderate)

PD pancreaticoduodenectomy, *DPPHR* duodenal-preserving pancreatic head resection, *NS* non significant, *NA* not available, *LOS* length of stay, *DGE* delayed gastric emptying, *PC* pulmonary complications, *PRT* prospective randomized trial pared to the DPPHR group (12 %) but not statistically significant. Pancreatic exocrine insufficiency, indicated by maldigestion and steatorrhea, was present in 100 % of patients in the PD group and in only 10 % of the DPPHR group 36–60 months after the respective procedures ($p<0.05$). Occupational rehabilitation was higher in the DPPHR group (75 %) than the PD group (50 %) but not statistically significant. Overall QoL was not assessed in the study. The study population was balanced with adequate definition of outcome parameters. The sample size calculation, allocation concealment, blinding of outcome assessment and intention to treat (ITT) analysis were not described. The quality of evidence is low according to the GRADE system.

The third listed randomized trial by Izbicki et al. [11] in 1998 consisted of 30 patients who underwent ppPD and 31 patients who underwent DPPHR (Frey). The ppPD group had no mortality while one patient (3.2 %) in the DPPHR group died of a myocardial infarction. Overall morbidity was significantly less in the DPPHR group due to the higher rate of delayed gastric emptying in patients undergoing ppPD ($p<0.05$). Delayed gastric emptying was defined as need for nasogastric tube decompression for more than 7 days postoperatively. After a median follow-up of 24 months, similar relief of symptoms was reported in each group (87 % and 90 % respectively). Additionally, patients were given a pain score that contained the following components: a visual analog scale, frequency of pain attacks, pain medications, and inability to work. The median pain score decreased 71 % in the ppPD group and 90 % in the DPPHR group. The postoperative pain scores were significantly lower in both groups when compared to their preoperative scores but were not different between groups. Pancreatic endocrine function was assessed by an oral glucose tolerance test, the treatment required (diet, oral agents, or insulin), fasting serum insulin, C-peptide, and HbA1C. Pancreatic exocrine function was assessed by measuring the fecal chymotrypsin concentration and the pancreolauryl test. Although no statistical analysis was provided to compare pancreatic endocrine and exocrine function between ppPD and DPPHR, the outcomes appear to be similar. Overall QoL, using the EORTC QLQ-30, was significantly higher for patients undergoing DPPHR compared to ppPD. Long-term follow-up of this trial was reported by Strate et al. [14] in 2008 at 84 months and by Bachman et al. [15] in 2013 at 180 months. Twenty four (80 %) and 14 (47 %) of the patients who underwent PD compared to 23 (74 %) and 21 (68 %) of patients who underwent DPPHR were available to be assessed. Neither follow-up report showed any significant difference in pain relief, pancreatic function or QoL. The study population was balanced with proper follow up reporting, adequate definition of outcome parameters, sample size calculation, and allocation concealment. Blinding of outcome assessment and intention to treat (ITT) analysis were not described. The quality of evidence is moderate according to the GRADE system.

The fourth listed randomized trial by Farkas et al. [16] in 2006 consisted of 20 patients who underwent ppPD and 20 patients who underwent DPPHR (modified Frey) with a median follow-up of 12 months. There was no perioperative mortality. The operative time and hospital LOS were significantly longer in the ppPD group. Additionally, overall morbidity was significantly higher in the ppPD group due to delayed gastric emptying and pulmonary complications. A pain frequency questionnaire demonstrated similar pain relief (ppPD 90 % versus DPPHR 85 %). Pancreatic endocrine function was assessed by the oral glucose tolerance test. Pancreatic exocrine function was evaluated by measuring stool elastase. There was no significance difference in either endocrine or exocrine function. The authors reported that QoL was superior in the DPPHR group, but no methodology for QoL assessment was described. The study population was balanced and all patients were available for follow-up. Outcome parameters were not well defined. Additionally, sample size calculation, allocation concealment, blinding of outcome assessment and intention to treat (ITT) analysis were not described. The quality of evidence is low according to the GRADE system.

The fifth listed randomized trial conducted by Keck et al. [17] reported short and long-term results comparing 45 patients who underwent ppPD and 47 patients who underwent DPPHR (Beger or Frey). There was no mortality in either group and the overall morbidity was similar (30 % versus 33 %). Pain relief was assessed using a visual analog scale and pain frequency questionnaire. At a median follow-up of 66 months, 67 % of patients in both groups were pain free. Pancreatic endocrine function was assessed preoperatively using the oral glucose tolerance test or a 24-h glucose profile. Postoperatively, pancreatic endocrine function was assessed using a questionnaire for the presence of diabetes and diabetes medication use. New onset diabetes developed in 19 % of patients in the PD group and 24 % of patients in the DPPHR group (p 0.56). Pancreatic exocrine function was determined by patient reported presence of steatorrhea or use of pancreatic enzyme supplementation. Postoperative de novo pancreatic exocrine insufficiency was 21 % in the PD group and 26 % in the DPPHR group (p 0.57). QoL was measured using the EORTC QLQ-30 questionnaire and was also similar in both groups. The study population was balanced with proper follow up reporting and adequate definition of outcome parameters. Examiners were blinded to QoL questionnaires but blinding of other outcome assessments was not described. Sample size calculation, allocation concealment, and intention to treat (ITT) analysis were not described. The quality of evidence is moderate according to the GRADE system.

Systematic Reviews and Meta-analysis

Three systematic reviews and meta-analyses were identified and summarized in Table 43.3. Diener et al. [18] included studies by Buchler, Klempa, Izbicki and Farkas. A total of 200 randomized patients were included with a range of 43–64 from each study. Mortality was 0 % in the PD group and 2.2 % in the DPPHR group. Although the PD group in the RCT by Izbicki et al. [11] had the highest morbidity rate of 53 % and the DPPHR group in the RCT by Klempa et al. [13] had the lowest morbidity rate of 18 %, no significant differences were found in the meta-analysis. When delayed gastric emptying rate was reviewed, a trend in favor of DPPHR was seen but this was not statistically significant. The analysis for pain relief consisted

Table 43.3 Outcomes of systematic reviews with meta-analysis comparing PD versus DPPHR

Study #	Author (year)	Patients PD/DPPHR	Median follow-up months	Postop morbidity type, p	Pain relief % pain free, p	Pancreatic endocrine function	Pancreatic exocrine function	Quality of life	Study type (quality of evidence)
1	Diener et al. (2008)	86/87	NA	Delayed gastric emptying in pylorus preserving PD	72/82, NS	NS	PD < DPPHR	PD < DPPHR	Meta-analysis (low)
2	Yin et al. (2012)	541/466	NA	NS	NS	NS	PD < DPPHR	PD < DPPHR	Meta-analysis (low)
3	Lu et al. (2013)	104/102	NA	NA	NS	NS	NS	PD < DPPHR	Meta-analysis (low)

PD pancreaticoduodenectomy, *DPPHR* duodenal-preserving pancreatic head resection, *NS* non significant, *NA* not available of 86 patients who underwent PD and 87 patients who underwent DPPHR. No significant differences were found in postoperative pain relief between the two groups. New onset diabetes mellitus showed a trend in favor of DPPHR while pancreatic exocrine impairment was significantly less with DPPHR. Pooled QoL from two RCT (Izbicki and Farkas) showed a significantly higher global QoL in the DPPHR group. The authors concluded that PD and DPPHR seem to be equally effective treatments for CP in terms of pain relief, overall morbidity and the incidence of endocrine insufficiency. Several peri-operative parameters and QoL seemed to favor DPPHR. Variations in study quality was noted in terms of sample size, allocation concealment, blinded outcome assessment, standardization of study interventions, definition of outcome parameters, and consistency of follow-up. For the primary outcome of pain relief, the authors found that a total sample size of 558 study patients (279 in each arm) would be needed for a RCT to be adequately powered (80 %). The quality of evidence is low according to the GRADE system.

The second systematic review and meta-analysis by Yin et al. [19] reported 541 patients in the PD group and 466 patients in the DPPHR from 15 studies. This review included the four randomized trials reported by Diener et al. as well as a randomized trial by Izbicki et al. that compared the Beger and Frey procedures. Also included were ten non-randomized or retrospective trials. Perioperative mortality was not reported. Pooled data for postoperative morbidity and pain relief were similar between the PD and DPPHR operations. However, subgroup analyses showed that the Beger procedure provided significantly better pain relief than PD while the Frey procedure had significantly lower postoperative morbidity than PD. Pancreatic endocrine insufficiency was similar in both groups but exocrine insufficiency outcomes significantly favored DPPHR. Pooled data showed that QoL was significantly better after DPPHR compared to PD. The five randomized trials were analyzed using the Cochrane Risk of Bias Tool in the meta-analysis and deemed of moderate quality by the authors. The ten observational studies were evaluated using the Newcastle-Ottawa Scale but the results were not described. These observational studies are at risk of allocation bias. None of the observational studies adequately described patient flow or methods for handling missing data. The quality of evidence is low.

The 2013 report from Lu et al. [20] included five RCT. Two RCT (Klempa and Farkas) were original trials and two (Strate and Muller) were follow-up reports of the original trials. The fifth trial included was a retrospective study by McClaine et al. that was incorrectly labeled as a prospective RCT. Perioperative mortality and morbidity were not analyzed. A total of 206 patients were available for meta-analysis: 104 patients in the PD group and 102 patients in the DPPHR group. Pain relief, pancreatic endocrine and exocrine functions were similar in both groups. Only global QoL was found to be significantly better in the DPPHR group. Heterogeneous study quality was reported with sample size, standardization of study interventions, consistency of follow-up and outcome assessment. Small sample size, inadequate allocation concealment, and loss of population during follow-up were limitations of the meta-analysis. The quality of evidence is low.

Recommendations

Either PD or DPPHR can provide pain relief for the majority of patients with CP who undergo these operations. Current evidence is inadequate to establish the superiority of either of these approaches over the other for pain relief.

Current evidence is inadequate to establish the superiority of either approach for post operative morbidity or mortality. Delayed gastric emptying has been noted more frequently following PD in several small RCTs. However, assessment of gastric emptying has not been standardized across studies and there has not been consistent distinction between PD with or without gastrectomy and pyloric preservation.

Current evidence is inadequate to clearly establish superiority of either approach for preservation of post operative pancreatic endocrine or exocrine function. The functional benefits of DPPHR observed in earlier reports of RCTs were diminished or nonexistent at longer term follow up. Methods for assessment of endocrine and exocrine function were not standardized.

Current evidence is inadequate to establish superiority of either approach for improved QoL. The suggestions that DPPHR may be associated with better QoL must be tempered by the differences in methodologies used for assessment and by the varied follow up intervals.

Based on this summary of the evidence available from RCTs and systematic reviews, we can recommend pancreatic head resection for patients with pancreatic head mass and intractable pain from CP. We can make no recommendation favoring either PD or DPPHR. All of the available RCTs are limited by sample size, by interventions that were similar but not identical (ppPD and/or PD vs. Frey and/or Beger), and by differences in the methodologies used for determining QoL and functional outcomes. In the sequential follow-up reports of Izbicki's study, a substantial proportion of the initial cohort was not included.

A Personal View of the Data

Pancreatic head resection is more beneficial for pain relief than non-operative treatment for selected patients with CP. We make the assumption that the typical patient suffering intractable pain from CP places higher value on pain relief and operative survival and lesser value on potentially undesirable side effects. This would be particularly true if the side effects are treatable and where the magnitude of differences in side effects between treatment options is limited. Furthermore, long term functional decline may more represent the natural history of disease progression rather than any operative sequela.

In our opinion, the surgeons' personal experience with peri -operative morbidity and mortality and clinically relevant pain relief is the key determinant for selecting PD or DPPHR in this circumstance, as it is for selection of the specific technical version of either approach. Surgeons will be biased by their training and practice. These may or may not involve a highly specialized center and may or may not include a substantial proportion of patients resected for CP rather than for pancreatic neoplasms. Objective interpretation of the current data will hopefully allow us to acknowledge that alternative operations may be equally reasonable. Evidence favoring one approach or another may waver. Observations from published studies may not apply to an individual patient, particularly to a patient suffering with CP with its varied morphologic, metabolic, social and medical nuances.

Recommendations

1. Patients with intractable pain associated with chronic pancreatitis and an inflammatory pancreatic head mass should undergo pancreatic head resection by PD or DPPHR (evidence quality high, strong recommendation).
2. DPPHR may have early advantages with respect to gastric emptying (evidence quality low, weak recommendation).
3. DPPHR may have advantages with respect to preservation of pancreatic exocrine function and quality of life (evidence quality low, weak recommendation).

References

1. Buchler M, Malfertheiner P, Friess H, et al. Chronic pancreatitis with inflammatory mass in the head of the pancreas: a special entity? In: Beger HG, Buchler M, Ditschuneit H, Malfertheiner P, editors. Chronic pancreatitis. New York: Springer; 1993. p. 41–6.
2. Beger HG, Schlosser W, Poch B, et al. Inflammatory mass in the head of pancreas. In: Beger HG et al., editors. The pancreas. London: Blackwell Science; 1998. p. 757–60.
3. Martin RF, Rossi RL, Leslie KA. Long-term results of pylorus-preserving pancreatoduodenectomy for chronic pancreatitis. Arch Surg. 1996;131:247–52.
4. Sakorafas GH, Farnell MB, Nagomey DM, et al. Pancreatoduodenectomy for chronic pancreatitis: long-term results in 105 patients. Arch Surg. 2000;135:517–23.
5. Bittner R, Butters M, Buchler M, et al. Glucose homeostasis and endocrine pancreatic function in patients with chronic pancreatitis before and after surgical therapy. Pancreas. 1994;9:47–53.
6. Malfertheiner P, Sarr MG, Nelson DK, Di Magno EP. Role of the duodenum in postprandial release of pancreatic and gastrointestinal hormones. Pancreas. 1994;9:13–9.
7. Creutzfeldt W, Ebert R, Arnold R, et al. Gastric inhibitory polypeptide (GIP), gastrin and insulin: response to a test meal in coeliac disease and after duodeno-pancreatectomy. Diabetologia. 1976;12:279–86.
8. Beger HG, Buchler MW. Duodenum-preserving resection of the head of the pancreas in chronic pancreatitis with inflammatory mass in the head. World J Surg. 1990;14:83–7.
9. Frey CF, Smith GJ. Description and rationale of a new operation for chronic pancreatitis. Pancreas. 1987;2:701–7.
10. Muller MW, Friess H, Martin DJ, Hinz U, Dahmen R, Buchler MW. Long-term follow-up of a randomized clinical trial comparing Beger with pylorus-preserving Whipple procedure for chronic pancreatitis. Br J Surg. 2008;95:350–6.

11. Izbicki JR, Bloechle C, Broeing DC, Knoefel WT, Kuechler T, Broelsch CE. Extended drainage versus resection in surgery for chronic pancreatitis. Ann Surg. 1998;228:771–9.
12. Buchler MW, Friess H, Muller MW, Wheatley AM, Beger HG. Randomized trial of duodenum-preserving pancreatic head resection versus pylorus-preserving Whipple in chronic pancreatitis. Am J Surg. 1995;169:65–70.
13. Klempa I, Spatny M, Zenzel J, et al. Pancreatic function and quality of life after resection of the head of the pancreas in chronic pancreatitis. A prospective, randomized comparative study after duodenum preserving resection of the head of the pancreas versus Whipple's operation. Chirurg. 1995;66:350–9.
14. Strate T, Bachmann K, Busch P, Mann O, Schneider C, Bruhn JP, Yekebas E, Kuechler T, Bloechle C, Izbicki JR. Resection vs drainage in treatment of chronic pancreatitis: long-term results of a randomized trial. Gastroenterology. 2008;134:1406–11.
15. Bachmann K, Tomkoetter L, Kutup A, Erbes J, Vashish Y, Mann O, Bockhorn M, Izbicki JR. Is the Whipple procedure harmful for long-term outcome in treatment of chronic pancreatitis? Ann Surg. 2013;258:815–21.
16. Farkas G, Leindler L, Daroczi M, Farkas Jr G. Prospective randomized comparison of organ-preserving pancreatic head resection with pylorus-preserving pancreaticoduodenectomy. Langenbecks Arch Surg. 2006;391:338–42.
17. Keck T, Adam U, Makowiec F, Riediger H, Wellner U, Tittelbach-Helmrich D, Hopt UT. Short- and long-term results of duodenum preservation versus resection for the management of chronic pancreatitis: a prospective, randomized study. Surgery. 2012;152:95–102.
18. Deiner MK, Rahbari NN, Fischer L, Antes G, Buchler MW, Seiler CM. Duodenum-preserving pancreatic head resection versus pancreatoduodenectomy for surgical treatment of chronic pancreatitis: a systematic review and meta-analysis. Ann Surg. 2008;247:950–61.
19. Yin Z, Sun J, Yin D, Wang J. Surgical treatment strategies in chronic pancreatitis: a meta-analysis. Arch Surg. 2012;147:961–8.
20. Lu WP, Shi Q, Zhang WZ, Cai SW, Jiang K, Dong JH. A meta-analysis of the long-term effects of chronic pancreatitis surgical treatments: duodenum-preserving pancreatic head resection versus pancreatoduodenectomy. Chin Med J. 2013;126:147–53.

Chapter 44
Is Total Pancreatectomy with Islet Autotransplantation Indicated in Hereditary/Genetic Pancreatitis?

Jeffrey B. Matthews

Abstract Total pancreatectomy with islet autotransplantation (TPIAT) has been used in selected centers to treat intractable hereditary/genetic forms of recurrent acute and chronic pancreatitis. It has theoretical advantages over continued medical management or traditional endoscopic and surgical interventions because it entails the complete removal of the inflamed and fibrotic organ to treat the symptoms of pain while both eliminating the long-term risk of pancreatic ductal adenocarcinoma and preserving islet mass and to limit post-pancreatectomy diabetes. While an emerging consensus favors TPIAT in this setting, the evidence base largely relies on retrospective patient series and expert opinion.

Keywords Chronic pancreatitis • Recurrent acute pancreatitis • Hereditary pancreatitis • Islet autotransplantation • PRSS1 • Total pancreatomy

Introduction

Recurrent acute pancreatitis (RAP) and chronic pancreatitis (CP) represent a spectrum of inflammatory and fibrotic conditions of the pancreas and their associated complications. Surgical intervention is most often considered for the indication of pain, which can occur as a pattern of recurrent episodes or persistent symptoms associated with progressive loss of pancreatic exocrine and endocrine function. The morphological consequences are highly variable and may include ductal stricture, dilation, ductal and parenchymal calcifications, focal mass effects, and extension to adjacent organs and vessels [1].

Treatment of the pain of chronic pancreatitis may be pharmacological, neuroablative, and endoscopic, but these are of variable success for short- and long-term

J.B. Matthews (✉)
Department of Surgery, University of Chicago Medical Center,
5841 S. Maryland Avenue, MC 5029, Chicago, IL 60637, USA
e-mail: jmatthews@surgery.bsd.uchicago.edu

J.M. Millis, J.B. Matthews (eds.), *Difficult Decisions in Hepatobiliary and Pancreatic Surgery*, Difficult Decisions in Surgery: An Evidence-Based Approach, DOI 10.1007/978-3-319-27365-5_44

control of symptoms. Surgical therapy may be an effective alternative in appropriately selected patients. The choice of operation generally reflects assumptions about the mechanism of pain. For example, duct decompression by lateral pancreaticojejunostomy may be recommended for patients with so-called large duct disease, whereas pancreatic resection by pancreaticoduodenectomy or duodenum-sparing pancreatic head resection may be indicated for patients with an inflammatory head mass [1].

Some patients have more complex situations, and the role of surgical therapy is controversial. For example, the patient with a non-dilated pancreatic duct (small-duct disease) may have no duct to decompress and no mass to resect. Others may have persistent or recurrent pain after prior pancreatic operation. Still others appear to have genetic/hereditary syndromes, some of which appear to be associated with increased risk of pancreatic cancer. Hereditary pancreatitis kindreds, over half of whom are found to have mutations in PRSS1 (the gene that encodes for cationic trypsinogen), are reported to have an over 50-fold increased risk of developing pancreatic cancer [2]. In smokers, the cumulative risk of cancer is 15 % by age 50 and exceeds 50 % by age 75 [2, 3], although in non-smokers the risk of cancer, while still elevated, appears to be considerably lower. Pancreatitis associated with PRSS1 gene mutations has an autosomal dominant pattern of inheritance with incomplete penetrance [4]. In contrast, RAP and CP associated with mutations in the CFTR or SPINK1 genes shows autosomal recessive inheritance and do not appear to carry an increased risk of pancreatic adenocarcinoma compared to other forms of CP [5].

The rationale for total pancreatectomy with islet autotransplantation (TPIAT) for hereditary/genetic forms of pancreatitis includes the complete removal of the inflamed and fibrotic organ to treat the symptoms of pain as well as to reduce or eliminate the long-term risk of pancreatic ductal adenocarcinoma, while preserving islet mass and preventing or limiting the extent of post-pancreatectomy type 3c diabetes [6, 7]. However, the consequences of total pancreatectomy in this setting are not trivial and include not only persistent pain (often attributed to central sensitization as well as narcotic bowel syndrome) but also the metabolic and nutritional impact of complete pancreatic exocrine insufficiency [6, 7]. For patients with severe and intractable symptoms, the main question is whether TPIAT truly improves short- and long-term quality of life. For less severely affected patients, the question is whether the long-term reduction in cancer risk sufficiently changes the risk-benefit ration to justify proceeding with TPIAT earlier, irrespective of the development of symptomatic incapacitation.

Search Strategy

A PubMed literature search of English language publications from 2000 to 2015 was used to identify series of patients with hereditary or genetic RAP or CP pancreatitis treated by TPIAT. Terms used in the search included "total pancreatectomy"

Table 44.1 PICO Table

P (Patients)	I (Intervention)	C (Comparator)	O (Outcomes)
Patients with hereditary/genetic recurrent acute and chronic pancreatitis	Total pancreatectomy with islet autotransplantation	Best medical management	Morbidity; diabetes; pain relief; QOL; durability

AND "islet autotransplantation" OR "autologous islet transplantation" AND "chronic pancreatitis", OR "recurrent acute pancreatitis" OR "hereditary pancreatitis" AND "genetic pancreatitis". Articles were excluded if patients with hereditary/genetic forms of RAP/CP were not specified, or for reports that addressed fewer than five TPIAT patients. A PICO approach was used to frame the relevant question, and the data were classified using the GRADE system (Table 44.1).

Results

Patient Selection

There was considerable heterogeneity in the patient populations selected to undergo TPIAT. Among the many factors that differed among the published series included the demographics and comorbidities of the patients as well as the type and number of prior pancreatic interventions. Several series did not specify the number of patients with genetic/familial/hereditary disease, and only two series reported the results of genetic testing for PRSS1 or other genes associated with RAP and CP. Because genetic testing is not routine (or routinely recommended), the total number of patients with PRSS1 gene mutations who have undergone TPIAT is unclear. An uncertain number of patients were included multiple times in various reports from the larger centers, notably the University of Minnesota and the University of Cincinnati series [8–15], complicating interpretation of the aggregate experience in hereditary/genetic RAP/CP. Some studies focused on pediatric populations; others focused on small-duct ("minimal change") chronic pancreatitis.

In the Minnesota series of 484 patients that underwent TPIAT, the 80 patients with hereditary/genetic forms of RAP and CP differed from those with non-hereditary forms in a number of respects: they were younger, had pancreatitis of longer duration, a higher pancreatic fibrosis score, and a trend toward lower islet yield [9]. Across all series, the vast majority of patients were described as having failed prior medical, endoscopic, and, in many instances, surgical therapy. Essentially all patients required substantial analgesic therapy and were in most instances dependent on narcotics.

Perioperative Morbidity and Mortality

The largest series, from the University of Minnesota, reported a 1 % in-hospital mortality rate [10], with other smaller series showing that postoperative mortality is below 2 % [12, 16]. A study based on data from the National Surgical Quality Improvement Program confirmed an approximately 1 % mortality rate and additionally identified that major morbidity occurred in found a 41 % of patient [17]. The most common significant early postoperative complication was hemorrhage, occurring in about 10 % of cases. Partial portal vein thrombosis is also noted, but this does not appear to adversely impact outcomes. Readmission rate was not consistently reported but in Wilson's series was 37 % [15]. Actuarial survival is 90 % at 5 years and 81 % at 10 years in the Minnesota series, although the cause of late deaths is not known in many instances [10].

Islet Function

Islet yield was highly variable between series, depending upon the age of the patients, duration of CP, the condition of the pancreas, and the type(s) of prior pancreatic operation. Prior lateral pancreaticojejunostomy was associated with dramatically lower islet yield. There was not a consistent correlation between the number of islet-equivalents isolated per kg body weight and ultimate insulin independence. Insulin independence within the first year was achieved in 20–41 % of patients (Table 44.2). Typically, daily insulin requirements were reported to be less than 20U/day in most patients. Although a measurable drop-off of C-peptide was demonstrated over time in some series, with a corresponding decrease in the rate of insulin-independence after 1 year, daily insulin requirements tended to otherwise remain stable out to 10 years and beyond [10, 14].

Data on the natural history of the development of endocrine insufficiency in patients with genetic/hereditary pancreatitis are sparse. In one study of patients carrying PRSS1 gene mutations, endocrine insufficiency was noted in 26 % of patients at a median age of 38 years [4]. A small series of children treated by modified Puestow procedure for intractable pain showed two out of nine patients developed insulin-dependent diabetes within 1 year of operation [18]. However, other small series have not shown such rapid progression [19].

Pain Relief/Narcotic Requirement

Following TPIAT, a significantly decrease in subjective assessment of pain and the need for narcotic pain medication was noted in all studies. Over 80 % of patients reported either no pain or only mild pain (Table 44.2). Some reports quantified the

Table 44.2 Series of TPIAT addressing hereditary/genetic etiology

Series (ref)	Total n	Hereditary/ genetic	PRSS1	Insulin independent	Narcotic-free	QOL
Sutton [12]	16	16	4	25 %	63 %	SF36
Bellin [11]	19 (pediatric)	12	9	37 %	74 %	SF36
Walsh [24]	20	2	n.s.	20 %	30 %	PDI VAS DASS
Morgan [23]	33	3	n.s.	24 %	24 %	SF12
Sutherland [10]	409	58	n.s.	30 %	59 %	SF36
Wilson [13]	14 (pediatric)	4	1	29 %	79 %	n.s.
Tai [22]	9	4	2	22 %	n.s.	n.s.
Georgiev [21]	53	8	n.s.	n.s.	n.s.	SF36 McGill pain
Wilson [15]	84 ("minimal change")	14	2	37 %	58 %	SF36
Chinnakotla [9]	80	80	38	~20 %	~80 %	SF36
Chinnakotla [8]	75 (pediatric)	41	n.s.	41 %	~80 %	SF36

n.s. not specified

reduction of pain medication requirements as morphine equivalents, although the details of reporting were highly variable. Achievement of the endpoint of narcotic-independence was inconsistent among the various series, ranging between 24 % and 80 % (Table 44.2).

QOL/Durability

A number of studies evaluated quality of life using several standard questionnaire-based surveys (Table 44.2), most commonly short-form 36 (SF36). These were administered at variable times after the procedure, and all published studies suffer from at least some patients being lost to follow up. Several of the larger series reported follow up over 5 years, and for some patients, over 10 years. These studies demonstrated that narcotic independence and islet function, as well as improvements in QOL are sustained for at least 10 years following operation. For example, Wilson [14] showed that the narcotic-independence rate rose from 55 % at 1 year to 73 % at 5 year follow up; although insulin-independence rates declined from 38 % at 1 year to 27 % after 5 years, daily insulin requirements remained relatively constant and glycemic control measured by HgA1C levels were stable in all patients evaluated.

Comparison to medical management is mostly implicit in that selection criteria included failure of non-operative therapy. One study addressed cost-effectiveness based on a series of indirect assumptions concluded that there was no cost disadvantage to TPIAT [16]. Wilson et al. [20] used a Markov model populated with data from a series of 46 patients with small duct chronic pancreatitis who underwent TPIAT to evaluate its cost-effectiveness compared to medical management. Significant reductions in the number of hospital admissions and the need for endoscopy and advanced imaging were noted following TPIAT, with significantly decreased cost per quality-adjusted life years. There are no data on long term nutritional status with respect to maintenance of body weight, anemia, vitamin deficiencies, complications due to diabetes, and other possible sources of morbidity after TPIAT.

Cancer Risk

TPIAT has been performed since 1977 and to date there have been no reports of a single instance of intrahepatic pancreatic adenocarcinoma [6]. In the Minnesota series of 80 patients with genetic/hereditary forms of pancreatitis, no cancers occurred during the 2936 patient-years of follow-up [9]. It is unclear whether the long-term risk of developing pancreatic cancer in hereditary CP in and of itself is sufficient justification for proceeding with TPIAT; risk modification by avoidance of tobacco may have a substantial impact. The value of surveillance imaging is unproven and may be difficult in a pancreas deformed by repeated damage and progressive fibrosis.

Expert Consensus

Given the limited number of series, the heterogeneity of patients, and uncertainties about both the natural history of RAP/CP (of any etiology) and the long term results of TPIAT, a working group of expert pancreatologists and pancreatic surgeons reviewed the relevant literature and compared their own clinical experiences to develop a series of consensus statements to guide patient selection. There is a high degree of consensus among these experts that TPIAT is indicated to treat intractable pain in patients with impaired quality of life due to CP or RAP when medical, endoscopic, or previous surgical therapy have failed [9]. Moreover, it was recommended by this group that special consideration be given to patients with genetic causes. The National Institute of Diabetes and Digestive and Kidney Disease (NIDDK) organized a workshop entitled "Total Pancreatectomy with Islet AutoTransplantation: Gaps, Needs and Opportunities" in July 2014 in Pittsburgh. One of the critical research gaps identified was the need for multicenter collaboration through a data registry [10].

Recommendations Based on the Data

Patients with intractable pain or significantly impaired quality of life due recurrent acute or chronic pancreatitis who have otherwise failed medical, endoscopic, or surgical therapy should be evaluated for TPIAT (evidence quality moderate; strong recommendation).

TPIAT is preferable to continued medical management in patients with symptomatic hereditary pancreatitis associated with a PRSS1 gene mutation and a family history of pancreatic cancer because of the virtual elimination of lifelong risk of pancreatic adenocarcinoma (evidence quality high, strong recommendation).

TPIAT should be performed in the setting of a multidisciplinary team experienced in patient selection and postoperative management, at or in collaboration with a center with experience in TPIAT (evidence quality high, strong recommendation).

A Personal View of the Data

TPIAT should be considered in patients who are severely affected by the pain of chronic pancreatitis and who have no conventional alternative. Patients with so-called "small duct" disease, or who have failed prior surgical interventions may be good candidates so long as they are not yet C-peptide negative diabetics. Patients with genetic predisposition (e.g., hereditary pancreatitis), particularly younger patients, are very well suited to this procedure. The outcomes for TPIAT are best when performed in a center that has deep, multidisciplinary experience in caring for the spectrum of benign and malignant pancreatic diseases. In addition to a significant institutional commitment to an islet isolation laboratory, a successful program requires close collaboration between medical pancreatologists, advanced endoscopists, and pancreatic surgeons in addition to experts in surgical nursing, nutrition, and pain management.

The published literature suffers from considerable selection bias, framing effects, and optimism bias. While earlier intervention may increase islet yield and the likelihood of insulin-independence, it eliminates the ability of the patient to benefit from future advances in islet isolation and preservation. This should temper enthusiasm for TPIAT in the pediatric population. Fears over the eventual development of cancer in patients with hereditary pancreatitis should be tempered by a number of considerations, including tobacco as a modifiable risk, and the possibility of the emergence of improved screening and treatment protocols for a disease that may not develop for decades.

It is difficult to generalize which patients will have the best outcome from TPIAT because of the high degree of variability in presentation, prior treatment, and anatomic circumstances. Potential patients differ not only in their clinical situations but also in adaptive emotional and physical responses to their illness. Substantial gaps in knowledge still remain, but due to patient heterogeneity and the relative infrequency of RAP/CP in the general population, it is unlikely that treatment decisions will be informed by randomized controlled trials in the foreseeable future. A multicenter registry that will track the most important characteristics of presentation, evaluation, postoperative course, and long-term outcomes is sorely lacking.

References

1. Ahmad SA, Wray C, Rilo HL, et al. Chronic pancreatitis: recent advances and ongoing challenges. Curr Prob Surg. 2006;43:127–238.
2. Rebours V, Levy P, Ruszniewski P. An overview of hereditary pancreatitis. Dig Liver Dis. 2012;44:8–15.
3. Rebours V, Boutron-Ruault MC, Schnee MF, et al. Risk of pancreatic adenocarcinoma in patients with hereditary pancreatitis: a national exhaustive series. Am J Gastroenterol. 2008;103:111–9.
4. Keim V, Bauer N, Teich N, et al. Clinical characterization of patients with hereditary pancreatitis and mutations in the cationic trypsinogen gene. Am J Med. 2001;111:622–6.
5. Matsubayashi H, Fukushima N, Sato N, et al. Polymorphisms of SPINK1 N34S and CFTR in patients with sporadic and familial pancreatic cancer. Cancer Biol Ther. 2003;2:652–5.
6. Bellin MD, Freeman ML, Gelrud A, et al. Total pancreatectomy and islet autotransplantation in chronic pancreatitis: recommendations from PancreasFest. Pancreatology. 2014;14:27–35.
7. Bellin MD, Gelrud A, Arreaza-Rubin G, et al. Total pancreatectomy with islet autotransplantation: summary of a National Institute of Diabetes and Digestive and Kidney Diseases workshop. Pancreas. 2014;43:1163–71.
8. Chinnakotla S, Bellin MD, Schwarzenberg SJ, et al. Total pancreatectomy and islet autotransplantation in children for chronic pancreatitis. Ann Surg. 2014;260:56–64.
9. Chinnakotla S, Radosevich DM, Dunn TB, et al. Long-term outcomes of total pancreatectomy and islet auto transplantation for hereditary/genetic pancreatitis. J Am Coll Surg. 2014;218:530–45.
10. Sutherland DER, Radosevich DM, Bellin MD. Total pancreatectomy and islet autotransplantation for chronic pancreatitis. J Am Coll Surg. 2012;214:409–26.
11. Bellin MD, Freeman ML, Schwarzenberg SJ, et al. Quality of life improves for pediatric patients after total pancreatectomy and islet autotransplant for chronic pancreatitis. Clin Gastroenterol Hepatol. 2011;9:793–9.
12. Sutton JM, Schmulewitz N, Sussman JJ, et al. Total pancreatectomy and islet cell autotransplantation as a means of treating patients with genetically linked pancreatitis. Surgery. 2010;148:676–86.
13. Wilson GC, Sutton JM, Salehi M, et al. Surgical outcomes after total pancreatectomy and islet cell autotransplantation in pediatric patients. Surgery. 2013;154:777–84.
14. Wilson GC, Sutton JM, Abbott DE, et al. Long-term outcomes after total pancreatectomy and islet cell autotransplantation: is it a durable operation? Ann Surg. 2014;260:659–67.
15. Wilson GC, Sutton JM, Smith MT. Total pancreatectomy and islet cell autotransplantation as the initial treatment for minimal-change chronic pancreatitis. HPB. 2014;17:232–8.
16. Garcea G, Pollard CA, Illouz S, et al. Patient satisfaction and cost-effectiveness following total pancreatectomy with islet cell transplantation for chronic pancreatitis. Pancreas. 2013;42:322–8.
17. Bhayani NH, Enomoto LM, Miller JL, et al. Morbidity of total pancreatectomy with islet cell auto-transplantation compared to total pancreatectomy alone. HPB. 2014;16:522–7.

18. Laje P, Adzick NS. Modified Puestow procedure for the management of chronic pancreatitis in children. J Ped Surg. 2013;48:2271–5.
19. Schmitt F, Le Henaff G, Piloquet H, et al. Hereditary pancreatitis in children: surgical implications with special regard to genetic background. J Ped Surg. 2009;44:2078–82.
20. Wilson GC, Ahmad SA, Schauer DP, et al. Cost-effectiveness of total pancreatectomy and islet cell autotransplantation for the treatment of minimal change pancreatitis. J Gastrointest Surg. 2015;19:46–55.
21. Georgiev G, Beltran del Rio M, Gruessner A, et al. Patient quality of life after autologous islet transplantation (AIT) for treatment of chronic pancreatitis: 53 patient series at the University of Arizona. Pancreatology. 2014;15:40–5.
22. Tai DS, Shen N, Szot GL, et al. Autologous islet transplantation with remote islet isolation after pancreas resection for chronic pancreatitis. JAMA Surg. 2014;150:118–24.
23. Morgan K, Owczarski SM, Borckardt J, et al. Pain control and quality of life after pancreatectomy with islet autotransplantation for chronic pancreatitis. J Gastrointest Surg. 2012;16:129–34.
24. Walsh RM, Aguilar-Saavedra JR, Lentz G, et al. Improved quality of life following total pancreatectomy and autoislet transplantation for chronic pancreatitis. J Gastrointest Surg. 2012;16:1469–77.

Chapter 45
Management of Blunt Pancreatic Trauma in Children

Grace Z. Mak

Abstract Pancreatic injury following blunt trauma in children is quite rare. Management of mild pancreatic injuries not involving the main duct is generally non-operative. However, the management of more severe injuries involving the main pancreatic duct is much more controversial with proponents for both non-operative as well as early operative intervention. Both treatment strategies have their advantages and disadvantages with no consistent findings allowing for a definitive best practice to be developed. While non-operative management generally leads to longer initial hospital stays and increased pseudocyst formation as well as multiple endoscopic or less invasive procedures, the child avoids a major abdominal operation and pancreatic resection. Operative management, on the other hand, generally leads to decreased hospital stay and quicker return to normal function but involves the inherent risks of a major abdominal surgery, long-term consequences of pancreatic resection and possible splenectomy, as well as increased incidence of pancreatic leak or fistulas. Furthermore, there have been no reported long-term differences between the two strategies. Due to the rarity of children with pancreatic duct injuries following blunt trauma, there have thus far been no randomized controlled studies comparing the two treatment modalities. The literature consists of only retrospective reviews making a strong recommendation for best practice impossible. Thus, both are viable options for the treatment of pancreatic duct injuries.

Keywords Pediatric pancreatic injury • Blunt pancreatic injury • Pancreatic duct transection • Early operative management

---

G.Z. Mak, MD (✉)
Department of Surgery and Pediatrics, Pritzker School of Medicine,
The University of Chicago, 5841 S. Maryland Avenue, MC4062, A426,
Chicago, IL 60637, USA
e-mail: gmak@surgery.bsd.uchicago.edu

J.M. Millis, J.B. Matthews (eds.), *Difficult Decisions in Hepatobiliary and Pancreatic Surgery*, Difficult Decisions in Surgery: An Evidence-Based Approach, DOI 10.1007/978-3-319-27365-5_45

Introduction

Blunt abdominal trauma in children is unfortunately quite common and can be due to motor vehicle collisions, pedestrian struck by car, bicycle accidents, falls, assault, all-terrain vehicle crashes, sports related injuries as well as nonaccidental trauma. The pancreas is the fourth most common solid organ injured in blunt trauma, occurring in 3–12 % of blunt traumas. Injury most commonly occurs at the junction between the neck and body of the pancreas where the pancreas directly overlies the vertebral body causing transection of the pancreatic parenchyma (grade 2) possibly including the pancreatic duct (grade 3) [1, 2]. Due to its retroperitoneal location, the nonspecific signs and symptoms following injury, as well as the poor sensitivity on common imaging modalities, diagnosis of pancreatic injury can be quite challenging. Many trauma centers utilize screening amylase and lipase upon admission though these values may be normal initially. Initial CT abdomen/pelvis may not show injury to the pancreas as abnormal findings often evolve with time as the edema increases the visualization of injury [1, 3]. Thus, one must maintain a high index of suspicion for pancreatic injury in settings of worsening epigastric pain, particularly following handlebar injuries from bicycle accidents. These patients should have repeat amylase and lipase levels drawn and may require repeat imaging.

Pancreatic injuries can be mild (grade 1 or 2) not involving the main pancreatic duct or severe/significant (grade 3 or 4) involving injury or transection of the main pancreatic duct. Most surgeons agree that mild injuries should be treated conservatively with NPO and pain control until the pain and hyperamylesemia resolve. There have been minimal complications reported with this treatment [1]. Severe injuries to the pancreatic duct, however, have been the source of significant debate particularly with the advent of endoscopic and minimally invasive treatment modalities. Multiple literature reviews, case reports, and retrospective reviews have been performed with no consistent findings reported such that both operative and nonoperative treatment approaches have been utilized [1, 4]. Overall mortality from pancreatic injury is rare unless associated with other significant injuries including head trauma, sepsis, and multiple organ injuries.

With the current ability to perform high quality MRCP as well as ERCP in the pediatric population, pancreatic injuries are being diagnosed with more accuracy following injury with the option to treat non-operatively with possible endoscopic intervention versus early operative management [5–7]. Historically, patients with distal pancreatic duct injuries have undergone distal pancreatectomy with sparing of the spleen. Proximal duct injuries have been more complicated being treated with enteric-pancreatic bypasses. Interventional radiology has also evolved such that pseudocysts and other intra-abdominal fluid collections can now be drained in a more minimally invasive fashion further allowing patients to be treated in a non-operative fashion. With these technological advances, and as more and more solid organ injuries have been treated non-operatively, the question of best practice regarding severe pancreatic injury treatment has been the source of heated debate and controversy.

Due to the small incidence of blunt pancreatic trauma in the pediatric population as well as the acute nature of the injury, it has been difficult to perform large randomized controlled studies. No randomized controlled trials were found comparing early operative intervention with non-operative therapy [1].Only retrospective reviews have been published and most have been small patient groups. In all these reviews, the outcomes measured include time to recovery (length of hospital stay, time to full feeds, time to return to normal activities), need for reintervention (repeat ERCP, surgery, or other interventions), and major morbidity (the development of complications including pseudocysts, pancreatic leak or fistula, infection, hospital readmissions) (Table 45.2). The long term complications from either an operative or non-operative approach rarely occur including significant chronic endocrine or exocrine dysfunction despite severe pancreatic injuries [1].

Search Strategy

Literature search of English language publications was performed extending from 1997 to 2014 with the greatest concentration from 2004 to 2014 to identify published data on the treatment of pancreatic injury following blunt trauma in children utilizing the PICO outline shown in Table 45.1. The following databases were searched: PubMed, SUM search, and Cochrane Evidence Based Medicine.

Search words included "blunt pancreatic trauma children", "pediatric pancreatic duct transection", "management blunt pancreatic trauma children", "management blunt pancreatic trauma," "pediatric pancreatic injury," "pediatric pancreatic duct injury", and "pediatric pancreatic trauma."

Articles not specifically addressing the treatment of pancreatic injury following blunt abdominal trauma as well as those not specifically discussing the management of children less than 18 years of age were excluded.

No randomized control trials were found. Four retrospective cohort studies, 1 systematic review, 12 retrospective reviews, 3 multi-institutional retrospective reviews, and 1 review article were included in the analysis. The data was classified using the GRADE system.

Results

Once a severe pancreatic injury is identified, it is important to classify the location of the injury within the pancreatic duct as well as the degree of injury to the duct. Based upon these parameters as well as the timing from injury to diagnosis and the

Table 45.1 PICO table for treatment of blunt pancreatic trauma in children

P (Patients)	I (Intervention)	C (Comparator Group)	O (Outcomes measured)
Children with significant pancreatic injury following blunt trauma	Early surgical therapy	Non-operative or endoscopic management	Time to recovery, need for reintervention, significant morbidity

degree of surrounding inflammation, a decision will need to be made regarding early operative intervention versus non-operative or endoscopic treatment. Most surgeons generally agree that operative intervention is indicated for patients with worsening clinical status, signs of peritonitis, or development of hemodynamic instability. Thus, late operative intervention is not included in the evaluation of operative versus non-operative treatment algorithms. Additionally, there have been reports that late operative intervention has increased risk of complications/post-operative morbidity including the development of pancreatic fistulas, other abdominal injuries during surgery, and a long recovery due to intra-abdominal adhesions and leakage of pancreatic enzymes within the abdominal cavity [1, 8]. However, the true consequences of this delay remain unclear [1, 9]. Thus, we will only compare early operative intervention to non-operative/endoscopic management.

Early operative intervention can involve wide surgical drainage, distal pancreatectomy (splenic sparing if possible), or enteric-pancreatic bypass for more proximal injuries such as Roux-en-Y pancreaticojejunostomy and rarely pancreaticoduodenectomy (whipple procedure) [1, 8, 10]. Most commonly, splenic-preserving distal pancreatectomy is performed as the location of injury is generally in the distal duct. Reported advantages include less recovery time with quicker return to normal activities, less repeat interventions required, and decreased overall morbidity with less secondary complications (pseudocyst development, TPN complications) [1, 8, 11–14]. Reported disadvantages include the requirement of surgical intervention with partial pancreatectomy, and possibly splenectomy including the infectious complications involved with OPSS. Post-operatively, these patients can have complications including pseudocyst, infection, pneumonia, sepsis, development of pancreatic leak or fistula. Additionally, the long-term consequences of partial pancreatectomy for children are largely unknown [1, 2].

Non-operative treatment entails initial treatment with NPO and TPN until the pancreatitis has resolved followed by the initiation of oral feeds. If the child is not able to tolerate oral feeds and develops pancreatitis, post-pyloric feeds are started. Surgery is reserved only for those patients who clinically deteriorate or become hemodynamically unstable [1]. Treatment can include endoscopic interventions such as ERCP with sphincterotomy and/or stent placement as well as drainage of fluid collections or pseudocysts under radiologic guidance [1, 6, 7]. Advantages of this treatment strategy include avoiding a major surgical procedure with pancreatic resection and possible splenectomy including the post-operative morbidity and complications. Disadvantages include the often prolonged hospital stay, need for multiple procedures and anesthetics, longer time until return to normal activity, and possible increased incidence of complications including post-ERCP pancreatitis, pancreatic pseudocysts with or without infection, pancreatic duct stricture following stent placement, TPN cholestasis, and line infections [1, 15–19]. There have been isolated reports of atrophy of the distal pancreas following non-operative management of pancreatic duct transections as well [20]. Recently, a group in Japan described the successful technique of delayed reconstruction of the pancreatic duct 6–8 weeks following the initial injury [21].

Table 45.2 Comparison of studies of operative and non-operative treatment for severe pancreatic injuries

Operative resection						Non-Operative resection					
Study	Patients	Pseudocyst formation	Pancreatic fistula or leak	Overall morbidity	Length of hospital stay	Patients	Pseudocyst formation	Pancreatic fistula or leak	Overall morbidity	Length of hospital stay	Quality of evidence
Iqbal et al. [2]	57	0[a]	7 %[a]	32 %	11.9±1	95	18 %[a]	0[a]	27 %	13.4±1.3	Retrospective cohort (low)
Beres [13]	15 (3 drainage only)	0[a]	2	4[a]	15.1±8.4[a]	24	13[a]	1	17[a]	27.5±19.8[a]	Retrospective cohort (low)
Paul [4]	20	3[a]	2	Not reported	16±13.4	23	8[a]	0	Not reported	14.2±12.8	Retrospective cohort (low)
Wood [11]	14	21 %[a]		Not reported	13	11	73 %[a]		Not reported	17	Retrospective cohort (low)
de Blaauw [15]	3	2	Not reported	Not reported	29	31	14	Not reported	Not reported	24	Retrospective cohort (low)
Mattix [12]	23	3	0	Not reported	9.7±8.4	27	6	Not reported	Not reported	13.8±10.1	Retrospective cohort (low)

[a]Statistically significant between the two groups

In the most recent multi-institutional review by Igbal, nonoperative treatment resulted in higher incidence of pseudocysts with 45 % requiring operative intervention for definitive treatment and overall increased morbidity with increased need for repeat interventions. However, this group had less pancreatic leaks compared to the operative group. Time to initial and full feeds was less in the operative group as was the time to complete resolution of pancreatic injury (defined as complete resolution of abdominal pain, full feeds, and discharge from follow-up). However, there was no significant difference in the initial length of hospitalization or rate of hospital readmission between the operative and non-operative treatment groups. Of note, in comparing operative drainage to resection, those patients treated by operative drainage alone had similar clinical courses as the nonoperative management group but even longer time until full feeds, hospitalization, and full recovery. When the patients were further analyzed comparing operative and non-operative treatment for patients specifically with grade 3 injuries, those patients treated with operative resection had less time to full feeds as well as decreased length of initial hospitalization [2].

Due to the rarity of severe pancreatic injuries from blunt trauma in children, there have been no randomized controlled studies evaluating early operative versus non-operative treatment. The only data available include retrospective reviews and patient reports with all but three reviews reporting on single center experiences. This makes it near to impossible to objectively conclude anything definitive about the best treatment for children with severe pancreatic injuries. Thus, we can only offer recommendations based upon the reported experience.

Recommendations

The most important consideration is the severity of injury and involvement of the pancreatic duct. For injuries not involving the pancreatic duct, general consensus is to treat these patients non-operatively. This has been further supported in the literature though the distinction between grade 2 and 3 injuries is not often well defined.

The clinical treatment of patients with pancreatic injuries involving the pancreatic duct remains controversial as the literature contains only patient reports and retrospective reviews with an overall low volume of reported cases. Additionally, given the overall low incidence of long-term complications with either early operative or non-operative treatment, the differences between the two operative strategies are less clinically relevant. The bottom line is that the decision can be made based on surgeon preference according to the complications/ramifications the surgeon and family are willing to accept.

For early operative treatment, you accept that the child will require a major abdominal operation with partial pancreatectomy and possibly splenectomy with the associated post-operative morbidity and complications. But, you also accept that the child will generally have a decreased length of stay and quicker return to normal activity. For non-operative treatment, you accept that the child will likely stay in the hospital longer with increased likelihood of developing pancreatic pseudocysts and requiring at least a few endoscopic/interventional radiologic procedures, but without the more morbid major abdominal operation retaining their pancreas and spleen. Additionally, there seems to be no utility in operative drainage since the outcomes are similar if not worse than the non-operative group. Drainage alone should be performed in as minimally invasive means as possible, i.e. under radiologic guidance rather than through an open procedure.

The definition of "early" operative intervention should not be based purely upon the time from injury to diagnosis as this may not be known with certainty particularly in cases of nonaccidental trauma. Rather, the distinction between "early" versus "late" should be based upon the degree of inflammation present which can lead to increased intra-operative complications including damage to surrounding structures, increased difficulty with the surgery as well as post-operative complications including development of pancreatic fistulas, ileus and pneumonia. Thus, the definition of "early" intervention should incorporate both time from injury to diagnosis as well as degree of inflammation seen on imaging.

A Personal View of the Data

The treatment plan should be individually based upon the child's specific pancreatic injury, associated injuries, and other comorbidities. Based upon the clinical history, imaging and the degree of surrounding inflammation as well as the child's clinical status, the surgeon can determine whether to proceed with early operative intervention or the non-operative approach. Again, as long as both the surgeon and the family understand the ramifications of both approaches and the inherent complications associated with each, either approach will ultimately treat the patient with little long-term consequences. Thus, there should be no set timeline to define "early" intervention. A decision should be made on an individual basis for each child. Personally, if there is minimal surrounding inflammation with a prompt diagnosis of transection of the pancreatic duct, I would favor splenic-preserving distal pancreatectomy. However, if there is surrounding inflammation, unclear diagnosis of pancreatic duct injury, or other clinically significant injuries or comorbidities, I would favor non-operative management.

Ultimately, a consortium capable of developing and implementing a randomized control trial to determine the best practice for this type of injury would be extremely helpful though the resources required are not insignificant. Perhaps, it could be a part of a larger blunt abdominal trauma study. Additionally, it will be extremely important to appropriately define the severe pancreatic injuries being studied, specifically differentiating grade 3 and 4 injuries. Treatment strategies should include non-operative with and without ERCP stent placement in addition to operative pancreatic resection. It would also be imperative to include the long-term follow-up of these patients specifically evaluating pancreatic exocrine and endocrine function.

Recommendations

- Following blunt trauma in children with mild pancreatic injury (grade 1 or 2) not involving injury or transection of the main pancreatic duct, non-operative management is indicated (evidence quality low; strong recommendation)
- Following blunt trauma in children with significant pancreatic injury involving injury or transection of the main pancreatic duct (grade 3 or 4), both nonoperative and early operative intervention are acceptable. (evidence quality low; weak recommendation)
- The definition of "early" intervention should incorporate both time from injury to diagnosis as well as degree of inflammation seen on imaging. (evidence quality low; weak recommendation)

References

1. Haugaard MV, Wettergren A, Hillingsø JG, Gluud C, Penninga L. Non-operative versus operative treatment for blunt pancreatic trauma in children. Cochrane Database Syst Rev. 2014 Feb 12;2.
2. Iqbal CW, St Peter SD, Tsao K, Cullinane DC, Gourlay DM, Ponsky TA, Wulkan ML, Adibe OO, Pancreatic Trauma in Children (PATCH) Study Group. Operative vs nonoperative management for blunt pancreatic transection in children: multi-institutional outcomes. J Am Coll Surg. 2014;218(2):157–62.
3. Maeda K, Ono S, Baba K, Kawahara I. Management of blunt pancreatic trauma in children. Pediatr Surg Int. 2013;29:1019–22.
4. Paul MD, Mooney DP. The management of pancreatic injuries in children: operate or observe. J Pediatr Surg. 2011;46:1140–3.
5. Houben CH, Ade-Ajayi N, Patel S, Kane P, Karani J, Devlin J, Harrison P, Davenport M. Traumatic pancreatic duct injury in children: minimally invasive approach to management. J Pediatr Surg. 2007;42:629–35.
6. Canty TG, Weinman D. Treatment of pancreatic duct disruption in children by an endoscopically placed stent. J Pediatr Surg. 2001;36(2):345–8.
7. Canty TG, Weinman D. Management of major pancreatic duct injuries in children. J Trauma. 2001;50(6):1001–7.
8. Meier DE, Coln CD, Hicks BA, Guzzetta PC. Early operation in children with pancreas transection. J Pediatr Surg. 2001;36(2):341–4.
9. Nadler EP, Gardner M, Schall L, Lynch J, Ford H. Management of blunt pancreatic injury in children. J Trauma: Inj Infect Crit Care. 1999;47(6):1098.
10. Thomas H, Madanur M, Bartlett A, Marangoni G, Heaton N, Rela M. Pancreatic trauma – 12-year experience from a tertiary center. Pancreas. 2009;38(2):113–6.
11. Wood JH, Patrick DA, Bruny JL, Sauaia A, Moulton SL. Operative vs nonoperative management of blunt pancreatic trauma in children. J Pediatr Surg. 2010;45:401–6.
12. Mattix KD, Tataria M, Holmes J, Kristoffersen K, Brown R, Groner J, Scaife E, Mooney D, Nance M, Scherer L. Pediatric pancreatic trauma: predictors of nonoperative management failure and associated outcomes. J Pediatr Surg. 2007;42(2):340–4.
13. Beres AL, Wales PW, Christison-Lagay ER, McClure ME, Fallat ME, Brindle ME. Non-operative management of high-grade pancreatic trauma: is it worth the wait? J Pediatr Surg. 2013;48:1060–4.

14. Snajdauf J, Rygl M, Kalousová J, Kucera A, Petrů O, Pýcha K, Mixa V, Keil R, Hríbal Z. Surgical management of major pancreatic injury in children. Eur J Pediatr Surg. 2007;17(5):317–21.
15. de Blaauw I, Winkelhorst JT, Rieu PN, van der Staak FH, Wijnen MH, Severijnen RS, van Vugt AB, Wijnen RM. Pancreatic injury in children: good outcome of nonoperative treatment. J Pediatr Surg. 2008;43(9):1640–3.
16. Abbo O, Lemandat A, Reina N, Bouali O, Ballouhey Q, Carfagna L, Lemasson F, Harper L, Sauvat F, Galinier P. Conservative management of blunt pancreatic trauma in children: a single center experience. Eur J Pediatr Surg. 2013;23(6):470–3.
17. Cigdem MK, Senturk S, Onen A, Siga M, Akay H, Otcu S. Nonoperative management of pancreatic injuries in pediatric patients. Surg Today. 2011;41(5):655–9.
18. Jurić I, Pogorelić Z, Biocić M, Todorić D, Furlan D, Susnjar T. Management of blunt pancreatic trauma in children. Surg Today. 2009;39(2):115–9.
19. Clark W, Paidas CN, Germain D, Guidi C, Pinkas H, Kayton ML. Delayed presentation of complete pancreatic ductal transection in children: management of two cases without resection. Pediatr Surg Int. 2013;29:401–5.
20. Klin B, Abu-Kishk I, Jeroukhimov I, Efrati Y, Kozer E, Broide E, Brachman Y, Copel L, Scapa E, Eshel G, Lotan G. Blunt pancreatic trauma in children. Surg Today. 2011;41(7):946–54.
21. Kawahara I, Maeda K, Ono S, Kawashima H, Deie R, Yanagisawa S, Baba K, Usui Y, Tsuji Y, Fukuta A, Sekine S. Surgical reconstruction and endoscopic pancreatic stent for traumatic pancreatic duct disruption. Pediatr Surg Int. 2014;30:951–6.

Chapter 46
Surgery or Surveillance for Asymptomatic Small Mucinous Pancreatic Head Cyst

J. Camilo Barreto and Mitchell C. Posner

Abstract Mucinous pancreatic cysts are now common incidental findings with the increased use and higher resolution of modern cross-sectional imaging, and surgeons are faced with the challenge of identifying those patients with premalignant or malignant lesions from those lesions with little chance of ever impacting patient survival. The risks of selecting to observe mucinous cystic lesions should be balanced against the morbidity and mortality of pancreatic resection, particularly when located in the head of the pancreas. Currently, the criteria for resection are based mainly on morphologic features or abnormal cytological findings. Most of the controversy revolves around the management of small branch-duct IPMN, given its relatively low malignant potential, high prevalence in older patients, and tendency to appear in the head of the gland. Thick/enhanced cyst wall, dilation of the pancreatic duct and mural nodules are consistent predictors of malignancy, while size alone remains controversial and a subject for continued debate.

Keywords IPMN • Mucinous • Cancer • Pancreaticoduodenectomy • Mortality

Introduction

The current widespread use of cross-sectional imaging has significantly increased the detection of small and often asymptomatic pancreatic lesions. In particular, pancreatic cystic lesions continue to represent a clinical challenge, and the

J.C. Barreto
Section of General Surgery, University of Chicago Medicine, Chicago, IL, USA

M.C. Posner (✉)
Section of General Surgery and Surgical Oncology, University of Chicago Medicine, 5841 S. Maryland Ave Room G209, MC 5094, Chicago, IL 60637, USA
e-mail: mposner@surgery.bsd.uchicago.edu

J.M. Millis, J.B. Matthews (eds.), *Difficult Decisions in Hepatobiliary and Pancreatic Surgery*, Difficult Decisions in Surgery: An Evidence-Based Approach, DOI 10.1007/978-3-319-27365-5_46

decision-making process that guides treatment of an asymptomatic cyst is focused on identification of those cysts with malignant potential or already harboring a malignancy. Among neoplastic lesions, there is a considerable spectrum of entities that range from benign (serous cystadenoma), dysplastic or premalignant (mucinous lesions) to frankly malignant (cystadenocarcinoma) [1]. The two main variants of mucinous lesions are mucinous cystic neoplasms (MCN) and intraductal papillary mucinous neoplasms (IPMN). The former are rare, they occur predominantly in perimenopausal women, have a characteristic ovarian-like stroma, and tend to arise in the body or tail of the pancreas [1, 2]. The focus of this chapter will be on IPMN, the most common neoplastic cystic lesion of the pancreas. These cysts can originate from either the main pancreatic duct (main-duct type), from secondary branches (branch-duct type) or from both (mixed variant). Main-duct IPMN has a higher incidence of invasive carcinoma, as will be discussed below. IPMN are more commonly located in the head of the pancreas, but can be multifocal in 30 % of cases, and can diffusely involve the entire gland in 5 % of cases. The full diagnostic approach to these lesions is beyond the scope of this chapter, but initially involves cross-sectional imaging in the form of CT scan or magnetic resonance imaging with cholangio-pancreatography (MRI/MRCP). Endoscopic ultrasound (EUS) with fine needle aspiration (FNA) is an invasive test but is often a critical tool to obtain fluid and tissue samples for cytological analysis and tumor markers. High levels of carcinoembryonic antigen (CEA) correlate with the presence of a mucinous neoplasm, but not with invasive carcinoma [3]. Despite these advanced imaging modalities, the definitive diagnosis frequently remains elusive, and clinical judgment is paramount to decide if the operative risks of a pancreaticoduodenectomy justify treating what may represent an indolent lesion. In this chapter, the evidence for current recommendations for treatment will be reviewed.

Search Strategy

A literature search of English language publications was used to identify data on risk of cancer in the presence of mucinous pancreatic head cysts (Table 46.1).

Table 46.1 PICO table for surgery or surveillance for asymptomatic small mucinous pancreatic head cysts

P (patients)	I (intervention)	C (comparator group)	O (outcomes measured)
Patients with small asymptomatic mucinous pancreatic head cyst	Resection	Observation	Cancer risk

Risk of Cancer Associated Mucinous Pancreatic Head Cysts

Main-Duct or Mixed Variant IPMN

The risk of malignancy, either invasive or non-invasive (in situ), in main duct IPMN ranges from 60 % to 90 %; in mixed variant the risk is similar at 60 %, with about two thirds found to be invasive [4–12]. Many studies have attempted to identify the critical variables associated with malignancy in main duct or mixed variant IPMN, including duct diameter or mural nodules. As expected, older or symptomatic patients had a higher risk of cancer; however, 29 % of patients with malignant main duct IPMN were asymptomatic [12]. Furthermore, there is evidence of a natural history of progression from benign to malignant histology IPMN [13]. Resected non-invasive lesions have an excellent survival, whereas lesions associated with carcinoma have a 5-year survival between 36 and 60 % [9, 11, 12, 14]. Therefore, the general expert consensus and current guidelines recommend resection of all main-duct and mixed variant IPMN in patients with acceptable surgical risk.

Branch-Duct IPMN

The risk of malignancy in branch-duct IPMN has been reported in the range of 6–46 %, with a mean of 25 %, [4–11] and management of these lesions, especially those less than 3 cm, remains highly controversial. International consensus guidelines for the management of mucinous neoplasms have been published. The collated results from seven previous series [4–11] specifically addressing risk of malignancy in IPMN have, during a consensus meeting in Sendai, Japan, produced currently accepted guidelines for resection based on identified high-risk criteria for malignancy [15]. Matsumoto et al. found no malignancy in a cohort of 57 patients, with lesions less than 30 mm in diameter without mural nodules. Most of these patients were asymptomatic, and had no progression during a mean follow-up of 33 months [7]. Sugiyama et al. found on multivariate analysis of 62 patients, that size greater than 30 mm and mural nodules were the strongest malignancy predictors in branch duct IPMN [10]. Retrospective studies utilizing the Sendai guidelines applied to surgically resected branch-duct IPMN demonstrated a high negative predictive value (meaning no cancers were missed), but a low positive predictive value (approximately 20 % of specimens found with cancer) [16–18]. The same consensus group updated their guidelines more recently in Fukuoka, Japan in 2012 [19]. They defined worrisome features as cyst size larger than 3 cm, thickened/enhanced cyst wall, pancreatic duct size of 5–9 mm, non-enhancing mural nodules, abrupt change in pancreatic duct caliber with distal pancreatic atrophy, and lymphadenopathy. In addition they described high risk stigmata that should prompt resection without further testing: obstructive jaundice with a cystic lesion in the pancreatic head, enhanced solid component, or pancreatic duct size equal or larger than 10 mm. They described a mean frequency of malignancy in branch-duct IPMN of 25 %, (and invasive malignancy of 17.7 %). But since IPMN tend to present in elderly patients, and data published after the first guidelines [20, 21] suggested an annual risk of malignancy of 2–3 % in branch-duct IPMN, the consensus group concluded that conservative management and follow up was supported in the absence of high-risk features for cancer. Therefore, in the 2012 guidelines, cyst size alone was de-emphasized and deemed a weaker risk factor compared to high-risk cytology or mural nodules. It was therefore recommended to consider observation as a reasonable option in lesions greater than 3 cm with no other risk factors. At the same time, a smaller size (2 cm) was suggested as the threshold for resection in younger, healthier patients [22].

However, recent publications have challenged the conclusion of observing branch-duct IPMN, even for smaller lesions. In a report from the University of Heidelberg [23], investigators described their experience in resected IPMN, and found that among branch-duct lesions smaller than 3 cm and with no malignant features according to the Sendai guidelines, 24.6 % had invasive carcinoma or carcinoma in situ upon histological examination. They concluded that cyst size is not a valid parameter to distinguish benign from malignant lesions and that resection should be considered, in principle, for all patients with branch-duct IPMN, although taking into account other factors like age, comorbidities and willingness to undergo follow-up studies. The reason for the higher incidence of carcinoma in their cohort is unclear, but it could be related to the inclusion of concomitant ductal adenocarcinomas not derived from IPMN, or different patient populations. In another report from Wong et al. at Moffitt Cancer Center [24], invasive carcinoma or carcinoma in situ was found in 60 % of patients with branch-duct IPMN smaller than 3 cm. However, the majority of patients in this cohort had either symptoms or concerning endosonographic morphologic features, which are typically associated with increased malignancy rates.

Adding to the evidence for more aggressive treatment in larger cysts, a recent meta-analysis [25] found that cyst size greater than 3 cm is substantially associated with increased risk of malignancy, with an odds ratio of 62, and size was the strongest predictor of malignancy in a multivariate analysis that included other factors like mural nodules, pancreatic duct size, and symptoms. This meta-analysis has the limitations of the individual studies it was based upon, with many of them being retrospective or flawed by selection bias.

Sahora et al. recently described their single institution experience with a cohort of 563 patients, aiming to address the controversy of size as criteria for resection of branch-duct IPMN, in the absence of worrisome features. They retrospectively reviewed their database of patients for high-risk stigmata and worrisome features according to the 2012 revised guidelines. In their entire cohort, they found invasive cancer arising in branch-duct IPMN in 4 % of cases, and an additional 3.7 % had or developed a distinct invasive ductal adenocarcinoma. The risk of high-grade dysplasia in lesions smaller than 3 cm with non-worrisome features was only 6.5 % with no invasive cancer found, in striking contrast with the Heidelberg report. If the threshold was increased to lesions greater than 3 cm, the high grade dysplasia incidence was 8.8 %, and one case of invasive cancer was found. Of note, most resected specimens where carcinoma was found had either high-risk stigmata or worrisome features in their preoperative work-up (76 % of carcinomas in situ and 95 % of invasive carcinomas) [26]. Importantly, no patient who underwent regular follow-up developed progression to unresectable carcinoma, nor were there any deaths from progressive cancer after undergoing resection for branch-duct IPMN initially under surveillance. They concluded that the old Sendai guidelines are adequate for selecting patients with incidental branch-duct IPMN for resection, and that eliminating the size threshold of 3 cm (as the new guidelines suggested), would double the rate of missed cases with high grade dysplasia [26].

Operative mortality in high volume centers after pancreaticoduodenectomy can be as low as 2 %, while in low volume centers is between 8 and 15 % [27, 28]. This risk should be factored in the decision making regarding resection for patients with IPMN. If a patient's risk of mortality from pancreaticoduodenectomy approaches the risk of premalignant or malignant pathology then the role of resection must be questioned since the potential benefit is outweighed by the inherent risk of intervening surgically.

Mucinous Cystic Neoplasm

Mucinous cystic neoplasms (MCN) occasionally present in the head of the pancreas, although as described above, the vast majority occur in the body and tail of the pancreas in relatively young women. The prevalence of invasive carcinoma is lower compared to IPMN, less than 15 %. Due to its higher frequency in younger patients, which translates to a higher lifetime risk of malignancy, resection is recommended in all fit surgical candidates. However, findings of malignancy are rare in MCNs smaller than 4 cm [2, 29] and as is the case with IPMN, observation may be reasonable in elderly or frail patients [29].

Recommendations

- For patients with main-duct IPMN, regardless of size, the risk of cancer is 60–90 %, and we recommend resection (pancreaticoduodenectomy) in all acceptable surgical candidates. (Evidence quality high, strong recommendation)
- For patients with small asymptomatic branch-duct IPMN (less than 3 cm), we recommend resection in the presence of mural nodules or suspicious or positive cytology in acceptable surgical candidates. We also recommend resection of branch-duct IPMN larger than 3 cm. (Evidence quality moderate, strong recommendation).

- MCN tends to present in young patients with long life expectancy, we therefore recommend resection in all surgical candidates. Observation can be considered in frail or elderly patients, especially with tumors smaller than 4 cm with no mural nodules. (Evidence quality moderate, weak recommendation)
- Patients with small branch-duct IPMN not undergoing resection and who are appropriate surgical candidates should undergo long term surveillance. The modality of choice is MRI/MRCP or CT scan. The optimal timing has not been well defined, but we recommend every 3–6 months, and then annually if stable. (Evidence quality low, weak recommendation)

References

1. Brugge WR, Lauwers GY, Sahani D, et al. Cystic neoplasms of the pancreas. N Engl J Med. 2004;351:1218–26.
2. Crippa S, Salvia R, Warshaw AL, et al. Mucinous cystic neoplasm of the pancreas is not an aggressive entity. Lessons from 163 resected patients. Ann Surg. 2008;247:571–9.
3. Nagula S, Kennedy T, Schattner MA, et al. Evaluation of cyst fluid CEA analysis in the diagnosis of mucinous cysts of the pancreas. J Gastrointest Surg. 2010;14:1997–2003.
4. Kobari M, Egawa S, Shibuya K, et al. Intraductal papillary mucinous tumors of the pancreas comprise 2 clinical subtypes: differences in clinical characteristics and surgical management. Arch Surg. 1999;134:1131–6.
5. Torris B, Ponsot P, Paye F, et al. Intraductal papillary mucinous tumors of the pancreas confined to secondary ducts show less aggressive pathologic features as compared with those involving the main pancreatic duct. Am J Surg Pathol. 2000;24:1372–7.
6. Doi R, Fujimoto K, Wada M, et al. Surgical management of intraductal papillary mucinous tumor of the pancreas. Surgery. 2002;132:80–5.
7. Matsumoto T, Aramaki M, Yada K, et al. Optimal management of the branch duct type intraductal papillary mucinous neoplasm of the pancreas. J Clin Gastroenterol. 2003;36:261–5.
8. Choi BS, Kim TK, Kim AY, et al. Differential diagnosis of benign and malignant intraductal papillary mucinous tumors of the pancreas: MR cholangio-pancreatography and MR angiography. Korean J Radiol. 2003;4:157–62.
9. Kitagawa Y, Unger TA, Taylor S, et al. Mucus is a predictor of better prognosis and survival in patients with intraductal papillary mucinous tumor of the pancreas. J Gastrointest Surg. 2003;7:12–9.
10. Sugiyama M, Izumisato Y, Abe N. Predictive factors for malignancy in intraductal papillary-mucinous tumors of the pancreas. Br J Surg. 2003;90:1244–9.
11. Sohn TA, Yeo CJ, Cameron JL, et al. Intraductal papillary mucinous neoplasms of the pancreas: an updated experience. Ann Surg. 2004;239:788–99.
12. Salvia R, Fernandez-del Castillo C, Basi C, et al. Main duct intraductal papillary mucinous neoplasms of the pancreas: clinical predictors of malignancy and long-term survival following resection. Ann Surg. 2004;239:678–87.
13. Wada K, Takada T, Yasuda H, et al. Does "clonal progression" relate to the development of intraductal papillary mucinous tumors of the pancreas? J Gastrointest Surg. 2004;8:289–96.
14. Chari S, Yadav D, Smyrk TC, et al. Study of recurrence after surgical resection of intraductal papillary mucinous neoplasm of the pancreas. Gastroenterology. 2002;123:1500–7.
15. Tanaka M, Chari S, Adsay V, et al. International consensus guidelines for management of intraductal papillary mucinous neoplasms and mucinous cystic neoplasms of the pancreas. Pancreatology. 2006;6:17–32.

16. Pelaez-Luna M, Chari ST, Smyrk TC, et al. Do consensus indications for resection in branch duct intraductal papillary mucinous neoplasm predict malignancy? A study of 147 patients. Am J Gastroenterol. 2007;102:1759–64.
17. Tang RS, Weinberg B, Dawson DW, et al. Evaluation of the guidelines for management of pancreatic branch-duct intraductal papillary mucinous neoplasm. Clin Gastroenterol Hepatol. 2008;6:815–9.
18. Nagai K, Doi R, Ito T, et al. Single-institution validation of the international consensus-guidelines for treatment of branch duct intraductal papillary mucinous neoplasms of the pancreas. J Hepatobiliary Pancreat Surg. 2009;16:353–8.
19. Tanaka M, Fernandez-del Castillo C, Adsay V, et al. International consensus guidelines 2012 for the management of intraductal papillary mucinous neoplasms and mucinous cystic neoplasms of the pancreas. Pancreatology. 2012;12:183–97.
20. Kang MJ, Jang JY, Kim SJ, et al. Cyst growth rate predicts malignancy in patients with branch duct intraductal papillary mucinous neoplasms. Clin Gastroenterol Hepatol. 2011;9:87–93.
21. Levy P, Jouannaud V, O'Toole D, et al. Natural history of intraductal papillary mucinous tumors of the pancreas: actuarial risk of malignancy. Clin Gastroenterol Hepatol. 2006;4:460–8.
22. Weinberg BM, Spiegel BM, Tomlinson JS, Farrell JJ. Asymptomatic pancreatic cystic neoplasms: maximizing survival and quality of life using Markov-based clinical nomograms. Gastroenterology. 2010;138:531–40.
23. Fritz S, Klauss M, Bergmann F, et al. Small (Sendai negative) branch-duct intraductal papillary mucinous neoplasms. Not harmless. Ann Surg. 2012;256:313–20.
24. Wong J, Weber J, Centeno BA, et al. High-grade dysplasia and adenocarcinoma are frequent in side-branch intraductal papillary mucinous neoplasm measuring less than 3 cm on endoscopic ultrasound. J Gastrointest Surg. 2012;17:78–85.
25. Anand NJ, Sampath K, Wu BU. Cyst features and risk of malignancy in intraductal papillary mucinous neoplasms of the pancreas: a meta-analysis. Clin Gastroenterol Hepatol. 2013;11:913–21.
26. Sahora K, Mino-Kenudson M, Brugge W, et al. Branch duct intraductal papillary mucinous neoplasms. Does cyst size change the tip of the scale? A critical analysis of the revised International Consensus Guidelines in a large single-institutional series. Ann Surg. 2013;258:466–75.
27. Yeo CJ, Cameron JL, Sohn TA, et al. Six hundred fifty consecutive pancreaticoduodenectomies in the 1990s. Pathology, complications and outcomes. Ann Surg. 1997;226:248–60.
28. Fong Y, Gonen M, Rubin D, et al. Long-term survival is superior after resection for cancer in high-volume centers. Ann Surg. 2005;242:540–7.
29. Reddy RP, Smyrk TC, Zapiach M, et al. Pancreatic mucinous cystic neoplasm defined by ovarian stroma: demographics, clinical features, and prevalence of cancer. Clin Gastroenterol Hepatol. 2004;2:1026–31.

Chapter 47
Management of Asymptomatic IPMN in the Elderly

Kimberly M. Brown

Abstract Intraductal papillary mucinous neoplasm (IPMN) comprises a spectrum of mucin-producing cystic neoplasms of pancreatic ductal origin that range from benign adenoma to invasive carcinoma. The 2012 Updated Consensus Guidelines recommend resection of all main duct IPMN (MD-IPMN) with a main pancreatic duct diameter of ≥10 mm, and for branch duct IPMN (BD-IPMN) with high-risk stigmata. These broad categories include many patients who do not harbor an invasive carcinoma, and additional investigations such as cyst fluid analysis, pancreatic juice cytology or FNA of associated solid components may be employed to further characterize the malignant nature of an asymptomatic IPMN. There are limited data on the natural history of patients falling within resection criteria who do not undergo surgery, but the available studies suggest comparable disease-specific and overall survivals in older patients who are managed with observation/surveillance versus resection. Mortality for major pancreatic resection is 0–4 % in high-volume centers, and morbidity ranges from 16 % to 53 %, both of which are increased in patients >70 years old. Quality of life data extrapolated from non-IPMN post-pancreatectomy patients suggests that most domains return to preoperative levels within 3 months, and that malignancy is associated with poor quality of life at 2 years. Non-operative management of IPMN meeting resection criteria may be appropriate for select older patients based on co-morbidities or patient preference.

Keywords Intraductal papillary mucinous neoplasm • IPMN • Morbidity • Mortality • Survival • Overall survival • Disease-specific survival • Pancreatectomy • Quality of life

K.M. Brown (✉)
Department of Surgery, University of Texas Medical Branch,
301 University Blvd, Galveston, TX 77555-0737, USA
e-mail: kim.brown@utmb.edu

J.M. Millis, J.B. Matthews (eds.), *Difficult Decisions in Hepatobiliary and Pancreatic Surgery*, Difficult Decisions in Surgery: An Evidence-Based Approach, DOI 10.1007/978-3-319-27365-5_47

Introduction

The ideal management of intraductal papillary mucinous neoplasm (IPMN) would be to offer safe resection to all symptomatic patients, and to medically fit patients with either known malignant tumors, or tumors that will progress to malignancy before the patient succumbs to another cause. This would avoid unnecessary surgery in those patients with benign IPMN, or in patients with other conditions that will be the limiting factors for their survival. The barrier to this ideal management is a lack of preoperative factors that accurately predict malignancy and behavior for an individual patient.

Based on literature review and expert opinion, the latest clinical guidelines recommend resection in the surgically fit patient with any of the following: (1) symptomatic IPMN, (2) IPMN with main duct diameter ≥10 mm, comprising main-duct IPMN (MD-IMPN) and mixed-type IPMN (MT-IPMN), or (3) branch-duct IPMN (BD-IPMN) with high-risk stigmata (HRS), which include an enhancing solid component, main pancreatic duct (MPD) diameter ≥10 mm, or obstructive jaundice in a patient with a pancreatic head BD-IPMN [1]. The presence of "worrisome features" (WF) such as cyst of ≥3 cm, thickened, enhanced cyst walls, non-enhanced mural nodules, MPD diameter 5–9 mm, abrupt change in MPD caliber with distal pancreatic atrophy, and lymphadenopathy are an indication for further evaluation or close surveillance, but not necessarily immediate resection. Treatment in these cases may be tailored based on patient characteristics and preferences.

However, even among patients meeting criteria for resection based on these updated guidelines, there is an ongoing search for preoperative characteristics that more precisely predict prognosis for an individual patient, and it is clear that our understanding of this tumor is not yet mature. In particular, an older patient with an asymptomatic IPMN that falls within criteria for resection may be less likely to benefit from surgery, and preoperative counseling for such a patient requires thoughtful review of imperfect literature. This chapter reviews the existing evidence comparing surgical resection to observation/surveillance in older patients with asymptomatic IPMN that meet criteria for resection, focusing on the risk of having or developing a malignant IPMN, procedural morbidity and mortality, survival and quality of life.

Search Strategy

A search of literature of publications from 2004 to 2014 was performed to assess studies on IPMN in the setting of asymptomatic elderly patients using the PICO format (Table 47.1). The following databases were queried: PubMed, Trip Database, and Science Citation Index/Social sciences Citation Index. The terms used in the search were "IPMN, asymptomatic/observation/surveillance," "IPMN/natural history," "elderly"; "pancreatectomy/pancreas surgery/quality of life,"

Table 47.1 PICO table for asymptomatic IPMN in the elderly

P (patients)	I (intervention)	C (comparator group)	O (outcomes measured)
Older patients with IPMN meeting criteria for resection	Major pancreatic resection	Observation/ surveillance	Morbidity/mortality
Older patients with IPMN meeting criteria for resection	Major pancreatic resection	Observation/ surveillance	Cancer risk
Older patients with IPMN meeting criteria for resection	Major pancreatic resection	Observation/ surveillance	Quality of life
Older patients with IPMN meeting criteria for resection	Major pancreatic resection	Observation/ surveillance	Overall survival, disease-specific survival

"pancreatectomy/complications," "pancreatectomy/morbidity," AND "IPMN," "Elderly." Articles were excluded if observational/surveillance arms did not meet 2006 Sendai Consensus Criteria or revised Sendai criteria for surgical resection (also referred to as the Fukuoka Consensus Guidelines) by study completion. Twenty-two retrospective cohort studies, four prospective cohort studies, two guidelines, and one time-series study were included for analysis. The GRADE system was used to grade the quality of evidence.

Results

Cancer Risk

A summary of studies from 2003 to 2010 describing the proportion of resected IPMNs containing malignancy is found in the International Consensus Guidelines 2012 manuscript [1]. Table 47.2 summarizes the studies that met search criteria for this manuscript. From these reports, the overall risk of malignant and invasive IPMN is approximately 40 % and 31 %, respectively. Malignant tumors include high-grade dysplasia, which has previously been referred to as carcinoma-in-situ, as well as invasive tumors. However, when evaluated by tumor type, MD-IPMN has a greater risk of malignant (62 %) and invasive (43.6 %) tumors compared to BD-IPMN (24.4 % and 16.6 %, respectively) [1]. Mixed-type tumors (MT-IPMN) tend to behave like MD-IPMN, with a 57.6 % and 45.3 % risk of malignant and invasive disease. The presence of WF and HRS are associated with an increased rate of malignant disease (no criteria: 4.3 %, WF 27 %, HRS 42 %) in a review of 362 surgical cases [2]. While several publications since the 2012 guidelines have further confirmed the increased risk of malignant tumors in MD-IPMN (72–74 %) compared to BD-IPMN (22–47 %) [2–7], there are also reports of malignant disease in smaller BD-IPMN [8, 9], further emphasizing the need for more precise patient-specific predictors of malignancy. There are no large series looking specifically at the risk of malignancy in asymptomatic IPMN; in one small study of 16

Table 47.2 Cancer risk

Study	Patients	Outcome classification	Resection	Observation	Quality of evidence
Roch 2014 [2]	362 resected tumors	Cancer risk by 2012 ICG criteria for resection	No criteria (70): 4.3 %/4.3 %		Low
			WF (185): 27 %/16 %		
			HRS (85): 57 %/42 % (malignant/ invasive)		
Kawakubo 2014 [24]	59 resected tumors	Cancer risk	20/59 (34 %) invasive		Low
Salvia 2004 [17]	140 resected tumors; 38 asymptomatic	Cancer risk	Benign 57 (41 %)		Low
			Malignant 83 (59 %)		
Sahora 2013 [32]	226 BD-IPMN	Cancer Risk	23 (10.2 %) invasive		Low
			LGD 74 (33 %)		
			MGD 100 (44 %)		
			HGD 29 (13 %)		
Abdeljawad 2014 [3]	16 asymptomatic pts with pure main duct IPMN	Cancer risk	HGD or invasive cancer 25 %		Low
Sohn 2004 [18]	136 resected tumors	Cancer risk	Non-invasive 84 (62 %)		Low
			Invasive 52 (38 %)		
Roch 2014 [33]	70 mixed-type IPMN	Progression to invasive carcinoma		9 (12.9 %) at a median of 2.7 years	Moderate
Aso 2014 [4]	30 MD-IPMN, 70 BD-IPMN stratified by WF and HRS	Cancer risk	MD: 67 % malignant		Moderate
			BD: 40 % malignant; 24 %, 77 % and 100 % for BD-IPMN with 0, 1 and 2 HRS		
Shimizu 2013 [7]	310 IPMN	Cancer risk	Benign 150 (48 %)		Moderate
			Malignant 160 (52 %)		
Correa-Gallego 2013 [5]	219 IPMN	Cancer risk	BD: 70 % benign		Moderate
			MD: 26 % benign		
Marchegiani 2015 [6]	173 MD-IPMN, 74 (43 %) Asymptomatic	Cancer risk	Malignant 125 (72 %)		Moderate
			Benign 48 (28 %)		

asymptomatic patients with MD-IPMN, the malignancy rate was lower than other published series at 25 %, suggesting an association between symptoms and malignancy [3].

Correa-Gallego and colleagues used data from 219 patients who underwent resection for IPMN to create a predictive nomogram for malignancy [5]. In MD-IPMN, significant factors for malignancy included male gender, past history of cancer, weight loss and a solid component. For BD-IPMN, maximum lesion diameter, weight loss and solid component were used to build the nomogram. Concordance index for each tumor type was 0.74.

Procedural Morbidity and Mortality

Operative mortality in patients over 70 years of age undergoing pancreaticoduodenectomy (PD) for all indications is 7–9 %, according to data from the Nationwide Inpatient Sample [10]. Clinical data from the American College of Surgeons National Surgical Quality Improvement Program (NSQIP) reveals 4.3 % mortality for PD in patients over 70 [11]. One study evaluating PD outcomes found an increase in morality from 1.7 % in patients <80 years old, to 4.1 % in patients 80–90, with 0 % morality in 10 patients >90. Morbidity was 41.6 % in patients <80, 52.8 % in 80–90 year olds, and 50 % in patients >90 [12]. Mortality in series describing laparoscopic and open distal pancreatectomy for all indications is 0–3 % and complications range from 20 to 57 % [13–16]. Single-institution series and multi-institutional pooled analyses of IPMN resections report mortality rates of 0–4.3 % and morbidities of 15–35 % [6, 17, 18]. A pancreatectomy risk calculator is available for patient-specific risk prediction, and age >74 was found to be a risk factor for increased morbidity and mortality [19]. These data are summarized in Table 47.3. There are no data on IPMN-specific risk factors for operative morbidity or mortality.

Survival

Survival following resection of IPMN is most consistently related to the histology of the resected specimen, with non-invasive tumors demonstrating improved overall 5-year survival compared to invasive carcinomas (77–92 % vs 31–43 %) (Table 47.4) [6, 17, 18, 20–22]. Histologic sub-type is also associated with survival; pancreaticobiliary subtype is associated with a 36 % 5-year overall survival compared to intestinal subtype (87 %) [23]. Given the challenges in patient-specific prediction of invasive malignancy, it may be difficult to assign a patient to one of these ranges for purposes of preoperative decision-making.

There have been relatively few studies directly comparing survival of patients who meet criteria for resection but have not undergone surgery to patients who do undergo surgery, and none specifically relating to asymptomatic IPMN. In an

Table 47.3 Survival

Study	Patients	Outcome classification	Resection	Observation	Quality of evidence
Piciucchi 2013 [27]	35 patients meeting resection criteria; 23 asymptomatic	Median OS		52 months;	Low
		5-year OS		35.2 %	
		Median DSS		55 months;	
		5-year DSS		48.5 %	
Wang 2005 [34]	39 resected; 13 resectable but observed; 5 unresectable	Median OS	21.5 months	14 months	Low
		5-year OS	69.8 %	59.8 %	
Ogura 2013 [26]	20 follow-up	3-year PFS		30 %	Low
	19 surgical	4-year PFS		47 %	
	MD-IPMN	DSS		95 %	
		OS		85 %	
Takuma 2011 [25]	MD-IPMN; 26 resection 15 (58 %) asx	DSS		85 %	Low
	20 observation 17 (85 %) asx	OS		60 %	
Waters 2011 [20]	113 invasive IPMN	Median OS	32 months;		Low
		5-year OS	31 %		
Sohn 2004 [18]	136 resected IPMN	5-year OS	Non-invasive 77 %		Low
			Invasive 43 %		
Uehara 2010 [28]	20 MD-IPMN with lower likelihood of malignancy	Progression to resection criteria (MN >10 mm or + cytology)		2/20 (10 %) 22–26 months	Low

Kawakubo 2014 [24]	48 resected propensity matched to 48 non-surgical	3-year DSS	95.3 %	98.3 %	Moderate
		5-yearDSS	88.5 %	80.7 %	
Distler 2013 [23]	103 resected tumors	5-year OS by histological subtype	PB 36 %		Low
			Intest 87 %		
			Oncocytic 75 %		
			Gastric 70 %		
Salvia 2004 [17]	140 resected MD-IPMN;	5-year DSS	Invasive: 60 % non-invasive 100 %		Low
	38 asymptomatic	OS	Invasive 75 % non-invasive 92 %		
Kang 2014 [21]	366 resected tumors	5-year OS	87 %		Low
		5-year DFS	79 %		
Marchegiani 2015 [6]	173 MD-IPMN	5-year OS	69 %		Low
		5-year DSS	83 %		
Nakagohri 2007 [22]	82 IPMN	5-year OS	Malignant: 47 %		Low
			Benign: 80 %		

Table 47.4 Morbidity and mortality

Study	Patients	Outcome classification	Resection	Quality of evidence
Are 2009 [10]	>70 years old; 8,060	Mortality from PD	7–9 %	Moderate
Salvia 2004 [17]	140 patients resected; 38 asx	M&M	0 mortality	Moderate
			31 % morbidity	
Haigh 2011 [11]	977 PD resections	M&M	40 % morbidity	Moderate
	>70 years old		4.3 % mortality	
Marchegiani 2015 [6]	173 MD-IPMN	M&M	0 30-day mortality	Moderate
			15.6 % major morbidity	
Sohn 2004 [18]	136 IPMN resections	M&M	3.7 % mortality	Moderate
			35 % morbidity	
Makary 2006 [12]	207 PD patients ≥80 years old; 2491 <80	Mortality	< 80: 1.7 %	Moderate
			80–90: 4.1 %	
			>90: 0 %	
Makary 2006 [12]	207 PD patients ≥80 years old; 2,491 <80	Morbidity	< 80: 41.6 %	Moderate
			80–90: 52.8 %	
			>90: 50 %	

attempt to address the inherent bias in observational studies of patients who do not undergo surgery for IPMN meeting criteria for resection, Kawakubo used 16 patient characteristics to perform propensity score matching of 48 patients with IPMN who did not undergo surgery to 48 patients who did undergo resection [24]. The non-surgical patients either refused surgery or had a contraindication to general anesthesia. Approximately 85 % of patients were asymptomatic in each group, and the mean ages were 68 and 66 years in the surgical and non-surgical groups. For the entire cohort, the overall survival at 3 and 5 years was 90 % and 78 %, and the 3- and 5-year disease-specific survival was 94 % and 88 %, respectively. Five-year disease-specific survival was 81 % in the surgery group and 89 % in the observation group. The only significant reduction in disease-specific mortality with surgical management was in the sub-group of patients with a hypo-attenuating lesion on CT, suggesting that a known invasive cancer may be unique factor when balancing survival risk with surgery compared to observation.

Wang reviewed 57 patients with IPMN, 39 of whom underwent resection, while 18 were observed. Five of the 18 were deemed unresectable, and the remainder had comorbidities or patient refusal that precluded operation. The mean age of the surgery patients was 70 compared to 76 in the observation group, and 8 % compared to 50 % were asymptomatic. The 5-year overall survival was 69.8 % in the surgical groups and 59.8 % in the observation group, with no statistical difference. Ogura studied 20 patients followed with MD-IPMN and compared them to 19 surgical patients. The mean age of the observation group was 76 compared to 65 in the surgical group, and there was no detail of the reasons for not undergoing resection. With a mean follow-up of around 5 years, the follow-up cohort had an overall survival of

85 % and a disease-specific survival of 95 %. Takuma reviewed 20 patients observed with MD-IPMN, 85 % of whom were asymptomatic, with a median age of 77 [25]. Most of these patients were observed because of second malignancies (n = 12), with advanced age, comorbidities and unresectable disease being the other reasons to not perform resection. Disease-specific survival in this group was 85 %, while overall survival was 40 %, with a range of 17–65 months of follow-up. Clearly survival in these studies is driven by comorbidities more so than IPMN-associated malignancy.

In case series reports describing patients who met resection criteria for IPMN but did not undergo surgery, 5-year overall survival of 35–85 %, and 5-year disease-specific survival of 49–95 % have been described [26, 27]. Other endpoints include a progression-free survival of 30 % at 3 years and 47 % at 4 years [26]. In a study of 20 MD-IPMN with mural nodules <10 mm and negative pancreatic juice cytology, two patients progressed to mural nodules greater than 10 mm or positive cytology at 22–26 months, and underwent resection, with one non-invasive and 1invasive carcinoma identified [28].

Quality of Life

Quality of life (QoL) after major pancreatic resection may be influenced by the presence and severity of post-operative complications, the development of exocrine or endocrine pancreatic insufficiency, recurrence of malignant disease, or anxiety about recurrence (Table 47.5). In asymptomatic patients who do not undergo surgery, QoL may be influenced by the nature and frequency of surveillance procedures and the anxiety associated with disease progression or developing symptoms. Given that many patients with IPMN who do not undergo surgery have significant co-morbidities or a second malignancy, QoL may also be influenced by these non-IPMN-related factors.

There is a paucity of literature addressing the question of what QoL differences an older patient with an asymptomatic IPMN might expect with operative versus non-operative management. The existing data from which one might piece together and/or extrapolate in an attempt to answer this question include QoL studies of patients who underwent pancreatic resection, which typically include predominantly pancreatic adenocarcinoma patients, QoL studies of patients who underwent total pancreatectomy, and a single QoL study comparing 16 patients who underwent partial pancreatectomy for IPMN to 16 patients who underwent surveillance, although none of the surveillance patients met criteria for resection and all were medically fit for surgery [29]. In this study, QoL was assessed by the Hospital Anxiety and Depression Scale, anxiety subscale (HADS-A) and the Functional Assessment of Cancer Therapy-Pancreas (FACT-P) instruments at variable intervals from surgery or diagnosis. The surgical group had a non-significant increase in anxiety score, and equivalent FACT-Pa scores when compared to the surveillance group. Only the functional well-being domain of the FACT-PA was significantly

Table 47.5 Quality of life

Study	Patients	Outcome classification	Resection	Observation	Quality of evidence
Lee 2010 [29]	16 IPMN resection (TP excluded) 16 IPMN surveillance (all Sendai neg)	Quality of life by HADS-A and FACT-Pa	HADS-A score 9.4	HADS-A score 7.4 (p=0.09)	Moderate
			FACT-Pa 113	FACT-Pa 123 (p=0.27)	
			Functional well-being domain 19	Functional well- being domain 23.5 (p=0.03)	
Belyaev 2013 [30]	31 resections for malignant indications	Quality of life by SF-36 at preop, 3 months and 24 months after surgery	PCS: 43.1 preop; 37 at 3 months; 34.5 at 24 months; MCS 43 preop; 44.8 at 3 months; 42.9 at 24 months		Low
Belyaev 2013 [30]	19 resections for benign indications	Quality of life by SF-36 at preop, 3 months and 24 months after surgery	PCS: 48.5 preop; 36.6 at 3 months; 47.5 at 24 months; MCS 49.4 preop; 47 at 3 months; 49.2 at 24 months		Low
Belyaev 2013 [30]	10 patients with total pancreatectomy	Quality of life by SF-36 at preop, 3 months and 24 months after surgery	PCS: 44.5 prepop; 35.2 3 months; 40.5 24 months; MCS 43.6 preop, 41.4 3 months; 46.4 24 months		Low
Park 2013 [31]	107 PD, 29 DP; 5 malignant IPMN, 18 benign IPMN	Quality of life by EORTC QLQ-C30	Decreased post-op but no difference from preop at 3, 6 and 12 months		Low

higher in the surveillance group compared with the surgical group. In other studies of post-pancreatectomy patients, QoL is decreased immediately post-operatively, but returns to preoperative levels by 3 months post-operatively in most patients, although physical functioning scores were noted to be lower at 3 and 24 months postoperatively in patients with malignant indications, which may reflect tumor recurrence [30, 31].

Recommendations

Older patients with asymptomatic IPMN falling within resection criteria based on the 2012 Updated International Consensus Guidelines:

- Can be further risk-stratified based on MD-IPMN vs BD-IPMN, maximum lesion diameter, weight loss, solid component, gender, and past history of cancer to give a patient-specific risk of harboring high-grade dysplasia or an invasive malignancy (evidence quality moderate, weak recommendation)
- Who have specific co-morbidities that pose a prohibitive surgical risk, or which present a reasonable risk of mortality within 5 years of IPMN diagnosis are likely to have similar overall and disease-specific survival with observation or resection and are appropriate candidates for observation (evidence quality low, weak recommendation)
- Who do no have specific co-morbidities that significantly increase pancreatectomy risk or co-morbidities limiting their survival should be offered resection with counseling that includes their risk of malignancy, risk of surgical complications, and survival ranges for invasive and non-invasive disease (evidence quality moderate, weak recommendation)

A Personal View of the Data

IPMN in an older patient presents challenging preoperative shared decision-making. Patients and their families often require education on the differences between IPMN and the more publicized ductal adenocarcinoma before a discussion on management options can begin, and some seem to harbor their emotional biases towards either aggressive resection or nilism, despite education. A poor surgical candidate is fairly easy to identify, and pancreatectomy-specific risk prediction tools can assist in presenting objective data to patients about surgical risk. A patient who refuses surgery makes the surgical decision more straight-forward, but makes the question of surveillance more complicated – the patient's preferences about undergoing surveillance, and whether surgery would be re-considered in light of disease progression should be thoroughly discussed, as older patients rarely become better surgical candidates with more time passing. The existing data on what outcomes an otherwise healthy older patient might expect by not choosing surgery are woefully inadequate to properly inform a shared decision-making process, and these patients should be offered resection based on current guidelines, and allowed to choose based on their preference.

References

1. Tanaka M, Fernandez-del Castillo C, Adsay V, et al. International consensus guidelines 2012 for the management of IPMN and MCN of the pancreas. Pancreatol: Off J Int Assoc Pancreatol. 2012;12:183–97.
2. Roch AM, DeWitt JM, Al-Haddad MA, et al. Nonoperative management of main pancreatic duct-involved intraductal papillary mucinous neoplasm might be indicated in select patients. J Am Coll Surg. 2014;219:122–9.
3. Abdeljawad K, Vemulapalli KC, Schmidt CM, et al. Prevalence of malignancy in patients with pure main duct intraductal papillary mucinous neoplasms. Gastrointest Endosc. 2014;79:623–9.
4. Aso T, Ohtsuka T, Matsunaga T, et al. "High-Risk Stigmata" of the 2012 international consensus guidelines correlate with the malignant grade of branch duct intraductal papillary mucinous neoplasms of the pancreas. Pancreas. 2014; 43(8):1239–43.
5. Correa-Gallego C, Do R, Lafemina J, et al. Predicting dysplasia and invasive carcinoma in intraductal papillary mucinous neoplasms of the pancreas: development of a preoperative nomogram. Ann Surg Oncol. 2013;20:4348–55.
6. Marchegiani G, Mino-Kenudson M, Sahora K, et al. IPMN involving the main pancreatic duct: Biology, epidemiology, and long-term outcomes following resection. Ann Surg. 2015; 261(5):976–83.
7. Shimizu Y, Yamaue H, Maguchi H, et al. Predictors of malignancy in intraductal papillary mucinous neoplasm of the pancreas: analysis of 310 pancreatic resection patients at multiple high-volume centers. Pancreas. 2013;42:883–8.
8. Fritz S, Klauss M, Bergmann F, et al. Small (Sendai negative) branch-duct IPMNs: not harmless. Ann Surg. 2012;256:313–20.
9. Wong J, Weber J, Centeno BA, et al. High-grade dysplasia and adenocarcinoma are frequent in side-branch intraductal papillary mucinous neoplasm measuring less than 3 cm on endoscopic ultrasound. J Gastrointest Surg: Off J Soc Surg Aliment Tract. 2013;17:78–84. discussion p -5.
10. Are C, Afuh C, Ravipati L, Sasson A, Ullrich F, Smith L. Preoperative nomogram to predict risk of perioperative mortality following pancreatic resections for malignancy. J Gastrointest Surg: Off J Soc Surg Aliment Tract. 2009;13:2152–62.
11. Haigh PI, Bilimoria KY, DiFronzo LA. Early postoperative outcomes after pancreaticoduodenectomy in the elderly. Arch Surg. 2011;146:715–23.
12. Makary MA, Winter JM, Cameron JL, et al. Pancreaticoduodenectomy in the very elderly. J Gastrointest Surg: Off J Soc Surg Aliment Tract. 2006;10:347–56.
13. Eom BW, Jang JY, Lee SE, Han HS, Yoon YS, Kim SW. Clinical outcomes compared between laparoscopic and open distal pancreatectomy. Surg Endosc. 2008;22:1334–8.
14. Kooby DA, Gillespie T, Bentrem D, et al. Left-sided pancreatectomy: a multicenter comparison of laparoscopic and open approaches. Ann Surg. 2008;248:438–46.
15. Velanovich V. Case-control comparison of laparoscopic versus open distal pancreatectomy. J Gastrointest Surg: Off J Soc Surg Aliment Tract. 2006;10:95–8.
16. Vijan SS, Ahmed KA, Harmsen WS, et al. Laparoscopic vs open distal pancreatectomy: a single-institution comparative study. Arch Surg. 2010;145:616–21.
17. Salvia R, Fernandez-del Castillo C, Bassi C, et al. Main-duct intraductal papillary mucinous neoplasms of the pancreas: clinical predictors of malignancy and long-term survival following resection. Ann Surg. 2004;239:678–85. discussion 85-7.
18. Sohn TA, Yeo CJ, Cameron JL, et al. Intraductal papillary mucinous neoplasms of the pancreas: an updated experience. Ann Surg. 2004;239:788–97. discussion 97-9.
19. Parikh P, Shiloach M, Cohen ME, et al. Pancreatectomy risk calculator: an ACS-NSQIP resource. HPB: Off J Int Hepato Pancreato Biliary Assoc. 2010;12:488–97.
20. Waters JA, Schnelldorfer T, Aguilar-Saavedra JR, et al. Survival after resection for invasive intraductal papillary mucinous neoplasm and for pancreatic adenocarcinoma: a multi-

institutional comparison according to American Joint Committee on Cancer Stage. J Am Coll Surg. 2011;213:275–83.
21. Kang MJ, Jang JY, Lee KB, Chang YR, Kwon W, Kim SW. Long-term prospective cohort study of patients undergoing pancreatectomy for intraductal papillary mucinous neoplasm of the pancreas: Implications for postoperative surveillance. Ann Surg. 2014; 260(2):356–63.
22. Nakagohri T, Kinoshita T, Konishi M, Takahashi S, Gotohda N. Surgical outcome of intraductal papillary mucinous neoplasms of the pancreas. Ann Surg Oncol. 2007;14:3174–80.
23. Distler M, Kersting S, Niedergethmann M, et al. Pathohistological subtype predicts survival in patients with intraductal papillary mucinous neoplasm (IPMN) of the pancreas. Ann Surg. 2013;258:324–30.
24. Kawakubo K, Tada M, Isayama H, et al. Disease-specific mortality among patients with intraductal papillary mucinous neoplasm of the pancreas. Clin Gastroenterol Hepatol: Off Clin Pract J Am Gastroenterol Assoc. 2014;12:486–91.
25. Takuma K, Kamisawa T, Anjiki H, et al. Predictors of malignancy and natural history of main-duct intraductal papillary mucinous neoplasms of the pancreas. Pancreas. 2011;40:371–5.
26. Ogura T, Masuda D, Kurisu Y, et al. Potential predictors of disease progression for main-duct intraductal papillary mucinous neoplasms of the pancreas. J Gastroenterol Hepatol. 2013;28:1782–6.
27. Piciucchi M, Crippa S, Del Chiaro M, et al. Outcomes of intraductal papillary mucinous neoplasm with "Sendai-positive" criteria for resection undergoing non-operative management. Dig Liver Dis: Off J Ital Soc Gastroenterol Ital Assoc Stud Liver. 2013;45:584–8.
28. Uehara H, Ishikawa O, Ikezawa K, et al. A natural course of main duct intraductal papillary mucinous neoplasm of the pancreas with lower likelihood of malignancy. Pancreas. 2010;39:653–7.
29. Lee MK, DiNorcia J, Pursell LJ, et al. Prophylactic pancreatectomy for intraductal papillary mucinous neoplasm does not negatively impact quality of life: a preliminary study. J Gastrointest Surg: Off J Soc Surg Aliment Tract. 2010;14:1847–52.
30. Belyaev O, Herzog T, Chromik AM, Meurer K, Uhl W. Early and late postoperative changes in the quality of life after pancreatic surgery. Langenbeck's Arch Surg/Deut Ges Chir. 2013;398:547–55.
31. Park JW, Jang JY, Kim EJ, et al. Effects of pancreatectomy on nutritional state, pancreatic function and quality of life. Br J Surg. 2013;100:1064–70.
32. Sahora K, Mino-Kenudson M, Brugge W, et al. Branch duct intraductal papillary mucinous neoplasms: does cyst size change the tip of the scale? A critical analysis of the revised international consensus guidelines in a large single-institutional series. Ann Surg. 2013;258:466–75.
33. Roch AM, Ceppa EP, Al-Haddad MA, et al. The natural history of main duct-involved, mixed-type intraductal papillary mucinous neoplasm: parameters predictive of progression. Ann Surg. 2014;260:680–90.
34. Wang SE, Shyr YM, Chen TH, et al. Comparison of resected and non-resected intraductal papillary mucinous neoplasms of the pancreas. World J Surg. 2005;29:1650–7.

Chapter 48
Minimally Invasive Surgery for Pancreatic Head Cancer

Deepa Magge and Amer H. Zureikat

Abstract An increasing number of reports on minimally-invasive pancreaticoduodenectomy (MIPD) have emerged over the last two decades. Morbidity, oncologic outcomes, and the impact of the learning curve for MIPD are being carefully scrutinized to ensure that safety and efficacy are not compromised, particularly in the setting of periampullary malignancies. Although many of the current adopters of MIPD are still within their learning curve, a number of single institutional series have recently confirmed the non-inferiority of the laparoscopic or robotic PD when performed by experienced pancreatic surgeons at high volume centers. In the absence of randomized controlled trials to address the safety, efficacy and potential advantages of the MIPD, this chapter will examine the available retrospective data on the safety and oncologic oncologic outcomes of the laparoscopic and robotic PD for pancreatic head malignancies.

Keywords Pancreatic adenocarcinoma • Peri-ampullary malignancies • Pancreaticoduodenectomy • Minimally invasive • Laparoscopic • Robotic

Introduction

Minimally invasive approaches have proven to be safe and feasible in the treatment of many complex GI malignancies [1–3]. Minimally invasive distal pancreatectomy for example, exhibits a favorable morbidity profile and equivalent short-term oncologic outcomes compared to its open counterpart [2, 3]. However, there remains no consensus regarding the safety and oncologic efficacy of minimally invasive

---

D. Magge • A.H. Zureikat (✉)
Division of Surgical Oncology, University of Pittsburgh Medical Center,
5150 Centre Ave, Suite 414, Pittsburgh, PA 15232, USA
e-mail: zureikatah@upmc.edu

J.M. Millis, J.B. Matthews (eds.), *Difficult Decisions in Hepatobiliary and Pancreatic Surgery*, Difficult Decisions in Surgery: An Evidence-Based Approach, DOI 10.1007/978-3-319-27365-5_48

pancreaticoduodenectomy (MIPD) for malignant lesions. An analysis of the National Cancer Database in 2007 revealed that 71.4 % of patients with clinical stage 1 pancreatic adenocarcinoma (PDA) chose not to undergo surgical resection, and consequently had shorter survival compared to patients treated with pancreatectomy ($p<0.001$) [4]. Although reasons for this are multifactorial, the morbidity associated with open pancreatic resections (particularly the PD) may substantially contribute to this nihilistic view of pancreatic surgery. A minimally invasive approach to PD has the potential to decrease post-operative morbidity, improve quality of life, facilitate the receipt of adjuvant therapy, and ultimately enhance the acceptance of this complex procedure.

Recently, two MIPD approaches have been popularized: laparoscopic and robotic. The laparoscopic pancreaticoudenectomy (LPD) was initially met with skepticism due to long operative times, but has now been established as safe and feasible when performed by select high volume surgeons at experienced centers [5]. The robotic pancreaticoduodenectomy (RPD) -first performed in 2007 -is now being increasingly utilized due to the perceived benefits of stereotactic vision, magnification, platform stability, and favorable ergonomics [6]. We present here a review of the two minimally invasive platforms for PD focusing on metrics of safety, morbidity and oncologic outcomes, as well as the impact of the learning curve.

Search Strategy

A literature search of English language publications from 2000 to 2013 was used to identity published data on minimally invasive pancreaticoduodenectomy (MIPD) and open pancreaticoduodenectomy (OPD). Databases searched were PubMed, Embase, Science Citation Index/Social sciences Citation Index and Cochrane Evidence Based Medicine. Terms used in the search were "pancreaticoduodenectomy," "minimally invasive pancreaticoduodenectomy," "minimally invasive versus open pancreaticoduodenectomy" AND "complications from pancreaticoduodenectomy." Only totally minimally invasive pancreaticoduodenectomies were included in the literature review, excluding any studies detailing a hand-assisted approach or use of a mini-laparotomy. English language was used as an exclusion criterion. Fifteen cohort studies, 3 systematic reviews, 4 review articles, and 1 guideline paper were included in our analysis. The data was classified using the GRADE system. The clinical issue is outlined in Table 48.1.

Table 48.1 PICO table

Patient	Intervention	Comparison	Outcome
Resectable pancreatic head adenocarcinoma	Robotic or laparoscopic pancreaticoduodenectomy	Open pancreaticoduodenectomy	Short-term complications

Results

Open Pancreaticoduodenectomy (OPD) Benchmarks

Significant improvements in operative technique and patient care over recent decades have improved the outcomes of open PD. In the modern era, a 2 % 30-day mortality can be expected at high volume centers, although this can be as high as 6–7 % when considering 90-day outcomes (a better surrogate of the true impact of PD) or cases that involve vascular resections [7–9]. Overall morbidity remains high at nearly 50 % [9]. Post-pancreatectomy hemorrhage, a potentially lethal complication that may be underreported, is typically around 6 % as published in large series [10]. Recently, a grading system (ISGPF) that takes into consideration the clinical impact of pancreatic fistulae (PF) (Grade A: no clinical sequlae, Grade B: mild-moderate clinical significance, Grade C: associated with sepsis, or end organ failure) was described by Bassi et al. The true incidence of PF after open PD when utilizing this grading system is approximately 15–20 %; about half of these being clinically significant (grade B/C leaks) [11]. Additionally, an average length of stay of 10 days with a readmission rate of between 15 and 30 % can be expected [9, 10, 12].

Oncologically, R2 resections should be avoidable if the preoperative staging workup is accurate. Microscopic margin positivity is around 5–20 % with the retroperitoneal margin being the most common R1 site [13]. When using a distance of >1 mm to define R0, most series have an increased R1 rate that ranges between 30 and 80 % [14, 15]. For PDA resections, resection of a minimum of 15 LNs is considered adequate for staging. Estimated median survival and 5-years OS for R0 resected PDA is around 19 months and 18 % respectively [9]. Receipt of adjuvant chemotherapy improves survival. Recently, two large analyses of resected PDA demonstrated no improvement in survival since the 1980s [9, 16]. One explanation may be that the morbidity associated with open PD renders a significant number of patients unfit to initiate or tolerate adjuvant chemotherapy.

Laparoscopic Pancreaticoduodenectomy (LPD)

The LPD is a technically challenging operation. Gagner and Pomp's initial report of ten LPDs in 1997 did not favor use of the laparoscopic technique over the open approach due to the high conversion rate (40 %) and lack of any perceived benefits [17]. Subsequently, several reports have emerged attempting to further characterize the safety and oncologic efficacy of the LPD (Table 48.2).

Two large reports (Table 48.2) by Palavinelu et al. (75 cases), and Kendrick et al. (62 cases), demonstrate that the LPD is safe and feasible when performed by skilled, high volume surgeons with reasonable operative times, minimal blood loss compared to historic reports, and a mortality and morbidity profile similar to open PD

Table 48.2 Largest series of open and minimally invasive pancreaticoduodenectomy

Author	Year	Technique	N (total) /N(malignancy)	EBL (mL)	Operative time (min)	Fistula rate (grade C)	Mortality rate	Oncologic outcomes (R0 rate, LN)	Evidence grade
Palanivelu [18]	2007	Lap	75/72	74	357	6.7 %	1.3 %	97.4 %, 14	Very low
Kendrick and Cusati [19]	2010	Lap	62/45	240	368	18 %	1.6 %	89 %,15	Low
Kim [20]	2013	Lap	100/12	–	474	6 %	–	100 %, 13	Very low
Guilianotti [24]	2010	Robot	60/45	394	421	31.6 %	3 %	90 %, 18	Very low
Zureikat [26]	2013	Robot	132/106	300	527	3.7 %	1.5 %	87.7 %,19	Low

Table 48.3 Comparative series of LPD vs OPD

	Zureikat [22] evidence grade: very low			Asbun/stauffer [21] evidence grade: low			Croome [23] evidence grade: low		
Series	LPD	OPD	P	LPD	OPD	P	LPD	OPD	P
N	14	14		53	215		108	214	
OR time (min)	456	372	0.01	541	401	<0.001	379.4	387.6	0.45
EBL(ml)	300	400	0.23	195	1,032	<0.001	492	866.7	<0.001
Transfusion N (%)	28.6 %	35.7 %	0.69	1.55	4.7 %	<0.001	19 %	33 %	0.01
Conversion N (%)	2 (4 %)			9 (17 %)			6.5 %		
R0 resection (%)	100 %	91.0.7 %	0.31	94.9 %	83 %	NS	77.8 %	76.6 %	0.81
Lymph nodes (N)	18.5	19.1	0.85	23.4	16.84	<0.001	21.4	20.1	0.15
Length of stay (d)	8	8.5	0.71	8	12.4	<0.001	6	9	<0.001
Morbidity (%)	21 %	7 %	NS	24.5 %	24.7 %	NS	5.6 %	13.6 %	0.17
Mortality (%)	7 %	0 %	NS	5.7 %	8.85	NS	1 %	2 %	0.5

[18, 19]. Additionally, the reoperation rate, length of stay, and readmission rates are comparable to previous OPD reports. Both of these reports however suffer from small numbers, selection bias, and lack of standardization in reporting pancreatic leaks, drain management and complication rates. Importantly, although both series contain a substantial cohort of pancreatic head malignancies, they do not report on those outcomes separately, making any conclusions difficult to formulate. Both series also lack long-term survival follow-up. More recently, Kim et al. described the outcomes of 100 laparoscopic pylorus preserving PDs, however the cancer subgroup was small (12 cases) and their outcomes were not detailed separately [20].

Several comparative studies between LPD and OPD are outlined in Table 48.3. In a study by Asbun and Stauffer, 53 LPDs (39 for malignant disease) were compared to 215 OPDs (141 for malignant disease). The authors noted significantly lower blood loss, transfusion rate, length of hospital stay, and length of ICU stay for the LPD group despite having no differences in patient demographics, ASA grade, or pathologic indications [21]. Operative time was significantly higher in the LPD group. The overall complication rate was 25 % in both groups with an equal occurrence of ISPGF grade B or C fistulae (9 %). Again, similar to previous LPD reports, cancer specific outcomes were not outlined separately, but with nearly two-thirds of each cohort having cancer, it is reasonable to infer that these results may be generalizable to the malignant group [21]. In another smaller comparative study, authors from the University of Pittsburgh noted operative times to be significantly higher in the LPD group, with all other perioperative metrics being equivalent [22].

Taken collectively, the aforementioned reports indicate that the LPD can be performed safely with a similar morbidity profile to OPD if done at high volume centers by experienced HPB/surgical oncologists. Importantly, many of the outcomes described above represent cases performed within the learning curve. Although the impact of the learning curve on outcomes of MIPD is significant (see later section), the above evidence suggests that – if performed in highly selected patients at high volume centers- outcomes are acceptable provided that the surgeon is well versed in the principles of open pancreatic surgery.

Regarding oncological efficacy, LPD has been shown to have comparable short-term outcomes of R0 resection rates and lymph node retrieval to the OPD (Tables 48.2 and 48.3). Unfortunately, all of the above-cited studies do not report on long-term survival, lack standardized definitions of R0 (0 mm distance versus >1 mm), and suffer from selection bias. Recently, Croome et al. compared the outcomes of LPD (N = 108) and OPD (N = 214) for PDA at the Mayo Clinic over a 5 years period [23]. Neoadjuvant therapy, tumor size, node positivity, and margin-positive resection were not significantly different between the two groups. There was a significantly higher proportion of OPD patients (12 %) that either had a delay in initiating chemotherapy of >90 days, or did not receive *any* adjuvant chemotherapy compared with that in the LPD group. Although there was no significant difference in overall survival between the two groups (LPD = 25.3 vs. OPD = 21.8 months) a significantly longer PFS was seen in the LPD cohort (P = 0.03).

Robotic Pancreaticoduodenectomy (RPD)

The LPD has been slow to adopt due to the technical and ergonomic challenges imposed by 2-D laparoscopy. The robotic approach, on the other hand, combines stereotactic vision with platform stability and favorable ergonomics, making it arguably better suited for complex pancreatic resections and reconstructions. Consequently, this platform may be easier to disseminate than its laparoscopic counterpart.

Giulianotti et al. are credited with the first reported RPD in 2010 [24]. Recently, the University of Pittsburgh (UPMC) reported the largest series of RPDs, detailing the safety and feasibility of this approach for 132 cases (106 of which were for malignancies) [25, 26]. Although, operative times were long (mean 527 min), conversion to open was required in only 11 patients (8 %). Thirty-day and 90-day mortality was 1.5 % and 3.8 %, respectively. The rate of Clavien 3 and 4 (major) complications was 22 %, the ISGPF Grade B + C fistula rate was 7 %, and the reoperation rate was 3 %. Average length of stay was 10 days, and 28 % of patients required readmissions.

A major concern for RPD is the lack of tactile feedback, and the potential for development of pseuodanuerysms due to inadvertent crush injury or heat dissipation during dissection. In the UPMC study, the authors described a PSA rate of 6 % (eight patients): three of the eight were confirmed by arteriography and resolved after stenting; the other five underwent arteriography due to a high index of clinical suspicion, but no PSA was found. When reviewing PSA rates in large OPD series, the occurrence rate can range between 4 and 6 %, with most authors agreeing that this feared complication is under-reported. Taken together, the UPMC series indicates that even when performed within its learning curve, initial safety and feasibility metrics support the robustness of this platform and suggest no unanticipated risks inherent to this new technology.

Several retrospective studies comparing the RPD to OPD are detailed in Table 48.4 [27–31]. Similar to comparative studies for LPD, the RPD data collectively implies that the procedure can be performed with acceptable safety metrics that are similar to OPD outcomes. Margin negative resection rates and lymph node harvest are also not compromised in these comparative studies; thus it may be reasonable to infer that early oncologic results are likely to yield the expected survival seen after OPD. Similar to LPD data however, all of these comparisons were performed within the implementation phase of RPD at each institution, and therefore represent 'learning curve' outcomes. Most of these reports also fail to document the outcomes of the cancer cohorts separately, suffer from low numbers and substantial selection bias, and lack long term follow-up.

Of particular interest will be the proportion of PDA patients able to receive and complete adjuvant chemotherapy. Recent data indicates that time to receipt of adjuvant chemotherapy may not be as important as the ability to complete all scheduled doses. Indeed, if RPD (or LPD) ultimately reduces morbidity and facilitates improved receipt and completion of scheduled adjuvant chemotherapy, a survival advantage may be detected.

Benefits of the MIPD

Recently, several meta-analyses comparing OPDs to MIPDs have demonstrated marginal benefits to the MI approach. A recent analysis of six retrospective studies comparing consecutive MIPDs (RPD and LPD) with either consecutive or matched OPD revealed that MIPD was associated with a significant reduction in intraoperative blood loss at the expense of longer operative times [32]. Clinically significant PF occurred in 8 % (MIPD) and 7 % (OPD) (P=NS). Overall morbidity and reoperations were comparable between the two groups and hospital stay was significantly reduced in the MIS group by 3.7 days. With regards to oncologic outcomes, the MIPD cohort had significantly higher lymph node retrieval rates ($p=0.03$) and fewer R1 resections, although tumor size was significantly larger in the OPDs ($p=0.02$).

In another meta-analysis by Nigri et al. eight studies encompassing 204 MIPD patients and 419 OPD patients were analyzed [33]. Patients in the two groups were similar with respect to age, sex, and histological diagnosis, but different with respect to tumor size, rate of pylorus preservation, and type of pancreatic anastomosis. There were no significant differences between MIPD and OPD regarding development of DGE, PF, wound infection, rates of reoperation and overall mortality. Although MIPD was associated with longer operative times, it was also associated-

Table 48.4 Comparative series of RPD versus OPD

	Buchs [31] evidence grade: low			Bao [29] evidence grade: low			Lai [28] evidence grade: low			Chalikonda [27] evidence grade: low			Zhou [30] evidence grade: low		
Series	RPD	OPD	P	RPD	OPD	P	RPD	OPD	P	RPD	OPD	P	RPD	OPD	P
N	44	39	NA	28	28	NA	20	67	NA	30	30	NA	8	8	NA
OR time(min)	444	559	0.0001	431	410	0.04	491	247	0.01	476	366	0.0005	718	420	0.011
EBL(ml)	387	827	0.0001	100	300	0.0001	247	774	0.03	485	775	0.13	153	210	0.045
Transfusion N (%)	10 (22.7)	12 (30.8)	0.46	32	50	0.17	NR	NR	NR	NR	NR	NR	NR	NR	NR
Conversion N (%)	2 (4.5)	NA	NA	14	NA	NA	5	NA	NA	10	NA	NA	NR	NA	NA
R0 resection (%)	90.9	81.5	0.45	63	88	0.070	73.3	64.1	0.92	0	13	0.02	100	83.3	0.05
Lymph nodes (N)	16.8	11	0.02	15	20	0.04	10	10	0.99	13.2	11.7	0.25	NR	NR	NR
Length of stay (d)	13	14.6	0.4	7.4	8.1	0.41	13.7	25.8	0.02	9.79	13.26	0.043	16.4	24.3	0.04
Morbidity (%)	36.4	48.7	0.27	28	28	NA	50	49.3	NS	30	43	0.14	NA	NA	NA
Mortality (%)	4.5	2.6	1	7 [1]	7 [1]	0.04	0	3	NS	4	1	0.09	7	7	NS

1: 90 day mortality

with lower post-operative complication rates, less intra-operative blood loss, shorter hospital stays, lower blood transfusion rates, higher numbers of harvested lymph nodes, and improved negative margin status rates.

Impact of the Learning Curve on MIPD Outcomes

Pancreatic surgery is technically complex and should be performed at high volume centers by high volume surgeons. Birkmeyer et al. used the Medicare claims database to show that PDs at high-volume hospitals had a superior 3-years survival compared to PDs at low-volume centers [34]. In 2002, Kotwall et al. used the Nationwide Inpatient Sample database to show a 50 % increased mortality in PDs performed at low-volume centers [35]. Additional data also indicates that a surgeon-based learning curve for PD also exists. Tseng et al. demonstrated that after 60 cases, surgeons achieved significantly decreased EBL, operative time and LOS, and carried out more margin-negative resections [36]. Similarly, Schmidt et al. noted that experienced surgeons performed PD with lower EBL, shorter operative time, and lower morbidity but no difference in quality of resection or mortality when compared with less experienced surgeons [37].

Similar data on the learning curve for MIPD is emerging. A recent RPD analysis from the University of Pittsburgh confirms that outcomes are optimized after an initial steep learning curve of approximately 80 cases [38]. In depth analysis of this learning curve revealed that blood loss and conversions were optimized after 20 cases (600 vs. 250, $p<0.05$, and 35 % vs. 3 %, $p<0.05$ respectively), incidence of pancreatic fistula after 40 cases (27 % vs. 14 %, $p<0.05$), and operative time after 80 cases (582 min vs. 417 min, $p<0.05$). Complication rates, length of stay and readmissions also improved but the sample size was underpowered to detect a significant difference. Importantly, a two attending approach was employed throughout the learning curve period to ensure patient safety and procedural efficacy. This data suggests that meaningful comparative effectiveness studies of minimally invasive and open PD should take into consideration the impact of the learning curve before any outcomes are assessed.

Recommendations

Based on the available evidence, the authors recommend cautious application of minimally invasive PD for pancreatic head malignancies. MIPD should only be performed by experienced pancreatic surgeons at high volume centers. In order to ensure patient safety and procedural efficacy, new adopters of MIPD should be well versed in open and laparoscopic pancreatic resections, utilize a two attending approach to the initial learning curve, and perform the 'learning curve cases' on carefully selected cohorts.

A Personal View of the Data

Due to the inherent difficulties in performing randomized controlled and the absence of large multi-institutional reports, the assessment of MIPD (or any surgical platform or technique) for pancreatic head malignancies will initially rely on single institutional reports of safety and feasibility; this was the case for the advent of many common surgical techniques embraced today such as the laparoscopic cholecystectomy. Consequently, the current evidence for MIPD is classified as 'low' or 'very low' according to the GRADE system. Despite this, an increasing number of reports support MIPD as an acceptable alternative to OPD in carefully selected patients. Two meta analyses suggest that MIPD is associated with reduced blood loss and marginally shorter lengths of hospital stay with no adverse effects on safety and oncologic results. This data must be interpreted with caution since all of these reports suffer from selection bias and reflect surgeons working through the early phases of implementation of MIPD. Regarding the two available platforms, RPD seems to be associated with fewer conversions than LPD. Additionally, the robotic approach may prove to be more disseminable due to the advantages afforded by a stereotactic, stable and highly ergonomic platform. Larger reports with longer follow-up, and those that reflect outcomes beyond the learning curve will allow more definitive conclusions to be made about the utility and impact of minimally invasive PD for pancreatic head cancer.

Recommendations

- In carefully selected patients, MIPD is a safe alternative to OPD if performed by skilled, experienced pancreatic surgeons at high volume centers (Evidence quality low; conditional (weak) recommendation).
- Safe conduct of robotic PD for pancreatic head cancer requires a learning curve of approximately 80 cases (Evidence quality low; conditional (weak) recommendation).
- When performed for pancreatic head cancer, MIPD cases should be carefully selected (resectable tumors, no vascular invasion), and preferably be performed by two experienced pancreatic surgeons (Evidence quality very low; conditional (weak) recommendation).

References

1. Mack MJ. Minimally invasive and robotic surgery. JAMA. 2001;285:568–72.
2. Magge D, Zeh 3rd HJ, Moser AJ, et al. Comparative effectiveness of minimally invasive and open distal pancreatectomy for ductal adenocarcinoma. JAMA Surg. 2013;148(6):525–31.

3. Daouadi M, Zureikat AH, Zenati MS, et al. Robot-assisted minimally invasive distal pancreatectomy is superior to the laparoscopic technique. Ann Surg. 2013;257(1):128–32.
4. Bilimoria KY, Bentrem DJ, Ko CY, et al. National failure to operate on early stage pancreatic cancer. Ann Surg. 2007;246(2):173–80.
5. Gagner M, Pomp A. Laparoscopic pylorus-preserving pancreatoduodenectomy. Surg Endosc. 1994;8(5):408–10.
6. Cadiere GB, Himpens J, Germay O, et al. Feasibility of robotic laparoscopic surgery: 146 cases. World J Surg. 2001;25:1467–77.
7. Fernandez-del Castillo C, Morales-Oyarvide V, McGrath D, et al. Evolution of the Whipple procedure at the Massachusetts General Hospital. Surgery. 2012;152(3):556–63.
8. Lieberman MD, Kilburn H, Lindsey M, et al. Relation of perioperative deaths to hospital volume among patients undergoing pancreatic resections for malignancy. Ann Surg. 1995;222:638–45.
9. He J, Ahuja N, Makary MA, Cameron JL, Eckhauser FE, Choti MA, Hruban RH, Pawlik TM, Wolfgang CL. 2564 resected periampullary adenocarcinomas at a single institution: trends over three decades. HPB (Oxf). 2014;16(1):83–90.
10. Yekebas EF, Wolfram L, Cataldegirmen G, et al. Postpancreatectomy hemorrhage: diagnosis and treatment: an analysis in 1669 consecutive pancreatic resections. Ann Surg. 2007;246(2):269–80.
11. Bassi C, Dervenis C, Butturini G, et al. Postoperative pancreatic fistula: an international study group (ISPGF) definition. Surgery. 2005;138(1):8–13.
12. Denbo JW, Orr WS, Behrman SW, et al. Toward defining grade C pancreatic fistula following pancreaticoduodenectomy: incidence, risk factors, management, and outcome. HPB (Oxf). 2012;14(9):589–93.
13. Merkow RP, Bilimoria KY, Bentrem DJ, et al. National assessment of margin status as a quality indicator after pancreatic cancer surgery. Ann Surg Oncol. 2014;21(4):1067–74.
14. Konstantinidis IT, Warshaw AL, Allen JN, et al. Pancreatic ductal adenocarcinoma: is there a survival difference for R1 resections versus locally advanced unresectable tumors? What is a "true" R0 resection? Ann Surg Oncol. 2013;257(4):731–6.
15. Esposito I, Kleeff J, Bermann F, et al. Most pancreatic cancer resections are R1 resections. Ann Surg Oncol. 2008;15(6):1651–60.
16. Winter JM, Brennan MF, Tang LH, et al. Survival after resection of pancreatic adenocarcinoma: results from a single institution over three decades. Ann Surg Oncol. 2012;19:169–75.
17. Gagner M, Pomp A. Laparoscopic pancreatic resection: is it worthwhile? J Gastrointest Surg. 1997;1(1):20–5.
18. Palanivelu C, Rajan PS, Rangarajan M, Vaithiswaran V, Senthilnathan P, Parthasarathi R, Praveen RP. Evolution in techniques of laparoscopic pancreaticoduodenectomy: a decade long experience from a tertiary center. J Hepatobiliary Pancreat Surg. 2009;16(6):731–40.
19. Kendrick ML, Cusati D. Total laparoscopic pancreaticoduodenectomy: feasibility and outcome in an early experience. Arch Surg. 2010;145(1):19–23.
20. Kim SC, Song KB, Jung YS, Kim YH, do Park H, Lee SS, et al. Short-term clinical outcomes for 100 consecutive cases of laparoscopic pylorus-preserving pancreatoduodenectomy: improvement with surgical experience. Surg Endosc. 2013;27(1):95–103.
21. Asbun HJ, Stauffer JA. Laparoscopic vs open pancreaticoduodenectomy: overall outcomes and severity of complications using the accordion severity grading system. J Am Coll Surg. 2012;215(6):810–9.
22. Zureikat AH, Breaux JA, Steel JL, Hughes SJ. Can laparoscopic pancreaticoduodenectomy be safely implemented? J Gastrointest Surg. 2011;15(7):1151–7.
23. Croome KP, Farnell MB, Que FG, Reid-Lombardo K, Truty MJ, Nagorney DM, Kendrick ML. Total laparoscopic pancreaticoduodenectomy for pancreatic ductal adenocarcinoma: oncologic advantages over open approaches? Ann Surg. 2014;260(4):633–40.
24. Giulianotti PC, Sbrana F, Bianco FM, Elli EF, Shah G, Addeo P, et al. Robot-assisted laparoscopic pancreatic surgery: single-surgeon experience. Surg Endosc. 2010;24(7):1646–57.

25. Zeh HJ, Zureikat AH, Secrest A, Dauoudi M, Bartlett D, Moser AJ. Outcomes after robot-assisted pancreaticoduodenectomy for periampullary lesions. Ann Surg Oncol. 2012;19(3):864–70.
26. Zureikat AH, Moser AJ, Boone BA, Bartlett DL, Zenati M, Zeh HJ. 250 robotic pancreatic resections: safety and feasibility. Ann Surg. 2013;258(4):554–9; discussion 559–62.
27. Chalikonda S, Aguilar-Saavedrea JR, Walsh RM. Laparoscopic robotic-assisted pancreatico-duodenectomy: a case-matched comparison with open resection. Surg Endosc. 2012;26:2397–402.
28. Lai EC, Yang GP, Tang CN. Robot-assisted laparoscopic pancreaticoduodenectomy versus open pancreaticoduodenectomy – a comparative study. Int J Surg. 2012;10:475–9.
29. Bao PQ, Mazirka PO, Watkins KT. Retrospective comparison of robot-assisted minimally invasive versus open pancreaticoduodenectomy for periampullary neoplasms. J Gastrointest Surg. 2014;18(4):682–9.
30. Zhou NX, Chen JZ, Liu Q, Zhang X, Wang Z, Ren S, et al. Outcomes of pancreatoduodenectomy with robotic surgery versus open surgery. Int J Med Robot. 2011;7:131–7.
31. Buchs NC, Addeo P, Bianco FM, Ayloo S, Benedetti E, Giulianotti PC. Robotic versus open pancreaticoduodenectomy: a comparative study at a single institution. World J Surg. 2011;35(12):2739–46.
32. Correa-Gallego C, Dinkelspiel HE, Sulimanoff I, Fisher S, Viñuela EF, Kingham TP, Fong Y, DeMatteo RP, D'Angelica MI, Jarnagin WR, Allen. Minimally-invasive vs open pancreatico-duodenectomy: systematic review and meta-analysis. J Am Coll Surg. 2014;218(1):129–39.
33. Nigri G, Petrucciani N, La Torre M, Magistri P, Valabrega S, Aurello P, Ramacciato G. Duodenopancreatectomy: open or minimally invasive approach? Surgeon. 2014;12(4):227–34.
34. Birkmeyer JD, Finlayson SR, Tosteson AN, Sharp SM, Warshaw AL, Fisher ES. Effect of hospital volume on in-hospital mortality with pancreaticoduodenectomy. Surgery. 1999;125(3):250–6.
35. Kotwall CA, Maxwell JG, Brinker CC, Koch GG, Covington DL. National estimates of mortality rates for radical pancreaticoduodenectomy in 25,000 patients. Ann Surg Oncol. 2002;9(9):847–54.
36. Tseng JF, Pisters PW, Lee JE, Wang H, Gomez HF, Sun CC, Evans DB. The learning curve in pancreatic surgery. Surgery. 2007;141(4):456–63.
37. Schmidt CM, Turrini O, Parikh P, et al. Effect of hospital volume, surgeon experience, and surgeon volume on patient outcomes after pancreaticoduodenectomy: a single-institution experience. Arch Surg. 2010;145:634–40.
38. Boone BA, Zenati M, Hogg ME, Steve J, Moser AJ, Bartlett DL, Zeh HJ, Zureikat AH. Assessment of Quality Outcomes for Robotic Pancreaticoduodenectomy: Identification of the Learning Curve. JAMA Surg. 2015;11. doi: 10.1001/jamasurg.2015.17.

Chapter 49
Advanced Pancreatic Cancer Discovered at Operation: The Role of Palliative Bypass

Ajay V. Maker

Abstract For the patient with advanced pancreatic cancer discovered to be unresectable at exploration, treatment revolves around minimizing disease related symptoms. The current chapter considers the patient who is found at operation to be unresectable and compares single/double bypass to expectant management in regards to the outcomes of jaundice, gastric outlet obstruction (GOO), overall survival, morbidity, mortality, and quality of life.

The level I/II data that have evaluated this question are of moderate quality and do recommend bypass over surveillance, and in some cases, over endoscopic stenting, especially for patients who have a predicted survival of over 2–6 months. Recent retrospective series have not recommended palliative surgical bypass as a routine practice, for high-risk patients, or patients with metastatic disease that are not obstructed, but define situations where it may be advantageous. These studies contain a low to moderate quality of level III data with important sources of selection bias.

Review of published studies of all levels of data, and taking into account that cross-sectional imaging, patient selection, and endoscopic techniques, experience, and equipment have all markedly improved since early trials; we conclude that palliative bypass is reasonable, certainly not contraindicated, and may provide prolonged biliary and gastric luminal patency in the patient found to be unresectable at exploration. However, the decision to bypass the patient can be individualized based on the surgeon's assessment of multiple factors including patient condition, an estimation of the pace and biology of the disease, the endoscopic expertise available locally, assessment of the level of impending GOO pre-operatively and intra-operatively, and cancer stage/expected OS. It is perhaps reasonable, then, to perform a palliative surgical bypass in highly selected patients in good condition, with localized or minimal metastatic disease, symptoms of jaundice not already stented, or for symptomatic GOO.

A.V. Maker (✉)
Department of Surgery, Division of Surgical Oncology, Department of Microbiology and Immunology, University of Illinois at Chicago, 835 S. Wolcott Ave. MC790, Chicago, IL 60612, USA

Creticos Cancer Center, Advocate Illinois Masonic Medical Center, Chicago, IL, USA
e-mail: amaker@uic.edu

J.M. Millis, J.B. Matthews (eds.), *Difficult Decisions in Hepatobiliary and Pancreatic Surgery*, Difficult Decisions in Surgery: An Evidence-Based Approach, DOI 10.1007/978-3-319-27365-5_49

Keywords Pancreatic cancer • Periampullary cancer • Bypass • Palliative by pass • Quality of life • Bilioenteric by pass • Gastrojejunostomy • Hepatojejunostomy • Biliary stent • Duodenal stent

Introduction

For the patient with advanced pancreatic cancer discovered to be unresectable at exploration, treatment revolves around minimizing disease related symptoms. From a procedural perspective, and to enable patients to be acceptable candidates for systemic therapy, palliative maneuvers may include operative biliary or duodenal bypass, celiac plexus blockade, endoscopic stenting, or best supportive care ± tube decompression. Routine palliative bypass has been advocated for palliation of patients with periampullary tumors who were explored with curative intent but found to be locally advanced or to have metastatic disease. This practice was supported by a randomized controlled trial (RCT) published in 1999 randomizing 87 patients at a single institution to undergo a biliary bypass ± a gastrojejunostomy (GJ), and revealed that 19 % of patients that did not receive a GJ required an operation for gastric outlet obstruction prior to death [1]. On the other hand, in a contemporaneous large retrospective single institution series of patients found to be unresectable at laparoscopy and not bypassed, only 2 % of patients later required a palliative surgical biliary or duodenal bypass [2]. Since the time of these reports, cross-sectional imaging, patient selection, and endoscopic techniques, experience, and equipment have all markedly improved, resulting in a decrease in the practice of palliative bypass, even at the same institution as the original RCT [3]. In the absence of new randomized controlled trials, we are reliant on recent single institution retrospective level III data, systematic reviews, and meta-analyses to guide patient management. The current chapter considers the patient who is found at operation to be unresectable and compares single/double bypass to expectant management in regards to the outcomes of jaundice, gastric outlet obstruction (GOO), overall survival (OS), morbidity, mortality, and quality of life (QOL).

Search Strategy

A literature search of English language publications from 2000 to 2014 was used to identify published data on palliative bypass using the PICO outline (Table 49.1). Databases searched were PubMed, Embase, Science Citation Index/Social sciences Citation Index, and Cochrane Evidence Based Medicine. Terms used in the search were "pancreas cancer AND bypass." The search strategy within PubMed was further enhanced to retrieve citations identified as systematic reviews, meta-analyses, reviews of clinical trials, evidence-based medicine, consensus development conferences, guidelines, and citations to articles from journals specializing in review

Table 49.1 PICO grid

P (patients)	I (intervention)	C (comparator)	O (outcomes)
Patients with locally advanced, unresectable pancreatic cancer	Single/double bypass	Expectant management	Jaundice or gastroduodenal obstruction, morbidity/mortality, and quality of life (QOL)

studies of value to clinicians. This filter was used in a systematic search [sb]: (systematic review [ti] OR meta-analysis [pt] OR meta-analysis [ti] OR systematic literature review [ti] OR (systematic review [tiab] AND review [pt]) OR consensus development conference [pt] OR practice guideline [pt] OR cochrane database syst rev [ta] OR acp journal club [ta] OR health technol assess [ta] OR evid rep technol assess summ [ta] OR drug class reviews [ti]) OR (clinical guideline [tw] AND management [tw])OR ((evidence based [ti] OR evidence-based medicine [mh] OR best practice* [ti] OR evidence synthesis [tiab]) AND (review [pt] OR diseases category[mh] OR behavior and behavior mechanisms [mh] OR therapeutics [mh] OR evaluation studies[pt] OR validation studies[pt] OR guideline [pt] OR pmcbook)) OR ((systematic [tw] OR systematically [tw] OR critical [tiab] OR (study selection [tw]) OR (predetermined [tw] OR inclusion [tw] AND criteri* [tw]) OR exclusion criteri* [tw] OR main outcome measures [tw] OR standard of care [tw] OR standards of care [tw]) AND (survey [tiab] OR surveys [tiab] OR overview* [tw] OR review [tiab] OR reviews [tiab] OR search* [tw] OR handsearch [tw] OR analysis [ti] OR critique [tiab] OR appraisal [tw] OR (reduction [tw]AND (risk [mh] OR risk [tw]) AND (death OR recurrence))) AND (literature [tiab] OR articles [tiab] OR publications [tiab] OR publication [tiab] OR bibliography [tiab] OR bibliographies [tiab] OR published [tiab] OR unpublished [tw] OR citation [tw] OR citations [tw] OR database [tiab] OR internet [tiab] OR textbooks [tiab] OR references [tw] OR scales [tw] OR papers [tw] OR datasets [tw] OR trials [tiab] OR meta-analy* [tw] OR (clinical [tiab] AND studies [tiab]) OR treatment outcome [mh] OR treatment outcome [tw] OR pmcbook)) NOT (letter [pt] OR newspaper article [pt] OR comment [pt]). In addition to the articles identified through this strategy, additional studies were hand-picked from the search results in the various databases and references. Studies used in systematic reviews prior to 2000 were included in the analysis. The data was classified using the GRADE system.

Results

Overall Survival, Morbidity, and Mortality of Palliative Bypass Surgery

Huser and colleagues performed a systematic review of the literature in 2009 and identified three large retrospective studies of over 4,000 patients with unresectable pancreatic cancer, and determined that the OS of patients undergoing GJ was not significantly different from those not bypassed, ranging from 5.8 to 6.7 months [4–7]. In these series, the mortality of surgical bypass was not different than surveillance and ranged from 12 to 17 %. In a more recent retrospective analysis of 50 patients undergoing various palliative bypass procedures for unresectable pancreatic cancer, patients lived longer that did not receive a bypass (6.6 vs. 15.4 months) and experienced significantly lower post-operative morbidity (56 % vs. 19 %) [8]. This was similar to the 6 month OS observed retrospectively in 553 patients that underwent palliative bypass with a morbidity of 37 % and mortality of 1.6 % at Johns Hopkins [3]. An additional large series of 124 patients evaluated retrospectively at MSKCC experienced a median OS of 11 months after palliative bypass, with a morbidity of 12 %, compared to 0 % for laparotomy only patients. Similar to the Johns Hopkins series, mortality was 2 % [9].

Additional prospective studies have also been reported. Overall survival of surgical bilioenteric bypass (BEB) from a single institution RCT and a 5 RCT meta-analysis comparing BEB to biliary stenting was 6.5 and 4 months, respectively, with a morbidity of 29–39 % and mortality of ~14 % [10, 11]. The low OS and high mortality rate may be a function of the patient population in these studies that presented with biliary obstruction; however, the trends are similar to the bypass vs. surveillance studies. Three studies, 2 RCTs and a systematic review, evaluated patients undergoing BEB ± GJ [1, 4, 12–14]. There was no difference in OS (HR 1.02 (0.84–1.25)), morbidity (OR 1.0, $p=0.99$), or mortality (OR2.72 (0.35–14), RR2.4 (0.1–58)) between the groups with an OS of ~7–8 months, comparable to the retrospective studies, and morbidity of ~30 %. The largest single database study on the topic, an analysis of 1,126 patients with pancreatic cancer undergoing palliative bypass and documented in the ACS NSQIP participant user file, revealed similar morbidity of bypass at 29 % compared to 18 % without bypass, and a mortality of 6.5 % with bypass compared to 5 % without (Table 49.2).

Taken together, OS of palliative bypass ranges from 4 months in prospectively randomized biliary obstructed patients to 14.6 months in highly selected patients in a modern series evaluated retrospectively. When OS is compared between bypassed and non-bypassed patients in a randomized fashion and in meta-analysis, there appears to be no difference in survival. Therefore, patients that undergo palliative bypass have a poor prognosis with median OS likely less than a year that is not significantly improved with bypass.

The morbidity of bypass in retrospective series ranged from 12 to 56 %, with RCTs averaging ~30 %. Though retrospective series with selected patients revealed increased morbidity with surgical bypass over laparotomy, level II evidence showed no significant increase in complications when evaluating all-comers, e.g., not selecting only for obstructed patients at presentation. Mortality is not insignificant after bypass and appears greater than in the no bypass groups, though meta-analyses and the large NSQIP data set support similar mortality rates.

Table 49.2 Survival, morbidity and mortality of palliative bypass

Reference (author/year)	N = bypass	N = no bypass	OS bypass	OS surveillance	Morbidity with bypass	Morbidity without bypass	Mortality with bypass	Mortality without bypass
Retrospective series and database analysis								
Bartlett 2014	1,126				29 %	18 %	6.50 %	5 %
Spanheimer 2014	34	16	6.6	15.4*	56 %	19 %*		
Lyons 2012	124	33	11		12 %	0 %	2 %	0 %
Ausania 2012	50		14.6		50 %		4 %	
Kneuertz 2011	553		6		37 %		1.60 %	
Single institution randomized controlled trial								
Van Heeck 2003	36	29	7.2	8.4	31 %	28 %	9 %	
Lillemoe 1999	44	43	8.3	8.3	32 %	33 %		
Smith 1994	101 (HJ)	100 (stent)	6.5	5.25	29 %	11 %	14 %	3 %
Systematic review, meta-analysis, cochrane review								
Glazer 2014 (5 RCTs)	191 (HJ)	188 (stent)	4	4.3	39 % major	21 % major	15 %	12 %
Guruswamy 2010 (2 RCTs)	80	72	HR 1.02 (0.84–1.25)		NS		RR 2.4 (0.1–58)	
Huser 2009	124	94			OR1.0		OR 2.72 (0.35–14)	

OS median overall survival (months), *$p < 0.05$

Quality of Life After Bypass Surgery

Quality of life was not formally addressed in most of the studies on the subject, however, in a RCT comparing double bypass to HJ, there was no difference between the groups in the early post-operative period or in the month prior to death based on the Pan26 and EORTC-C30 QOL questionnaires [14]. In multiple trials, hospital stay was longer after bypass, and retrospective data revealed equivalent numbers of post-operative procedures required after bypass [4, 9]. Furthermore, in patients with GOO treated with a duodenal stent compared to bypass, though there was no difference in QOL, there was quicker return to per oral intake and an improvement in physical health with stenting as measured by the short-form 26 questionnaire ($p<0.01$) [15, 16].

Should We Perform a Biliary Bypass?

The data on prophylactic biliary bypass is difficult to determine clearly, as the enrollment of patients on these trials varies, and retrospective series include patients without obstruction, with impending obstruction, and with acute obstruction. Furthermore, some patients were already endoscopically stented prior to surgery. Most of the RCTs evaluating palliative bypass randomized to BEB ± GJ, thereby limiting the ability to determine the morbidity and mortality secondary to the BEB alone. The outcome most helpful, in this regard, is evaluation of jaundice after BEB (Table 49.3).

From retrospective single institution case series, in 34 patients that underwent a palliative operation that included a BEB, 14.3 % experienced recurrent biliary obstruction compared to 4 % in the 124 patient MSKCC experience, and 2.3 % in the 553 patient Johns Hopkins series [3, 8, 9]. Of the 33 patients not bypassed in the MSKCC experience, 36 % eventually encountered biliary obstruction. It is also important to note that in the Iowa series, the infectious complications of bypass were 21 % greater compared to laparotomy alone, and not-insignificant morbidity was experienced even with the addition of palliative cholecystectomy to the laparotomy.

Systematic reviews and RCTs have addressed groups randomized to BEB or endoscopic stenting. This may be a more useful measure of the success of BEB, especially since, in the main, the morbidity and mortality of stenting was not found to be different than surgery. The difference, however, lies in durability of the bypass. Smith et al. found a 7 % incidence of jaundice after bypass compared to 17 % with stenting, and Glazer et al., in a review of five RCTs, found a 29 % recurrence of jaundice with stenting compared to only 3.1 % after BEB (RR 0.14, $p=0.01$) [10, 11]. This was consistent with a systematic review of 24 RCTs, of which three focused on biliary bypass compared to plastic stenting [17]. As expected, there was no difference in the technical success of both procedures; however, the relative risk

Table 49.3 Risk of obstruction after bypass

Reference (author/year)	N=bypass	N=no bypass	Jaundice after bypass	Jaundice without bypass	GOO with bypass	GOO without bypass	Authors recommend bypass (Y/N)	Level of evidence	Grade
Retrospective series and database analysis									
Bartlett 2014	1,126						N, in high risk patients	II/III	Moderate quality
Spanheimer 2014	34	16	14.3 %		11 %	6.3 %	N	III	Low quality
Lyons 2012	124	33	4 %	36 %	1 %	29 %	N, unless asymptomatic and no access to medical care, or if impending obstruction	III	Low quality
Ausania 2012	50						Only in specialized centers	III	Low quality
Kneuertz 2011	553		2.3 %		3.10 %		N, if have metastatic disease and not obstructed	III	Low quality
Single institution randomized controlled trial									
Van Heeck 2003	36	29			5.5 %	41 %	Y	I/II	Moderate quality
Lillemoe 1999	44	43			0	19 %	Y	I/II	Moderate quality
Smith 1994	101 (HJ)	100 (stent)	7 %	17 %	36 %	2 %	Bypass and stenting are both effective	I/II	Moderate quality
Systematic review, meta-analysis, cochrane review									
Glazer 2014 (5 RCTs)	191 (HJ)	188 (stent)	3.1 % RR 0.14 p=0.01	29 %			Y, if survival >months	II	Moderate quality

(continued)

Table 49.3 (continued)

Reference (author/ year)	N = bypass	N = no bypass	Jaundice after bypass	Jaundice without bypass	GOO with bypass	GOO without bypass	Authors recommend bypass (Y/N)	Level of evidence	Grade
Guruswamy 2010 (2 RCTs)	80	72			2.5 % RR 0.1 ($p < 0.01$)	28 %	Y	I/II	Moderate quality
Huser 2009	124	94			OR 0.06 (0.02–0.21) $p < 0.001$		Y	III	Moderate quality
Moss 2007	153 (HJ)	153 (stent)	RR 18.59*				N	II	Moderate quality

GOO gastric outlet obstruction, *HJ* hepatojejunostomy/biliary bypass

*$p<0.05$

of jaundice after stenting was 18.6 times greater than after surgical bypass. It should be noted, though, that in the same review, seven RCTs compared plastic stents to metal stents, and found metal stents to have significantly improved patency compared to plastic stents at both 4 months after the procedure and prior to death. Therefore, it can be inferred that the modern day risk of recurrent biliary obstruction after stenting with self-expanding metallic stents is less than published in this study. Based on contemporary series, it appears that when recurrent biliary obstruction does occur, it is treated endoscopically 82 % of the time in previously stented patients and 75 % of the time in previously bypassed patients. In bypassed patients, repeat surgery is performed <1 % of the time and medical management is utilized 25 % of the time [10]. This highlights the point that recurrent biliary obstruction is likely a symptom of aggressive tumor biology and progressive disease where obviating biliary obstruction may not impact OS, though this was not addressed in these trials.

Evidently, surgical BEB appears to be a more robust solution to biliary obstruction and is more durable than stenting without significant addition of morbidity to laparotomy alone, however, it may not affect the number of post-operative treatments needed for the patient globally, and in the majority of cases, biliary obstruction can be relieved with rescue or repeat endoscopy.

Should We Perform a Duodenal Bypass?

The landmark RCT addressing this question randomized patients to BEB ± GJ and found no recurrent obstruction in the surgical group and 19 % gastric outlet obstruction (GOO) in the non-bypass group [1]. This was supported by a later RCT revealing 5.5 % GOO in the GJ bypass group compared to 41 % in the non-bypassed group [14]. A Cochrane review of the two trials established a RR of GOO of 0.1 ($p<0.01$) with GJ [12]. A meta-analysis by Huser et al. included these two RCTs in addition to a prospective study by Shyr et al., determining an OR of 0.06 (0.02–0.21, $p<0.001$) for GOO in bypassed patients [4, 13]. More recent retrospective analyses have both supported and refuted these findings, showing a 5 % increase in procedures required for GOO after bypass compared to laparotomy alone in one study, yet a 28 % increase in non-bypassed patients in another (Table 49.3) [8, 9].

To directly address this question in the modern era, one can evaluate trials that compare surgical bypass to duodenal stenting, which is the non-invasive rescue strategy for non-bypassed patients that choose bypass over palliative decompression or supportive care. Though the total number of patients is small, the SUSTENT RCT compared 18 patients undergoing surgical GJ to 21 patients receiving a duodenal stent for GOO [15]. There was no difference in OS, stented patients had a more rapid return of per oral intake, and recurrent GOO was over four times more prevalent in the stented patients. These findings were recapitulated in another small RCT where one of three patients with a GJ experienced recurrent GOO compared to five of ten patients in the duodenal stent group [16].

Should We Perform an R2 Resection as the Bypass?

The question of whether an R2 resection, as opposed to an attempted R0 or R1 resection for locally advanced cancer [18], may offer advantages over palliative bypass was addressed by systematic review of four cohort studies consisting of 261 patients in the bypass group and 138 patients in the palliative resection group [19]. This is an interesting group of patients to study since attempted aggressive resections for locally advanced lesions may impart a survival advantage even if an R1 resection results [20]. Overall survival was quite heterogeneous, but pooled median survival time was 6.7 months in the bypassed patients compared to 8.2 months in the resected patients. Morbidity and mortality were increased in the R2 resected group with pooled risk ratios of 1.75 (1.35–2.26) and 2.98 (1.31–6.75), respectively. The authors concluded that purposeful R2 resection was not supported by the data available.

Recommendations Based on the Data

Recent retrospective series have not recommended palliative surgical bypass as a routine practice [8, 9], for high-risk patients [21] or patients with metastatic disease that are not obstructed [3], but define situations where it may be advantageous, including in asymptomatic patients without access to medical care, with impending obstruction [9], or in specialized medical centers that treat pancreatic diseases [22]. These studies contain a low to moderate quality of level III data with important sources of selection bias. The level I/II RCT data that have evaluated this question do recommend bypass over surveillance, and in some cases, over endoscopic stenting, especially for patients who have a predicted survival of over 2–6 months [1, 4, 10, 12–15, 19]. These studies contain a moderate quality of data. Based on the available data, palliative bypass is recommended (weak) in the patient found to be unresectable at exploration.

A Personal View of the Data

Palliative surgical bypass may not significantly improve OS or QOL and offers improved luminal patency at the expense of increased hospital stay, complications, and in some studies, mortality, without decreasing the total number of post-operative procedures required, or the ability to perform rescue endoscopic stenting. Furthermore, the majority of the sentinel RCTs used in the systematic reviews were performed in an era before advanced endoscopic materials and experience were readily utilized, and critically, before high-resolution cross-sectional imaging and the widespread use of neoadjuvant therapy for borderline locally advanced pancreatic cancers were employed; both of which have aided in the selection of patients for exploration. Additionally, the data on surgical bypass compared to surveillance is skewed since there are no randomized trials of surgical intervention compared to best available chemotherapy ± radiation, palliative or hospice care, nor will there ever likely be. Therefore, there is inherent bias the retrospective studies as a large number of the patients that underwent intervention were likely already obstructed, and even in the prospective studies evaluated, obstructed patients were chosen for bypass, perhaps selecting for larger or more aggressive tumors.

Most of the studies evaluated the utility of GJ bypass and not HJ. Currently, if the patient is already significantly jaundiced upon presentation, then they will likely receive a preoperative stent. On the other hand, if the patient proceeds directly to operation, then it is reasonable to perform a biliary bypass at the time given the increased patency rate. The question of how to manage the stented patient at the time of surgery remains to be addressed in a clinical trial, though one would likely exclude patients found to have metastatic disease, and it would be difficult to randomize a completely asymptomatic patient to a procedure that carries increased morbidity and, specifically, infectious complications. Part of the concern for percutaneous drainage in the past was that it used to be permanent and a continued nidus for infection seeding the biliary tree both from the gastrointestinal tract and from the skin, however, now these drains are often able to internalized.

Surgical bypass may be more durable, however, in an era where we have not only improved endoscopic techniques, but improved systemic and local palliative measures, clinical trials need to be performed evaluating OS in non-obstructed patients randomized at laparotomy to bypass or endoscopic treatment when symptomatic, especially since there are no robust studies on the role of palliative bypass compared to endoscopic stenting [23]. In light of historical data from MSKCC that found that only 2 % of all patients who were found to have unresectable pancreatic cancer needed a subsequent bypass operation, universal application of palliative bypass may be subjecting patients who will not experience malignant obstruction to unnecessary morbidity [2].

What if palliative operative bypass delays the time to palliative chemotherapy, which is the only intervention that may increase OS, and in some cases, improve QOL? This is a possibility since bypass patients appear to require additional hospital days, may have an increased incidence of delayed gastric emptying, and in recent retrospective series, experienced increased morbidity [8, 9, 14, 21]. With improved chemotherapy regimens, radiation planning, and endoluminal stents, patients may succumb to metastatic disease before obstruction. Furthermore, by the time these patients obstruct, they may be physically deconditioned and less able to tolerate laparotomy and an anastomosis.

Based on the available data, palliative bypass is reasonable, certainly not contraindicated, and may provide prolonged biliary and gastric luminal patency in the patient found to be unresectable at exploration. However, the available tools and the management of these patients has evolved and the decision to bypass the patient can be individualized based on the surgeon's assessment of multiple factors including patient condition, an estimation of the pace and biology of the disease, the endoscopic expertise available locally, assessment of the level of impending GOO pre-operatively and intra-operatively, and cancer stage/expected OS. It is perhaps reasonable, then, to perform a palliative surgical bypass in highly selected patients in good condition, with localized or minimal metastatic disease, symptoms of jaundice not already stented, or for symptomatic GOO.

Recommendations

1. Based on the available data, palliative bypass is recommended in the patient found to be unresectable at exploration (evidence quality moderate; weak recommendation)
2. It is reasonable to perform a palliative surgical bypass at exploration in highly selected patients in good condition, with localized or minimal metastatic disease, symptoms of jaundice not already stented, or for symptomatic GOO (evidence quality very low, very weak recommendation)

References

1. Lillemoe KD, Cameron JL, Hardacre JM, et al. Is prophylactic gastrojejunostomy indicated for unresectable periampullary cancer? – A prospective randomized trial. Ann Surg. 1999;230:322–30.
2. Espat NJ, Brennan MF, Conlon KC. Patients with laparoscopically staged unresectable pancreatic adenocarcinoma do not require subsequent surgical biliary or gastric bypass. J Am Coll Surg. 1999;10:649–57.
3. Kneuertz PJ, Cunningham SC, Cameron JL, et al. Palliative surgical management of patients with unresectable pancreatic adenocarcinoma: trends and lessons learned from a large, single institution experience. J Gastrointest Surg. 2011;15:1917–27.
4. Huser N, Michalski CW, Schuster T, Friess H, Kleeff J. Systematic review and meta-analysis of prophylactic gastroenterostomy for unresectable advanced pancreatic cancer. Br J Surg. 2009;96:711–9.
5. Sarr MG, Cameron JL. Surgical palliation of unresectable carcinoma of the pancreas. World J Surg. 1984;8:906–18.
6. Watanapa P, Williamson RCN. Surgical palliation for pancreatic cancer: developments during the past two decades. Br J Surg. 1992;79:8–20.
7. Sarr MG, Cameron JL. Surgical management of unresectable carcinoma of the pancreas. Surgery. 1982;91:123–33.
8. Spanheimer PM, Cyr AR, Liao J, et al. Complications and survival associated with operative procedures in patients with unresectable pancreatic head adenocarcinoma. J Surg Oncol. 2014;109:697–701.
9. Lyons JM, Karkar A, Correa-Gallego CC, et al. Operative procedures for unresectable pancreatic cancer: does operative bypass decrease requirements for postoperative procedures and in-hospital days? HPB (Oxf). 2012;14:469–75.
10. Glazer ES, Hornbrook MC, Krouse RS. A meta-analysis of randomized trials: immediate stent placement vs. surgical bypass in the palliative management of malignant biliary obstruction. J Pain Symptom Manage. 2014;47:307–14.

11. Smith AC, Dowsett JF, Russell RCG, Hatfield ARW, Cotton PB. Randomised trial of endoscopic stenting versus surgical bypass in malignant low bileduct obstruction. Lancet. 1994;344:1655–60.
12. Gurusamy KS, Kumar S, Davidson BR. Prophylactic gastrojejunostomy for unresectable periampullary carcinoma. Cochrane Database Syst Rev. 2010;2:CD008533.
13. Shyr YM, Su CH, Wu CW, Lui WY. Prospective study of gastric outlet obstruction in unresectable periampullary adenocarcinoma. World J Surg. 2000;24:60–5.
14. Van Heek NT, De Castro SMM, Van Eijck CH, et al. The need for a prophylactic gastrojejunostomy for unresectable periampullary cancer: a prospective randomized multicenter trial with special focus on assessment of quality of life. Ann Surg. 2003;238:894–905.
15. Jeurnink SM, van Eijck CHJ, Steyerberg EW, Kuipers EJ, Siersema PD. Stent versus gastrojejunostomy for the palliation of gastric outlet obstruction: a systematic review. BMC Gastroenterol. 2007;7:18.
16. Mehta S, Hindmarsh A, Cheong E, et al. Prospective randomized trial of laparoscopic gastrojejunostomy versus duodenal stenting for malignant gastric outflow obstruction. Surg Endosc. 2006;20:239–42.
17. Moss AC, Morris E, Mac Mathuna P. Palliative biliary stents for obstructing pancreatic carcinoma. Cochrane Database Syst Rev. 2006;63:986–95. DOI: 10.1002/14651858.CD004200.pub4
18. Gurusamy KS, Kumar S, Davidson BR, Fusai G. Resection versus other treatments for locally advanced pancreatic cancer. Cochrane Database Syst Rev. 2014;2:CD010244.
19. Gillen S, Schuster T, Friess H, Kleeff J. Palliative resections versus palliative bypass procedures in pancreatic cancer – a systematic review. Am J Surg. 2012;203:496–502.
20. Tseng JF, Raut CP, Lee JE, et al. Pancreaticoduodenectomy with vascular resection: margin status and survival duration. J Gastrointest Surg. 2004;8:935–49. discussion 49–50.
21. Bartlett EK, Wachtel H, Fraker DL, et al. Surgical palliation for pancreatic malignancy: practice patterns and predictors of morbidity and mortality. J Gastrointest Surg. 2014;18:1292–8.
22. Ausania F, Vallance AE, Manas DM, et al. Double bypass for inoperable pancreatic malignancy at laparotomy: postoperative complications and long-term outcome. Ann R Coll Surg Engl. 2012;94:563–8.
23. Mann CD, Thomasset SC, Johnson NA, et al. Combined biliary and gastric bypass procedures as effective palliation for unresectable malignant disease. ANZ J Surg. 2009;79:471–5.

Chapter 50
Neoadjuvant Therapy for Borderline Resectable Pancreatic Head Cancer

Susan M. Sharpe and Mark S. Talamonti

Abstract Borderline resectable pancreatic head cancer represents a relatively new classification for patients with intermediate tumors between those that are well-localized with no radiographic evidence of significant mesenteric vascular involvement and those considered to have locally advanced and technically unresectable disease based on the inability to safely perform a vascular resection and reconstruction of the vital blood vessels. These tumors can be removed but are likely to require major vascular resection and reconstruction and the incidence of margin-positive resections is high. Clinical trials with adjuvant therapy after resection of pancreatic head cancers have demonstrated survival benefits for multi-modality therapy compared to surgery alone. Because of the high likelihood of a margin-positive resection, neoadjuvant strategies employing chemotherapy with and without radiation therapy have been used in single institution or limited clinical trials. Biologic considerations and clinical justifications exist to support this approach, but to date, there are no sufficiently powered randomized clinical trials that demonstrate significant improvements in local control rates, disease-free survival and overall survival rates compared to a surgery-first approach. Clinical trials employing novel chemotherapy combinations and modified radiation approaches are underway and may provide more definitive evidence in the near future.

Keywords Neoadjuvant therapy • Borderline resectable • Pancreatic cancer • Chemoradiation • Clinical trials

S.M. Sharpe
Division of Surgical Oncology, Department of Surgery,
University of Chicago Pritzker School of Medicine, Chicago, IL, USA

M.S. Talamonti (✉)
Department of Surgery, NorthShore University Health System,
2650 Ridge Ave., Evanston, IL 60201, USA
e-mail: mtalamonti@northshore.org

J.M. Millis, J.B. Matthews (eds.), *Difficult Decisions in Hepatobiliary and Pancreatic Surgery*, Difficult Decisions in Surgery: An Evidence-Based Approach, DOI 10.1007/978-3-319-27365-5_50

Introduction

Borderline resectable pancreatic head cancer represents a relatively new classification for patients with intermediate tumors between those that are well-localized with no radiographic evidence of significant mesenteric vascular involvement and those considered to have locally advanced and technically unresectable disease based on the inability to safely perform a vascular resection and reconstruction of the vital blood vessels. Traditional clinical and radiographic classifications of pancreatic head tumors have consisted of localized cancer with no evidence of metastatic disease and no evidence of mesenteric venous or arterial involvement, locally advanced disease in which there is no evidence of metastatic disease but the extent of vascular involvement was thought to preclude a safe and complete resection of local disease, and finally, patients with clear evidence of peritoneal or visceral metastases. With advances in three-dimensional imaging and improved operative techniques resulting in decreased morbidity and mortality of superior mesenteric/portal venous resections (SMV/PV) and limited arterial resections, the term "borderline resectable pancreatic cancer" has evolved. Surgical resection of these tumors is likely to require major vascular resection and reconstruction and oftentimes these vascular resection margins will demonstrate microscopic extension to within a millimeter of the transection (R1 resections). Whether the patient with a borderline resectable tumor should undergo a surgery-first approach, followed by adjuvant therapies, versus a neoadjuvant course of combined modality therapy preceding an attempt at surgical resection is currently one of the most controversial topics in pancreatic surgery. Because of the high likelihood of a margin-positive resection and the potential for early tumor recurrence, neoadjuvant strategies employing chemotherapy with and without radiation therapy have been used in an attempt to "down-stage" tumors to margin-negative resections and to biologically select those patients who develop progressive disease while on neoadjuvant therapy and can then be spared the morbidity of surgery. Furthermore, large randomized clinical trials in the United States and Europe have demonstrated survival benefits for multi-modality therapy compared to surgery alone for resected cancers. While not specifically designed to address the issue of treatment sequencing for borderline resectable tumors, combined modality therapy for resectable pancreatic cancer has become the current standard of care. The theoretical advantages of a neoadjuvant approach to these high-risk borderline tumors are rational and logical; however, the potential increase in operative complications and the delay in surgical resection and subsequent adjuvant treatments are legitimate concerns and have served to heighten the current controversy. This chapter describes the current radiographic definition of borderline resectable pancreatic head cancer, outlines the potential benefits of a neoadjuvant strategy for these tumors, and reviews the results of existing series and trials employing neoadjuvant therapy relative to post-operative therapy.

Search Strategy

A computerized literature search of English language publications from 2000 to 2014 was done to identify published data on neoadjuvant therapy for borderline resectable pancreatic head cancers using the PICO outline (Table 50.1). Databases searched were PubMed, Embase, and Cochrane Evidence Based Medicine. The searches were done using the following terms: "borderline resectable pancreatic cancer," "locally advanced pancreatic cancer," "neoadjuvant therapy," "neoadjuvant chemotherapy," "neoadjuvant chemoradiation," "adjuvant therapy," "pancreatic cancer," "pancreatic ductal adenocarcinoma." A summary table was crafted and each publication was graded by the authors following the Grading Recommendations Assessment, Development, and Evaluation guidelines (GRADE system).

Results

Radiographic Staging and Definition of Borderline Resectable Pancreatic Head Cancer

It is important to emphasize the borderline resectable classification is a radiographic determination using precise three-dimensional imaging and applying defined criteria to categorize the extent of mesenteric and portal venous and arterial involvement [1]. Early studies on neoadjuvant therapy for resectable cancers were flawed by the use of suboptimal scanning technology and limited vascular imaging. More recent studies are limited by the lack of a universally accepted definition of borderline resectable cancer [1]. Two major definitions have been proposed. The MD Anderson anatomic definition differs from that proposed by the American Hepato-Pancreatico-Biliary Association (AHPBA), Society of Surgical Oncology (SSO), and Society for Surgery of the Alimentary Tract (SSAT) in terms of mesenteric vein involvement [2]. Minimal abutment without distortion of the SMV or PV is considered potentially resectable in the MD Anderson criteria while the AHPBA/SSO/SSAT definition considers any vein involvement that may require even a small vein resection as borderline resectable. The International Study Group of Pancreatic Surgery

Table 50.1 PICO table

P (Patients)	I (Intervention)	C (Comparator)	O (Outcome)
Pancreatic cancer of the head	Neoadjuvant chemotherapy	Surgery + adjuvant chemotherapy	Down-staging
Borderline resectable	Neoadjuvant chemoradiation		Morbidity
			Mortality
			Delay to adjuvant chemotherapy
			Overall survival

(ISGPS) recently published a consensus statement to address these differences on the definition and subsequent treatment recommendations for borderline resectable cancers [3]. In an attempt to reconcile these subtle but important differences and to underscore the importance of accurate assessment of arterial involvement, the ISGPS has recommended the adoption of the following definitions when reporting institutional series outcomes and when designing future clinical trials.

- Determination of borderline resectability should be done using a specialized pancreatic protocol and a multidetector CT with high-resolution, multiplanar reconstructions.
- The radiographic findings supporting the designation of a borderline tumor in the head of the pancreas are: venous distortion of the SMV/portal venous axis even including short-segment venous occlusion with proximal and distal sufficient vessel length allowing safe reconstruction; encasement of the gastroduodenal artery up to the hepatic artery, with either short-segment encasement or direct abutment of the hepatic artery without extension to the celiac axis; and tumor abutment of the SMA but with no greater than 180° of the vessel wall circumference.

Failure to apply these definitions or the lack of stated inclusion criteria compromise many of the neoadjuvant series. Heterogeneous patient groups likely included localized tumors and locally advanced, unresectable lesions. Retrospectively analyzing the groups to find the subset of patients with borderline resectable tumors is questionable and further diminishes the strength of the evidence. More recent series have reported findings for better defined and more carefully selected patients and should form the basis for comparisons to standard surgery-first strategies [4]. Ongoing clinical trials now use these definitions and patients are deemed borderline resectable and included in the study group only after central review of the CT scans.

Rationale and Current Evidence for Neoadjuvant Therapy for Borderline Resectable Disease

Clinical trials examining combined modality therapy for resected pancreatic cancer were justified given the high risk of systemic and locoregional recurrence following surgery alone. Early clinical trials of adjuvant therapy for resected patients were limited by their small size, lack of standardized patient entry criteria, and less than rigorous quality controls [5]. Over the past decade, several adjuvant therapy trials were completed and have established a survival benefit for combined therapy versus surgery alone. The ESPAC-1 study, while criticized for its enrollment criteria, analytical design, and radiation therapy techniques, concluded that adjuvant chemotherapy with 5-FU administered for 6 months offered an overall survival advantage over no post-surgical therapy. Excluding patients who received any radiation, the patients receiving adjuvant chemotherapy alone had a median survival of 21.6 months compared to 16.9 months for the observation group [6]. An important modern adjuvant therapy study, noteworthy for its rigorous trial design, is the CONKO-001 trial, which compared six cycles of gemcitabine to observation alone after surgery in 354 patients [7]. Disease-free survival and overall survival were 6.9 months and 20.5 months for the observation arm and 13.4 months ($p<0.001$) and 24.2 ($p<0.06$) months for the treatment arm. After the initial publication of this trial, gemcitabine became an accepted and standard recommendation for adjuvant therapy. The Radiation Therapy Oncology Group (RTOG) 97.04 study examined the role of adjuvant chemotherapy combined with modern radiation planning and stringent treatment quality controls. A 5-year update of the trial reported by Regine et al. demonstrated a trend toward improved survival ($p=0.08$) for those patients receiving adjuvant gemcitabine versus conventional 5-FU [8]. More importantly, and more relevant to the current discussion of borderline tumors, the local failure rates were 25 % for the gemcitabine arm and 30 % for the 5-FU arm; both markedly improved from earlier studies using lower doses of radiation and without contemporary three-dimensional image planning, and data used to justify the inclusion of radiation therapy in most series examining neoadjuvant therapy for borderline tumors at high risk for local recurrence. Finally, Johns Hopkins University and Mayo Clinic recently reported large series of patients who had undergone surgical resection for pancreatic cancer and received postoperative 5-FU-based chemoradiation with a median dose of 50.4 Gy [9, 10]. Both series found chemoradiation associated with improved survival and increased locoregional control compared to surgery alone. While these adjuvant trials and large institutional series do not specifically address borderline resectable cancers, collectively they provide justification to employ combined modality therapy for these high-risk tumors and serve as high quality standards for comparison purposes.

There are several theoretical and potential advantages of neoadjuvant therapy for borderline resectable disease [11]. These include the potential to decrease tumor volume such that borderline resectable disease may become more easily resectable and to sterilize the peripheral extent of tumor infiltration, resulting in fewer R1 resections and reducing locoregional recurrences. Patients who receive neoadjuvant therapy may be more likely to complete the full course of treatments since 20–30 % of patients undergoing resection may not complete adjuvant treatments due to postoperative morbidity and frailty [9, 10]. Lastly, and perhaps most importantly, patients who exhibit disease progression during neoadjuvant therapy self-select themselves as poor responders who are least likely to gain benefit from resection and may forgo the morbidity of pancreatic resection.

Despite these biologic considerations and clinical justifications, to date, there are no sufficiently powered randomized clinical trials that demonstrate significant improvements in local control rates or disease-free survival and overall survival rates for neoadjuvant therapy for resectable or borderline resectable cancers compared to a surgery-first approach. Retrospective single institution series or reviews of combined centers' experiences have similar design issues and statistical limitations that diminish the GRADE of their conclusions and recommendations (Table 50.2). Patients were not randomized to a surgery-first versus neoadjuvant strategy, thereby interjecting obvious selection bias in any group comparisons. The determination of borderline resectable status was often done retrospectively using poorly defined or inconsistent criteria but clearly including patients ranging from localized disease to minimal venous distortion to those with significant arterial abutment and partial encasement. Neoadjuvant treatments were variable and not controlled for the use of radiation. Early studies employed 5-FU-based protocols while more recent investigations either added or replaced 5-FU with gemcitabine [11]. Surgical techniques for vascular resection and reconstruction and the dissection of the critical uncinate margin on the right lateral wall of the superior mesenteric artery are not reported or not standardized. And the currently recommended guidelines for standard pathology handling of the specimens and critical margin determinations were not performed or poorly documented [3, 4].

Prospective trials analyzing only patients with borderline resectable pancreas cancer are rare and limited by extremely small patient numbers, inconsistent inclusion criteria, and short follow-up times. The safest conclusions from these trials are that neoadjuvant therapy was relatively safe and associated with acceptable resection rates. Follow-up times are short, survival data are inconsistently reported, and conclusions regarding the effects on median survival and overall survival cannot be consistently determined. Marti et al. reported a phase I/II trial of induction gemcitabine and cisplatin followed by concurrent radiation in borderline resectable disease with 4 of 26 patients (15 %) undergoing resection [12]. Median survival was 13 months. A randomized phase II trial comparing two different gemcitabine-based protocols in borderline resectable disease was terminated early due to poor accrual, but toxicities were considered acceptable and 5 of 21 patients (24 %) underwent resection [13]. Kim et al. reported a recent multi-institutional phase II trial using full dose gemcitabine, oxaliplatin, and radiation, and included 39 patients with borderline resectable disease. The overall resection rate was 63 % and the R0 resection rate was 53 % in the borderline resectable group [14]. Based on the small size of the study populations, the variability in treatment schemes and the relatively short follow-up times of the phase II trials for neoadjuvant therapy for borderline resectable tumors, the quality of this line of evidence would have to be considered very low-to-low.

Single institution reports represent by far the largest number of reports examining neoadjuvant therapy for borderline resectable cancers. In the largest, 84 patients with anatomically borderline resectable tumors were treated at MD Anderson with 5-FU- or gemcitabine-based chemoradiation, typically preceded by systemic chemotherapy prior to planned resection [15]. Of this group, 38 % underwent resection and 97 % of these had R0 resections. The median survival of all patients was 21 months: 40 months for resected patients and 15 months for patients who did not undergo resection [15]. Patel et al. prospectively examined 17 patients with borderline disease treated with gemcitabine-docetaxel-capecitabine induction chemotherapy and 5-FU-based chemoradiation. Resections were successful in 64 % and 89 % had an R0 resection [16]. Stokes et al. prospectively examined 40 borderline resectable cases treated with capecitabine and concurrent radiation. The resection rate was 40 %, the R0 resection rate was 88 % and the reported median survival was 23 months [17]. McClain et al. reported 26 borderline resectable patients treated at

Table 50.2 Neoadjuvant therapy for borderline resectable pancreatic cancer

Author	Year	Journal	Study type	Conclusion	Quality of evidence
Sultana et al.	2014 [22]	Cochrane Database of Systematic Reviews	Systematic review of cohort studies	Protocol stage	Very low
Tempero et al.	2014 [21]	J Natl Compr Canc Netw	Review of cohort studies	Neoadjuvant therapy increases R0 rate	Low
Sen et al.	2014 [23]	Clin Oncol (R Coll Radiol)	Systematic review of cohort studies	None	Very low
Tsvetkova et al.	2014 [24]	Curr Oncol	Systematic review of cohort studies	Recommend neoadjuvant CT	Very low
Bittoni et al.	2014 [25]	Gastroenterol Res Pract	Review of cohort studies	Neoadjuvant CT may downsize tumors, become resectable, increase R0 rate, identify subgroups with early progression	Very low
Bockhorn et al.	2014 [3]	Surgery	Consensus statement: Systematic review of cohort studies	Neoadjuvant treatment may have a favorable outcome in the future	Very low
Cooper et al.	2014 [26]	J Amr Coll Surg	Single institutional retrospective review	Role for neoadjuvant CT in elderly	Very low
Papavasiliou et al.	2014 [27]	HPB (Oxford)	Single institutional retrospective review	Neoadjuvant CRT increases DFS	Very low
Motoi et al.	2013 [28]	Ann Surg Oncol	Multi-institutional prospective cohort study	Neoadjuvant CT is safe and well-tolerated	Low
Oettle et al.	2013 [7]	JAMA	Randomized controlled clinical trial	Increased DFS & OS with adjuvant gemcitabine	High
Heinemann et al.	2013 [29]	Ann Oncol	Review of cohort studies	Neoadjuvant CT increases R0 rate	Very low
Belli et al.	2013 [30]	Cancer Treat Rev	Systematic review of cohort studies	None (too little data)	Very low
Kim et al.	2013 [14]	Cancer	Prospective cohort study	Neoadjuvant CT is feasible, high number of R0 rate	Low
Papavasiliou et al.	2013 [31]	Surg Clin North Am	Review of cohort studies	None: data lacking	Very low
Paulson et al.	2013 [32]	Gastroenterology	Review of cohort studies	None: data lacking	Very low

(continued)

Table 50.2 (continued)

Author	Year	Journal	Study type	Conclusion	Quality of evidence
Tsuruga et al.	2013 [33]	World J Gastroenterol	Case report	Suspect association between portal venous stenosis and neoadjuvant CRT	Very low
Galindo et al.	2013 [34]	World J Surg Oncol	Case report	Neoadjuvant downstages, enables R0	Very low
Katz et al.	2012 [4]	J Am Coll Surg	Case report	Vascular resection with pancreaticoduodenectomy can be performed safely	Very low
Chatterjee et al.	2012 [35]	Cancer	Single institutional retrospective review	Increase in OS with ypCR than Stage I/II s/p neoadjuvant CRT + surgery	Low
Wolff	2012 [36]	Curr Drug Targets	Review of cohort studies	Neoadjuvant therapy increases R0 rate, identifies patients who will benefit from surgery	Very low
Satoi et al.	2012 [37]	J Gastrointest Surg	Single institution comparative prospective cohort	Neoadjuvant CRT increases R0 rate, decreases nodal metastases	Moderate
Lim et al.	2012 [38]	Oncologist	Review of cohort studies	Neoadjuvant therapy downstages, increases R0 rate	Very low
Zhao et al.	2012 [39]	Ann Diagn Pathol	Single institutional retrospective review	Increases OS with ypCR than Stage I/II s/p neoadjuvant CRT + surgery	Very low
Estrella et al.	2012 [40]	Cancer	Single institutional retrospective review	Post-therapy tumor staging after neoadjuvant therapy is a prognostic factor in OS; increases OS and decreases nodal metastases with neoadjuvant CT/CRT	Low
Laurence et al.	2011 [20]	J Gastrointest Surg	Systematic review of prospective cohort studies; meta-analysis	Neoadjuvant CRT increased R0 rate	Low
Assifi et al.	2011 [19]	Surgery	Systematic review of prospective cohort studies; meta-analysis	Neoadjuvant therapy may downstage patients to resectable	Low
Patel et al.	2011 [16]	J Surg Oncol	Prospective cohort study	Neoadjuvant CRT may improve R0 rate	Very low

Takahashi et al.	2011 [41]	J Hepatobiliary Pancreat Sci	Single institutional retrospective review	Recommend neoadjuvant CT	Low
Palta et al.	2011 [42]	Oncologist (Williston Park)	Review of cohort studies	Neoadjuvant CRT has potential advantages	Very low
Regine et al.	2011 [8]	Ann Surg Oncol	Randomized controlled clinical trial	Pre-and post-CRT with gemcitabine did not improve OS compared to 5-FU	High
Stokes et al.	2011 [17]	Ann Surg Oncol	Single institutional retrospective review, not all borderline	Neoadjuvant CT identifies subgroup that benefits from resection	Very low
van Tienhoven et al.	2011 [43]	Ther Adv Med Oncol	Review of cohort studies	Potential benefit of neoadjuvant CT	Very low
Katz et al.	2010 [44]	Oncologist	Review of cohort studies	Recommend neoadjuvant CT	Very low
Brunner and Scott-Brown	2010 [45]	Radiat Oncol	Systematic review of cohort studies	None	Very low
Landry et al.	2010 [13]	J Surg Oncol	Prospective cohort study	Neoadjuvant CT is a tolerable regimen	Low
Gillen et al.	2010 [46]	PLoS Med	Systematic review of cohort studies	Neoadjuvant CT should be given on protocol	Very low
Abbott et al.	2010 [11]	J Surg Oncol	Review of cohort studies	Neoadjuvant CRT is well-tolerated with improved survival	Very low
McClaine et al.	2010 [18]	HPB (Oxford)	Single institutional retrospective review	Similar R0 and OS to resectable	Low
Morganti et al.	2010 [47]	Ann Surg Oncol	Systematic review of cohort studies	Recommend neoadjuvant CRT for locally advanced, high R0 rate	Very low
Callery et al.	2009 [1]	Ann Surg Oncol	Expert consensus	Definition of borderline resectable tumors	Very low
Satoi et al.	2009 [48]	Pancreas	Single institutional comparative prospective cohort	Neoadjuvant CRT increases R0 rate and decreases nodal metastases	Low
Crane et al.	2009 [49]	Cancer Radiother	Review of cohort studies	Recommend neoadjuvant CT	Very low
Marti et al.	2008 [12]	Ann Surg Oncol	Prospective cohort study	Neoadjuvant CRT is well-tolerated	Moderate

(continued)

Table 50.2 (continued)

Author	Year	Journal	Study type	Conclusion	Quality of evidence
Varadhachary et al.	2008 [50]	J Clin Oncol	Prospective cohort study	Neoadjuvant gemcitabine-RT basis for future studies	Moderate
Evans et al.	2008 [51]	J Clin Oncol	Prospective cohort study	Neoadjuvant gemcitabine-radiation identifies patients who will benefit from surgery	Moderate
Herman et al.	2008 [9]	J Clin Oncol	Single institutional retrospective review	Adjuvant CRT had improved OS compared to no CRT	Very low
Corsini et al.	2008 [10]	J Clin Oncol	Single institutional retrospective review	Adjuvant CRT had improved OS compared to no CRT after R0	Very low
Katz et al.	2008 [15]	J Am Coll Surg	Prospective cohort study	Neoadjuvant therapy identifies patients who will benefit from surgery	Moderate
Brown et al.	2008 [52]	Am J Surg	Single institutional retrospective review	Increase R0/R1 rates	Low
Gnaneh et al.	2008 [53]	Eur J Surg Oncol	Review of cohort studies	Neoadjuvant therapy as part of clinical trial	Very low
Varadhachary et al.	2006 [2]	Ann Surg Oncol	Single institutional expert opinion	Definition and management of borderline resectable tumors	Very low
Mornex et al.	2005 [54]	Semin Radiat Oncol	Review of cohort studies	Neoadjuvant therapy should be used in clinical trials (too little data)	Very low
Neoptolemos et al.	2004 [6]	N Engl J Med	Randomized controlled clinical trial	Adjuvant CT has an OS benefit over surgery alone	Moderate
Wayne et al.	2002 [55]	Oncologist	Review of cohort studies	Neoadjuvant therapy on protocol	Very low
White et al.	2001 [56]	Ann Surg Oncol	Single institutional retrospective review	Neoadjuvant CRT downstages, identifies patients who will benefit from surgery	Low
Breslin et al.	2001 [57]	Ann Surg Oncol	Single institutional retrospective review	Neoadjuvant CRT maximizes survival	Low

CT chemotherapy, *CRT* chemoradiation, *DFS* disease-free survival, *OS* overall survival, *pCR* pathologic complete response the University of Cincinnati who completed neoadjuvant chemotherapy (gemcitabine) and then underwent exploration. Surgical resections were completed in 12 patients (46 %) with 67 % R0 resections and a median survival in the resected patients of 23.3 months [18]. The quality of this line of evidence would also have to be graded as very low-to-low with the exception of the tightly controlled MD Anderson series, which is graded as moderate quality.

Systematic reviews and meta-analyses of neoadjuvant therapy for pancreatic cancer have been performed but recommendations from these reviews are limited by the inconsistencies of the individual studies and the variability of the treatment schemes. Assifi et al. reviewed a total of 14 phase II clinical trials including 536 patients with resectable and/or borderline resectable disease [19]. After treatment, resectability was 65.8 % (95 % CI, 55.4–75.6 %) in patients with localized, resectable tumors compared with 31.6 % in patients with borderline disease (95 % CI, 14.0–52.5 %). A partial response was observed in patients with borderline/unresectable tumors; 31.8 % (95 % CI, 24.2–39.8 %) compared to 9.5 % (95 % CI, 2.9–19.4 %) in the resectable group ($p=.003$). Progressive disease was seen in 17.0 % (95 % CI, 11.9–22.7) of patients with resectable tumors versus 21.8 % (95 % CI, 10.1–36.5 %) in the borderline group ($p=.006$). Median survival in resected patients was 23 months for the resectable group and 22 months for borderline patients [19]. Laurence et al. reviewed prospective trials and retrospective series with a focus on complication rates, surgical morbidity and survival [20]. The meta-analysis found that patients with "unresectable" (criteria not well-described) pancreatic cancer who underwent neoadjuvant chemoradiotherapy achieved similar survival outcomes to patients with resectable disease, even though only 40 % were ultimately resected. Neoadjuvant chemoradiotherapy was not associated with a statistically significant increase in the rate of pancreatic fistula formation or total complications. Patients receiving neoadjuvant chemoradiotherapy were less likely to have a positive resection margin, although there was an increased risk of peri-operative death [20]. While these meta-analyses and reviews serve to summarize the current approaches and reported outcomes for neoadjuvant therapy for pancreatic cancer, the quality of the included studies and the limited power of the statistical analysis would qualify the strength of these studies as very low to low.

Recommendations

There have been two expert consensus statements on borderline resectable pancreas cancer crafted in the last 5 years and the 2014 NCCN guidelines for pancreatic cancer are now published [1, 3, 21]. All acknowledge the limitations of the currently available data. All unequivocally emphasize the need for high quality radiographic imaging to accurately categorize these cancers and clearly delineated and stringently applied definitions of vascular involvement for appropriate treatment recommendations. The NCCN guidelines recommend that patients with borderline resectable cancer should be treated first with chemotherapy, and then consolidated with chemoradiation and surgery if appropriate. The basis for this recommendation was not data driven but rather on the authors' perspectives that patients with pancreatic cancer should be selected for a surgery-first approach based on the likelihood of obtaining margin-negative resections. Patients with borderline resectable tumors are at high risk for margin-positive resections that are associated with poorer outcomes in most surgical series. The use of neoadjuvant therapy in borderline cases was recommended because of the potential to increase R0 resections [21]. Clinical trials employing novel chemotherapy combinations found to be active in advanced, metastatic disease and modified radiation approaches are underway and referral to large volume centers participating in these trials is strongly encouraged. In the United States, Katz et al. have initiated a multi-institutional feasibility trial with FOLFIRINOX (5-FU, leucovorin, oxaliplatin, irinotecan) followed by a capecitabine-based chemoradiotherapy protocol (Alliance trial A0201102). A comparable study has been initiated by high-volume German centers (NEOPA-Trial; 1.8 Gy in 28 fractions with concurrent gemcitabine 300 mg/m; registered at EudraCT [European Union Drug Regulating Authorities Clinical Trials] www.eudract.ema.europa.eu), Reg-No. 2012-003669-17).

Surgeons operating on patients with borderline resectable cancers should anticipate portal and mesenteric venous involvement and extension of the cancer to arterial margins. Only surgeons experienced with advanced techniques of vascular resection and reconstruction should therefore undertake these operations [4, 21].

Recommendations

1. Patients with suspected borderline resectable pancreatic head cancers should have high-quality three-dimensional imaging performed to precisely define the extent of mesenteric and portal vein involvement and the degree of arterial abutment and encasement (evidence quality high; strong recommendation).
2. Patients with borderline resectable tumors, as defined by the ISGPS, will likely require PV/SMV resection and reconstruction and should be referred to high volume centers with surgeons experienced in advanced vascular techniques (evidence quality high; strong recommendation).
3. A surgery-first approach versus a neoadjuvant strategy should be individualized for each patient, and whenever possible, participation in a prospective clinical trial is encouraged (evidence quality low; conditional recommendation).

A Personal View of the Data

In summary, there are no proven protocols for neoadjuvant therapy for borderline resectable pancreatic head cancers. Reports include both 5-FU-based and gemcitabine-based chemotherapy protocols and nearly all of the series include concurrent radiation. Complications rates are not markedly increased relative to traditional surgery-first approaches and median survival rates are at best comparable to those reported in large primary surgical series. Conversely, there are no large, well-controlled, prospective, multi-institutional series or even high-quality single institution reports sufficiently powered to prove that a surgery-first approach results in a better outcome than when a neoadjuvant strategy is utilized for this particular subset of patients. There are certainly no randomized phase III trials that have compared neoadjuvant therapy for borderline resectable disease versus surgery without initial therapy. There is simply no data that irrefutably supports one approach over the other. Regardless of therapeutic strategy, these are particularly challenging and potentially dangerous cases that should be cared for by experienced surgeons at high-volume centers.

References

1. Callery MP, Chang KJ, Fishman EK, et al. Pretreatment assessment of resectable and borderline resectable pancreatic cancer: expert consensus statement. Ann Surg Oncol. 2009;16:1727–33.
2. Varadhachary GR, Tamm EP, Abbruzzese JL, et al. Borderline resectable pancreatic cancer: definitions, management, and role of preoperative therapy. Ann Surg Oncol. 2006;13:1035–46.
3. Bockhorn M, Uzunoglu FG, Adham M, International Study Group of Pancreatic Surgery, et al. Borderline resectable pancreatic cancer: a consensus statement by the International Study Group of Pancreatic Surgery (ISGPS). Surgery. 2014;155:977–88.
4. Katz MH, Lee JE, Pisters PW, et al. Retroperitoneal dissection in patients with borderline resectable pancreatic cancer: operative principles and techniques. J Am Coll Surg. 2012;215:e11–8.
5. Gastrointestinal Tumor Study Group. Further evidence of effective adjuvant combined radiation and chemotherapy following curative resection of pancreatic cancer. Cancer. 1987;59:2006–10.
6. Neoptolemos JP, Stocken DD, Friess H, European Study Group for Pancreatic Cancer, et al. A randomized trial of chemoradiotherapy and chemotherapy after resection of pancreatic cancer. N Engl J Med. 2004;350:1200–10.
7. Oettle H, Neuhaus P, Hochhaus A, et al. Adjuvant chemotherapy with gemcitabine and long-term outcomes among patients with resected pancreatic cancer: the CONKO-001 randomized trial. JAMA. 2013;310:1473–81.
8. Regine WF, Winter KA, Abrams R, et al. Fluorouracil-based chemoradiation with either gemcitabine or fluorouracil chemotherapy after resection of pancreatic adenocarcinoma: 5-year analysis of the U.S. Intergroup/RTOG 9704 phase III trial. Ann Surg Oncol. 2011;18:1319–26.
9. Herman JM, Swartz MJ, Hsu CC, et al. Analysis of fluorouracil-based adjuvant chemotherapy and radiation after pancreaticoduodenectomy for ductal adenocarcinoma of the pancreas: results of a large, prospectively collected database at the Johns Hopkins Hospital. J Clin Oncol. 2008;26:3503–10.
10. Corsini MM, Miller RC, Haddock MG, et al. Adjuvant radiotherapy and chemotherapy for pancreatic carcinoma: the Mayo Clinic experience (1975–2005). J Clin Oncol. 2008;26:3511–6.

11. Abbott DE, Baker MS, Talamonti MS. Neoadjuvant therapy for pancreatic cancer: a current review. J Surg Oncol. 2010;101:315–20.
12. Marti JL, Hochster HS, Hiotis SP, et al. Phase I/II trial of induction chemotherapy followed by concurrent chemoradiotherapy and surgery for locoregionally advanced pancreatic cancer. Ann Surg Oncol. 2008;15:3521–31.
13. Landry J, Catalano PJ, Staley C, et al. Randomized phase II study of gemcitabine plus radiotherapy versus gemcitabine, 5-fluorouracil, and cisplatin followed by radiotherapy and 5-fluorouracil for patients with locally advanced, potentially resectable pancreatic adenocarcinoma. J Surg Oncol. 2010;101:587–92.
14. Kim EJ, Ben-Josef E, Herman JM, et al. A multi-institutional phase 2 study of neoadjuvant gemcitabine and oxaliplatin with radiation therapy in patients with pancreatic cancer. Cancer. 2013;119:2692–700.
15. Katz MH, Pisters PW, Evans DB, et al. Borderline resectable pancreatic cancer: the importance of this emerging stage of disease. J Am Coll Surg. 2008;206:833–46; discussion 846–8.
16. Patel M, Hoffe S, Malafa M, et al. Neoadjuvant GTX chemotherapy and IMRT-based chemoradiation for borderline resectable pancreatic cancer. J Surg Oncol. 2011;104:155–61.
17. Stokes JB, Nolan NJ, Stelow EB, et al. Preoperative capecitabine and concurrent radiation for borderline resectable pancreatic cancer. Ann Surg Oncol. 2011;18:619–27.
18. McClaine RJ, Lowy AM, Sussman JJ, et al. Neoadjuvant therapy may lead to successful surgical resection and improved survival in patients with borderline resectable pancreatic cancer. HPB (Oxf). 2010;12:73–9.
19. Assifi MM, Lu X, Eibl G, et al. Neoadjuvant therapy in pancreatic adenocarcinoma: a meta-analysis of phase II trials. Surgery. 2011;150:466–73.
20. Laurence JM, Tran PD, Morarji K, et al. A systematic review and meta-analysis of survival and surgical outcomes following neoadjuvant chemoradiotherapy for pancreatic cancer. J Gastrointest Surg. 2011;15:2059–69.
21. Tempero MA, Malafa MP, Behrman SW, et al. Pancreatic adenocarcinoma, version 2.2014: featured updates to the NCCN guidelines. J Natl Compr Canc Netw. 2014;12:1083–93.
22. Sultana A, Jackson RJ, Cox T, et al. Chemotherapy, radiotherapy, chemoradiotherapy and combination therapy in localised and locally advanced pancreatic cancer. Cochrane Database Syst Rev. 2014, Issue 8. Art. No.: CD011044. doi: 10.1002/14651858.CD011044.
23. Sen N, Falk S, Abrams RA. Role of chemoradiotherapy in the adjuvant and neoadjuvant settings for resectable pancreatic cancer. Clin Oncol (R Coll Radiol). 2014;26:551–9.
24. Tsvetkova EV, Asmis TR. Role of neoadjuvant therapy in the management of pancreatic cancer: is the era of biomarker-directed therapy here? Curr Oncol. 2014;21:e650–7.
25. Bittoni A, Santoni M, Lanese A, et al. Neoadjuvant therapy in pancreatic cancer: an emerging strategy. Gastroenterol Res Pract. 2014:183852 doi: 10.1155/2014/183852. Epub Jul 1 2014.
26. Cooper AB, Holmes HM, des Bordes JK, et al. Role of neoadjuvant therapy in the multimodality treatment of older patients with pancreatic cancer. J Am Coll Surg. 2014;219:111–20.
27. Papavasiliou P, Hoffman JP, Cohen SJ, et al. Impact of preoperative therapy on patterns of recurrence in pancreatic cancer. HPB (Oxf). 2014;16:34–9.
28. Motoi F, Ishida K, Fujishima F, et al. Neoadjuvant chemotherapy with gemcitabine and S-1 for resectable and borderline pancreaticductal adenocarcinoma: results from a prospective multi-institutional phase 2 trial. Ann Surg Oncol. 2013;20:3794–801.
29. Heinemann V, Haas M, Boeck S. Neoadjuvant treatment of borderline resectable and non-resectable pancreatic cancer. Ann Oncol. 2013;24:2484–92.
30. Belli C, Cereda S, Anand S, et al. Neoadjuvant therapy in resectable pancreatic cancer: a critical review. Cancer Treat Rev. 2013;39:518–24.
31. Papavasiliou P, Chun YS, Hoffman JP. How to define and manage borderline resectable pancreatic cancer. Surg Clin North Am. 2013;93:663–74.
32. Paulson AS, Tran Cao HS, Tempero MA, et al. Therapeutic advances in pancreatic cancer. Gastroenterology. 2013;144:1316–26.

33. Tsuruga Y, Kamachi H, Wakayama K, et al. Portal vein stenosis after pancreatectomy following neoadjuvant chemoradiation therapy for pancreatic cancer. World J Gastroenterol. 2013;19:2569–73.
34. Galindo J, Gabrielli M, Guerra JF, et al. Neoadjuvant chemoradiation therapy for borderline pancreatic adenocarcinoma: report of two cases. World J Surg Oncol. 2013;11:37.
35. Chatterjee D, Katz MH, Rashid A, et al. Histologic grading of the extent of residual carcinoma following neoadjuvant chemoradiation in pancreatic ductal adenocarcinoma: a predictor for patient outcome. Cancer. 2012;118:3182–90.
36. Wolff RA. Neoadjuvant therapy for resectable and borderline resectable adenocarcinoma of the pancreas. Curr Drug Targets. 2012;13:781–8.
37. Satoi S, Toyokawa H, Yanagimoto H, et al. Neoadjuvant chemoradiation therapy using S-1 followed by surgical resection in patients with pancreatic cancer. J Gastrointest Surg. 2012;16:784–92.
38. Lim KH, Chung E, Khan A, et al. Neoadjuvant therapy of pancreatic cancer: the emerging paradigm? Oncologist. 2012;17:192–200.
39. Zhao Q, Rashid A, Gong Y, et al. Pathologic complete response to neoadjuvant therapy in patients with pancreatic ductal adenocarcinoma is associated with a better prognosis. Ann Diagn Pathol. 2012;16:29–37.
40. Estrella JS, Rashid A, Fleming JB, et al. Post-therapy pathologic stage and survival in patients with pancreatic ductal adenocarcinoma treated with neoadjuvant chemoradiation. Cancer. 2012;118:268–77.
41. Takahashi S, Kinoshita T, Konishi M, et al. Borderline resectable pancreatic cancer: rationale for multidisciplinary treatment. J Hepatobiliary Pancreat Sci. 2011;18:567–74.
42. Palta M, Willett C, Czito B. Role of radiation therapy in patients with resectable pancreatic cancer. Oncology (Williston Park). 2011;25:715–21.
43. van Tienhoven G, Gouma DJ, Richel DJ. Neoadjuvant chemoradiotherapy has a potential role in pancreatic carcinoma. Ther Adv Med Oncol. 2011;3:27–33.
44. Katz MH, Fleming JB, Lee JE, et al. Current status of adjuvant therapy for pancreatic cancer. Oncologist. 2010;15:1205–13.
45. Brunner TB, Scott-Brown M. The role of radiotherapy in multimodal treatment of pancreatic carcinoma. Radiat Oncol. 2010;5:64.
46. Gillen S, Schuster T, Meyer Zum Büschenfelde C, et al. Preoperative/neoadjuvant therapy in pancreatic cancer: a systematic review and meta-analysis of response and resection percentages. PLoS Med. 2010;7:e1000267.
47. Morganti AG, Massaccesi M, La Torre G, et al. A systematic review of resectability and survival after concurrent chemoradiation in primarily unresectable pancreatic cancer. Ann Surg Oncol. 2010;17:194–205.
48. Satoi S, Yanagimoto H, Toyokawa H, et al. Surgical results after preoperative chemoradiation therapy for patients with pancreatic cancer. Pancreas. 2009;38:282–8.
49. Crane CH, Varadhachary G, Settle SH, et al. The integration of chemoradiation in the care of patient with localized pancreatic cancer. Cancer Radiother. 2009;13:123–43.
50. Varadhachary GR, Wolff RA, Crane CH, et al. Preoperative gemcitabine and cisplatin followed by gemcitabine-based chemoradiation for resectable adenocarcinoma of the pancreatic head. J Clin Oncol. 2008;26:3487–95.
51. Evans DB, Varadhachary GR, Crane CH, et al. Preoperative gemcitabine-based chemoradiation for patients with resectable adenocarcinoma of the pancreatic head. J Clin Oncol. 2008;26:3496–502.
52. Brown KM, Siripurapu V, Davidson M, et al. Chemoradiation followed by chemotherapy before resection for borderline pancreatic adenocarcinoma. Am J Surg. 2008;195:318–21.
53. Ghaneh P, Smith R, Tudor-Smith C, et al. Neoadjuvant and adjuvant strategies for pancreatic cancer. Eur J Surg Oncol. 2008;34:297–305.

54. Mornex F, Girard N, Delpero JR, et al. Radiochemotherapy in the management of pancreatic cancer – part I: neoadjuvant treatment. Semin Radiat Oncol. 2005;15:226–34.
55. Wayne JD, Abdalla EK, Wolff RA, et al. Localized adenocarcinoma of the pancreas: the rationale for preoperative chemoradiation. Oncologist. 2002;7:34–45.
56. White RR, Hurwitz HI, Morse MA, et al. Neoadjuvant chemoradiation for localized adenocarcinoma of the pancreas. Ann Surg Oncol. 2001;8:758–65.
57. Breslin TM, Hess KR, Harbison DB, et al. Neoadjuvant chemoradiotherapy for adenocarcinoma of the pancreas: treatment variables and survival duration. Ann Surg Oncol. 2001;8:123–32.

Chapter 51
Neoadjuvant Therapy for Resectable Pancreatic Adenocarcinoma

Heather L. Lewis and Syed A. Ahmad

Abstract For the subset of patients with pancreatic cancer who have been deemed to have resectable disease at the time of diagnosis, complete surgical resection offers the only chance of long-term cure. More recently, the addition of adjuvant therapy has been shown to offer a survival advantage over those patients who undergo resection alone, and multimodality therapy represents the widely accepted treatment paradigm. Neoadjuvant therapy in the setting of a multimodality approach to treating resectable pancreatic head adenocarcinoma may allow for: (1) early treatment of occult micometastatic disease and testing of the biology of the tumor to minimize the risk of unnecessary surgical resection in patients who would not benefit from surgery, (2) increasing the rate of margin negative resections, (3) increasing the likelihood of completing adjuvant therapy, and (4) possibly reducing surgical morbidity.

Keywords Pancreatic cancer • Neoadjuvant • Resectable • Chemotherapy • Chemoradiation

Introduction

Pancreatic adenocarcinoma is the fourth leading cause of cancer related deaths amongst both men and women in the United States [1]. Unlike many other malignancies, the incidence of pancreatic cancer has remained stable over the past decade [2]. The diagnosis remains one which is associated with a poor long-term prognosis, with an estimated overall 5-year survival of 5 %. Because of the insidious nature of the disease process, most patients have advanced or unresectable disease at the time

H.L. Lewis
Department of Surgery, The University of Cincinnati Medical Center, Cincinnati, OH, USA
e-mail: lewishh@ucmail.uc.edu

S.A. Ahmad (✉)
Pancreas Disease Center, University Cincinnati Cancer Institute,
231 Albert Sabin Way, ML 0558, SRU Room 1466, Cincinnati, OH 45267, USA
e-mail: ahmadsy@uc.edu

J.M. Millis, J.B. Matthews (eds.), *Difficult Decisions in Hepatobiliary and Pancreatic Surgery*, Difficult Decisions in Surgery: An Evidence-Based Approach, DOI 10.1007/978-3-319-27365-5_51

of diagnosis. Even in the one fifth of patients with pancreatic cancer who are deemed to have resectable disease, roughly 85 % who undergo resection will ultimately suffer from recurrence, a fact which points towards what appears to be the systemic nature of pancreatic cancer at diagnosis [3].

The introduction of a multimodality approach to the treatment of pancreatic cancer allows for a more effective strategy in an effort to treat both local and systemic disease. In patients with resected pancreatic cancer, adjuvant therapy using chemotherapy and/or chemoradiation have been postulated as a means to improve overall survival. The ESPAC-1 and CONKO-001 trials established a survival advantage in those patients who underwent administration of adjuvant chemotherapy [4–6]. The value of radiation therapy continues to be debated and is currently being investigated in the current RTOG 0848 study [7]. However, despite the survival advantage associated with the receipt of adjuvant therapy, approximately one quarter of patients with resected pancreatic cancer do not ultimately undergo treatment with adjuvant therapy due to decreased performance status and/or complications associated with surgical recovery [5]. As a result, continued study into additional strategies for improved outcomes has resulted in the evaluation of different neoadjuvant therapies, including both chemotherapy and chemoradiation based regimens.

Incorporation of neoadjuvant therapy into the multimodality regimen for the treatment of pancreatic cancer has been shown to be feasible, with many potential advantages. The proposed rationale behind neoadjuvant therapy includes an increased probability of margin negative resection, increased probability of completion of a multimodality treatment regimen, allowing for declaration of distant metastasis, and possibly improved surgical outcomes. However, others have argued that using neoadjuvant therapy in patients with resectable disease may lead to a loss of "the window" for surgical resectability, and the associated difficulty of obtaining a pre-treatment tissue diagnosis. The aim of this chapter is to address the data behind the use of neoadjuvant therapy in the setting of resectable pancreatic head adenocarcinoma, specifically assessing morbidity and mortality, overall survival, and cost effectiveness.

Search Strategy

A literature search of English language publications from 1990 to 2014 was used to identity published data on neoadjuvant therapy for resectable pancreatic head cancer using the PICO outline (Table 51.1). Databases searched were PubMed and Cochrane Evidence Based Medicine. Terms used in the search were "pancreatic adenocarcinoma AND resectable," "pancreatic adenocarcinoma neoadjuvant chemoradiation," "pancreatic adenocarcinoma adjuvant therapy," "pancreatic adenocarcinoma neoadjuvant chemotherapy" "pancreatic adenocarcinoma" AND ("resectable") AND ("neoadjuvant chemoradiation" OR "neoadjuvant chemotherapy"). The data was classified using the GRADE system.

Table 51.1 PICO table

(P) Patients	(I) Intervention	(C) Comparator group	(O) Outcome measured
Patients with resectable pancreatic adenocarcinoma	Neoadjuvant therapy	Surgery first with adjuvant therapy	Overall survival, morbidity/ mortality, cost effectiveness

Results

Resectable Pancreatic Cancer

Utilization of a standardized definition for what is considered resectable pancreatic head adenocarcinoma allows for treatment strategies to be more uniformly evaluated. Importantly, accurate determination of resectability also saves the morbidity associated with laparotomy and pancreaticoduodenectomy in those patients whose disease stage would not allow them to derive benefit from that therapy. A consensus statement has been developed in order to establish set criteria for tumors which may be considered resectable [8].

Advancements in imaging have further facilitated accurate pretreatment staging of pancreatic adenocarcinoma. Currently, a MRI, or a multidetector 64-slice CT scanner with advanced volumetric processing capacity is considered the optimal radiographic imaging modality. For CT imaging, both arterial and portal venous phase IV contrast with administration of water as PO contrast should be employed. In addition, endoscopic ultrasound may be used as an adjunct for further evaluation of major vascular structures, assessment of atypical lesions, and as a means for tissue diagnosis. Major criteria for resectability include (1) the absence of distant metastasis (2) portal vein and superior mesenteric vein free of any tumor distortion, abutment, tumor thrombus, or encasement and (3) no tumor involvement of arterial vascular structures, including the hepatic artery, celiac axis and superior mesenteric artery.

Neoadjuvant Therapy

Establishing Feasibility

Use of neoadjuvant chemoradiation for resectable pancreatic adenocarcinoma was first shown to be feasible, and with a low rate of complication and toxicity by Evans et al. in 1992. In their study of 28 patients, a regimen of 5-FU and 50.4 Gy radiation was given and completed in the preoperative setting by all patients. A total of 17 patients were then able to undergo resection, the remaining excluded due to progression of disease. Evidence of tumor cell injury was seen in all resected specimens [9]. Yeung et al. subsequently published their results using neoadjuvant chemoradiation in a phase II trial out of Fox Chase Cancer Center in 1993. In this study, 26 patients with pancreatic cancer were treated with a regimen, which consisted of 50.4 Gy radiation in combination with 5-FU and Mitomycin C. They demonstrated a decreased rate of lymph node positive disease and an R0 resection in all of the 38 % of patients who ultimately underwent resection [10]. Shortly thereafter, Spitz et al. categorized 142 patients with radiographically resectable pancreatic head adenocarcinoma to receive either preoperative chemoradiation followed by surgery or surgery first followed by adjuvant therapy. While the overall survival difference between the two groups (19.2 months vs 22 months) did not reach statistical significance, they did note a lower rate of locoregional recurrence in the group who received preoperative chemoradiation. Additionally, it is important to note that 24 % of the patients who underwent surgery first did not ultimately receive adjuvant therapy [11]. This subset represents the group spared unnecessary surgery.

Historical Review

Over the course of the following years after these initial studies, multiple other phase II trials and multi-institutional studies of neoadjuvant chemoradiation have been completed, utilizing several different modifications in treatment regimens (Table 51.2). Recognizing the increased GI toxicity associated with the 50.4 Gy radiation regimen, the group at MD Anderson Cancer Center introduced a 30 Gy multi-fractionated radiation therapy regimen given in conjunction with infusional 5-FU. This regimen was well tolerated, as 35 out of 35 patients completed all assigned therapy and underwent successful surgery. Median survival in this study was 25 months [12]. During this time, additional research was done that demonstrated the benefit of gemcitabine in the setting of advanced pancreatic cancer, as well as, its ability to act as a potent radiosensitizer. Thus, this agent was subsequently investigated in conjunction with radiation therapy in the neoadjuvant setting. A small multi-institutional study which evaluated 20 patients with potentially resectable pancreatic adenocarcinoma who received full dose preoperative gemcitabine-based chemoradiation (1000 mg/m2 gemcitabine + 36 Gy fractionated radiation therapy) was reported on by Talamonti et al. in 2006. In their study, 85 % of patients underwent successful pancreaticoduodenectomy with a resultant median overall survival of 26 months [13].

In order to further decrease toxicity and improve delivery of chemotherapeutic agents, the group from the MD Anderson Cancer Center enrolled 86 patients to receive reduced dose gemcitabine chemotherapy (400 mg/m2) in combination with 30 Gy fractionated radiation therapy in a neoadjuvant fashion [14]. Disease progression or a decline in performance status excluded 13 patients from surgery, but of the 73 patients who ultimately went to surgery 64 underwent successful pancreaticoduodenectomy. Median overall survival in those patients who completed chemoradiation with surgical resection was 34 months, and for all patients 22.7 months [14]. Concomitant to that study, investigation of the addition of a gemcitabine-cisplatin chemotherapy regimen prior to receipt of gemcitabine-based chemoradiation was also undertaken by the researchers at the MD Anderson Cancer Center. Unfortunately,

Table 51.2 Neoadjuvant therapy for pancreatic adenocarcinoma

Author	N	Regimen	% Resected	Survival resected (mo)	Margin negative (%)	Characteristics	Notes
Pisters et al. [12]	35	30 Gy + 5-FU (300 mg/m2)	74	25	90	Resectable	Institutional
Talamonti et al. [13]	20	36 Gy + gemcitabine (1000 mg/m2)	85	26	94	Resectable	Multi institutional, phase II
Palmer et al. [19]	50	Gemcitabine (1000 mg/m2) vs gemcitabine (1000 mg/m2) + cisplatin (25 mg/m2)	54	28.4	75	Resectable	Phase II, randomized
Heinrich et al. [18]	28	Gemcitabine (1000 mg/m2) + cisplatin (50 mg/m2)	89	19.1	unk	Resectable	Phase II, randomized
Vradachahary et al. (15)	90	[Gemcitabine (750 mg/m2) + cisplatin (30 mg/m2)] + [30 Gy + gemcitabine (400 mg/m2)]	66	31	96	Resectable	Single institution, phase II
Evans et al. [14]	86	30 Gy + gemcitabine (400 mg/m2)	74	34	89	Resectable	Single institution, phase II
Turrini et al. [17]	34	45 Gy + docetaxel (30 mg/m2)	50	32	100	Resectable	Multi institutional, phase II
Kim et al. [16]	68	30Gy + gemcitabine + oxaliplatin	63	27.1	84	Resectable/borderline/unresectable	Multi institutional, phase II
O'Reilly et al. [20]	38	Gemcitabine + oxaliplatin	63	27.2	74	Resectable	Single institution, phase II

this regimen did not demonstrate any superiority to gemcitabine-based chemoradiation alone [15].

Another combination regimen that has been utilized was full dose gemcitabine (1000 mg/m2) and oxaliplatin (85 mg/m2) with multi fractionated radiation therapy (30 Gy total). In this multi institutional study, 68 patients with either resectable, borderline resectable, or unresectable pancreatic adenocarcinoma were evaluated. Of the 23 patients with potentially resectable disease, 13 (57 %) ultimately underwent resection and median overall survival for all resected patients was 27.1 months [16]. Finally, another alternative regimen that has been studied was the combination of docetaxel-based chemoradiation along with infusional docetaxel therapy (30 mg/m2/week) over 5 weeks. The authors reported tumor progression in 32 % of patients which precluded resection, however, all 17 patients who underwent successful pancreaticoduodenectomy were noted to have an R0 resection, and three patients had a complete pathological response. Median survival in resected patients was 32 months [17]. A smaller subset of studies have been done addressing neoadjuvant chemotherapy alone, most utilizing a gemcitabine or gemcitabine + platinum based regimen [18, 19]. Recently, a prospective phase II single institution trial out of Memorial Sloan Kettering Cancer Center evaluated 38 patients who received gemcitabine (1000 mg/m2) and oxaliplatin (80 mg/m2) for four cycles, of which 27 underwent successful surgical resection (71 %). At the conclusion of the study, 63 % of patients remained alive with a median survival of 27 months [20].

The collective body of evidence regarding the use of neoadjuvant therapy demonstrates a range of overall survival between 26 and 34 months in recent studies [13–17, 20]. This is compared to a median overall survival of 22–23 months in the major studies evaluating patients who undergo surgery plus adjuvant therapy alone [4, 6]. It is important to note that the survival data for patients receiving neoadjuvant therapy is influenced by a strong selection bias as most results do not denote an intent to treat analysis. Additionally, comparison of the different neoadjuvant regimens is difficult as they have utilized different algorithms, dosing of radiation, and dosing of chemotherapeutic regimens. Finally, the patterns of failure following a neoadjuvant approach seem to be similar to that seen after an adjuvant approach, and an overall analysis of the data would suggest that outcomes following neoadjuvant treatment is at least equivalent to an adjvuant approach. The rational for a neoadjuvant approach, therefore, lies with the theoretical advantages that are discussed in the sections below.

Rationale for Administration of Neoadjuvant Therapy

As the understanding of the biology of pancreatic cancer continues to evolve, new research continues to drive the rationale behind of the advantages which may be provided through the incorporation of neoadjuvant therapy into the multimodality treatment sequence. Through use of DNA sequencing in tissue from patients with pancreatic cancer, the presence of metastatic subclones which live within the primary tumor have been identified, and mathematical modeling has been used to predict a timeframe of multiple years over which these cells may disseminate and eventually cause metastatic disease [21]. More recently however, evidence has emerged which may indicate even earlier metastatic capabilities of neoplastic pancreatic cells, even in the setting of pancreatic intraepithelial neoplasia (PanIN) [22]. Further, cells with very high metastatic capacity may be generated during early and exponential tumor growth [23]. Collectively, this data points towards the concept of pancreatic adenocarcinoma as a systemic disease process, regardless of the size or appearance of the primary tumor or presence of clinically evident metastasis. As such, systemic therapy which is initiated in the neoadjuvant setting addresses occult micrometastatic disease that could lead to recurrence.

In those patients that undergo a surgery first approach, margin negative resections have been associated with an overall improved median survival. The margin that is most likely to be positive following pancreaticoduodenectomy (PD) is the superior mesenteric artery/uncinate (SMA/uncinate) margin. The SMA/uncinate margin comprises the tissue that connects the uncinate process to the right lateral border of the proximal 3–4 cm of the SMA. Because tumors in the pancreatic head lie in close proximity to the SMA and because the SMA cannot be removed and reconstructed at surgery, the SMA/uncinate margin is the margin that is most often positive following PD. Numerous studies have demonstrated inferior survival when this margin is positive during a surgery first approach. In a study by Yeo et al. the survival of 201 patients undergoing PD were analyzed. A positive margin was observed in 29 % of patients, patients with negative margins had a median survival of 18 months compared to 10 months for patients with positive margins [24]. A similar result was found by Neoptolemos et al. in analysis of the ESPAC-1 Study results. In this study of 541 patients, those with negative resection margins had superior overall survival [25]. Utilization of a neoadjuvant approach may offer the advantage of improved negative margin resection. This was highlighted in the study by Talamonti et al.[13] utilizing a full dose Gemcitabine and reduced dose radiation strategy. In this study, 94 % of patients underwent a margin negative resection. In addition to decreasing overall margin positivity, a neoadjuvant approach may decrease the significance of a positive margin. In a study by Raut et al. margin analysis was undertaken in 360 patients undergoing PD following a neoadjuvant strategy. The resection margins were negative in 83 % of patients. Patients who underwent a margin negative resection had a median survival of 28 months compared to 22 months for those with positive margins (p = NS) [26]. This indicates that after neoadjuvant therapy, the negative impact of a positive margin may be diminished.

The ability to downstage pancreatic adenocarcinoma with neoadjuvant therapy has been evaluated in both the setting of resectable as well as locally advanced disease. Evans et al. [14] demonstrated that 58 % of patients who underwent neoadjuvant gemcitabine based chemoradiation had a partial response to therapy, with two patients noted to have a pathologic complete response, and 89 % of patients noted to have an R0 resection. Response to therapy may also help the surgeon predict long term survival. In the setting of locally advanced pancreatic adenocarcinoma, despite only 12 % of patients meeting radiographic criteria for downstaging, Katz et al. were able to achieve an 80 % margin negative (R0) resection rate in their study of 122 patients [27]. Notably, in both of these studies, patients who completed therapy and underwent resection were noted to have a median overall survival of 34 months and 33 months, respectively. In contrast, those patients who had progression of disease while undergoing neoadjuvant therapy and were not ultimately able to undergo resection, had a median overall survival of 7.1 months and 12 months [14, 27]. In the French multi-instituional Phase II FFCD 9704-SFRO trial, histopathologic response to neoadjuvant chemoradiation was measured in patients receiving a regimen of infusional 5-FU and cisplatin along with 50 Gy radiation. In 41 patients with potentially resectable pancreatic adenocarcinoma who underwent chemoradiation, 26 (63 %) completed therapy and went on to surgery, with an R0 resection rate of 80.7 % [28]. One complete pathologic response was noted in this group, with that patient still alive at 64 months following resection, emphasizing the additional survival advantage that has been noted in the small subset of patients who do achieve a pathologic complete response (pCR). In a large, retrospective review of 442 patients who underwent neoadjuvant chemoradiation therapy, only 2.5 % of patients were noted to have a pCR, however, those patients had a significantly better disease specific survival than their counterparts [29].

Patients who undergo neoadjuvant therapy are more likely to complete trimodality therapy, in contrast to the often-poor rates of completion in patients who undergo surgery first followed by adjuvant therapy [30]. Notably, in the recent ESPAC-3 study for adjuvant therapy comparing 5-FU and folinic acid with gemcitabine, only 68 % of patients were able to complete all six cycles of therapy, with a median overall survival difference of 28 months vs 14.6 months when those who completed therapy were compared with those who did not [31]. In those patients greater than 70 years old there was a further decreased rate of completion of postoperative therapy, and a higher risk for morbidity associated with surgical resection [32]. In contrast, a recent study at MD Anderson Cancer Center demonstrated that receipt of neoadjuvant therapy in patients who were greater than 70 years of age with resectable pancreatic head adenocarcinoma resulted in 85 % completion rate of trimodality therapy [33]. Neoadjuvant therapy also is able to select out those patients whose performance status does not allow them to tolerate that regimen preoperatively, therefore excluding them from the morbidity related to pancreaticoduodenectomy [34, 35].

It is clear that neoadjuvant therapy does not contribute to increased post operative morbidity. Cooper et al. demonstrated in their review of data from the NSQIP Pancreatectomy Demonstration Project over 2011–2012, a total of 1562 patients with pancreatic adenocarcinoma undergoing neoadjuvant therapy (chemotherapy alone or chemotherapy + radiation) vs surgery first, that postoperative morbidity and 30-day mortality rates were similar between groups [36]. Similarly, in an institutional review of 167 patients with resectable pancreatic head adenocarcinoma who underwent either neoadjuvant therapy or surgery first, the group at MD Anderson Cancer Center, demonstrated a similar rate of postoperative major complications when the groups were compared [27]. While the toxicity profile for neoadjuvant therapy has been demonstrated to be low overall, there have been several factors that critics have cited in order to support a surgery first approach. One of those is the need for tissue diagnosis prior to initiation of neoadjuvant therapy, something that is not requisite for a surgery first approach in resectable pancreatic head adenocarcinoma. However, in the current era in which the diagnostic work up of pancreatic cancer includes endoscopic ultrasound for the vast majority of patients, obtaining a biopsy is increasingly less a complicating component. Similarly, the need for endobiliary stenting, while some have shown a potentially increased risk of post-operative wound infection [37], was not a factor accounting for increased morbidity and mortality overall, and is associated with an overall low rate of complications [38]. In a recent review of 1302 patients undergoing pancreaticoduodenectomy, endobiliary stenting did not increase risk of 30- or 90-day readmission [39]. In favor of a neoadjuvant approach, many studies have demonstrated a lower leak rate at the pancreaticojejunal anastomosis in those patients who received neoadjuvant therapy, further enforcing an optimal surgical benefit for this group of patients [14, 15]. While some still argue that the "window of opportunity" for resection may be lost during the period of time during which neoadjuvant therapy is administered, it is significant to note that those patients who do progress during neoadjuvant therapy are most often noted to have systemic disease and not local progression. A recent retrospective review comparing patients who underwent a surgery first approach versus neoadjuvant therapy first noted distant spread of disease in all patients who progressed while on therapy [30]. This again underlines both the biology of pancreatic adenocarcinoma as a frequently systemic disease at the time of diagnosis, as well as the benefit that may be derived in identifying those patients who may have occult micrometastatic disease at the time of diagnosis. Finally, emerging data also suggests that neoadjuvant therapy may in fact be more cost effective as well, with a recent review using data from the American College of Surgeons National Cancer Database and the National Surgical Quality Improvement Program (NSQIP) demonstrating a cost savings of approximately $10,000 per patient-case compared to those who underwent a surgery first approach [40].

Emerging Strategies

No prospective, randomized, controlled trials have yet been published in order to directly compare neoadjuvant therapy plus surgery with surgery and adjuvant therapy. However, there are several ongoing trials that seek to address this question. The Interdisciplinary Working Group of Gastrointestinal Tumors of the German Cancer Aid has undertaken a multicenter randomized phase II trial for patients with resectable pancreatic adenocarcinoma to be randomized to one of two arms: (A) conventional, fractionated radiation therapy (50.4 Gy) combined with gemcitabine (300 mg/m2) and cisplatin (30 mg/m2) followed by surgery and adjuvant gemcitabine or (B) surgical resection alone followed by gemcitabine [41].

The NEOPA trial (NCT 01900327) is a randomized, two armed, multicenter, open label, phase III trial whose aim is to investigate low dose (300 mg/m2) gemcitabine-based radiation therapy (50.4 Gy) with surgical resection alone.

Accrual is currently ongoing [42]. The NEOPAC trial (NCT 01314027) is a prospective randomized phase III trial whose primary study endpoint is progression free survival between patients with resectable pancreatic adenocarcinoma who undergo surgery first followed by adjuvant full dose gemcitabine (1000 mg/m2) versus neoadjuvant chemotherapy with gemcitabine (1000 mg/m2) and oxaliplatin (100 mg/m2) followed by surgery and the same adjuvant regimen as the surgery first group [43]. Finally, the NEOPANC trial is a prospective one-armed single center phase I/II trial (NCT 01372735) which will evaluate feasibility of neoadjuvant short course intensity modulated radiation therapy (5 Gy × 5) in combination with intraoperative radiation therapy (15 Gy), followed by adjuvant chemotherapy [44]. One year local recurrence rates will also be assessed.

Based on the recent literature demonstrating a survival advantage for those patients with metastatic pancreatic adenocarcinoma using the FOLFIRINOX (oxaliplatin, irinotecan, leucovorin, fluorouracil) regimen compared to gemcitabine alone [45], studies are additionally underway to assess the role that these agents may play in the neoadjuvant setting. Although this regimen is not currently being investigated for patients with resectable pancreatic adenocarcinoma, the Alliance for Clinical Trials in Oncology group is evaluating the use of FOLFIRINOX followed by 50.4 Gy radiation + capecitabine in the neoadjuvant setting for patients with borderline resectable tumors (Alliance A021101). Goals of this study will be to assess survival and toxicity of this regimen [46]. Other agents which have shown antitumor activity in the setting of metastatic or locally advanced pancreatic adenocarcinoma are also being evaluated in the neoadjuvant setting. The agent S-1, an oral fluoropyrimidine derivative that has previously been used in conjunction with gemcitabine in metastatic pancreatic adenocarcinoma, was studied in a group of 36 patients with resectable and borderline resectable disease [47] with a 87 % R0 resection rate and good overall tolerance, indicating potential for continued future study and application in the neoadjuvant setting.

Recommendations

Pancreatic cancer remains a disease with a dismal long term prognosis, because of the formation of early micrometastatic disease. When possible, multimodality therapy incorporating surgery, systemic therapy, and radiation therapy can improve survival. Based on the literature to date, we may conclude that utilization of a neoadjuvant approach to deliver chemotherapy and radiation in the setting of potentially resectable pancreatic adenocarcinoma is a reasonable and safe alternate to a surgery first approach, with similar overall morbidity and mortality. It allows for identification of patients with favorable biology that may benefit from surgery, it may downstage tumors and, therefore, enhances margin negative resection rates. Finally, it allows for evaluation of treatment response, and improves the rate of completion of multimodality therapy.

A Personal View of the Data

It is now clear that in the overwhelming majority of patients pancreas cancer is a systemic disease at diagnosis. This has been demonstrated by both pre-clinical and clinical data. Historically, our approach in managing pancreas cancer has focused on aggressive local regional therapy, and despite increasingly aggressive surgery median survival for pancreas cancer has not improved. This is reflected in the analysis of randomized clinical studies that have been completed. The median survival in the treatment arm of the 1995 GITSG study was 21 months, and despite two decades of effort, the median survival for the 2010 ESPAC-3 study remained at 23 months. Continued progress in pancreas cancer will depend on development of effective systemic therapy and early treatment of micrometastic disease. The neoadjuvant approach to pancreas cancer offers theoretical and common sense advantages for both the clinician and the patient. For example, it allows clinicians to assess treatment response in order to determine effectiveness of therapy. It also establishes a model in which researchers can study the tumor response to therapy at a molecular level. For the patients, it allows surgeons to reserve the most morbid part of multimodality therapy (i.e. surgery) for the subset of people most likely to benefit from it. It increases the likelihood of complete tumor extirpation, and potentially decreased post operative morbidity.

Recommendations

- Neoadjuvant therapy in the setting of pancreatic head adenocarcinoma is a reasonable first line alternate with equivalent morbidity and mortality rates compared to a surgery first approach (Evidence quality high; strong recommendation).
- Neoadjuvant therapy helps to identify a subset of patients for which surgical resection would not offer survival benefit (Evidence quality high; strong recommendation).
- Neoadjuvant therapy is cost effective (Evidence quality moderate; weak recommendation).
- Neoadjuvant therapy may improve R0 resection rates and decrease local recurrence (Evidence quality moderate; weak recommendation).

References

1. Siegal R, Ma J, Zou Z, Ahmedin J. Cancer statistics, 2014. CA Cancer J Clin. 2014;64(1):9–29.
2. Ma J, Siegal R, Ahmedin J. Pancreatic cancer death rates by race among US men and women, 1970–2009. J Natl Cancer Inst. 2013;105:1694–00.

3. Lowy A. Neoadjuvant therapy for pancreatic cancer. J Gastrointest Surg. 2008;12:1600–8.
4. Oettle H, Neuhaus P, Hochhaus A, Hartmann JT, Gellert K, Ridwelski K, Niedergethman M, Zulke C, Fahlke J, Arning MB, Sinn M, Hinke A, Riess H. Adjuvant therapy with gemcitabine and long term outcome among patients with resected pancreatic cancer: the CONKO-001 randomized trial. JAMA. 2013;310(14):1473–81.
5. Neoptolemos JP, Dunn JA, Stocken DD, Almond J, Link K, Beger H, Bassi C, Flaconi M, Pederzoli P, Dervenis C, Fernandez-Cruz L, Lacaine F, Pap A, Spooner D, Kerr DJ, Friess H, Buchler MW, European Study Group for Pancreatic Cancer. Adjuvant chemoradiotherapy and chemotherapy in resectable pancreatic cancer: a randomized controlled trial. Lancet. 2001;358(9293):1576–85.
6. Neoptolemos JP, Stocken DD, Bassi C, Ghaneh P, Cunningham D, Goldstein D, Padbury R, Moore MJ, Gallinger S, Mariette C, Wente MN, Izbicki JR, Friess H, Lerch MM, Dervenis C, Olah A, Butturini G, Doi R, Lind PA, Smith D, Valle JW, Palmer DH, Buckels JA, Thompson J, McKay CJ, Rawcliffe CL, Buchler MW, European Study Group for Pancreatic Cancer. Adjuvant chemotherapy with fluorouracil plus folinic acid vs gemcitabine following pancreatic cancer resection: a randomized controlled trial. JAMA. 2010;304(10):1073–81.
7. Regine WF, Winter KA, Abrams R, Safran H, Hoffman JP, Konski A, Benson AB, Macdonald JS, Rich TA, Willett CG. Fluorouracil-based chemoradiation with either gemcitabine or fluorouracil chemotherapy after resection of pancreatic adenocarcinoma: 5-year analysis of the US Intergroup/RTOG 9704 phase III trial. Ann Surg Oncol. 2011;18(5):1319–26.
8. Callery MP, Chang KJ, Fishman EK, Talamonti MS, William Traverso L, Linehan DC. Pretreatment assessment of resectable and borderline resectable pancreatic cancer: expert consensus statement. Ann Surg Oncol. 2009;16(7):1727–33.
9. Evans DB, Rich TA, Byrd DR, Cleary KR, Connelly JH, Levin B, Charnsangavej C, Fenoglio CJ, Ames FC. Preoperative chemoradiation and pancreaticoduodenectomy for adenocarcinoma of the pancreas. Arch Surg. 1992;127(11):1335–9.
10. Yeung RS, Weese JL, Hoffman JP, Solin LJ, Paul AR, Engstrom PF, Litwin S, Kowalyshyn MJ, Eisenberg BL. Neoadjuvant chemoradiation in pancreatic and duodenal carcinoma. A Phase II Study. Cancer. 1993;72(7):2124–33.
11. Spitz FR, Abbruzzese JL, Lee JE, Pisters PW, Lowy AM, Fenoglio CJ, Cleary KR, Janjan NA, Goswitz MS, Rich RA, Evans DB. Preoperative and postoperative chemoradiation strategies in patients treated with pancreaticoduodenectomy for adenocarcinoma of the pancreas. J Clin Oncol. 1997;15(3):928–37.
12. Pisters PW, Abbruzzese JL, Janjan NA, Cleary KR, CHarnsangavej C, Goswitz MS, Rich TA, Raijman I, Wolff RA, Lenzi R, Lee JE, Evans DB. Rapid-fractionation preoperative chemoradiation, pancreaticodudenectomy, and intraoperative radiation therapy for resectable pancreatic adenocarcinoma. J Clin Oncol. 1998;16(12):3848–50.
13. Talamonti MS, Small Jr W, Mulcahy MF, Wayne JD, Attaluri V, Colletti LM, Zalupski M, Hoffman JP, Freedman GM, Kinsella TJ, Philip PA, McGinn CJ. A multi-institutional phase II trial of preoperative full-dose gemcitabine and concurrent radiation for patients with potentially resectable pancreatic cancer. Ann Surg Oncol. 2006;13(2):150–8.
14. Evans DB, Varadhachary GR, Crane CH, Sun CC, Lee JE, Pisters PW, Vauthey JN, Wang H, Cleary KR, Staerkel GA, Charnsangavei C, Lano EA, Ho L, Lenzi R, Abbruzzese JL, Wolff RA. Preoperative gemcitabine-based chemoradiation for patients with resectable adenocarcinoma of the pancreatic head. J Clin Oncol. 2008;26(21):3496–502.
15. Varadhachary GR, Wolff RA, Crane CH, Sun CC, Lee JE, Pisters PW, Vauthey JN, Abdulla E, Wang H, Staerkel GA, Lee JH, Ross WA, Tamm EP, Bhosale PR, Krishnan S, Das P, Ho L, Xiong H, Abbruzzese JL, Evans DB. Preoperative gemcitabine and cisplatin followed by gemcitabine-based chemoradiation for resectable adenocarcinoma of the pancreatic head. J Clin Oncol. 2008;26(21):3487–95.
16. Kim EJ, Ben-Josef E, Herman JM, Bekaii-Saab T, Dawson LA, Griffith KA, Francis IR, Greenson JK, Simeone DM, Lawrence TS, Laheru D, Wolfgang CL, Williams T, Bloomston M, Moore MJ, Wei A, Zalupski MM. A multi-institutional phase 2 study of neoadjuvant gem-

citabine and oxliplatin with radiation therapy in patients with pancreatic cancer. Cancer. 2013;119(15):2692–700.
17. Turrini O, Ychou M, Moureau-Zabotto L, Rouanet P, Giovannini M, Moutardier V, Azria D, Delpero JR, Viret F. Neoadjuvant docetaxel-based chemoradiation for resectable adenocarcinoma of the pancreas: new neoadjuvant regimen was safe and provided an interesting pathologic response. Eur J Surg Oncol. 2010;36(10):987–92.
18. Heinrich S, Petalozzi BC, Schafer M, Weber A, Bauerfeind P, Knuth A, Clavien PA. Prospective phase II trial of neoadjuvant chemotherapy with gemcitabine and cisplatin for resectable adenocarcinoma of the pancreatic head. J Clin Oncol. 2008;26(15):2526–31.
19. Palmer DH, Stocken D, Hewitt H, Markham CE, Hassan AB, Johnson PJ, Buckels JA, Bramhall SR. A randomized phase 2 trial of neoadjuvant chemotherapy in resectable pancreatic cancer: gemcitabine alone versus gemcitabine combined with cisplatin. Ann Surg Oncol. 2007;14(7):2088–96.
20. O'Reilly EM, Perelshteyn A, Jarnagin WR, Schattner M, Gerdes H, Capanu M, Tang LH, LaValle J, Winston C, DeMatteo RP, D'Angelica M, Kurtz RC, Abou-Alfa GK, Klimstra DS, Lowery MA, Brennan MF, Coit DG, Reidy DL, Kingham TP, Allen PJ. A single-arm, nonrandomized phase II trial of neoadjuvant gemcitabine and oxliplatin in patients with resectable pancreas adenocarcinoma. Ann Surg. 2014;260(1):142–8.
21. Yachida S, Jones S, Bozic I, Antal T, Leary R, Fu B, Kamiyama M, Hruban RH, Eshleman JR, Nowak MA, Velculescu VE, Kinzler KW, Vogelstein B, Iacobuzio-Donahue CA. Distant metastasis occurs late during the genetic evolution of pancreatic cancer. Nature. 2010;467(7319):1114–7.
22. Rhim AD, Mirek ET, Aiello NM, Maitra A, Bailey JM, McAllister F, Reichert M, Beatty GL, Rustgi AK, Vonderheide RH, Leach SD, Stanger BZ. EMT and dissemination precede pancreatic tumor formation. Cell. 2012;148(1–2):349–61.
23. Haeno H, Gonen M, Davis MB, Herman JM, Iacobuzio-Donahue CA, Michor F. Computational modeling of pancreatic cancer reveals kinetics of metastasis suggesting optimum treatment strategies. Cell. 2012;148(1–2):362–75.
24. Yeo CJ, Cameron JL, Lillemoe KD, Sitzmann JV, Hruban RH, Goodman SN, Dooley WC, Coleman J, Pitt HA. Pancreaticoduodenectomy for cancer of the head of the pancreas. 201 patients. Ann Surg. 1995;221(6):721–31.
25. Neoptolemos JP, Stocken DD, Dunn JA, Almond J, Beger HG, Pederzoli P, Bassi C, Dervenis C, Fernandez-Cruz L, Lacaine F, Buckels J, Deakin M, Adab FA, Sutton R, Imrie C, Ihse I, Tihanyi T, Olah A, Pedrazzoli S, Spooner D, Kerr DJ, Friess H, Buchler MW, European Study Group for Pancreatic Cancer. Influence of resection margins on survival for patients with pancreatic cancer treated by adjuvant chemoradiation and/or chemotherapy in the ESPAC-1 randomized controlled trial. Ann Surg. 2001;234(6):758–68.
26. Raut CP, Tseng JF, Sun CC, Wang H, Wolff RA, Crane CH, Hwang R, Vauthey JN, Abdalla EK, Lee JE, Pisters PW, Evans DB. Impact of resection status on pattern of failure and survival after pancreaticoduodenectomy for pancreatic adenocarcinoma. Ann Surg. 2007;246(1):52–60.
27. Katz MH, Wang H, Balachandran A, Bhosale P, Crane CH, Wang X, Pisters PW, Lee JE, Vauthey JN, Abdalla EK, Wolff R, Abbruzzese J, Varadhachary G, Chopin-Laly X, Charnsangavej C, Fleming JB. Effect of neoadjuvant chemoradiation and surgical technique on recurrence of localized pancreatic cancer. J Gastrointest Surg. 2012;16(1):68–78.
28. Le Scodan R, Mornex F, Partensky C, Mercier C, Valette PJ, Ychou M, Roy P, Scoazec JY. Histopathological response to preoperative chemoradiation for resectable pancreatic adenocarcinoma: the French Phase II FFCD 9704-SFRO Trial. Am J Clin Oncol. 2008;31(6):545–52.
29. Zhao Q, Rashid A, Gong Y, Katz MH, Lee JE, Wolf R, Balachandran A, Varadhachary GR, Pisters PW, Wang H, Gomez HF, Abruzzese JL, Fleming JB, Wang H. Pathologic complete response to neoadjuvant therapy in patients with pancreatic ductal adenocarcinoma is associated with a better prognosis. Ann Diagn Pathol. 2012;16(1):29–37.

30. Tzeng CW, Tran Cao HS, Lee JE, Pister PW, Varadhachary GR, Wolff RA, Abbruzzese JL, Crane CH, Evans DB, Wang H, Abbott DE, Vauthey JN, Aloia TA, Fleming JB, Katz MH. Treatment sequencing for resectable pancreatic cancer: influence of early metastases and surgical complications on multimodality therapy completion and survival. J Gastrointest Surg. 2014;18(1):16–24.
31. Valle JW, Palmer D, Jackson R, Cox T, Neoptolemos JP, Ghaneh P, Rawcliffe CL, Bassi C, Stocken DD, Cunningham D, O'Reilly D, Goldstein D, Robinson BA, Karapetis C, Scarfe A, Lacaine F, Sand J, Izbicki JR, Mayerle J, Dervenis C, Oláh A, Butturini G, Lind PA, Middleton MR, Anthoney A, Sumpter K, Carter R, Büchler MW. Optimal duration and timing of adjuvant chemotherapy after definitive surgery for ductal adenocarcinoma of the pancreas: ongoing lessons from the ESPAC-3 study. Clin Oncol. 2014;32(6):504–12.
32. Amin S, Lucas AL, Frucht H. Evidence for treatment and survival disparities by age in pancreatic adenocarcinoma: a population-based analysis. Pancreas. 2013;32(2):249–53.
33. Cooper AB, Holmes HM, des Bordes JK, Fogelman D, Parker NH, Lee JE, Aloia TA, Vauthey JN, Fleming JB, Katz MH. Role of neoadjuvant therapy in the multimodality treatment of older patients with pancreatic cancer. J Am Coll Surg. 2014;219(1):111–20.
34. Aloia TA, Lee JE, Vauthey JN, Abdalla EK, Wolff RA, Varadhachary GR, Abbruzzese JL, Crane CH, Evans DB, Pisters PW. Delayed recovery after pancreaticoduodenectomy: a major factor impairing the delivery of adjuvant therapy? J Am Coll Surg. 2007;204(3):347–55.
35. Tzeng CW, Katz MH, Fleming JB, Lee JE, Pisters PW, Holmes HM, Varadhachary GR, Wolff RA, Abbruzzese JL, Vauthey JN, Aloia TA. Morbidity and mortality after pancreaticoduodenectomy in patients with borderline resectable type C clinical classification. J Gastrointest Surg. 2014;18(1):146–55.
36. Cooper AB, Parmar AD, Riall TS, Hall BL, Katz MH, Aloia TA, Pitt HA. Does the use of neoadjuvant therapy for pancreatic adenocarcinoma increase postoperative morbidity and mortality rates? J Gastrointest Surg. 2015;19(1):80–6.
37. Sohn TA, Yeo CJ, Cameron JL, Pitt HA, Lillemoe KD. Do preoperative biliary stents increase postpancreaticoduodenectomy complications? J Gastrointest Surg. 2000;4(3):258–67.
38. Pisters PW, Hudec WA, Lee JE, Raijman I, Lahoti S, Janjan NA, Rich TA, Crane CH, Lenzi R, Wolff RA, Abbruzzese JL, Evans DB. Preoperative chemoradiation for patients with pancreatic cancer: toxicity of endobiliary stents. J Clin Oncol. 2000;18(4):860–7.
39. Ahmad SA, Edwards MJ, Sutton JM, Grewal SS, Hanseman DJ, Maithel SK, Patel SH, Bentram DJ, Weber SM, Cho CS, Winslow ER, Scoggins CR, Martin RC, Kim HJ, Baker JJ, Merchant NB, Parikh AA, Kooby DA. Factors influencing readmission after pancreaticoduodenectomy: a multi-institutional study of 1302 patients. Ann Surg. 2012;256(3):529–37.
40. Abbott DA, Tzeng CW, Merkow RP, Cantor SB, Chang GJ, Katz MH, Bentrem DJ, Bilimoria KY, Crane CH, Varadhachary GR, Abbruzzese JL, Wolff RA, Lee JE, Evans DB, Fleming JB. The cost-effectiveness of neoadjuvant chemoradiation is superior to a surgery-first approach in the treatment of pancreatic head adenocarcinoma. Ann Surg Oncol. 2013;20(Suppl3):S500–8.
41. Brunner TB, Grabenbauer GG, Meyer T, Golcher H, Sauer R, Hohenberger W. Primary resection versus neoadjuvant chemoradiation followed by resection for locally resectable or potentially resectable pancreatic carcinoma without distant metastasis. A multi-centre prospectively randomized phase II study of the Interdisciplinary Working Group Gastrointestinal Tumours (AIO, ARO, and CAO). BMC Cancer. 2007;7:41.
42. Tachezy M, Gebauer F, Peterson C, Arnold D, Trepel M, Wegscheider K, Schafhausen P, Bockhorn M, Izbicki JR, Yekebas E. Sequential neadjuvant chemoradiotherapy (CRT) followed by curative surgery vs surgery alone for resectable, non-metastasized pancreatic adenocarcinoma: NEOPA-a randomized multicenter phase III study (NCT01900327, DRKS00003893, ISRCTN82191749). BMC Cancer. 2014;14:411.
43. Heinrich S, Pestalozzi B, Lesurtel M, Berrevoet F, Laurent S, Delpero JR, Raoul JL, Bachellier P, Dufour P, Moehler M, Weber A, Lang H, Rogiers X, Clavien PA. Adjuvant gemcitabine versus NEOadjuvant gemcitabine/oxaliplatin plus adjuvant gemcitabine in resectable pancre-

atic cancer: a randomized multicenter phase III study (NEOPAC study). BMC Cancer. 2011;11:346.
44. Roeder F, Timke C, Saleh-Ebrahimi L, Schneider L, Hackert T, Hartwig W, Kopp-Schneider A, Hensley F, Buechler M, Debus J, Huber P, Werner J. Clinical phase I/II trial to investigate neoadjuvant intensity-modulated short term radiation therapy (5x5Gy) and intraoperative radiation therapy (15Gy) in patients with primarily resectable pancreatic cancer-NEOPANC. BMC Cancer. 2012;12:112.
45. Conroy T, Desseigne F, Ychou M, Bouche O, Guimbaud R, Becouarn Y, Adenis A, Raoul JL, Gourgou-Bourgade S, de la Fouchardiere C, Bennouna J, Bachet JB, Khemissa-Akouz F, Pere-Verge D, Delbaldo C, Assenat E, Chauffert B, Michel P, Montoto-Grillot C, Ducreaux M, Groupe Tumeurs Digestives of Unicancer, PRODIGE Intergroup. FOLFIRINOX versus gemcitabine for metastatic pancreatic cancer. N Engl J Med. 2011;364(19):1817–25.
46. Katz MH, Marsh R, Herman JM, Shi Q, Collison E, Venook AP, Kindler HL, Alberts SR, Philip P, Lowy AM, Pisters PW, Posner MC, Berlin JD, Ahmad SA. Borderline resectable pancreatic cancer: need for standardization and methods for optimal clinical trial design. Ann Surg Oncol. 2013;20(8):2787–95.
47. Motoi F, Ishida K, Fujishima F, Ottomo S, Oikawa M, Okada T, Shimamura H, Takemura S, Ono F, Akada M, Nakagawa K, Katayose Y, Egawa S, Unno M. Neoadjuvant chemotherapy with gemcitabine and S-1 for resectable and borderline pancreatic ductal adenocarcinoma: results from a prospective multi-institutional phase 2 trial. Ann Surg Oncol. 2013;20(12):3794–801.

Chapter 52
Management of Borderline Resectable Pancreatic Cancer

Gareth Morris-Stiff and R. Mathew Walsh

Abstract Conventional definitions of resectability for pancreatic cancer would suggest that approximately 20 % are suitable for resection. Over recent years, the concept of borderline resectable pancreatic cancer (BRPC) has evolved to describe the cohort comprising around 25 % of patients with tumors involving either the portovenous confluence or mesenteric arteries in which a curative resection is technically feasible. The technical feasibility should correspond with acceptable perioperative and oncologic outcomes, both of which may be improved with neoadjuvant therapy. It is crucial that high quality cross-sectional imaging be performed during the evaluation, and that patients fitting internationally accepted criteria for BRPC be discussed in a multidisciplinary setting where neoadjuvant therapy should be considered. In order to comprehensively evaluate outcomes, and allow comparison with other contemporary series, an adopted standardized system of intra-operative evaluation and vascular resection is required. It is also of great importance that a standardized means of pathological assessment of resected specimens be used to allow accurate definition of curative resections in the technically challenging BRPC cohort.

Keywords Pancreatic cancer • Borderline resection • Chemotherapy • Radiotherapy • Surgery

Introduction

While surgical resection is the only curative option for pancreatic cancer, only 10–20 % of patients have clearly resectable disease, and 30–40 % have locally advanced disease often deemed 'inoperable' due to involvement of surrounding major vessels. The remaining 50–60 % have metastatic disease [1]. Recent improvements in pre-operative assessment and operative technique has challenged the

G. Morris-Stiff • R.M. Walsh (✉)
Department of General Surgery, Division of Hepato-Pancreato-Biliary Surgery, Digestive Disease Institute, A100 Cleveland Clinic Foundation, Cleveland, OH 44195, USA
e-mail: walshm@ccf.org

J.M. Millis, J.B. Matthews (eds.), *Difficult Decisions in Hepatobiliary and Pancreatic Surgery*, Difficult Decisions in Surgery: An Evidence-Based Approach, DOI 10.1007/978-3-319-27365-5_52

'inoperability' of tumors involving the portovenous confluence or encroaching on the superior mesenteric artery/celiac axis, and such tumors are now termed borderline resectable pancreatic cancer (BRPC).

At present, there is no uniform agreement as to specific definitions of BRPC and there are two classifications systems whose merits are the subject of significant debate [2, 3]. To add further confusion, the American Joint Committee on Cancer (AJCC) does not currently recognize BRPC and defines venous occlusion and arterial encasement as unresectable disease [4].

The aim of this chapter is to present an overview of current understanding and debate and to indicate areas in which further evaluation is required.

Search Strategy

A comprehensive text-word and MeSH-based electronic search of English language literature up until October 2014 was used to identity manuscripts published on the topic of BRPC using the PICO outline (Table 52.1). Databases searched included PubMed, Embase, Science Citation Index/Social sciences Citation Index and Cochrane Evidence Based Medicine. Terms used in the search were "pancreatic cancer," "borderline resectable," "superior mesenteric vein," "portal vein," "celiac axis," "superior mesenteric artery," "common hepatic artery," "neoadjuvant chemotherapy," "neoadjuant radiotherapy," and "neoadjuvant chemoradiotherapy." Additionally, the bibliographies of relevant articles were hand searched for additional material.

Articles were excluded if they included related to resectable or unresectable disease rather than specifically addressing BRPC. After evaluating the manuscripts, the data was classified using the GRADE system and recommendations are classified using this approach.

Results

Defining BRPC

Agreement is required to obtain a uniformly accepted definition of BRPC. Although numerous classification systems have been proposed over the past decade, there are two that are widely referenced: the National Comprehensive Cancer Network (NCCN) [2], and the Alliance for Clinical Trials in Oncology group [3].

Table 52.1 PICO table for borderline resectable pancreatic cancer

P (Patients)	I (Intervention)	C (Comparator group)	O (Outcomes measured)
Patients with borderline resectable pancreatic cancer	Surgical resection	Non-operative therapy including chemotherapy and radiotherapy	Morbidity and mortality

The origin of the NCCN guidelines was a series of expert statements made on behalf of the American Hepato-Pancreato-Biliary Association, the Society of Surgical Oncology, and the Society of the Alimentary Tract in 2009 [5–7]. The guideline, which subjectively describes the relationship between the tumor and the vessels (Table 52.1), was adopted by the NCCN, and the guidelines now bear its name [2]. The Alliance criteria [3], which arose from the MD Anderson definition [8], differ from those of the NCCN as they assign degrees of contact between tumor and specific vessels. The International Study Group of Pancreatic Surgery [9] also recently endorsed the NCCN definition of BPRC.

Diagnosing BRPC

The diagnosis and classification of by computed tomography cross-sectional imaging is the modality used by NCCN and Alliance criteria [2, 3]. The ISGPS guidelines recommend scanning within the 4-week period prior to resection using a high-resolution multidetector CT, with multiplanar reconstruction capabilities to accurately assess the precise relationship between the tumor and the mesenteric vessels (Tables 52.2 and 52.3) [9]. The ISGPS also stipulate that all cases should be discussed in a multidisciplinary team (MDT) setting and management be carried out in high volume centers.

A second area requiring clarification is the fact that the American Joint Committee on Cancer (AJCC) does not currently recognize BRPC and defines venous occlu-

Table 52.2 Definition of borderline resectable pancreatic cancer (BRPC) based on NCCN 2014 [4]

Localized and resectable	Borderline resectable	Unresectable*
No distant metastasis	No distant metastasis	Distant metastasis
No radiographic evidence of SMV or PV distortion	Venous involvement of the SMV or PV with distortion or narrowing of the vein or occlusion of the vein with suitable vessel proximal and distal, allowing for safe resection and replacement	Unreconstructable SMV/portal occlusion or IVC encasement
Clear fat planes around CA, HA, and SMA	GDA encasement up to the hepatic artery with either short segment encasement or direct abutment of the HA without extension to the CA Tumor abutment of the SMA not to exceed 180° of the circumference of the vessel wall	CA abutment Greater than 180° SMA encasement Aortic invasion or encasement

CA Celiac axis, *GDA* gastroduodenal artery, *HA* hepatic artery, *IVC* inferior vena cava, *NCCN* National Comprehensive Cancer Network, *PV* portal vein, *SMA* superior mesenteric artery, *SMV* superior mesenteric vein

*Applies to head cancers only

Table 52.3 ISGPS classification if venous resections [11]

Classification	Nature of resection/reconstruction
Type 1	Partial venous excision with direct closure (venorraphy) by suture closure
Type 2	Partial venous excision using a patch
Type 3	Segmental resection with primary venovenous anastomosis
Type 4	Segmental resection with interposed venous conduit and at least two anastomoses

sion and arterial encasement as unresectable disease [4]. This will need addressing in the next revision to take account of changes in practice.

Venous Involvement

There is a large volume of contemporary evidence regarding venous resection for curative resection. Zhou et al. in a recent meta-analysis examined 2,247 patients from 19 non-randomized trials undergoing pancreatic resection during the period 1994–2010, including 661 in whom a venous resection (VR) was performed [10]. They reported no difference in morbidity (OR: 0.95; 95 % CI: 0.74–1.21; P=0.67), peri-operative mortality (OR: 1.19; 95 % CI: 0.73–1.96; P=0.48), or 5-year overall survival (OR: 0.57; 95 % CI: 0.32–1.02; P=0.06) between patients undergoing VR and those undergoing standard resection. The authors concluded that resection was justified in the presence of venous involvement when considering surgical outcomes.

In a second meta-analysis, Yu and co-workers examined 2,890 patients from 22 series, including 794 undergoing VR [11]. In this analysis, the morbidity (OR: 1.01; 95 % CI: 0.82–1.24; P=0.93), and peri-operative mortality (OR: 1.49; 95 % CI: 0.97–2.31; P=0.07), were comparable for pancreatoduodenectomy (PD) and PD VR cohorts. However, they noted that while there was no difference in 1-year (OR: 1.00; 95 % CI: 0.65–1.53; P=0.99) or 3-year (OR: 0.78; 95 % CI: 0.54–1.14; P=0.20) survival between the groups, the 5-year survival was inferior when vein resection was required (OR: 0.69; 95 % CI: 0.49–0.97; P=0.03). An additional factor noted in this meta-analysis was that the R0 resection rates were significantly inferior following PDVR (OR: 0.6; 95 % CI: 0.48–0.74; P<0.001).

The relationship between vascular resection and negative microscopic margins is not clear. Kelly and colleagues evaluated 492 patients undergoing PD from a single center where neoadjuvant therapy was not performed, compared 422 undergoing PD alone to 70 undergoing PD VR [12]. They reported no difference in R0 resection (66 % versus 75 %, P=NS), and noted that vein involvement was not predictive of disease-free or overall survival (OR: 1.00; 95 % CI: 0.91–2.76; P=0.07). The ISGPS guidelines note that the extent of venous resection and the method of reconstruction are not accurately documented and they propose a classification for comparison between series (Table 52.2).

Arterial Involvement

The evidence for arterial resection in BRPC is less compelling. A meta-analysis by Mollberg et al. of 26 studies between 1977 and 2010 contained 366 undergoing arterial resection during various types of pancreatic resection [13]. In contrast to venous resection, arterial resection was associated with a significantly increased peri-operative morbidity (OR: 2.17; 95 % CI: 1.26–3.75; P=0.006) and mortality (OR: 5.04; 95 % CI: 2.69–9.45; P=0.002). Furthermore, the 1-year (OR: 0.49; 95 % CI: 0.31–0.78; *P*=0.002) and 3 years (OR: 0.39; 95 % CI: 0.17–0.86; P=0.02) were significantly inferior, leading the authors to conclude arterial resection should be performed in only highly selected patients.

Neoadjuvant Therapy

There is good rationale to believe that neoadjuvant therapy (NAT) may be beneficial in patients with BRPC.

(i) Progression of disease during NAT may select patients with poor natural history. It is presumed that tumors that progress on therapy would have done poorly with upfront resection.
(ii) Systematic treatment is justified based on the high incidence of metastatic disease at presentation.
(iii) The use of a treatment modality that could increase the R0 margin rate by removing the tumor from the major vasculature would appear logical [14].
(iv) NAT may result in fewer pancreatic fistulae following radiotherapy-induced fibrosis [15].

The evidence for NAT in BRPC is summarized in Table 52.4. All studies are single center, retrospective series using a variety of NATs. There was a variation in the resectability rates, but the negative margin status was generally high, providing a median survival a little over 20 months in most of the studies.

The heterogeneity of treatment regimens and mix of definitions of BRPC, has lead the ISGPS to not recommend BAT as standard of care. The ESPAC 5F study that randomizes patients with BRPC to surgery versus NAT followed by surgery should add to the quality of the evidence [25].

Standardized Radiology

The importance of accurate documentation of the radiological appearance of pancreatic carcinoma was highlighted in a recent consensus statement behalf of the Society of Abdominal Radiology and the American Pancreatic Association [26] that

Table 52.4 Neoadjuvant therapy in BRPC for studies published 2010–2014

Authors	Number BRPC	Definition of BRPC	Neoadjuvant	Resected	Negative margins	Median OS (months)
Chun et al. [16]	109	Ishikawa [22]	5FU or Gemcitabine CRT	100 %	59 %	23
Stokes et al. [17]	40	MDA	Capecitabine CRT	46 %	75 %	23
Kang et al. [18]	35	NCCN	Gemcitabine CRT	91 %	87 %	26.3
Katz et al. [19]	129	NCCN 115 MDA 72	Gemcitabine and CRT or CRT alone	84 % vs. 75 %	95 %	33
Cho et al. [20]	30	MDA	Gemcitabine CRT	100 %	96.7 %	21.1
Chuong et al. [21]	57	NCCN	Gemcitabine CRT	56 %	96 %	16.4
Christans et al. [22]	18	Milwaukee[a]	FOLFIRINOX followed by gemcitabine or capecitabine CRT	67 %	100 %	22
Chakraborty et al. [23]	13	MDA	Capecitabine CRT	38 %	80 %	9.1
Rose et al. [24]	64	NCCN	Gemcitabine and docetaxel	48 %	87 %	21.6

MDA MD Anderson, *NCCN* National comprehensive cancer network; *CRT* chemoradiotherapy

[a]Classification

advocated a dedicated protocol for CT evaluation of the cancer location, as well as the degree of vascular contact of the tumor. Al-Hawary and colleagues also recommended the use of a standardized reporting protocol with the aim of improving preoperative staging and surgical decision making, as well as facilitating comparison of imaging results between centers for purposes of research and clinical study design.

Standardized Histopathology

The importance of meticulous pathological assessment of resection specimen was highlighted following the seminal work of Verbeke and colleagues which re-defined the way in which specimen are processed [27] Verbeke later published a detailed account of the technique that became the basis of the Royal College of Pathologists standards for reporting periampullary cancers [28, 29]. This revised approach shows a significantly lower R0 resection rate, and a change in frequencies of the origin of periampullary cancers. The ISGPS guidelines recommend the use of the protocol to allow accurate comparison between sites.

A Personal View of The Data

The recently published ISPGS guidelines have gone a long way towards setting standards against which future data on BRPC may be assessed. A clear, globally acceptable definition of BRPC needs to be adopted, and the use of other terminology should be discontinued. Assessment of operability should be made on the basis of high quality imaging in a multi-disciplinary team setting. There are good data to support the safety and efficacy of resection of the superior mesenteric and portal veins by experienced teams, however, there is no compelling evidence to recommend arterial resection, and this should be considered on a highly selective basis. Although there are some encouraging studies indicating the potential value of various different NATs in BRPC, there is not yet high-level evidence indicating they should be uniformly applied, and data from randomized trials of NAT and surgery versus surgery alone are awaited. For patients undergoing resection, a classification of the procedure performed, using a system such as that proposed by the ISPGS will allow a more reliable comparison of published series. To-date, the majority of published series have not utilized the Royal College of Pathologists guidelines to assess resection margins suggesting the majority of series report artificially high R0 resection rates. A reproducible assessment of treatment effect on the primary tumor should also be incorporated into the results. Widespread application of these guidelines and subsequent long-term follow-up are required in order to better assess the true effect of treatment of BRPC.

Recommendations

- The definition of borderline resectable pancreatic head adenocarcinoma should be based on the NCCN criteria (evidence quality moderate, strong recommendation).
- Histopathological reporting should be standardized according to the RCPath guidelines (evidence quality moderate, strong recommendation).
- Decision planning for borderline resectable pancreatic cancer should be multidisciplinary (evidence quality moderate, strong recommendation).
- Surgical resection should include portal, superior mesenteric, and splenic vein reconstruction (according to anatomic circumstances) to achieve an R0 outcome (evidence quality moderate, strong recommendation).
- Surgical resection should not be undertaken for locally invasive disease involving the superior mesenteric and/or hepatic arterial system (evidence quality weak, weak recommendation).
- Neoadjuvant chemotherapy ± radiotherapy should be considered prior to surgical resection for locally invasive disease (evidence quality weak, weak recommendation).

References

1. Gillen S, Schuster T, Meyer Zum Büschenfelde C, Friess H, Kleeff J. Preoperative/neoadjuvant therapy in pancreatic cancer: a systematic review and meta-analysis of response and resection percentages. PLoS Med. 2010;7:e1000267.
2. Tempero MA, Malafa MP, Behrman SW, Benson III AB, Casper ES, Chiorean EB, et al. Pancreatic adenocarcinoma, version 2.2104. J Natl Compr Canc Netw. 2014;12:1083–93.
3. Katz MH, Marsh R, Herman JM, Shi Q, Collison E, Venook AP, et al. Borderline resectable pancreatic cancer: need for standardization and methods for optimal clinical trial design. Ann Surg Oncol. 2013;20:2787–95.
4. Edge SB, Byrd DR, Compton CC, Fritz AG, Greene FL, Trotti A, editors. AJCC cancer staging manual. 7th ed. New York: Springer-Verlag; 2010.
5. Callery MP, Chang KJ, Fishman EK, Talamonti MS, Treverso WL, Linehan DC. Pretreatment assessment of resectable and borderline resectable pancreatic cancer: expert consensus statement. Ann Surg Oncol. 2009;16:1727–33.
6. Evans DB, Farnell MB, Lillemoe KD, Vollmer Jr C, Strasberg SM, Schulick RD. Surgical treatment of resectable and borderline resectable pancreas cancer: expert consensus statement. Ann Surg Oncol. 2009;16:1736–44.
7. Pisters PW. Combined modality treatment of resectable and borderline resectable pancreas cancer: expert consensus statement. Ann Surg Oncol. 2009;16:1751–6.
8. Varadhachary GR, Tamm EP, Crane C, Evans DB, Wolff RA. Borderline resectable pancreatic cancer. Curr Treat Options Gastroenterol. 2005;8:377–84.
9. Bockhorn M, Uzunoglu FG, Adham M, Imrie C, Milicevic M, Sandberg AA, et al. Borderline resectable pancreatic cancer: a consensus statement by the International Study Group of Pancreatic Surgery (ISGPS). Surgery. 2014;155:977–88.

10. Zhou Y, Zhang Z, Liu Y, Li B, Xu D. Pancreatectomy combined with superior mesenteric vein-portal vein resection for pancreatic cancer: a meta-analysis. World J Surg. 2012;36:884–91.
11. Yu XZ, Li J, Fu DL, Di Y, Yang F, Hao SJ, Jin C. Benefit from synchronous portal-superior mesenteric vein resection during pancreaticoduodenectomy for cancer: a meta-analysis. Eur J Surg Oncol. 2014;40:371–8.
12. Kelly KJ, Winslow E, Kooby D, Lad NL, Parikh AA, Scoggins CR, et al. Vein involvement during pancreaticoduodenectomy: is there a need for redefinition of "borderline" resectable disease? J Gastrointest Surg. 2013;17:1209–17.
13. Mollberg N, Rahbari NN, Koch M, Hartwig W, Hoeger Y, Buchler MW, et al. Arterial resection during pancreatectomy for pancreatic cancer: a systematic review and meta-analysis. Ann Surg. 2011;254:882–93.
14. Laurence JM, Tran PD, Morarji K, Eslick GD, Lam VW, Sandroussi C. A systematic review and meta-analysis of survival and surgical outcomes following neoadjuvant chemoradiotherapy for pancreatic cancer. J Gastrointest Surg. 2011;15:2059–69.
15. Lowy AM, Lee JE, Pisters PW, Davidson BS, Fenoglio CJ, Stanford P, et al. Prospective, randomized trial of octreotide to prevent pancreatic fistula after pancreaticoduodenectomy for malignant disease. Ann Surg. 1997;226:632–41.
16. Chun YS, Milestone BN, Watson JC, Cohen SJ, Burtness B, Engstrom PF, et al. Defining venous involvement in borderline resectable pancreatic cancer. Ann Surg Oncol. 2010;17:2832–8.
17. Stokes JB, Nolan NJ, Stelow EB, Walters DM, Weiss GR, de Lange EE, et al. Preoperative capecitabine and concurrent radiation for borderline resectable pancreatic cancer. Ann Surg Oncol. 2011;18:619–27.
18. Kang CM, Chung YE, Park JY, Sung JS, Hwang HK, Choi HJ, et al. Potential contribution of preoperative neoadjuvant concurrent chemoradiation therapy on margin-negative resection in borderline resectable pancreatic cancer. J Gastrointest Surg. 2012;16:509–17.
19. Katz MH, Fleming JB, Bhosale P, Varadhachary G, Lee JE, Wolff R, et al. Response of borderline resectable pancreatic cancer to neoadjuvant therapy is not reflected by radiographic indicators. Cancer. 2012;118:5749–56.
20. Cho IR, Chung MJ, Bang S, Park SW, Chung JB, Song SY, et al. Gemcitabine based neoadjuvant chemoradiotherapy therapy in patients with borderline resectable pancreatic cancer. Pancreatology. 2013;13:539–43.
21. Chuong MD, Springett GM, Freilich JM, Park CK, Weber JM, Mellon EA, et al. Stereotactic body radiation therapy for locally advanced and borderline resectable pancreatic cancer is effective and well tolerated. Int J Radiat Oncol Biol Phys. 2013;86:516–22.
22. Christians KK, Tsai S, Mahmoud A, Ritch P, Thomas JP, Wiebe L, et al. Neoadjuvant FOLFIRINOX for borderline resectable pancreas cancer: a new treatment paradigm? Oncologist. 2014;19:266–74.
23. Chakraborty S, Morris MM, Bauer TW, Adams RB, Stelow EB, Petroni G, Sanoff HK. Accelerated fraction radiotherapy with capecitabine as neoadjuvant therapy for borderline resectable pancreatic cancer. Gastrointest Cancer Res. 2014;7:15–22.
24. Rose JB, Rocha FG, Alseidi A, Biehl T, Moonka R, Ryan JA, et al. Extended neoadjuvant chemotherapy for borderline resectable pancreatic cancer demonstrates promising postoperative outcomes and survival. Ann Surg Oncol. 2014;21:1530–7.
25. European Study Group for Pancreatic Cancer (ESPAC) Study 5f http://public.ukcrn.org.uk/search/StudyDetail.aspx?StudyID=16201.
26. Al-Hawary MM, Francis IR, Chari ST, Fishman EK, Hough DM, Lu DS, et al. Pancreatic ductal adenocarcinoma radiology reporting template: consensus statement of the society of abdominal radiology and the American Pancreatic Association. Gastroenterology. 2014;146:291–304.

27. Verbeke CS, Leitch D, Menon KV, McMahon MJ, Guillou PJ, Anthoney A. Redefining the R1 resection in pancreatic cancer. Br J Surg. 2006;93:1232–7.
28. Verbeke CS. Resection margins and R1 rates in pancreatic cancer – are we there yet? Histopathology. 2008;52:787–96.
29. The Royal College of Pathologists: standards and datasets for reporting cancers. Dataset for the histopathological reporting of carcinomas of the pancreas, ampulla of Vater and common bile duct. The Royal College of Pathologists; London; 2010.

Chapter 53
Peritoneal Drain Placement at Pancreatoduodenectomy

Matthew T. McMillan and Charles M. Vollmer Jr.

Abstract Routine peritoneal drainage has traditionally accompanied pancreatoduodenectomy, yet its efficacy has been questioned in recent years. The first randomized, controlled trial to evaluate this practice reported an association between drainage and intra-abdominal abscess, fluid collection, and fistula following major pancreatic resections. Since that study, several retrospective works have also found little to no advantage from routine drainage. Conversely, a recent randomized, controlled trial suggested that eliminating drains increases the frequency and severity of complications. A deeper analysis of that trial demonstrated a benefit to selective drainage based on the degree of risk for developing clinically relevant pancreatic fistula, as assessed by the Fistula Risk Score. Drainage appeared to confer no benefit to patients with negligible and low fistula risk, while drain placement in moderate and high fistula risk patients was associated with significantly lower rates of intra-abdominal abscess, clinically relevant pancreatic fistula, and IR-guided percutaneous drainage. The Fistula Risk Score can identify patients who benefit from peritoneal drainage at pancreatoduodenectomy. The highest quality evidence on this topic suggests calculating the Fistula Risk Score intraoperatively, at the point of reconstruction, and placing drains in only patients with moderate or high clinically relevant pancreatic fistula risk.

Keywords Intraoperative drain • Pancreatoduodenectomy • Pancreatic fistula • Risk assessment • Fistula Risk Score (FRS)

M.T. McMillan • C.M. Vollmer Jr. (✉)
Department of Surgery, University of Pennsylvania Perelman School of Medicine, Philadelphia, PA 19104, USA
e-mail: Charles.Vollmer@uphs.upenn.edu

J.M. Millis, J.B. Matthews (eds.), *Difficult Decisions in Hepatobiliary and Pancreatic Surgery*, Difficult Decisions in Surgery: An Evidence-Based Approach, DOI 10.1007/978-3-319-27365-5_53

Introduction

Routine peritoneal drainage has traditionally accompanied pancreatoduodenectomy (PD), with the rationale being to evacuate blood, bile, chyle, or pancreatic juices that may collect during the postoperative period. Additionally, proponents of routine drainage suggest that it may serve as an early warning system for the development of clinically relevant postoperative pancreatic fistulas (CR-POPF) and their sequelae (e.g., hemorrhage). Despite these purported benefits, routine drainage for major pancreatic resections has been questioned in recent years; particularly, since it had demonstrated no benefit following other abdominal operations [1–5].

A major concern associated with routine drainage is that it may serve as a pathway for retrograde infection. Such a process could potentially transform a benign fluid collection into an abscess [6]. Another common concern is that high-pressure, closed-suction drainage may cause trauma to visceral tissues; erosion at the anastomotic site could lead to fistula formation. These points, as well as advances in abdominal imaging and image-guided drain placement, have led some surgeons to advocate drainage in only the minority of patients who demonstrate clinical symptoms.

This chapter will comprehensively assess the peer-reviewed literature comparing drainage versus no drainage at pancreatoduodenectomy. Each approach will be evaluated in terms of pancreatic fistula and/or intra-abdominal abscess formation, need for interventional radiology (IR) guided percutaneous drainage, and mortality. The quality of evidence derived from each study will be graded and subsequently used to develop recommendations for clinical practice.

Search Strategy

A search of English language, peer-reviewed literature was conducted to identify data on peritoneal drain placement at PD. This approach was carried out in accordance with the PICO framework (Table 53.1) using the following databases: PubMed, EMBASE, Cochrane Library, SUMSearch 2, and Trip. Search terms included "drain," "peritoneal drainage," "suction," AND ("postoperative complications," OR "fistula," OR "clinically relevant fistula," OR "clinically relevant postoperative pancreatic fistula," OR "abscess," OR "IR-guided drainage," OR "mortality"), "pancreatectomy," "pancreaticoduodenectomy," "pancreatoduodenectomy." Studies eligible for inclusion in the analysis had to meet several requirements: (i) patients

Table 53.1 PICO table for peritoneal drain placement at pancreatoduodenectomy

P (Patients)	I (Intervention)	C (Comparisons)	O (Outcomes measured)
Patients undergoing pancreatoduodenectomy	Intraoperative peritoneal drain placement	Drainage vs. no drainage vs. selective drainage	Pancreatic fistula, intra-abdominal abscess, IR-guided drainage, mortality

underwent major pancreatic resection, including PD; (ii) reported a high-volume series (>75 cases); and (ii) comparisons were made between drain and no drain cohorts in terms of postoperative pancreatic fistula (POPF)/intra-abdominal abscess formation, IR-guided percutaneous drainage, or mortality. Application of these criteria identified five observational and two randomized, controlled studies for analysis. The quality of evidence was classified using the GRADE (Grades of Recommendation, Assessment, Development, and Evaluation) system [7, 8].

Grading the Quality of Evidence

The efficacy of peritoneal drainage at PD has been evaluated in prospective, retrospective, and randomized studies. Study design plays a critical role in the GRADE framework. With this approach, reported evidence from observational cohorts is initially rated as low quality; conversely, randomized trial evidence is considered high quality from the outset. Other factors such as very large reported effects, special factors, and serious limitations can increase or decrease the quality of evidence accordingly.

Results

Observational Studies

Heslin and colleagues reported the first retrospective review of prophylactic drainage versus no drainage at PD [9]. Eighty-nine patients underwent PD and drains were placed 57 % of the time. There were no significant differences in the frequency of POPF, intra-abdominal abscess, or IR drainage (Table 53.2). As a result, the authors concluded that routine drainage may be unnecessary and should be tested in a randomized trial. The quality of evidence from Heslin's study is very low, due to several major limitations.

First, no data was provided regarding the texture of the pancreatic parenchyma and main pancreatic duct diameter. Both factors have been strongly associated with POPF/abscess formation and the need for IR-guided drainage [10]. Secondly, cohort comparisons of disease pathology were limited to malignancy, node positivity, and surgical margin; a more useful comparison would have contrasted the presence of high-risk pathologies that are associated with major morbidity following PD. In fact, high-risk pathologies such as ampullary, bile duct, and duodenal cancers appeared twice as frequently in the drain cohort (36 vs. 18 %), perhaps indicating bias in drain placement. In spite of this disparity, neither a direct comparison nor p-value was provided. Another source of bias was the prolonged anesthesia time in

Table 53.2 Efficacy of peritoneal drain placement at major pancreatic resections

Author (year)	Study type (quality of evidence)	Study group (N)	Overall fistula (%)		CR-POPF (%)		Abscess (%)		IR Drain (%)		Mortality (%)	
			D	ND	D	ND	D	ND	D	ND	D	ND
Heslin (1998)	Retrospective (very low)	PD (89)	6	3	–	–	6	0	4	3	–	–
Conlon (2001)	RCT (low/moderate)	Proximal and distal (179)	13	0	–	–	7	7	9	5	2	2
Fisher (2011)	Prospective (very low)	Proximal and distal (226)	44*	11*	12	11	6	4	2*	11*	1	1
Mehta (2013)	Retrospective (very low)	PD (709)	24*	11*	16*	8*	–	–	8	6	2	3
Adham (2013)	Retrospective (very low)	Proximal, distal, central, and enucleation (242)	16	13	9	11	12	13	5	4	5	5
Correa-Gallego (2013)	Retrospective (moderate/very low[a])	PD (739)	27*	17*	19	15	–	–	18	14	1*	3*
Van Buren (2013)	RCT (high)	PD (137)	31	20	12	20	12*	26*	9*	23*	3	12
McMillan (2014)	RCT (high)	PD – negligible/low CR-POPF risk (52)	15	5	15	5	11	16	15	12	0	4
		PD – moderate/high CR-POPF risk (85)	42	30	12*	30*	12*	32*	5*	30*	5	16

D drain, *ND* no drain, *CR-POPF* clinically relevant pancreatic fistula, *PD* pancreatoduodenectomy, *RCT* randomized controlled trial

*$P \leq 0.05$

[a]The multivariable findings were of moderate quality; however, the study's conclusion focused on heavily biased univariate analyses. The evidence supporting the conclusion is very low in quality

the drained patients (386 vs. 292 min, P = 0.0001); extended operative time has been correlated with CR-POPF development.

Additional concerns with Heslin's analysis include the use of outdated POPF nomenclature and methodological ambiguity. The study defined a POPF as ≥30 mL of pancreatic fluid not resolved by POD7, which resembles thresholds used to identify biochemical POPFs. This definition is susceptible to bias as biochemical leaks, in the absence of clinical symptoms, cannot be detected without a drain. Conversely, modern classifications of POPF—using the 2005 International Study Group on Pancreatic Fistula (ISGPF) nomenclature—delineate between biochemical and clinically relevant fistulas [11]. Lastly, the authors did not clarify which specific complications were compared between cohorts in a multivariable analysis; furthermore, it was not apparent whether the reported p-values were derived from a multivariable or univariate analysis.

A single-center, prospective study by Fisher et al. in 2011 evaluated routine drainage in 226 consecutive patients who underwent either proximal (N = 153) or distal (N = 73) pancreatectomy [6]. As expected, the incidence of overall POPFs was greater in the drain cohort; however, rates of the more pertinent CR-POPFs were nearly identical (drain vs. no drain: 12 vs. 11 %). Notably, IR-guided drainage was required more frequently in the no drain cohort (11 vs. 2 %, P = 0.001). Similarly to the review by Heslin and colleagues, the study was not without bias; patients with drains experienced greater intraoperative blood loss (400 vs. 250 mL, P = 0.006), required more operative transfusions (19 vs. 6 %, P = 0.038), and had fewer patients with low-risk pathologies (pancreatic adenocarcinoma/pancreatitis). Alternatively, patients without drains were more likely hypertensive (55 vs. 26 %, P < 0.0001); a condition associated with reduced CR-POPF risk [10, 12]. Although the study attempted to ameliorate discrepancies in CR-POPF risk by comparing a subset of patients deemed 'high-risk' (soft pancreas and/or small duct [<3 mm]), it controlled for neither disease pathology nor blood loss. A multivariable analysis would have been the optimal approach; nevertheless, differences in CR-POPF occurrence were non-significant in the subset analysis.

In 2013, Mehta and colleagues reviewed 709 patients to assess the efficacy of drainage at PD [13]. The reported findings demonstrated higher rates of overall POPF and CR-POPF in the presence of drains; in spite of these differences, routine drainage was not associated with an increased incidence of IR-guided drainage or mortality. The authors concluded that routine drainage is unnecessary and may lead to excess morbidity. Analogous to earlier observational studies, the findings were derived from inherently biased data.

Patients who were selectively drained (N = 251, 35 %) were often at a higher risk for complications in terms of operative and endogenous POPF risk factors. Drain placement was associated with longer operative time (294 vs. 201 min, P = 0.021), elevated operative blood loss (572 vs. 282 mL), blood transfusions (10 vs. 2 %, P < 0.0001), and portal vein resections (14 vs. 9 %, P = 0.022). Additionally, pancreatitis (a low-risk pathology) was more prevalent in the no drain group (15 vs. 7 %, P = 0.002). This pathological discrepancy also suggests a greater proportion of the no drain cohort was characterized by hard pancreatic parenchyma, although gland texture was not reported. While the majority of risk factors for major morbidity—particularly CR-POPFs—were present in the drain cohort, interestingly, patients without drains did have a smaller mean pancreatic duct diameter (2.2 vs. 3.8 mm, $P<0.0001$).

One approach to control for a surgeon's proclivity to drain in high risk patients would be to conduct comparisons using a multivariable or propensity score-matched analysis. Mehta reported the former approach, but compared cohorts in terms of overall POPF, rather than CR-POPF incidence. As mentioned by Fisher [6] and others, biochemical fistulas are impossible to detect when drain(s) are absent; therefore, Mehta's comparison of overall POPF between cohorts offered skewed results. Discrepancies in patient risk and questionable statistical methodology greatly weaken the quality of evidence from Mehta and colleagues' study.

Another retrospective review of routine drainage was reported by Adham et al. [14]. That study evaluated 242 patients (148 PDs) who underwent a major pancreatic resection, excluding total pancreatectomy. The authors did not find significant differences between drain and no drain cohorts in terms of overall POPF, CR-POPF, intra-abdominal abscess, IR-guided drainage, or 90-day mortality. Comparable outcomes between cohorts reinforced the authors' conclusion, which favored a no-drainage approach; however, confounding factors were clearly present that may have acted as a source of bias. First, the use of drains positively correlated with central pancreatectomy and enucleations; these forms of pancreatic resection have been associated with higher rates of fistula compared to proximal resections [15]. Secondly, operative time was longer in drained patients ($P=0.016$). Inconsistencies in surgical practice could have also influenced outcomes; one surgeon always used a drain, while the other changed from practicing as a routine drainer to no-drainer after gaining surgical expertise later in the study period. These confounding factors obfuscate Adham's findings, particularly when multivariable analyses were not conducted for the comparisons of outcomes such as fistula, abscess, IR-guided drainage, and mortality.

The most recent retrospective evaluation of routine drainage was carried out by Correa-Gallego et al. [16]. The single-center experience evaluated 739 PDs, of which 386 (52 %) were routinely drained. Patients with prophylactic drainage experienced elevated rates of overall POPF (27 vs. 17 %, $P=0.001$), yet differences in the occurrence of clinically significant fistula (19 vs. 15 %, $P=0.1$) were non-significant. IR-guided drainage was employed more frequently in drained patients ($P=0.2$), but mortality rates were higher in the absence of drains (3 vs. 1 %, $P=0.02$). Despite higher mortality rates in the absence of prophylactic drainage, Correa-Gallego and colleagues concluded that routine drainage could be safely abandoned.

The univariate findings of Correa-Gallego should be minimized since risk factors for CR-POPF and other major morbidities were more prevalent in patients with prophylactic drainage. The imbalance of risk factors encompassed soft pancreatic parenchyma, elevated operative blood loss, extended operative time, high-risk pathology, and small pancreatic duct diameter; however, in contrast to other observational studies, Correa-Gallego compared cohorts using a regression analysis, which comprehensively compared cohorts while only focusing on fistulas with clinical relevance. The risk-adjusted analysis reported no correlation between drainage and CR-POPF occurrence ($P=0.8$). Although the work by Correa-Gallego and colleagues reported several forms of unbiased regression analyses, the results described in the manuscript's conclusion focus on univariate findings. Therefore, the quality of the multivariable findings should be considered low/moderate as it was a well designed observational analysis. Conversely, the quality of the focused conclusion is very low as biased univariate findings were emphasized.

Randomized Controlled Studies

The first randomized, controlled trial to assess routine drainage was a single-center study by Conlon et al. in 2001 [17]. One hundred seventy-nine patients underwent either proximal ($N=139$) or distal ($N=40$) pancreatectomy, with drains placed 49 % of the time. No differences were noted in terms of mortality, IR-guided drainage, overall POPF, or abscess formation; however, clustering overall POPF and abscess formation revealed a significantly greater incidence in the drained cohort ($P<0.02$). Since biochemical fistulas cannot be detected in the absence of a drain, the value of this categorization is questionable. In light of these outcomes, the authors declared that drains should not be considered mandatory after standard pancreatic resections.

The quality of evidence derived from Conlon's study is low/moderate. The randomization process eliminated much of the selection bias that is characteristic of many observational studies, but the study had other limitations. First, the single-center nature of the study makes it difficult to generalize the findings. Secondly, two major risk factors for the development of CR-POPF—soft pancreatic parenchyma and small duct diameter—were not described in the manuscript. Substratification based on approximated gland texture would have been preferable. Furthermore, distal pancreatectomies were performed more often in the drain cohort; this form of pancreatic resection has been associated with elevated rates of CR-POPF compared with proximal pancreatectomy. Lastly, though no fault of the authors, the study predated the advent of the ISGPF nomenclature, which importantly delineated between innocuous biochemical fistulas and those with clinical relevance. The definition used by Conlon most closely resembles that of a biochemical fistula. Despite these shortcomings, this study laid the groundwork for future multicenter, randomized studies on routine drainage.

The first multicenter, randomized study to evaluate routine drainage was conducted with two primary endpoints: (1) report associations between routine drainage and the frequency and severity of complications; (2) ascertain the efficacy of selective drainage based on calculated Fistula Risk Score (FRS) CR-POPF risk [18, 19]. The findings of the first endpoint were recently reported by Van Buren et al. [18]. Comparing randomizations in the overall patient population ($N=137$) revealed non-significant differences in the occurrence of overall POPF and CR-POPF; how-

Table 53.3 Fistula risk score for the prediction of clinically-relevant pancreatic fistula (CR-POPF) after pancreatoduodenectomy

Risk factor	Parameter	Points
Gland texture	Firm	0
	Soft	2
Pathology	Pancreatic adenocarcinoma or pancreatitis	0
	Ampullary, duodenal, cystic, islet cell, etc.…	1
Pancreatic duct diameter	≥5 mm	0
	4 mm	1
	3 mm	2
	2 mm	3
	≤1 mm	4
Intraoperative blood loss	≤400 ml	0
	401–700 ml	1
	701–1,000 ml	2
	>1,000 ml	3
		Total 0–10 points

Callery et al. [20], with permission from Elsevier

ever, patients without routine drainage experienced a greater incidence of intra-abdominal abscess (26 vs. 12 %, P=0.033) and required IR-guided drainage more frequently (23 vs. 9 %, P=0.022). The study, with an accrual of 137 patients, was pre-maturely stopped by the Data Safety Monitoring Board since no drainage trended towards greater mortality (12 vs. 3 %, P=0.097).

The second endpoint of the randomized study was addressed by McMillan and colleagues [19]. This analysis assessed the value of selective drainage based on FRS CR-POPF risk. The FRS (0–10) is predicated on the weighted influence of four risk factors for the development of CR-POPF: soft pancreatic parenchyma, small pancreatic duct diameter, operative blood loss, and high risk pathology (anything other than pancreatic adenocarcinoma or pancreatitis) (Table 53.3) [20, 21]. After assigning FRS values to each patient, scores were then discretized into negligible/low (FRS: 0–2) and moderate/high (FRS: 3–10) risk groups. Next, randomizations were compared within each cohort to determine whether drains were beneficial or harmful in various scenarios of risk.

Among negligible/low patients, there were no significant differences in the rates of overall POPF, CR-POPF, intra-abdominal abscess, IR-guided drainage, or mortality. Though non-significant, the rates of CR-POPF and mortality were 10 % and 4 % higher in the drain cohort. While routine drainage did not minimize major morbidity in negligible/low risk patients, drainage appeared to be beneficial in moderate/high risk patients. Drained patients matching this risk profile had significantly fewer CR-POPFs, intra-abdominal abscesses, and IR-guided percutaneous drain placement procedures (P ≤ 0.05 for each). Mortality differences also trended towards significance.

The works by Van Buren and McMillan had several notable limitations. First, the protocol for the postoperative day of drain removal was not standardized. Secondly, the study was underpowered due to early stoppage by the Data Safety Monitoring Board. Despite these shortcomings, the quality of the study's evidence is high. It was the first multi-center (nine institutions and 15 surgeons) randomized trial to evaluate routine drainage, and its multivariable analyses of POPF only focused on those with clinical significance—per the current ISGPF standards. Furthermore, patients were substratified based on expected gland texture during the randomization process. Though the study was terminated early, it was because patients without drains, largely those with moderate/high CR-POPF risk, experienced much higher morbidity and mortality.

Recommendations

The only multicenter, level I evidence to date has demonstrated a benefit to routine drainage for patients with moderate or high (Fistula Risk Score 3–10) clinically relevant pancreatic fistula risk. Additionally, that study reported that drains confer no benefit to negligible and low fistula risk patients (Fistula Risk Score 0–2). Therefore, we recommend calculating the Fistula Risk Score operatively, at the point of reconstruction, and only placing drains in patients with moderate or high CR-POPF risk.

A Personal View of the Data

Most of the reported evidence on the value of routine drainage is very low to low in quality due to numerous shortcomings. These biases typically manifest in retrospective studies where drains are intuitively placed in higher risk patients; most of those studies do not control for this disparity in risk when comparing complications such as intra-abdominal abscess formation, IR-guided drainage, and mortality. Additionally, multivariable analyses of fistula incidence often include biochemical fistulas, which can only be detected with a drain present and confer little to no burden on the patient.

An oft-cited fear surrounding routine drainage involves the risk of fistula through suction-induced erosion of the anastomotic connection [17, 22]; this claim was recently discredited in a randomized trial comparing closed-suction versus gravity drainage [23]. That study found no significant differences between randomizations in terms of CR-POPF, intra-abdominal abscess, mortality, overall complications, and duration of stay. In fact, each complication occurred less frequently with closed-suction drainage, even though differences were non-significant. Another common source of angst is the fear that drains may act as a portal of entry for bacteria; [6, 16]

however, this retrograde infection theory was recently disproven in a study by Nagakawa et al. [24].

An important component that was missing in all of the observational and randomized studies comparing prophylactic drainage was a standardized protocol for early drain removal (POD3). Randomized studies by Bassi and Kawai showed early drain removal to be associated with reduced morbidity [22, 25]. Furthermore, POD1 drain fluid amylase cut-offs have been shown to reliably rule-out subsets of patients who will not develop a fistula; these cut-offs have been used to identify patients who qualify for early drain removal. Given the quality of evidence presented in this review, future prospective studies should evaluate the practice of early drain removal in moderate and high CR-POPF risk patients.

Drains may not mitigate the physical process of fistula formation, but they might dampen the severity of a fistula by allowing for earlier detection and evacuation of degradative fluids. This may serve to not only minimize the complication burden experienced by patients, but also reduce healthcare costs associated with reoperation, IR-guided drainage, and readmission. Given the current level I evidence, we believe the surveillance benefit offered by placing drains in patients with moderate and high fistula risk outweighs any purported disadvantages.

Recommendations

- We recommend routine drainage for patients with moderate and high (Fistula Risk Score 3–10) clinically relevant pancreatic fistula risk (evidence quality high; strong recommendation).
- We do not recommend routine drainage at PD for patients with negligible and low (Fistula Risk Score 0–2) clinically relevant pancreatic fistula risk (evidence quality high; weak recommendation).

References

1. Fong Y, Brennan MF, Brown K, Heffernan N, Blumgart LH. Drainage is unnecessary after elective liver resection. Am J Surg. 1996;171(1):158–62.
2. Merad F, Yahchouchi E, Hay JM, Fingerhut A, Laborde Y, Langlois-Zantain O. Prophylactic abdominal drainage after elective colonic resection and suprapromontory anastomosis: a multicenter study controlled by randomization. French Associations for Surgical Research. Arch Surg. 1998;133(3):309–14.
3. Merad F, Hay JM, Fingerhut A, Yahchouchi E, Laborde Y, Pelissier E, et al. Is prophylactic pelvic drainage useful after elective rectal or anal anastomosis? A multicenter controlled randomized trial. French Association for Surgical Research. Surgery. 1999;125(5):529–35.
4. Kim J, Lee J, Hyung WJ, Cheong JH, Chen J, Choi SH, et al. Gastric cancer surgery without drains: a prospective randomized trial. J Gastrointest Surg. 2004;8(6):727–32.

5. Alvarez Uslar R, Molina H, Torres O, Cancino A. Total gastrectomy with or without abdominal drains. A prospective randomized trial. Rev Esp Enferm Dig. 2005;97(8):562–9.
6. Fisher WE, Hodges SE, Silberfein EJ, Artinyan A, Ahern CH, Jo E, et al. Pancreatic resection without routine intraperitoneal drainage. HPB (Oxf). 2011;13(7):503–10.
7. Brozek JL, Akl EA, Compalati E, Kreis J, Terracciano L, Fiocchi A, et al. Grading quality of evidence and strength of recommendations in clinical practice guidelines part 3 of 3. The GRADE approach to developing recommendations. Allergy. 2011;66(5):588–95.
8. Brozek JL, Akl EA, Alonso-Coello P, Lang D, Jaeschke R, Williams JW, et al. Grading quality of evidence and strength of recommendations in clinical practice guidelines. Part 1 of 3. An overview of the GRADE approach and grading quality of evidence about interventions. Allergy. 2009;64(5):669–77.
9. Heslin MJ, Harrison LE, Brooks AD, Hochwald SN, Coit DG, Brennan MF. Is intra-abdominal drainage necessary after pancreaticoduodenectomy? J Gastrointest Surg. 1998;2(4):373–8.
10. McMillan MT, Vollmer Jr CM. Predictive factors for pancreatic fistula following pancreatectomy. Langenbeck's Arch Surg/Deut Ges Chirurgie. 2014;399(7):811–24.
11. Bassi C, Dervenis C, Butturini G, Fingerhut A, Yeo C, Izbicki J, et al. Postoperative pancreatic fistula: an international study group (ISGPF) definition. Surgery. 2005;138(1):8–13.
12. Lermite E, Pessaux P, Brehant O, Teyssedou C, Pelletier I, Etienne S, et al. Risk factors of pancreatic fistula and delayed gastric emptying after pancreaticoduodenectomy with pancreaticogastrostomy. J Am Coll Surg. 2007;204(4):588–96.
13. Mehta VV, Fisher SB, Maithel SK, Sarmiento JM, Staley CA, Kooby DA. Is it time to abandon routine operative drain use? A single institution assessment of 709 consecutive pancreaticoduodenectomies. J Am Coll Surg. 2013;216(4):635–42; discussion 42–4.
14. Adham M, Chopin-Laly X, Lepilliez V, Gincul R, Valette PJ, Ponchon T. Pancreatic resection: drain or no drain? Surgery. 2013;154(5):1069–77.
15. Pratt W, Maithel SK, Vanounou T, Callery MP, Vollmer Jr CM. Postoperative pancreatic fistulas are not equivalent after proximal, distal, and central pancreatectomy. J Gastrointest Surg. 2006;10(9):1264–78; discussion 78–9.
16. Correa-Gallego C, Brennan MF, D'Angelica M, Fong Y, Dematteo RP, Kingham TP, et al. Operative drainage following pancreatic resection: analysis of 1122 patients resected over 5 years at a single institution. Ann Surg. 2013;258(6):1051–8.
17. Conlon KC, Labow D, Leung D, Smith A, Jarnagin W, Coit DG, et al. Prospective randomized clinical trial of the value of intraperitoneal drainage after pancreatic resection. Ann Surg. 2001;234(4):487–93; discussion 93–4.
18. Van Buren 2nd G, Bloomston M, Hughes SJ, Winter J, Behrman SW, Zyromski NJ, et al. A randomized prospective multicenter trial of pancreaticoduodenectomy with and without routine intraperitoneal drainage. Ann Surg. 2014;259(4):605–12.
19. McMillan MT, Fisher WE, Van Buren 2nd G, McElhany A, Bloomston M, Hughes SJ, et al. The value of drains as a fistula mitigation strategy for pancreatoduodenectomy: something for everyone? Results of a randomized prospective multi-institutional study. J Gastrointest Surg. 2015;19(1):21–30.
20. Callery MP, Pratt WB, Kent TS, Chaikof EL, Vollmer Jr CM. A prospectively validated clinical risk score accurately predicts pancreatic fistula after pancreatoduodenectomy. J Am Coll Surg. 2013;216(1):1–14.
21. Miller BC, Christein JD, Behrman SW, Drebin JA, Pratt WB, Callery MP, et al. A multi-institutional external validation of the fistula risk score for pancreatoduodenectomy. J Gastrointest Surg. 2014;18(1):172–9; discussion 9–80.
22. Bassi C, Molinari E, Malleo G, Crippa S, Butturini G, Salvia R, et al. Early versus late drain removal after standard pancreatic resections: results of a prospective randomized trial. Ann Surg. 2010;252(2):207–14.
23. Lee SE, Ahn YJ, Jang JY, Kim SW. Prospective randomized pilot trial comparing closed suction drainage and gravity drainage of the pancreatic duct in pancreaticojejunostomy. J Hepatobiliary Pancreat Surg. 2009;16(6):837–43.

24. Nagakawa Y, Matsudo T, Hijikata Y, Kikuchi S, Bunso K, Suzuki Y, et al. Bacterial contamination in ascitic fluid is associated with the development of clinically relevant pancreatic fistula after pancreatoduodenectomy. Pancreas. 2013;42(4):701–6.
25. Kawai M, Tani M, Terasawa H, Ina S, Hirono S, Nishioka R, et al. Early removal of prophylactic drains reduces the risk of intra-abdominal infections in patients with pancreatic head resection: prospective study for 104 consecutive patients. Ann Surg. 2006;244(1):1–7.

Chapter 54
Management of Villous Adenoma of the Ampulla of Vater

Ashley N. Hardy, David J. Bentrem, and Jeffrey D. Wayne

Abstract Adenomas are the most common benign tumor of the ampulla of Vater and are thought to follow a similar adenoma-carcinoma sequence as seen in colonic adenocarcinomas. This is particularly the case for the villous subtype. Because of this potential for malignant degeneration, when identified, ampullary adenomas should be considered for resection. There is controversy however, on how to best treat these lesions with options including endoscopic or open ampullectomy or pancreaticoduodenectomy. Although there is increased morbidity and mortality with a pancreaticoduodenectomy procedure, the rates of incomplete resection and recurrence are higher with endoscopic and open ampullectomy. Lesion characteristics that support a full oncologic resection with a pancreaticoduodenectomy as opposed to the other procedures include ones that are >3 cm in size; firm, ulcerated, or friable; with intraductal extension; and with evidence of high-grade dysplasia, carcinoma in situ, or invasion.

Keywords Villous adenoma • Ampulla of Vater • Pancreaticoduodenectomy • Transduodenal ampullectomy • Endoscopic ampullectomy

Introduction

Adenomas are the most common benign tumor of the ampulla of Vater (Fig. 54.1), with an incidence ranging from 0.04 to 0.12 % in autopsy series [1]. Ampullary adenomas, which may occur sporadically or more commonly, in association with familial polyposis syndromes, are classified histologically as tubular, villous, or

A.N. Hardy (✉)
Department of Surgical Oncology, Fox Chase Cancer Center,
333 Cottman Avenue, Philadelphia, PA 19111, USA
e-mail: Ashley.Hardy@fccc.edu

D.J. Bentrem • J.D. Wayne
Department of Surgery, Northwestern University Feinberg School of Medicine,
676 Saint Clair St, Arkes Pavilion, Suite 6-650, Chicago, IL 60611, USA
e-mail: dbentrem@northwestern.edu; jwayne@northwestern.edu

J.M. Millis, J.B. Matthews (eds.), *Difficult Decisions in Hepatobiliary and Pancreatic Surgery*, Difficult Decisions in Surgery: An Evidence-Based Approach, DOI 10.1007/978-3-319-27365-5_54

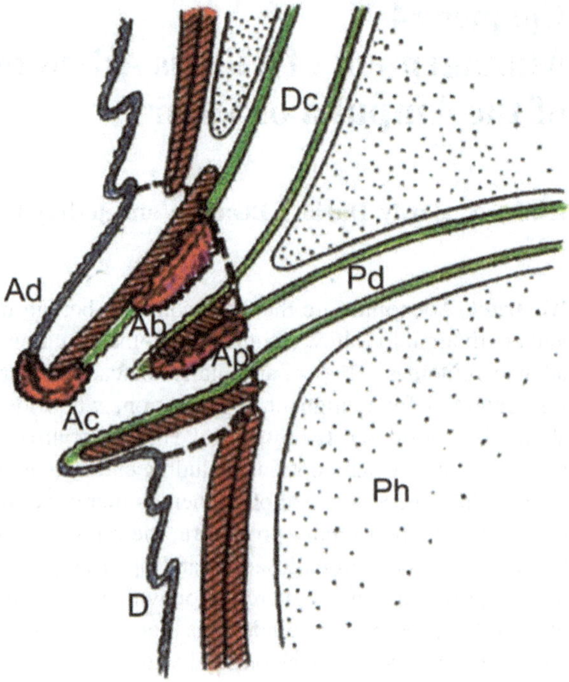

Fig. 54.1 Diagrammatic illustration of the papilla of Vater. Different primary sites of neoplastic lesions are shown: ampullo-biliary segment (*Ab*), ampullo-pancreatic segment (*Ap*), ampullo-pancreatico-biliary segment of the common channel (*Ac*), ampulloduodenum (*Ad*). Neighboring structures are the choledochal duct (*Dc*), pancreatic duct (*Pd*), pancreatic head (*Ph*), and duodenum (*D*) (Reproduced with the permission of Springer Science + Business Media. Zhou et al. J Hepatobiliary Pancreat Surg. 2004;11:301–309)

tubulovillous. As they are thought to follow a similar adenoma-carcinoma sequence well-established in colonic adenocarcinomas [2], when identified, ampullary adenomas should be considered for resection. This is particularly the case for the villous subtype, which tend to be more aggressive and more prone to malignant degeneration with a reported incidence of such ranging between 22 and 56 % [1].

Although pancreaticoduodenectomy is considered standard treatment for ampullary carcinomas, controversy exists regarding the most appropriate method for treating ampullary adenomas, with several studies suggesting that many of these tumors may be successfully treated with open transduodenal or endoscopic excision.

Studies in support of pancreaticoduodenectomy cite the risk of occult malignancy and the risks of recurrence as two major reasons to pursue a more radical resection [3]. In addition to decreased morbidity and mortality compared with pancreaticoduodenectomy, proponents of transduodenal ampullectomy and in particular endoscopic resection insist that the risks of recurrence is relatively low and that in the event of recurrence or the presence of occult malignancy, that the majority of these lesions can subsequently be treated with open or endoscopic re-excision or pancreaticoduodenectomy [4–6].

Therefore, the aim of this chapter is to compare the morbidity and mortality and risk of recurrence between pancreaticoduodenectomy, transduodenal resection, and endoscopic ampullectomy in the treatment of villous adenomas of the ampulla of Vater. This chapter will focus on sporadic ampullary adenomas and attempts will be made to identify those factors that may assist in determining which method of treatment would provide the most benefit for each individual patient.

Search Strategy

A literature search of English language publications from 1994 to 2014 was used to identify published data on the management of villous adenomas of the ampulla of Vater with either pancreaticoduodenectomy or open or endoscopic ampullectomy. This was accomplished using the PICO outline (Table 54.1). Databases searched were PubMed, Embase, and Web of Science. Terms used individually and in combination in the search were "ampullary villous adenoma," "ampulla of Vater adenoma," "pancreaticoduodenectomy," "transduodenal ampullectomy," and "endoscopic ampullectomy." Articles that addressed the differences in morbidity and mortality, risk of recurrence, and factors that influence the success of each treatment modality were of particular interest. Case reports, publications written in languages other than English, and those that fell out of the aforementioned date range were excluded. Fourteen retrospective cohort studies, two prospective cohort studies, and one systematic review were included in our analysis. The data was classified using the GRADE system.

Morbidity and Mortality

Although historically pancreaticoduodenectomy was the mainstay of treatment for ampullary adenomas, there has been a push towards using transduodenal or endoscopic resection as a primary means of treating these benign lesions. This shift in treatment paradigm was influenced by the increased morbidity and mortality associated with pancreaticoduodenectomy. Although perioperative mortality associated with pancreaticoduodenectomies in experienced hands at high-volume centers is less than 2 %, the procedure continues to have an operative morbidity ranging from 30 to 50 %. Furthermore, these complications, which include delayed gastric emptying, pancreatic fistulas, and biliary leak, tend to be more severe and of longer duration in comparison to those encountered with open or endoscopic ampullectomy [7].

Table 54.1 PICO table for management of villous adenomas of the ampulla of Vater

P (Patients)	I (Intervention)	C (Comparator group)	O (Outcomes measured)
Patients with villous adenomas undergoing resection	Pancreaticoduodenectomy	Transduodenal or endoscopic ampullectomy	Differences in morbidity/mortality, and recurrence

A number of studies have shown that transduodenal ampullectomy is associated with lower rates of morbidity compared to pancreaticoduodenectomies (Table 54.2). In a study by de Castro et al. which compared the short-term outcomes and long-term survival in 145 patients undergoing either local or transduodenal (LR) resection versus pancreaticoduodenectomy (PD) for ampullary neoplasms, the mean operative time (LR 141 min ± 34.7 vs. PD 278 min ± 81.9, $p<0.001$) and hospital length of stay (LR 13 days ± 6.7 vs. PD 23 days ± 21.8, $p=0.032$) were significantly shorter for those undergoing local resection. Furthermore, although mortality was nearly equal for both modalities, perioperative morbidity was found to be significantly lower in the local resection group (LR 27 % vs. PD 52 %, $p=0.035$) [4].

These findings were similar to a retrospective review by Clary and colleagues, for which mean operative times (LR 169 min vs. PD 268 min, $p=0.04$), estimated blood loss (LR 192 mL vs. PD 727 mL), average length of stay (LR 10 days vs. 25 days, $p<0.01$), and overall complication rates (LR 29 % vs. PD 78 %, $p<0.01$) were lower for those patients undergoing transduodenal resection for ampullary neoplasms [5].

Endoscopic mucosal resection (EMR) and the use of ablative therapies like argon plasma coagulation, laser, and bipolar electrocautery, are among the techniques employed for the endoscopic removal of ampullary adenomas. Even when performed by the most experienced endoscopists, the complications seen after endoscopic papillectomy are higher compared to other endoscopic procedures and include acute pancreatitis, bleeding and less commonly cholangitis, papillary stenosis, and perforation [6]. In an effort to reduce some of these complications, pancreatic or biliary sphincterotomy is often performed after papillectomy along with placement of a pancreatic stent. In a prospective randomized study of prophylactic stent placement following papillectomy, there was a statistically significant decrease in the rate of pancreatitis in patients who received a stent (unstented 33 % vs. 0 % stented, $p=0.02$) [8].

Table 54.2 Overview of the morbidity, mortality, and risk of recurrence with transduodenal resection of ampullary adenomas

Author (year)	No.	Morbidity (%)	Mortality (%)	Follow-up (years)	Recurrence (%)	Study type (quality of evidence)
de Castro (2004) [4]	25	27	4	5.6	8	Retrospective cohort (low)
Clary (2000) [5]	16	29	0	4.2	0	Retrospective cohort (low)
Onkendi (2014) [9]	9	58*	0	4.4	33	Retrospective cohort (moderate)
Farnell (2004) [12]	53	21	0	5.6	34	Retrospective cohort (low)
Rattner (2001) [14]	14	14	0	1.3	0	Retrospective cohort (low)

*Includes morbidity rate for patients undergoing pancreaticoduodenectomy and pancreas-sparing total duodenectomy

Studies comparing endoscopic excision to operative resection with either transduodenal resection or pancreaticoduodenoctomy consistently show that endoscopy is associated with lower rates of morbidity and mortality (Table 54.3). Furthermore, although not without risk, the periprocedural complications of endoscopy are typically mild and short-lived.

In a study by Onkendi and colleagues, there was a 58 % complication rate in those undergoing open resection with either transduodenal ampullectomy or pancreaticoduodenectomy compared to only 29 % in those undergoing endoscopic excision ($p<0.001$). In addition, these complications were less severe with the most common being that of gastrointestinal bleeding for which all were managed conservatively. Of the 130 patients treated endoscopically, only 2 sustained more significant complications of ampullary obstruction or perforation, both of which were successfully managed nonoperatively as well [9].

Recurrence

Despite a mean success rate of 82.2 % [10] and lower morbidity, systematic reviews of endoscopic ampullectomy continue to demonstrate higher rates of recurrence, ranging from 0 % to 30 % [11]. These findings are summarized in Table 54.3. The same holds true for transduodenal excisions as illustrated in Table 54.2. In this study, among the 50 patients with benign adenomas managed by transduodenal excision, 17 (32 %) experienced a recurrence at 5 years and 43 % at 10 years compared to none of the patients in the pancreaticoduodenectomy group. Although the majority of the recurrences were benign and amendable to endoscopic resection, 4 of the 17 were characterized by invasion, requiring subsequent pancreaticoduodenectomy [12].

Table 54.3 Overview of the morbidity, mortality, and risk of recurrence with endoscopic resection of ampullary adenomas

Author (year)	No.	Morbidity (%)	Mortality (%)	Follow-up (years)	Complete resection (%)	Recurrence (%)	Study type (quality of evidence)
Onkendi (2014) [9]	130	29	0	4.4	93	32	Retrospective cohort (moderate)
Laleman (2013) [10]	79	22.8	0	5	78.4	14.5	Retrospective cohort (moderate)
Ridtitid (2014) [13]	151	18.7	0	5	70.8	15	Retrospective cohort (low)
Cheng (2004) [15]	45	14.3	0	2.5	74	33	Retrospective cohort (low)
Desilets (2001) [16]	13	8	0	1.6	92	0	Retrospective cohort (low)
Catalano (2004) [17]	72	9.7	0	3	86	4	Retrospective cohort (low)

Onkendi et al. found a fivefold greater risk of recurrence after endoscopic resection compared to operative resection with either approach (32 vs. 6 %, $p=0.006$) but when comparisons were only made between those patients undergoing open versus endoscopic ampullectomy, there was no difference in the rate of recurrence (33 vs. 32 %, $p=0.49$). Furthermore, the majority of recurrences occurred in adenomas greater than 3.6 cm in size, ones containing foci of high-grade dysplasia, carcinoma in situ, and those cases in which more than one endoscopic procedure was required to obtain a complete excision [9].

These findings emphasize the necessity for repeat endoscopic examinations although the exact frequency and duration of surveillance endoscopy has yet to be established.

Risk Factors

As previously eluded to, certain factors may decrease the likelihood of achieving a complete excision and increase the incidence of recurrence in those undergoing less invasive means of resection.

Ridtitid and colleagues discovered that for those patients undergoing endoscopic ampullectomies between 1995 and 2012 at a large tertiary medical center, that the presence of jaundice (27.7 % vs. 4.5 %, $p<0.0001$) and intraductal extension were associated with higher rates of incomplete resection (31.3 % vs. 9 %, $p=0.0002$). In addition, tumors that were able to be removed en bloc as opposed to piecemeal had a significantly higher probability of being completely excised (57.5 % vs. 22.9 %, $p<0.001$) [13]. Although there was no significant difference in this study with regards to tumor size, this may have been affected by the piecemeal fashion in which many of the tumors were removed.

There are no definitive guidelines as to the size above which an attempt at endoscopic excision should be avoided. Although it has been advised by many that open or endoscopic excision should not be attempted for lesions greater than 3 cm [9, 14] there have been reports of endoscopic success for tumors greater than 4–5 cm and up to 7.5 cm with transduodenal resection [15, 16]. However, the majority of tumors presenting with pancreaticobiliary symptoms, intraductal extension, and ones not amendable to en bloc resection, tend to be large in size [13]. Furthermore, size is an important predictor of endoscopic success with the highest rates achieved for lesions less than 24 mm in a large, multicenter study by Catalano et al. [17].

These characteristics, along with adenomas that are firm, ulcerated, and friable are more commonly seen in tumors harboring high-grade dysplasia, carcinoma in situ, and foci of invasive malignancy. These findings therefore suggest that the most appropriate treatment for such ampullary tumors may be that of a full oncologic resection with a pancreaticoduodenectomy [9].

Although a few, small series have reported technical success in the endoscopic removal of adenomas with high-grade dysplasia and foci of well-differentiated T1 adenocarcinoma [18–21], the reality remains that such lesions have higher rates of incomplete resection and recurrence when managed endoscopically.

This notion is supported by a study by Kim et al. which demonstrated a co-existence of cancer in 50 % of patients with pre-procedural high-grade dysplasia undergoing endoscopic ampullectomy, compared to only 15.7 % in those with low-grade dysplasia. Likewise, the rates of recurrence in the high versus low-grade dysplasia groups were 80 % and 5.2 % respectively [22].

The same argument can be made for invasive malignancies treated with transduodenal resection. In fact, Roggin et al. showed a 0 % recurrence-free survival after 2 years in the open ampullectomy group versus 48 % in those undergoing pancreaticoduodenectomy (95 % CI 37–60 %). In addition, the 2-year estimated disease free survival was 58 % versus 78 % (95 % CI 22–95 %) in the open ampullectomy and pancreaticoduodenectomy groups respectively [23]. This is likely due to the presence of lymphovascular invasion and intraductal infiltration observed in 20–40 % of T1 tumors [21].

Recommendations

Adenomas of the ampulla of Vater are rare tumors with tremendous potential for malignant degeneration into ampullary carcinomas. Therefore, when encountered, effort should be made to excise these lesions prior to the development of dysplasia or invasive cancer. Despite the three available treatment options available, the fact that we lack a clear consensus on how to approach ampullary adenomas was the inspiration for this chapter.

Based on a thorough review of current literature available on this topic, we recommend surgical excision rather than endoscopic excision for the following:

1. Lesions >3 cm in size (evidence quality moderate; weak recommendation).
2. Evidence of high-grade dysplasia, carcinoma in situ, or foci of invasion (evidence quality moderate; strong recommendation).
3. Lesions that are firm, ulcerated, or friable on endoscopic evaluation (evidence quality moderate; strong recommendation).
4. Presence of intraductal extension (evidence quality low; weak recommendation).
5. Lesions accompanied by pre-procedural jaundice or pancreatitis (evidence quality low; weak recommendation).

Furthermore, in the absence of endoscopists skilled in performing ampullectomies and in which there is failure of complete resection with endoscopic attempts, surgical excision is advised. Although there is significantly less morbidity associated with transduodenal resection, we favor surgical resection with pancreaticoduodenectomy as a result of the high recurrence rate observed with open ampullectomy. Endoscopic resection should be attempted therefore, in smaller lesions including those with evidence of low-grade dysplasia and which lack the aforementioned high-risk characteristics. Limiting endoscopic excision to adenomas 3 cm or less will ensure successful removal with a decreased risk of recurrence. Open or endoscopic ampullectomies may prove to be better options, however for patients whose underlying health and comorbidities render them incapable of tolerating more extensive surgery. If either approach is taken, patients should be followed closely for recurrence with surveillance endoscopy (Fig. 54.2).

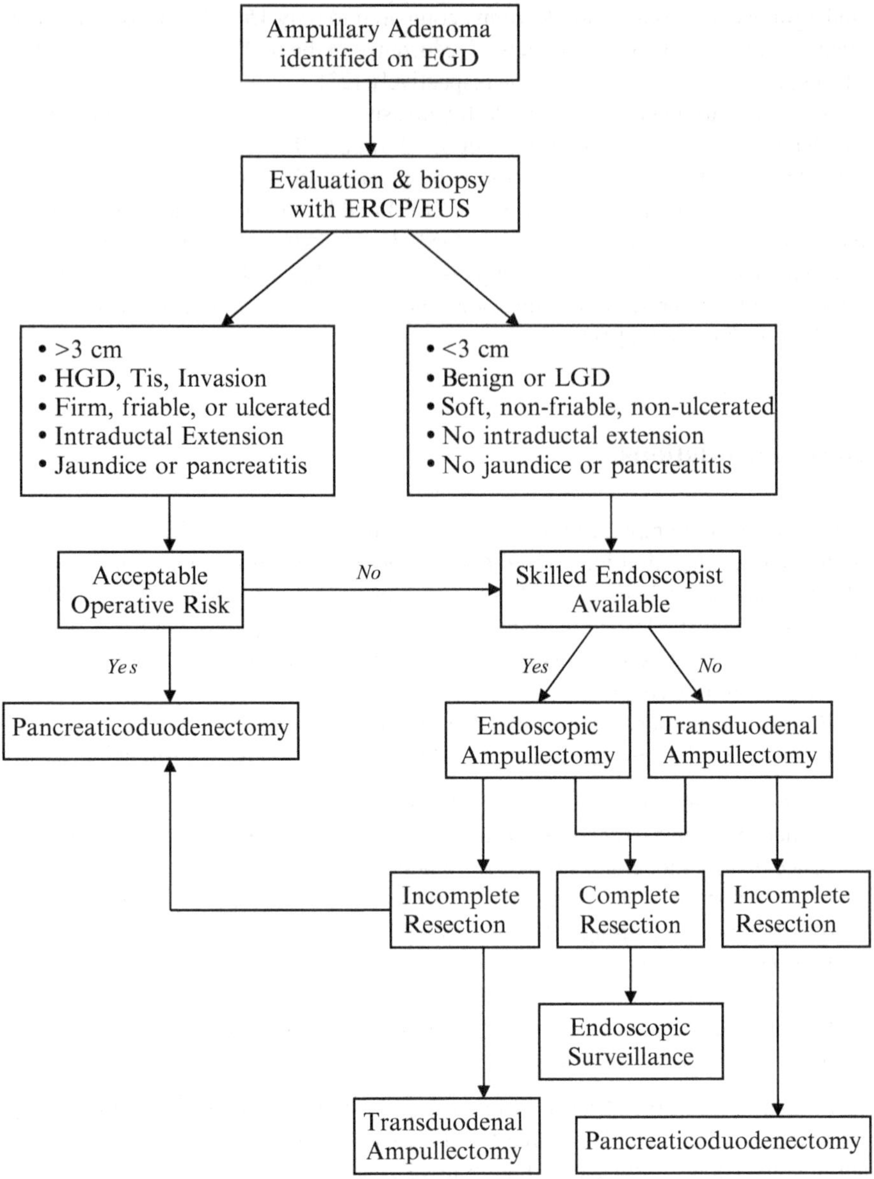

Fig. 54.2 Algorithm for the management of ampullary adenomas. *EGD* Esophagogastroduodenoscopy, *ERCP* Endoscopic Retrograde Cholangiopancreatography, *EUS* Endoscopic Ultrasound, *HGD* High-grade dysplasia, *LGD* Low-grade dysplasia, *Tis* Carcinoma in situ

While there are no established guidelines on the frequency and duration of endoscopic surveillance, we support the recommendations made by the Standards of Practice Committee of the American Society for Gastrointestinal Endoscopy. The committee suggests an initial surveillance exam 1–6 months following the initial ampullectomy followed by repeat endoscopies every 3–12 months for at least 2 years with periodic exams thereafter based on symptoms [24]. If feasible, it may be of benefit to extend this surveillance period beyond 2 years in consideration of the findings by Farnell et al. who observed recurrences 5–10 years after initial treatment [12].

Finally, if the lesion appears amendable to endoscopic excision, consideration should be made towards the placement of prophylactic pancreatic stents to decrease the incidence of post-procedural pancreatitis [8].

References

1. Rosenberg J, Welch JP, Pyrtek LJ, Walker M, Trowbridge P. Benign villous adenomas of the ampulla of Vater. Cancer. 1986;58(7):1563–8.
2. Martin JA, Haber GB. Ampullary adenoma: clinical manifestations, diagnosis, and treatment. Gastrointest Endosc Clin N Am. 2003;13(4):649–69.
3. Hoyuela C, Cugat E, Veloso E, Marco C. Treatment options for villous adenoma of the ampulla of Vater. HPB Surg. 2000;11(5):325–30.
4. de Castro SM, van Heek NT, Kuhlmann KF, Busch OR, Offerhaus GJ, van Gulik TM, Obertop H, Gouma DJ. Surgical management of neoplasms of the ampulla of Vater: local resection or pancreatoduodenectomy and prognostic factors for survival. Surgery. 2004;136:994–1002.
5. Clary BM, Tyler DS, Dematos P, Gottfried M, Pappas TN. Local ampullary resection with careful intraoperative frozen section evaluation for presumed benign ampullary neoplasms. Surgery. 2000;127(6):628–33.
6. Chini P, Draganov V. Diagnosis and management of ampullary adenoma: the expanding role of endoscopy. World J Gastrointest Endosc. 2011;3(12):241–7.
7. Winter JM, Cameron JL, Campbell KA, Arnold MA, Chang DC, Coleman J, Hodgin MB, Sauter PK, Hruban RH, Riall TS, Schulick RD, Choti MA, Lillemoe KD, Yeo CJ. 1423 pancreaticoduodenectomies for pancreatic cancer: a single-institution experience. J Gastrointest Surg. 2006;10:1199–210.
8. Harewood GC, Pochron NL, Gostout CJ. Prospective, randomized, controlled trial of prophylactic pancreatic stent placement for endoscopic snare excision of the duodenal ampulla. Gastrointest Endosc. 2005;62(3):367–70.
9. Onkendi EO, Naik ND, Rosedahl JK, Harmsen SW, Gostout CJ, Baron Sr TH, Sarr MR, Que FG. Adenomas of the ampulla of Vater: a comparison of outcomes of operative and endoscopic resections. J Gastrointest Surg. 2014;18(9):1588–96.
10. Laleman W, Verreth A, Topa B, Aerts R, Komuta M, Roskams T, Van der Merwe S, Cassiman D, Nevens F, Verslype C, Van Steenbergen W. Endoscopic resection of ampullary lesions: a single-center 8-year retrospective cohort study of 91 patients with long-term follow-up. Surg Endosc. 2013;27:3865–76.
11. Han J, Kim MH. Endoscopic papillectomy for adenomas of the major duodenal papilla (with video). Gastrointest Endosc. 2006;63(2):292–301.
12. Farnell MB, Sakorafas GH, Sarr MG, Rowland CM, Tsiotos GG, Farley DR, Nagorney DM. Villous tumors of the duodenum: reappraisal of local vs. extended resection. J Gastrointest Surg. 2000;4:13–21; discussion 22–13.

13. Ridtitid W, Tan D, Schmidt SE, Fogel EL, McHenry L, Watkins JL, Lehman GA, Sherman S, Coté GA. Endoscopic papillectomy: risk factors for incomplete resection and recurrence during long-term follow-up. Gastrointest Endosc. 2014;79(2):289–96.
14. Rattner DW, Fernandez-del Castillo C, Brugge WR, Warshaw AL. Defining the criteria for local resection of ampullary neoplasms. Arch Surg. 1996;131(4):366–71.
15. Cheng CL, Sherman S, Fogel EL, et al. Endoscopic snare papillectomy for tumors of the duodenal papillae. Gastrointest Endosc. 2004;60:757–64.
16. Desilets DJ, Dy RM, Ku PM, Hanson BL, Elton E, Mattia A, Howell DA. Endoscopic management of tumors of the major duodenal papilla: refined techniques to improve outcome and avoid complications. Gastrointest Endosc. 2001;54(2):202.
17. Catalano MF, Linder JD, Chak A, Sivak MV, Raijman I, Geenen JE, Howell DA. Endoscopic management of adenoma of the major duodenal papilla. Gastrointest Endosc. 2004;59:225–32.
18. Yamao T, Isomoto H, Kohno S, Mizuta Y, Yamakawa M, Nakao K, Irie J. Endoscopic snare papillectomy with biliary and pancreatic stent placement for tumors of the major duodenal papilla. Surg Endosc. 2010;24(1):119.
19. Ito K, Fujita N, Noda Y, Kobayashi G, Obana T, Horaguchi J, Koshita S, Kanno Y, Ogawa T, Kato Y, Yamashita Y. Impact of technical modification of endoscopic papillectomy for ampullary neoplasm on the occurrence of complications. Dig Endosc. 2012;24(1):30–5.
20. Yoon SM, Kim MH, Kim MJ, Jang SJ, Lee TY, Kwon S, Oh HC, Lee SS, Seo DW, Lee SK. Focal early stage cancer in ampullary adenoma: surgery or endoscopic papillectomy? Gastrointest Endosc. 2007;66(4):701–7.
21. Yoon YS, Kim SW, Park SJ, Lee HS, Jang JY, Choi MG, Kim WH, Lee KU, Park YH. Clinicopathologic analysis of early ampullary cancers with a focus on the feasibility of ampullectomy. Ann Surg. 2005;242(1):92–100.
22. Kim JH, Kim JH, Han JH, Yoo BM, Kim MW, Kim WH. Is endoscopic papillectomy safe for ampullary adenomas with high-grade dysplasia? Ann Surg Oncol. 2009;16(9):2547–54.
23. Roggin KK, Yeh JJ, Ferrone CR, Riedel E, Gerdes H, Klimstra DS, Jaques DP, Brennan MF. Limitations of ampullectomy in the treatment of nonfamilial ampullary neoplasms. Ann Surg Oncol. 2005;12(12):971–80.
24. Standards of Practice Committee, Adler DG, Qureshi W, Davila R, Gan SI, Lichtenstein D, Rajan E, Shen B, Zuckerman MJ, Fanelli RD, Van Guilder T, Baron TH. The role of endoscopy in ampullary and duodenal adenomas. Gastrointest Endosc. 2006;64(6):849–54.

Chapter 55
Splenic Preservation at Distal Pancreatectomy

Benjamin D. Ferguson and Jeffrey B. Matthews

Abstract There is currently debate as to whether splenic preservation should be attempted during distal pancreatectomy, as splenectomy brings with it the risk of overwhelming post-splenectomy sepsis as well as hematologic aberrations such as thrombocytosis and leukocytosis. Little clarity has been established in understanding the differential benefits and disadvantages of spleen preservation at distal pancreatectomy as compared to those of splenectomy. After review, there are few differences between the two techniques regarding outcomes and postoperative complications. Splenic preservation should be attempted when it is technically feasible and not otherwise contraindicated.

Keywords Distal pancreatectomy • Splenectomy • Splenic preservation

Introduction

Splenectomy is often performed in conjunction with distal pancreatectomy for a variety of reasons. First, the close anatomical relationship of the splenic vessels to the dorsal aspect of the pancreas often makes for difficult dissection of the pancreas off of these structures, especially in the event of pancreatic inflammation such as pancreatitis or of neoplasms in the pancreatic body or tail involving adjacent structures. This is compounded by the variable anatomy of the splenic vessels themselves, particularly the splenic artery [1], and their branches and confluences. Furthermore, the anatomical relationship between the pancreatic tail and the splenic hilum is often such that dissecting these from each other is technically challenging and often prone to risk of intraoperative and/or postoperative complications. Splenectomy is commonly performed in operations for left-sided pancreatic cancer in order to clear lymph nodes in the splenic hilum that may be sites of early nodal

B.D. Ferguson • J.B. Matthews (✉)
Department of Surgery, University of Chicago Medical Center,
5841 S. Maryland Avenue, MC 5029, Chicago, IL 60637, USA
e-mail: jmatthews@surgery.bsd.uchicago.edu

J.M. Millis, J.B. Matthews (eds.), *Difficult Decisions in Hepatobiliary and Pancreatic Surgery*, Difficult Decisions in Surgery: An Evidence-Based Approach, DOI 10.1007/978-3-319-27365-5_55

metastasis from the pancreas. Additionally, the spleen is not a vital organ in the sense that living without one is not typically life-threatening.

However, splenectomy at distal pancreatectomy does predispose patients to the typical risks of asplenia, particularly hematologic abnormalities, such as thrombocytosis, leukocytosis, and thrombotic events, and infectious complications including overwhelming postsplenectomy infection (OPSI) and significantly increased risk for infections involving encapsulated or intraerythrocytic organisms. While OPSI is a major concern following splenectomy given its potentially devastating outcomes, its incidence is exceedingly low even over long periods of follow-up [2–4], probably owing at least in part to scrupulous peri- and postoperative immunization.

Mallet-Guy and Vachon first described spleen-preserving distal pancreatectomy in 1943. Warshaw in 1988 was the first to rigorously demonstrate the feasibility and safety of splenic preservation in patients undergoing distal pancreatectomy through ligation of the splenic vessels beyond the pancreatic tail, leaving the spleen to be supplied by the left gastroepiploic and short gastric vessels [5]. The so-called Warshaw technique and its associated modifications (most frequently division of the splenic artery and vein at the origin from the celiac trunk and at the confluence with the superior mesenteric vein, respectively) have become the most common method of splenic salvage during distal pancreatectomy, though preservation of the splenic vessels is another widely used operative technique [6, 7]. Soper et al. later demonstrated in a porcine model the feasibility of laparoscopic distal pancreatectomy [8], which since its inception has become an increasingly common and oft-preferred technique for distal pancreatectomy both with and without splenectomy.

Attempts have been made to clarify the benefits and disadvantages of spleen preservation at distal pancreatectomy as compared to those of splenectomy during these procedures in situations allowing for such a nuanced decision. We review the available data here.

Search Strategy

A Medline search was performed using the following search strings based on PICO elements (Table 55.1): "(distal pancreatectomy OR left pancreatectomy) AND (splenectomy OR splenic OR spleen)". The search was limited to studies on human subjects written in the English language and those that specifically addressed

Table 55.1 PICO table for splenic preservation at distal pancreatectomy

P (patients)	I (intervention)	C (comparator group)	O (outcomes measured)
Patients undergoing distal pancreatectomy for any indication	Splenic preservation	Splenectomy	Splenic function/perfusion, OPSS, hemorrhage/transfusion requirement, other complications, postoperative pain, oncological efficacy

outcomes of interest, particularly feasibility, postoperative complications, risk for infection, and oncologic efficacy. All results were read and reviewed, and irrelevant results were excluded from the analysis. Single-case reports, systematic and other reviews, and editorials and commentaries were also excluded.

Results

We identified a number of prospective observational and other non-randomized studies, large retrospective case reviews, and meta-analyses with our search. The vast majority have been published within the past 5 years, underscoring the recent intensity of the debate. These are discussed below based on the focus of their findings. We did not find any prospective randomized controlled trials comparing splenectomy and splenic preservation at distal pancreatectomy, unfortunately.

Physiologic Considerations

A retrospective case series review of 180 patients undergoing distal pancreatectomy with or without splenectomy at a single institution over an 11-year period was reported by Lee et al. [9]. This group found that there were no statistically significant differences between groups in intraoperative blood loss or need for intraoperative transfusion, operative time, or postoperative complications. However, the authors did find that white blood cell and platelet counts were significantly higher on postoperative day 7 ($p=0.008$ and $p<0.001$, respectively) and at 6 months of follow-up ($p<0.001$ and $p=0.002$, respectively) in patients who underwent splenectomy compared to those with splenic preservation. One patient who had splenic salvage was noted to have splenic infarction but has not suffered symptoms of hyposplenism. One patient who underwent splenectomy developed symptoms consistent with OPSI on postoperative day 9. It is worth noting that this group did not routinely pre- or perioperatively vaccinate patients against *Pneumococcus*, meningococcus, or *Haemophilus*, though these commonly are administered later in the postoperative course than the point at which this patient developed sepsis, and none of these organisms were found to be causative in this patient's sepsis.

Tezuka et al. [10] reviewed 53 patients who underwent distal pancreatectomy with or without splenectomy over a 12-year period at a single institution and examined early postoperative changes in hematologic function, among other outcomes. As expected, patients undergoing concomitant splenectomy had significantly higher platelet count and leukocyte count than patients with splenic preservation; these peaked at 2 weeks and 2 days postoperatively, respectively, and later normalized, though the differential effect between groups remained significant at 3 months following surgery. Hemoglobin, CRP, and albumin levels generally followed identical trends between groups and were largely statistically indistinct from one another, differing significantly only at single time points over 3 months of follow-up assessments. There were no statistical differences between groups in postoperative pancreatic fistulae or infections, and there were no splenic vein thromboses, splenic thromboses or torsion (among those with splenic salvage), or deaths in either group.

A similar review of 78 patients undergoing distal pancreatectomy with either splenic preservation using the Warshaw technique or splenectomy over a 14-year period at a single institution was published by Tsiouris et al. [11]. Spleen-preserving operations were performed laparoscopically more often than those with concomitant splenectomy (33.3 % versus 6.3 %, $p = 0.004$) and required significantly shorter operative time (154 versus 204 min, $p = 0.003$). Neither infectious nor non-infectious complications were significantly different between groups. However, advanced patient age and length of stay were independently associated with non-infectious complications, while intraoperative transfusion (but not operative blood loss) was associated with infectious and non-infectious complications. Leukocyte and platelet counts were higher in the splenectomy group at postoperative day 7 and postoperative month 6, and this effect persisted at postoperative day 7 after controlling for postoperative infections. There was no mortality or incidence of OPSI in either group.

Kohan et al. [12] conducted a prospective study to examine changes in gastrosplenic circulation and other measures of splenic function following spleen-preserving distal pancreatectomy with splenic vessel ligation. A total of 35 patients undergoing spleen-preserving distal pancreatectomy were studied. Each patient had a preoperative CT with IV contrast to define celiac, superior mesenteric, and splenic vascular anatomy and identify the presence of splenic vein thrombosis. No patients had preoperative splenic vein thrombosis or portal hypertension. Postoperatively, 26 % of patients developed pancreatic fistula. On the seventh postoperative day, all patients again underwent CT with IV contrast, and only 37 % were found to have normal splenic perfusion without evidence of infarction; 46 % had grade 1 and 17 % had grade 2 perfusion defects. At 6 months postoperatively, 81 % of those with early grade 1 and 50 % of those with early grade 2 perfusion defects had no remaining evidence of hypoperfusion, and the other 50 % of those with early grade 2 defects improved to grade 1 defects. CT at 6 months also revealed that 74 % of patients had perigastric varices. A subset of these patients underwent upper endoscopy; 73 % had gastric varices that were radiographically apparent on CT. There were two patients with variceal bleeding complications at 3 and 4 years of follow-up that were managed endoscopically. Postoperative splenic dysfunction was noted in 59 % of patients at 6 months postoperatively, with 19 % of these demonstrating functional asplenia (greater than 15 % of erythrocytes with pitted membrane morphology on peripheral smear). No patients developed OPSI over a mean follow-up time of 3.7 years. These data suggest that splenic function and perfusion is impaired following spleen-preserving distal pancreatectomy with splenic vessel ligation (Warshaw technique), though the clinical consequences of these findings are not entirely clear.

Complications and Postoperative Course

A number of retrospective studies have examined differential complications and outcomes following distal pancreatectomy with or without splenectomy. Among 11 relevant studies, none reported any instances of overwhelming post-splenectomy infection or splenic infarction or necrosis following splenic preservation. Most found no differences in the rates of pancreatic fistula. Only two studies found that overall complications were significantly different between groups, which in these studies were more common in patients undergoing splenectomy (Table 55.2).

Technical Considerations

In a retrospective study of 43 patients undergoing laparoscopic distal pancreatectomy and splenectomy with or without splenic vessel preservation at a single institution over an 8-year period, Butturini et al. [24] found that among 36 patients with preservation of the splenic vessels (84 % of study cohort) and 7 patients who underwent a Warshaw-type distal pancreatectomy with splenic salvage (16 % of study cohort), there were no significant differences in operative time, any perioperative complication studied, need for reoperation, or hospital length of stay. One patient in each group developed splenic infarction and required subsequent splenectomy. There were also no differences in rates of hematologic aberrations, splenic vascular patency, or the development of gastric or perigastric varices at long-term follow-up.

Beane et al. [25] compared splenic-preserving distal pancreatectomy with and without splenic vessel salvage in a retrospective study of 86 patients at a single institution over a 7-year period; these patients were also compared to a matched group of 86 patients who underwent distal pancreatectomy with splenectomy. Intraoperative blood loss was significantly less in the vessel-preserving group compared to both the vessel-ligating group and the splenectomy group (224 mL, 507 mL, and 646 mL, respectively; $p<0.05$ for each). There were no other statistically sig-

Table 55.2 Studies primarily reporting on complications and postoperative course following distal pancreatectomy with splenectomy or splenic preservation. Statistically significant differences in outcomes ($p<0.05$) are highlighted in bold/gray

		Splenectomy						Splenic preservation					
Study	Total N	N	Fistula	Abscess/ infection	OPSI	Overall complications	LOS (days)	N	Fistula	Abscess/ infection	Splenic infarct/ necrosis	Overall complications	LOS (days)
Richardson (1989)	21	10	20 %	10 %	NR	40 %	18.8	11	9 %	9 %	9 %	36 %	17.5
Aldridge (1991)	77	42	12 %	NR	0 %	24 %	NR	35	11 %	NR	NR	20 %	NR
Benoist (1999)	40	25	12 %	4 %	0 %	20 %	12.5	15	**24 %**	**16 %**	4 %	40 %	**19**
Lillemoe (1999)	235	198	NR	NR	NR	30 %	13	37	NR	NR	NR	30 %	**21**
Shoup (2002)	125	79	8 %	**28 %**	NR	49 %	**9**	46	7 %	9 %	NR	39 %	7
Rodriguez (2006)	259	185	33 %	14 %	NR	58 %	7	74	36 %	8 %	1 %	54 %	6
Kleeff (2007)	302	231	11 %	5 %	NR	34 %	11	71	5 %	0 %	NR	27 %	10
Nau (2009)	24	17	12 %	0 %	0 %	41 %	7.0	7	29 %	0 %	0 %	71 %	7.1
Choi (2012)	72	32	**56 %**	16 %	NR	**59 %**	**12.5**	40	25 %	5 %	NR	28 %	7.1
Tang (2014)	160	82	**21 %**	**7 %**	NR	**41 %**	**13.5**	78	9 %	3 %	NR	26 %	12.4
Dumitrascu (2014)	66	33	24 %	6 %	NR	33 %	8	33	33 %	12 %	3 %	36 %	9

References for table in order: [13–23]

nificant differences in the operative characteristics studied. Patients with vessel preservation experienced significantly fewer splenic infarctions, postoperative drainage procedures, and total complications and had significantly shorter lengths of stay compared to the vessel-ligating and splenectomy groups. These findings suggest that while outcomes for distal pancreatectomy with splenectomy or splenic preservation with ligation of the splenic vessels are comparable, distal pancreatectomy with spleen and splenic vessel preservation has superior outcomes with respect to intraoperative blood loss and postoperative considerations.

Adam et al. [26] compared splenic vessel preservation to ligation at laparoscopic spleen-preserving distal pancreatectomy in a retrospective study of 140 patients over a 14-year period across two institutions. All patients had benign or low-grade malignant pancreatic tumors. There were no statistical differences between the two groups in operative time, intraoperative blood loss, conversion to laparotomy, or intraoperative complications. No significant differences were noted in postoperative fistulae or in the number of patients with any complication. However, length of stay was significantly shorter (8.2 versus 10.5 days) and there were significantly fewer spleen-related complications (none versus 10.5 %) in the splenic vessel preservation group as compared to the Warshaw technique group. Among patients with spleen-related complications, all had symptomatic splenic infarctions, and 44 % of these required subsequent splenectomy. An additional seven patients across both groups (5 % of total) were found to have splenic infarction on imaging that was asymptomatic. Reoperation was required in 5 % of the splenic vessel preservation group and in 6 % of the Warshaw technique group (four aforementioned patients undergoing splenectomy with one additional patient developing hemorrhagic shock related to pancreatic fistula). These data suggest that splenic vessel preservation in laparoscopic spleen-preserving distal pancreatectomy is associated with less frequent splenic infarction and shorter hospital length of stay than the Warshaw technique.

Outcomes following robotic distal pancreatectomy with or without splenic preservation were described by Suman et al. [27]. In a retrospective review of 40 patients successfully undergoing robotic resection at a single institution over a 4-year-period, this group found no statistical differences between splenic preservation and splenectomy groups in postoperative complication rates or length of stay. In this series, 30 % of distal pancreatectomies were accomplished with splenic preservation, and in 92 % of these, the splenic vessels were also preserved. Of 49 total patients who underwent attempted robotic distal pancreatectomy, 81.6 % of cases were completed robotically, while 18.4 % required open conversion, most commonly due to technically difficult vascular dissections and bleeding complications.

Oncologic Considerations

Kim et al. [28] employed a multicenter retrospective review of 85 patients undergoing radical antegrade modular distal pancreatectomy (that is, an "extended" Warshaw procedure involving division of the pancreas and splenic vessels near the confluence of the superior mesenteric vein and splenic vein and including regional dissection of common hepatic, celiac, and superior mesenteric artery lymph nodes) for pancreatic body or tail adenocarcinomas without clinical evidence of invasion into the spleen or splenic hilum. This group also performed en bloc splenectomy and specifically dissected perihilar soft tissue and lymph nodes for pathologic analysis, which would ordinarily be left in place during a spleen-preserving Warshaw procedure. In a pilot study involving 12 patients, none were found to have splenic hilar lymph node metastasis on microscopic examination. It should be noted that 7 out of 12 patients had T3 tumors, 6 out of 12 had N1 disease (with spread to sites other than the splenic hilum, 4 out of 12 had undergone preoperative chemoradiation, and 10 out of 12 had tumors located in the pancreatic body, with one in the body and tail, and one in the tail. In a subsequent validation study in which 85 patients from three additional centers were retrospectively reviewed, 4.7 % (4/85) were found to have splenic hilar lymph node metastasis on microscopic examination. Each of these patients had tumors located in the pancreatic tail or in the body and tail within 1.5 cm of the splenic hilum. Splenic hilar metastasis was significantly more frequent in patients with primary tumors greater than 3 cm ($p=0.032$). This group concluded that spleen preservation for oncologic pancreatectomy is reasonable in selected patients with tumors located in the pancreatic neck or body and spanning less than 3 cm.

Recommendations

1. For patients in which splenic preservation is technically feasible and is not otherwise contraindicated, spleen-preserving distal pancreatectomy is recommended (evidence quality moderate, weak recommendation).
2. Splenic vessel preservation is the preferred method of spleen-preserving distal pancreatectomy when technically feasible (evidence quality low, weak recommendation).
3. Spleen preservation should be attempted during laparoscopic and robotic distal pancreatectomy when technically feasible (evidence quality low, weak recommendation).

A Personal View of the Data

Upon review, there seem to be few differences between splenectomy and splenic preservation at distal pancreatectomy regarding outcomes and postoperative complications. Splenic preservation should be attempted when it is technically feasible, and in these cases, splenic vessel preservation should be attempted when it is technically easy, though there should be a low threshold to convert to Warshaw technique. During entrance into the lesser sac and exposure of the pancreas, care should be taken to avoid division of the most caudal short gastric vessels. Situations that should preclude consideration of splenic preservation include disease involving the splenic hilum and tenuous vascular anatomy or other structural challenges that would necessitate technically difficult dissection. Careful inspection of the lower tip of the spleen following distal pancreatectomy is often useful to estimate the likelihood of partial or early splenic infarction. If more than a minimal amount of the spleen tip appears dusky, then there should be a low threshold for splenectomy and appropriate postoperative immunization.

References

1. Pandey SK, Bhattacharya S, Mishra RN, Shukla VK. Anatomical variations of the splenic artery and its clinical implications. Clin Anat. 2004;17(6):497–502.
2. Gwilliam NR, Lazar DA, Brandt ML, Mahoney DH, Wesson DE, Mazziotti MV, Nuchtern JG, Lee TC. An analysis of outcomes and treatment costs for children undergoing splenectomy for chronic immune thrombocytopenia purpura. J Pediatr Surg. 2012;47(8):1537–41.
3. Davies IL, Cho J, Lewis MH. Splenectomy results from an 18-year single centre experience. Ann R Coll Surg Engl. 2014;96(2):147–50.
4. Holdsworth RJ, Irving AD, Cuschieri A. Postsplenectomy sepsis and its mortality rate: actual versus perceived risks. Br J Surg. 1991;78(9):1031–8.
5. Warshaw AL. Conservation of the spleen with distal pancreatectomy. Arch Surg. 1988;123(5):550–3.
6. Scott-Conner CE, Dawson DL. Technical considerations in distal pancreatectomy with splenic preservation. Surg Gynecol Obstet. 1989;168(5):451–2.
7. Kimura W, Inoue T, Futakawa N, Shinkai H, Han I, Muto T. Spleen-preserving distal pancreatectomy with conservation of the splenic artery and vein. Surgery. 1996;120(5):885–90.
8. Soper NJ, Brunt LM, Dunnegan DL, Meininger TA. Laparoscopic distal pancreatectomy in the porcine model. Surg Endosc. 1994;8(1):57–60; discussion 60–1.
9. Lee SE, Jang J-Y, Lee KU, Kim S-W. Clinical comparison of distal pancreatectomy with or without splenectomy. J Korean Med Sci. 2008;23(6):1011–4.
10. Tezuka K, Kimura W, Hirai I, Moriya T, Watanabe T, Yano M. Postoperative hematological changes after spleen-preserving distal pancreatectomy with preservation of the splenic artery and vein. Dig Surg. 2012;29(2):157–64.
11. Tsiouris A, Cogan CM, Velanovich V. Distal pancreatectomy with or without splenectomy: comparison of postoperative outcomes and surrogates of splenic function. HPB (Oxf). 2011;13(10):738–44.
12. Kohan G, Ocampo CG, Zandalazini HI, Klappenbach R, Quesada BM, Porras LTC, Rodriguez JA, Oria AS. Changes in gastrosplenic circulation and splenic function after distal pancreatectomy with spleen preservation and splenic vessel excision. J Gastrointest Surg. 2013;17(10):1739–43.
13. Richardson DQ, Scott-Conner CE. Distal pancreatectomy with and without splenectomy. A comparative study. Am Surg. 1989;55(1):21–5.
14. Aldridge MC, Williamson RC. Distal pancreatectomy with and without splenectomy. Br J Surg. 1991;78(8):976–9.
15. Benoist S, Dugué L, Sauvanet A, Valverde A, Mauvais F, Paye F, Farges O, Belghiti J. Is there a role of preservation of the spleen in distal pancreatectomy? J Am Coll Surg. 1999;188(3):255–60.

16. Lillemoe KD, Kaushal S, Cameron JL, Sohn TA, Pitt HA, Yeo CJ. Distal pancreatectomy: indications and outcomes in 235 patients. Ann Surg. 1999;229(5):693–8; discussion 698–700.
17. Shoup M, Brennan MF, McWhite K, Leung DHY, Klimstra D, Conlon KC. The value of splenic preservation with distal pancreatectomy. Arch Surg. 2002;137(2):164–8.
18. Rodríguez JR, Madanat MG, Healy BC, Thayer SP, Warshaw AL, Fernandez-del CC. Distal pancreatectomy with splenic preservation revisited. Surgery. 2007;141(5):619–25.
19. Kleeff J, Diener MK, Z'graggen K, Hinz U, Wagner M, Bachmann J, Zehetner J, Müller MW, Friess H, Büchler MW. Distal pancreatectomy: risk factors for surgical failure in 302 consecutive cases. Ann Surg. 2007;245(4):573–82.
20. Nau P, Melvin WS, Narula VK, Bloomston PM, Ellison EC, Muscarella P. Laparoscopic distal pancreatectomy with splenic conservation: an operation without increased morbidity. Gastroenterol Res Pract. 2009;2009:846340.
21. Choi SH, Seo MA, Hwang HK, Kang CM, Lee WJ. Is it worthwhile to preserve adult spleen in laparoscopic distal pancreatectomy? Perioperative and patient-reported outcome analysis. Surg Endosc. 2012;26(11):3149–56.
22. Tang CW, Feng WM, Bao Y, Fei MY, Tao YL. Spleen-preserving distal pancreatectomy or distal pancreatectomy with splenectomy?: perioperative and patient-reported outcome analysis. J Clin Gastroenterol. 2014;48(7):e62–6.
23. Dumitrascu T, Dima S, Stroescu C, Scarlat A, Ionescu M, Popescu I. Clinical value of spleen-preserving distal pancreatectomy: a case-matched analysis with a special emphasis on the postoperative systemic inflammatory response. J Hepatobiliary Pancreat Sci. 2014;21(9):654–62.
24. Butturini G, Inama M, Malleo G, Manfredi R, Melotti GL, Piccoli M, Perandini S, Pederzoli P, Bassi C. Perioperative and long-term results of laparoscopic spleen-preserving distal pancreatectomy with or without splenic vessels conservation: a retrospective analysis. J Surg Oncol. 2011;105(4):387–92.
25. Beane JD, Pitt HA, Nakeeb A, Schmidt CM, House MG, Zyromski NJ, Howard TJ, Lillemoe KD. Splenic preserving distal pancreatectomy: does vessel preservation matter? J Am Coll Surg. 2011;212(4):651–7.
26. Adam J-P, Jacquin A, Laurent C, Collet D, Masson B, Fernandez-Cruz L, Sa-Cunha A. Laparoscopic spleen-preserving distal pancreatectomy: splenic vessel preservation compared with the Warshaw technique. JAMA Surg. 2013;148(3):246–52.
27. Suman P, Rutledge J, Yiengpruksawan A. Robotic distal pancreatectomy. JSLS. 2013;17(4):627–35.
28. Kim SH, Kang CM, Satoi S, Sho M, Nakamura Y, Lee WJ. Proposal for splenectomy-omitting radical distal pancreatectomy in well-selected left-sided pancreatic cancer: multicenter survey study. J Hepatobiliary Pancreat Sci. 2013;20(3):375–81.

Chapter 56
Management of Small Nonfunctional Pancreatic Neuroendocrine Tumors

Gabriella Grisotti and Sajid A. Khan

Abstract Pancreatic neuroendocrine tumors (PNETs) are rare, accounting for only 2 % of pancreatic tumors. Traditional dogma dictates that nonfunctional PNETs are static in size and a correlation between size and malignant potential exists. However, improvements in radiographic technology have pointed to the contrary. Modern imaging is responsible for a rising incidence of PNET diagnoses and for observations that even small tumors may grow. With a steep rise in the diagnosis of small PNETs, the controversial question in modern hepatopancreaticobiliary surgery of appropriate management for small nonfunctional PNETs has never been more important, and this chapter explores the role of surgery.

The small size of incidental, nonfunctional PNETs may belie metastatic potential. Review of the data does not guarantee that small size precludes metastasis and clear predictors of malignant potential are not consistently defined. There is moderate evidence that supports that surgical resection, as opposed to observation, should remain the standard of care. Future prospective studies, a constellation of biomarkers, or genetic findings may improve prognostication to supplement histopathology and better aid in a selective treatment approach. Special consideration to a nonsurgical approach should be afforded to patients with poor lifetime expectancy or those with cancer susceptibility syndromes that include Multiple Endocrine Neoplasia Type 1, von Hippel-Lindau disease, neurofibromatosis Type 1, and tuberous sclerosis.

Keywords Small nonfunctional pancreatic neuroendocrine tumor • Pancreatic tumors • Pancreatic surgery • Surgical resection • Observation

G. Grisotti
Department of Surgery, Yale University School of Medicine, New Haven, CT, USA

S.A. Khan (✉)
Department of Surgery, Section of Surgical Oncology, Yale University School of Medicine, PO Box 208062, New Haven, CT 06520-8062, USA
e-mail: Sajid.khan@yale.edu

J.M. Millis, J.B. Matthews (eds.), *Difficult Decisions in Hepatobiliary and Pancreatic Surgery*, Difficult Decisions in Surgery: An Evidence-Based Approach, DOI 10.1007/978-3-319-27365-5_56

Introduction

Pancreatic neuroendocrine tumors (PNETs) are rare clinical entities. They are diagnosed in approximately 1 in 100,000 people and comprise 2 % of pancreatic tumors [1]. They are notably found with relatively high frequency in individuals with the hereditary cancer syndromes of Multiple Endocrine Neoplasia Type 1 (MEN-1) [2], von Hippel-Lindau disease (vHL), neurofibromatosis Type 1 (NF-1), and tuberous sclerosis (TS). PNETs are either functional or nonfunctional. Functional tumors synthesize a hormone (e.g. insulin, gastrin, vasoactive intestinal peptide, glucagon, somatostatin) that elicits a sign or symptom related to the hormone; this clinical response relates to an individual's tumor burden in addition to the secretory hormone status. Nonfunctional tumors do not cause a clinical syndrome though they may secrete proteins, such as pancreatic polypeptide or chromogranins [3]. The presentation of these less common, nonfunctional PNETs is often incidental discovery on cross-sectional imaging. Mass effect of primary or metastatic tumors may also cause biliary or gastric obstruction, pain secondary to celiac plexus involvement, and hepatomegaly from liver metastases [4].

Traditional dogma has been that nonfunctional PNETs are static in size and a correlation between size and malignancy exists. However, improvements in radiographic technology have pointed to the contrary [5]. Modern imaging is responsible for a rising incidence of PNET diagnoses and has suggested that small PNETs grow in size. As a corollary, a controversial question in modern hepatopancreaticobiliary surgery is how best to manage small pancreatic neuroendocrine tumors. The National Comprehensive Cancer Network's (NCCN) guideline for management of nonfunctional PNETs is that surgical resection is indicated, except in cases <10 mm where observation may be appropriate [6]. The North American NeuroEndocrine Tumor Society (NANETS), while acknowledging controversy, recommends resection of all sporadic, nonfunctional tumors, unless in the setting of prohibitive surgical risk from comorbidity. In a background of vHL and MEN-1, indications for surgical resection are based on tumor size with a threshold of 3 cm and 2 cm, respectively [7]. A consensus on management and indications for surgery of these small, sporadic tumors remains elusive [8].

With a steep rise in the diagnosis of small PNETs, the question of the appropriate management for small nonfunctional PNETs has never been more important [9]. A recent retrospective analysis of the Surveillance, Epidemiology, and End Results (SEER) database found that the diagnosis of individuals with PNETs ≤2 cm had increased 710 % from 1988 to 2009 [10], likely an underestimate given that this database omits benign disease. A common postulate is that widespread use of abdominal axial imaging (i.e., computed tomography (CT), magnetic resonance imaging (MRI), somatostatin receptor scintigraphy) is responsible for increased detection, yet endoscopic ultrasound (EUS) is also partly responsible for this trend [11].

Central to the work up and evaluation of PNETs, is a high-quality triple phase CT of the pancreas to determine tumor resectability. MRI should be considered with contraindications to CT. EUS is an excellent study because it affords the opportunity for a tissue diagnosis (i.e., fine needle aspiration (FNA)) and is the most sensitive modality for tumors ≤1 cm [11]. For those with genetic syndromes, it affords for preoperative localization for multifocal disease and for surveillance of patients predisposed to developing nonfunctional PNETs. Somatostatin receptor scintography can be considered (except for insulinomas) but is not always indicated in preoperative evaluation [12]. Serum tumor markers such as chromogranin A (CgA), neuron specific enolase (NSE), and pancreatic polypeptide (PP) can be considered for future surveillance.

Different organizations, such as the American Joint Committee on Cancer (AJCC) and the World Health Organization (WHO) have compiled varying classification systems for PNETs. The AJCC staging system (Table 56.1) relies on tumor size and nodal or distant spread. The WHO grading system divides tumors into well-differentiated (Grades 1–2) or poorly differentiated (Grade 3) based on mitotic count and Ki-67 proliferation index (Table 56.2) [13].

Surgical resection is considered the basis of treatment for nonfunctional PNETs. Tumor encasement (greater than 180°) of the superior mesenteric artery or celiac axis, or occlusion of the portal vein-superior mesenteric vein (PV-SMV) confluence without ability for venous reconstruction, indicate unresectability. For small tumors that are completely resectable, surgical approaches include enucleation, subtotal pancreatectomy, or pancreaticoduodenectomy. We believe loco-regional lymphadenectomy is indicated for prognostic and potential therapeutic purposes. There is no standardized number of lymph nodes advised for resection, but it has been noted that procedures reliant on enucleation often suffer from minimal lymph node sampling [14].

Table 56.1 AJCC PNET staging [40]

Stage 0	**Tis** Carcinoma in situ	**N0** No regional lymph node metastasis	**M0** No distant metastasis
Stage Ia	**T1** Tumor limited to the pancreas, ≤2 cm		
Stage Ib	**T2** Tumor limited to the pancreas, >2 cm		
Stage IIa	**T3** Tumor extends beyond the pancreas, without involvement of the celiac axis or the superior mesenteric artery		
Stage IIb	**T1, T2, or T3**	**N1** Regional lymph node metastasis	
Stage III	**T4** Tumor involves the celiac axis or the superior mesenteric artery	**Any N**	
Stage IV	**Any T**		**M1** Distant metastasis

Used with permission of the American Joint Committee on Cancer (AJCC), Chicago, Illinois. The original and primary source for this information is the AJCC Cancer Staging Manual, 7th Edition (2010) published by Springer Science + Business Media

Table 56.2 WHO grading system for PNET

Grade	Differentiation	Mitotic Count (per 2 mm^2)	Ki-67 index (%)
Grade 1 (low grade)	Well differentiated	<2	≤2
Grade 2 (intermediate grade)	Well differentiated	2–20	3–20
Grade 3 (high grade)	Poorly differentiated	>20	>20

Table 56.3 PICO table for surgical intervention for small nonfunctional pancreatic neuroendocrine tumors

P (Patients)	I (Intervention)	C (Comparator group)	O (Outcomes measured)
Small nonfunctional pancreatic neuroendocrine tumors	Resection	Observation	Morbidity, mortality, cancer risk, risk of progression, overall survival

Five-year and 10-year overall survivals for all nonfunctional PNETs are 55 % and 30 %, respectively. Five-year survival in one study of 274 patients, when stratified by TNM staging (Table 56.1) revealed 100 % survival for stage I, 93 % for stage II, 65 % for stage III, and 35 % for stage IV [15]. Adverse prognostic indicators include poor differentiation of the tumor, lack of resection of the primary tumor, and liver metastases, especially if not treated aggressively. Surgery is recommended for locally advanced disease where the nonfunctional PNET has spread beyond the pancreas to the surrounding tissues or local lymph nodes. The value of surgical resection for small, nonfunctional PNETs is controversial [16, 17].

Search Strategy

A literature search of English language publications from 2007 to 2014 was used to identity published data on surgical resection for small nonfunctional neuroendocrine tumors of the pancreas using the PICO outline (Table 56.3). Databases searched were Pubmed, SUMSearch, Cochrane Library, OVID, Web of Science, SCOPUS, and EMBASE.

The literature search relied on the terms: "nonfunctional pancreatic neuroendocrine tumors", "nonfunctioning pancreatic neuroendocrine tumors", "nonfunctional pancreatic endocrine tumors", "nonfunctioning pancreatic endocrine tumors", "surgery/resection/observation AND small nonfunctional pancreatic neuroendocrine tumors", "surgery/resection/observation AND nonfunctioning pancreatic neuroendocrine tumors", "surgery/resection/observation AND nonfunctional pancreatic endocrine tumors", "surgery/resection/observation AND nonfunctioning pancreatic endocrine tumors".

Papers were excluded if they were solely focused on metastases of pancreatic neuroendocrine tumors, published prior to 2007, or published in a non-English language.

There were no randomized control trials published. Eighteen cohort studies, four database studies, and one systematic review were included in our analysis. The data was classified using the GRADE system.

Results

Predictors of Survival

One observational study of 41 patients with small (<2 cm), nonfunctional PNETs found no loco-regional spread or distant metastasis over a 34-month median follow-up [18]. Average tumor growth was 0.12 mm per year, only one tumor grew beyond 2 cm, and of eight patients that underwent resection, all had low grade, lymph node negative disease. Statistical analysis was unable to identify any statistically significant patient or tumor characteristics that predicted growth rate. The short clinical follow-up and the lack of statistically significant variables to forecast tumor progression are obvious criticisms of this study.

A retrospective study of 151 patients who underwent resection of nonfunctional PNETs with a 2.6 cm median diameter evaluated prognostic factors for survival [19]. The 10-year overall survival, disease-specific survival, and disease-free survival rates were 72.6 %, 85.1 %, and 57.2 % respectively. Based on the WHO classification schema, survival was inversely related to tumor grade. Further validating the WHO classification, on multivariate analysis, Ki-67 index, mitotic count, and lymph node metastasis were all indicators of poor prognosis. This study did not provide data stratified based on tumor size, and as the range in size was 2–15 cm, it is hard to infer the natural history of truly small tumors, but it does provide insight into predictive clinical variables for PNETs in general.

Tumor size alone does not predict its biology and there is data to support the presence of loco-regional and distant spread in small PNETs. In a recent review of the National Cancer Database (NCDB) from 1998 to 2011, Gratian et al. reported interesting data on 1,854 patients with PNETs ≤2 cm [20]. Among tumors ≤0.5 cm, one-third of patients presented with loco-regional lymph node disease and 11 % had distant disease. Furthermore the 5-year overall survival in patients with small nonfunctional PNETs who did not undergo surgery was markedly decreased compared to those who did have surgery (27.6 % vs 72.0–86.0 %, $P<0.01$). This was after excluding those patients with distant metastases, prohibitive comorbidities, or death before reaching surgery. The type of surgery, ranging from enucleation to pancreaticoduodenectomy, was not found to have a significant impact on survival, leading the authors to recommend that the type of surgery be left to the surgeon's discretion. Lymphadenectomy also did not affect overall survival, but this may be colored by a lack of standards for extent of lymphadenectomy. Other limitations, based on the nature of the database, include that all PNETs included were coded as malignant, some functional PNETs may have been included, and as with all databases, the results may have been tainted by miscoding.

Nodal involvement has been used as a surrogate marker for survival in some studies. Several studies found that tumor size is predictive of nodal metastasis and overall survival [21]. A large retrospective study (Curran et al.), of PNETs in the SEER database, from 1988 to 2010, which did not differentiate functional from nonfunctional tumors, found that tumor size ≥2 cm and increased grade significantly increased the chances of nodal involvement [22]. They further substratified lesions, again, both functional and not, and those ≤2 cm had a 22 % chance of nodal metastasis and those ≤1 cm had a 17 % chance of nodal metastasis in the absence of grade data. With grade data, not yet regularly recorded for every patient, the authors hypothesize that these small PNETs, both functional and nonfunctional, may be able to be risk-stratified for nodal metastasis with greater accuracy.

A study that looked at nonfunctional PNETs in both the SEER database from 1988 to 2009 and an institutional database from 1996 to 2012, with 1,371 and 79 cases each (Kuo et al.), found two interesting, significant predictors of survival for tumors ≤2 cm [10]. Minority race (black or Asian, compared to white (Asian, HR 30.2, 95 % CI 3.1–291.7; black, HR 60.1, 95 % CI 2.1–1,027.9)) and tumor grades of moderate (HR 37.2, 95 % CI 2.7–518.8) and poor (HR 94.2, 95 % CI 4.9–1,794.4) differentiation were associated with decreased disease-specific survival. Disease-specific survival was not related to nodal involvement. Nodal involvement was negatively associated with small tumor size. However, in those tumors ≤2 cm which did have nodal involvement, it was associated with extra-pancreatic spread and was less likely in patients 65 years of age, or older, compared to those younger than 45 years of age. It is unclear if the relationship between race and survival is due to genetics or to other socio-economic factors. The caveat remains, as with other SEER studies, that benign disease is excluded, thus skewing results and requiring caution in generalizing.

A single institution retrospective study (Toste et al.) from 1989 to 2012 found a different relationship between tumor size, dichotomizing at 2 cm, and nodal involvement, but not survival [21]. Again, a small minority of tumors ≤2 cm did have nodal metastasis. Acknowledging the limitations of the study size and retrospective nature, they concluded that in certain high risk patients, observation of tumors ≤2 cm may be appropriate. These findings were echoed in another small case series with less than 20 patients [23].

Resection of Tumors ≤2 cm

A strong multi-institutional study supporting resection was reported by Cherefant et al. in 2013 [24]. This study included 128 patients who had undergone resection for nonfunctional PNET. Three patients with tumors ≤2 cm developed distant metastasis and two of those patients died of disease, prompting the authors to argue that it was unsafe to differentiate based on tumor size.

A single institution retrospective study (Haynes et al.) from 1977 to 2009 of 139 patients with a nonfunctional PNET, found that of the 39 tumors ≤2 cm which were resected, 7.7 % of patients had late metastasis or recurrence [25]. Disease progression or recurrence was even found to develop in a patient classified as "benign" tumor. Without a prospective randomized trial, deemed unfeasible due to lack of clinical equipoise by the authors, they recommend resection for all surgically fit patients with nonfunctional PNETs without distinction based on size.

A retrospective study of the NCDB database, with 380 patients identified to have nonmetastatic, nonfunctional PNETs ≤2 cm from 1998 to 2006 evaluated the effect of observation on survival [26]. Nineteen percent of those patients were observed, but the reasoning behind the nonoperative approach was not available. Seventy-five percent of the observed patients did not undergo any other therapy (e.g. chemotherapy or radiation). On a multivariate analysis of the overall 5-year survival rates (82.2 % for resection and 34.3 % for observation, $P<0.0001$) resection conferred an overall survival advantage independent of the patient's health status or the tumor's pathology, reinforcing the findings of Gratian et al. [22], as described above, who also used the NCDB database.

A different retrospective study of PNETs in the SEER database (Hill et al.) did not stratify patients based on the size of the tumor but also found that resection improved survival across all stages in patients who were advised to undergo surgery [27]. They evaluated 728 patients from 1988 to 2002, 84 % of whom had nonfunctional tumors. Patients who underwent resection had significantly increased overall survival compared to those who were advised to undergo resection, but did not (114 months vs 35 months, $P<0.0001$). Although functional PNETs were included in this study, on a subgroup analysis of functional status, adjusted Cox model showed no effect of functional status.

Observation of Tumors ≤2 cm

A two center study in Italy (Crippa et al.) was done with 355 patients with nonfunctional PNETs who underwent resection and 12 patients with nonfunctional PNETs who were observed [28]. In the latter group, median tumor size was 14 mm, and none of the tumors enlarged or progressed over a median follow up of 3 years. Albeit with a small observation population and relatively short term follow up, the authors conclude that observation of tumors ≤2 cm is safe when operative risks are prohibitive, for example in an older population with more comorbidities. The same Italian group also published on a retrospective study from 1990 to 2008 (Bettini et al.) of resected nonfunctional PNETs [29]. While they saw an inverse relationship between tumor size and malignancy, and went so far as to say that tumors ≤2 cm might be safely observed, they admitted that only 60 % of their tumors ≤2 cm were benign.

In Japan, another single institution study (Kishi et al.) from 1981 to 2013, followed 90 patients with nonfunctional PNETs [30]. Seventy-five patients underwent resection and 19 patients, with a median tumor size of 12 mm, were followed by serial imaging. The institutional guidelines were to observe tumors ≤10 mm, and any patients with larger tumors who were in the observation arm, were patients who had refused surgery. Five-year progression-free survival for the observed patients was 83 %. Of the patients who underwent resection, no patients with tumors ≤15 mm had recurrence or late metastasis. With a less than 4-year median follow-up, this study advised that patients with tumors ≤10 mm could be observed, but once the tumor was ≥15 mm, resection was indicated.

A single institution, retrospective study with a much larger proportion of observed patients was reported by Lee et al. [31]. Seventy-seven patients with non-functional PNETs (median size 1 cm, range 0.3–3.2 cm) diagnosed with or without a tissue diagnosis were observed for a mean radiologic follow up of only 35 months without increase in tumor size, disease progression, or disease related mortality. Fifty-six patients (with a median tumor size of 1.8 cm) underwent resection with pathology revealing that all patients were AJCC Stage I, except for five patients with lymph node involvement and four patients who did not have a PNET. Using the WHO criteria, 73 % were low grade, 21 % were intermediate grade, there were no high grade cases, and 6 % did not have this data available. This study recommended observation and serial imaging for patients with tumors ≤2 cm. This recommendation did not restrict nonoperative management to those patients with prohibitive risks for surgery, as other studies had. The short term follow-up and lack of confirmatory tissue for diagnosis of the nonoperative group calls into question the generalizability of these findings.

Another case series of 108 patients who underwent resection of a nonfunctional PNET from 1994 to 2010 (Birnbaum et al.) discriminated based on whether the nonfunctional PNET was discovered incidentally or based on patient symptoms [32]. Significant findings included that incidental tumors were more likely to be ≤2 cm (65 % compared to 42 %), T1 stage (62 % vs 33 %, $P=0.0001$), node negative (85 % vs 60 %; $P=0.005$), and grade 1 (66 % vs 33 %, $P=0.0001$). Five-year disease-free survival was 92 % in the incidentally discovered group and 82 % in the symptomatic group. They also reported no significant difference in disease-free survival between those with incidentally discovered ($N=36$) and symptomatic ($N=16$) tumors <2 cm. This led the authors to cautiously agree that observation may be suitable for patients with tumors ≤2 cm.

Tumors in the Background of vHL or MEN I

Individuals with hereditary cancer syndromes present a distinct patient population with more frequent occurrence of nonfunctional PNETs. A unique prospective study by Blansfield et al. examined 633 patients with vHL from 1988 to 2006 and found that 108 patients had a nonfunctional PNET [33]. This rate coincides with the occurrence of PNET in 12–17 % of patients with vHL. The tumors were resected (in 39 patients) if >3 cm without evidence of metastatic disease, or if laparotomy was performed for another reason and tumor resection was considered feasible with minimal morbidity. The rest of the patients were followed with serial imaging. The recommendations were that patients with vHL should be evaluated by three criteria: size ≥3 cm, presence of a specific mutation in exon 3, and tumor size doubling time less than 500 days. With no criteria fulfilled, a patient can be managed nonoperatively with serial imaging every 2–3 years. With one criterion, the frequency of imaging is increased to every 6 months. With two or three criteria, the patient should be evaluated for surgery.

Nonfunctional PNETs are diagnosed in 70–80 % of individuals with MEN 1, with almost all patients demonstrating pancreatic hyperplasia on autopsy. PNETs are a significant cause of mortality in patients with MEN I, as compared to parathyroid or pituitary lesions [34, 35]. Nonfunctional PNETs may even present as early as the second decade [36] and disease is often multicentric [37]. In a study of 11 patients with MEN 1 (D'Souza et al.), 18 tumors were found ranging in size from 5 mm to 2.4 cm with a mean of 10.3 mm [38]. Over a mean follow up period of 79 months, the initial tumors grew an average of 1.32 mm per year. However, 12 new lesions were found with an accelerated rate of growth of 3 mm per year. This led the authors and an editorial related to this study [39], to support surveillance of nonfunctional PNETs in the setting of MEN-1, until growth beyond 2 cm, in conjunction with a slow rate of growth per year (≤15 % initial diameter).

Recommendations

There has been a sharp rise in the proportion of patients presenting with small, nonfunctional PNETs. While advanced tumor grade, mitotic rate, and Ki-67 indices portend a poorer prognosis for all diagnosed PNETs, size does not necessarily predict tumor biology. For small tumors, the incidence of loco-regional lymphatic and distant metastasis is not trivial and malignant potential may still exist (evidence quality moderate). Until prospective studies provide clarity to predicted clinical outcome, surgical resection must remain the standard of care. Individuals in whom surgery presents a prohibitive risk may be observed with serial imaging with the understanding that the possibility to develop metastasis is possible. Those with a limited life expectancy and low tumor grade may also be considered for observation because data suggests a slow progression of disease. Though recommendations for management in a background of vHL and MEN-1 are not clear, surgical resection should be considered for tumor sizes of 3 cm and 2 cm, respectively.

Personal View

Improvements to radiographic imaging, in addition to their overutilization, have increased the incidence of incidentalomas for various solid tumors. This is of critical relevance to the hepatopancreatobiliary surgeon because of the surge of newly discovered small PNETs. There are no large, prospective, high quality studies that support observation over resection in the treatment of this disease. However, multiple retrospective studies have shown that loco-regional lymphatic and distant metastasis is possible in small tumors ≤2 cm. An incidental finding on abdominal imaging of a small nonfunctional PNET should prompt referral to a surgeon. A recent patient treated by our surgical oncology service reinforces the concept that small tumors are capable of spread. An asymptomatic 75 year-old woman with an excellent performance status presented with a 1 cm, hypervascular, pancreatic tail lesion on CT. This was radiographically stable in size for 4 years, not amenable to biopsy, and she underwent a laparoscopic distal subtotal pancreatectomy. Pathologic examination revealed that while the tumor was only 1.1 cm in largest dimension, well differentiated, and had a Ki-67 index <2 %, it had already metastasized to two of seven resected lymph nodes (Fig. 56.1). Until better data point to the contrary, pancreatectomy is superior to observation for small, nonfunctional PNETs.

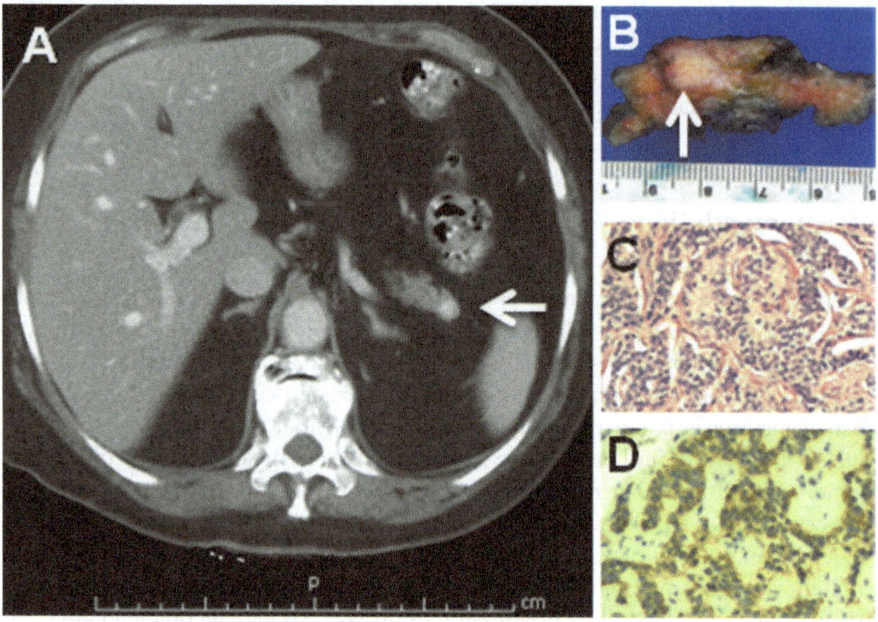

Fig. 56.1 Imaging and pathology from a case of a small, nonfunctional PNET. (**a**) A transverse image from a computed tomography (CT) scan with intravenous contrast. White arrow points to the 1 cm enhancing lesion in the tail of the pancreas. On comparison to CT scans over the past 4 years (not shown), the size of the lesion was stable. No evidence of liver metastasis or lymphadenopathy in the rest of the scan (not shown). (**b**) Gross specimen of the same 1 cm pancreatic lesion seen in **a**, removed during a laparoscopic distal pancreatectomy. It was noted to be a 1.1 × 1.0 × 1.0 cm, tan-white, and slightly granular tumor (*white arrow*) with negative margins. The remainder of the pancreas was unremarkable. Tumor was present in two of seven lymph nodes (not shown). (**c**) Hematoxylin and eosin stain of a section of the same pancreatic lesion, under high power resolution. Cells are in a festooning, trabecular pattern, with round nuclei with granular chromatin. Mitotic figures are less than 2 per 10 high power fields. Ki-67 index <2 %. (**d**) Chromogranin stain of a section of the same pancreatic lesion, under high power resolution. Cells were positive for both chromogranin and synaptophysin (not shown)

Recommendations

- For medically fit patients with sporadic, small, nonfunctional PNETs, we recommend surgical resection over observation (evidence quality moderate; weak recommendation).
- We favor resection over enucleation partly because the latter often suffers from minimal lymph node sampling (evidence quality moderate; weak recommendation).
- In a background of vHL and MEN-1, indications for surgical resection are tumor size greater than 3 cm and 2 cm, respectively (evidence quality low; weak recommendation).

References

1. Kuo JH, Lee JA, et al. Nonfunctional pancreatic neuroendocrine tumors. Surg Clin N Am. 2014;94(3):689–708.
2. Botsios D, Vasiliadis K, et al. Management of nonfunctioning pancreatic endocrine tumors in the context of multiple endocrine neoplasia type 1 syndrome. J Gastrointest Liver Dis. 2007;16(3):257–62.
3. Metz DC, Jensen RT. Gastrointestinal neuroendocrine tumors: pancreatic endocrine tumors. Gastroenterology. 2008;135(5):1469–92.
4. Libutti SK. Evolving paradigm for managing small nonfunctional incidentally discovered pancreatic neuroendocrine tumors. J Clin Endocrinol Metab. 2013;98(12):4670–2.
5. Fischer L, Bergmann F, et al. Outcome of surgery for pancreatic neuroendocrine neoplasms. Br J Surg. 2014;101(11):1405–12.
6. Neuroendocrine tumors. Version 2. 2414. NCCN Clinical Practice Guidelines in Oncology. http://www.nccn.org/professionals/physician_gls/pdf/neuroendocrine.pdf.
7. Kunz PL, Reidy-Lagunes D, et al. Consensus guidelines for the management and treatment of neuroendocrine tumors. Pancreas. 2013;42(4):557–77.
8. Cheema A, Weber J, et al. Incidental detection of pancreatic neuroendocrine tumors: an analysis of incidence and outcomes. Ann Surg Oncol. 2012;19(9):2932–6.
9. Yao JC, Hassan M, et al. One hundred years after "carcinoid": epidemiology of and prognostic factors for neuroendocrine tumors in 35,825 cases in the United States. J Clin Oncol. 2008;26(18):3063–72.
10. Kuo EJ, Salem RR. Population-level analysis of pancreatic neuroendocrine tumors 2 cm or less in size. Ann Surg Oncol. 2013;20(9):2815–21.
11. Rustagi T, Farrell JJ. Endoscopic diagnosis and treatment of pancreatic neuroendocrine tumors. J Clin Gastroenterol. 2014;48(10):837–44.
12. Minter RM, Simeone DM. Contemporary management of nonfunctioning pancreatic neuroendocrine tumors. J Gastrointest Surg. 2012;16(2):435–46.
13. Klimstra DS, Arnold R, Capella C, et al. Neuroendocrine neoplasms of the pancreas. In: Bosman F, Carneiro F, Hruban RH, Theise N, editors. WHO classification of tumours of the digestive system. Lyon: IARC Press; 2010. p. 322–6.
14. Haugvik SP, Labori KJ, et al. Surgical treatment of sporadic pancreatic neuroendocrine tumors: a state of the art review. Sci World J. 2012;2012. Article ID 357475, 9 pages. doi: 10.1100/2012/357475.
15. Scarpa A, Mantovani W, et al. Pancreatic endocrine tumors: improved TNM staging and histopathological grading permit a clinically efficient prognostic stratification of patients. Mod Pathol. 2010;23(6):824–33.

16. Dickson PV, Behrman SW. Management of pancreatic neuroendocrine tumors. Surg Clin N Am. 2013;93(3):675–91.
17. Karakaxas D, Gazouli M, et al. Pancreatic neuroendocrine tumors: current opinions on a rare, but potentially curable neoplasm. Eur J Gastroenterol Hepatol. 2014;26(8):826–35.
18. Gaujoux S, Partelli S, et al. Observational study of natural history of small sporadic nonfunctioning pancreatic neuroendocrine tumors. J Clin Endocrinol Metab. 2013;98(12):4784–9.
19. Song, K. B., S. C. Kim, et al. (2014). Prognostic factors in 151 patients with surgically resected non-functioning pancreatic neuroendocrine tumours. ANZ J Surg. doi: 10.1111/ans.12738.
20. Gratian L, Pura J, et al. Impact of extent of surgery on survival in patients with small nonfunctional pancreatic neuroendocrine tumors in the United States. Ann Surg Oncol. 2014;21(11):3515–21.
21. Toste PA, Kadera BE, et al. Nonfunctional pancreatic neuroendocrine tumors <2 cm on preoperative imaging are associated with a low incidence of nodal metastasis and an excellent overall survival. J Gastrointest Surg. 2013;17(12):2105–13.
22. Curran T, Pockaj BA, et al. Importance of lymph node involvement in pancreatic neuroendocrine tumors: impact on survival and implications for surgical resection. J Gastrointest Surg. 2015;19(1):152–160.
23. Nomura N, Fujii T, et al. Nonfunctioning neuroendocrine pancreatic tumors: our experience and management. J Hepato-Biliary-Pancreat Surg. 2009;16(5):639–47.
24. Cherenfant J, Stocker SJ, et al. Predicting aggressive behavior in nonfunctioning pancreatic neuroendocrine tumors. Surgery. 2013;154(4):785–93.
25. Haynes AB, Deshpande V, et al. Implications of incidentally discovered, nonfunctioning pancreatic endocrine tumors: short-term and long-term patient outcomes. Arch Surg. 2011;146(5):534–8.
26. Sharpe SM, In H, et al. Surgical resection provides an overall survival benefit for patients with small pancreatic neuroendocrine tumors. J Gastrointest Surg. 2015;19(1):117–123.
27. Hill JS, McPhee JT, et al. Pancreatic neuroendocrine tumors: the impact of surgical resection on survival. Cancer. 2009;115(4):741–51.
28. Crippa S, Partelli S, et al. Incidental diagnosis as prognostic factor in different tumor stages of nonfunctioning pancreatic endocrine tumors. Surgery. 2014;155(1):145–53.
29. Bettini R, Partelli S, et al. Tumor size correlates with malignancy in nonfunctioning pancreatic endocrine tumor. Surgery. 2011;150(1):75–82.
30. Kishi Y, Shimada K, et al. Basing treatment strategy for non-functional pancreatic neuroendocrine tumors on tumor size. Ann Surg Oncol. 2014;21(9):2882–8.
31. Lee LC, Grant CS, et al. Small, nonfunctioning, asymptomatic pancreatic neuroendocrine tumors (PNETs): role for nonoperative management. Surgery. 2012;152(6):965–74.
32. Birnbaum DJ, Gaujoux S, et al. Sporadic nonfunctioning pancreatic neuroendocrine tumors: prognostic significance of incidental diagnosis. Surgery. 2014;155(1):13–21.
33. Blansfield JA, Choyke L, et al. Clinical, genetic and radiographic analysis of 108 patients with von Hippel-Lindau disease (VHL) manifested by pancreatic neuroendocrine neoplasms (PNETs). Surgery. 2007;142(6):814–8.
34. Kunstman JW, Carling T. Multiple endocrine neoplasias. Chichester: eLS, Wiley; 2001.
35. Goudet P, Murat A, et al. Risk factors and causes of death in MEN1 disease. A GTE (Groupe d'Etude des Tumeurs Endocrines) cohort study among 758 patients. World J Surg. 2010;34(2):249–55.
36. Goncalves TD, Toledo RA, et al. Penetrance of functioning and nonfunctioning pancreatic neuroendocrine tumors in multiple endocrine neoplasia type 1 in the second decade of life. J Clin Endocrinol Metab. 2014;99(1):E89–96.
37. Partelli S, Maurizi A, et al. Surgical management of pancreatic neuroendocrine neoplasms. Ann Saudi Med. 2014;34(1):1–5.

38. D'Souza SL, Elmunzer BJ, et al. Long-term follow-up of asymptomatic pancreatic neuroendocrine tumors in multiple endocrine neoplasia type I syndrome. J Clin Gastroenterol. 2014;48(5):458–61.
39. Tonelli F. How to follow up and when to operate asymptomatic pancreatic neuroendocrine tumors in multiple endocrine neoplasia type 1? J Clin Gastroenterol. 2014;48(5):387–9.
40. Edge SB, Byrd DR, Compton CC, editors. AJCC cancer staging handbook. 7th ed. New York: Springer; 2010.

Chapter 57
Management of Pancreatic Gastrinoma

Shady F. Gad and Jason K. Sicklick

Abstract Pancreatic gastrinoma is a functional pancreatic neuroendocrine tumor that secretes gastrin and leads to Zollinger-Ellison Syndrome (ZES), a disorder characterized by hypergastrinemia and gastric acid hypersecretion. These tumors may be either sporadic or part of multiple endocrine neoplasia type 1 (MEN-1) syndrome. At present, surgical management remains the first-line treatment for cases of sporadic or hereditary gastrinomas while medical therapy is utilized to ameliorate the effects of hypergastrinemia and resultant gastric acid hypersecretion. Together, these approaches improve survival and reduce disease-related complications in these patients. As such, multi-disciplinary, personalized care is critical for optimizing outcomes in these patients.

Keywords Zollinger-Ellison syndrome • MEN-1 • Gastrinoma • Pancreatic surgery • Morbidity

Introduction

Pancreatic gastrinoma is a functional pancreatic neuroendocrine tumor that secretes gastrin and leads to Zollinger-Ellison Syndrome (ZES) characterized by hypergastrinemia and gastric acid hypersecretion. Patients with gastrinomas can develop ulcers in the stomach, duodenum, and small bowel. Gastrinomas most commonly arise within the "gastrinoma triangle" bordered by the junction of the cystic-common bile duct, the junction of the second-third portions of the duodenum, and the junction of the neck-body of the pancreas. They may also arise within the pancreatic body/tail, esophagus, stomach, jejunum, omentum, liver, ovaries, and kidneys [1]. The reported incidence of all gastrinomas is 1–3 per 1,000,000 [2]. These tumors may be either sporadic or part of multiple endocrine neoplasia type 1

S.F. Gad • J.K. Sicklick (✉)
Division of Surgical Oncology and Department of Surgery, Moores Cancer Center, University of California San Diego, UC San Diego Health System, 3855 Health Sciences Drive, Mail Code 0987, La Jolla, CA 92093-0987, USA
e-mail: jsicklick@ucsd.edu

J.M. Millis, J.B. Matthews (eds.), *Difficult Decisions in Hepatobiliary and Pancreatic Surgery*, Difficult Decisions in Surgery: An Evidence-Based Approach, DOI 10.1007/978-3-319-27365-5_57

(MEN-1) syndrome. At present, surgical management remains the first line treatment for cases of sporadic or hereditary gastrinomas while medical therapy remains an indispensable part of the treatment algorithm in order to abrogate the effects of hypergastrinemia and resultant gastric acid hypersecretion. As such, medical therapy should be utilized in patients with sporadic disease following failure to localize a tumor, when disease is unresectable, or when disease recurs. On the other hand, lifelong medical management is warranted in all cases of MEN-1 syndrome-associated gastrinomas because of the high risk of multifocal disease. This chapter addresses the management and outcomes of both sporadic and familial pancreatic gastrinoma.

Search Strategy

A literature search of English language publications ending in September 2014 was used to identity published data on pancreatic gastrinoma management and outcomes. The PubMed, Scopus, and Embase databases were searched. Terms used in the searches were "gastrinoma," "pancreatic gastrinoma," "Zollinger-Ellison syndrome," "MEN-1," "MEN 1," "metastatic gastrinoma," "surgical treatment of gastrinoma," "pancreaticoduodenectomy and gastrinoma," and "medical treatment of gastrinoma." Case reports, case series, review articles, and clinical trials were included in our literature review.

Presentation of Pancreatic Gastrinoma

Gastrinoma is the second most common functional pancreatic neuroendocrine tumor (PNET) and the most common functional NET in MEN-1 patients [2]. Patients may present with gastroesophageal reflux, dyspepsia, dysphagia, esophagitis, esophageal strictures, recurrent or multiple gastric/duodenal/jejunal ulcerations, or secretory diarrhea [3–6]. In turn, this is the underlying cause of peptic ulcer disease (PUD) in approximately 0.1–1 % of all PUD patients [7]. The mean age of presentation has been reported around 50 years old [8–10]. However, the disease probably occurs earlier in life since the mean time from symptoms to diagnosis has been reported to be as long as 8 years [11]. The delay to diagnosis may be further exacerbated in cases of sporadic gastrinomas by the increased availability of medications to control gastric acid hypersecretion (e.g., proton pump inhibitors, histamine H2 receptor antagonists, and antacids) [12]. In contrast, patients with a personal or family history of MEN-1, hypercalcemia, recurrent nephrolithiasis, parathyroid adenomas, recurrent peptic ulcers at a young age, and/or pituitary tumors should raise suspicion for a gastrinoma in the setting of MEN-1 syndrome [2].

The diagnosis of ZES associated with pancreatic and non-pancreatic gastrinoma is defined by several factors, including elevated gastrin levels and elevated basal gastric acid levels. More specifically, patients must have a fasting serum gastrin greater than 100 pg/mL and basal acid output greater than 15 mEq/h [4]. Furthermore, an increase of 200 pg/mL of gastrin after secretin injection confirms the diagnosis of ZES. It is important to note that patients should cease taking anti-secretory medications for at least 3 days prior to measurement of hormone levels.

Tumor Localization

Pancreatic gastrinomas may occur anywhere within the pancreas, including the tail (48 %), head (30 %), and body (22 %) [2, 13]. In order to define the tumor location(s) and evaluate for metastatic disease, non-invasive imaging studies should be utilized. These include abdominal ultrasonography (20–30 % sensitivity to detect any gastrinoma), abdominal/pelvic computed tomography (CT) scan (80–100 % sensitivity) and magnetic resonance imaging (MRI, 83 % sensitivity to detect liver metastases) [2, 14]. Additionally, functional nuclear studies, including 68Ga-DOTA-Tyr3-octreotide positron emission tomography (PET) scan and 111In-DTPA-octreotide scintigraphy can be utilized for localization based upon tumor expression of the somatostatin receptor [15]. The combined use of PET and CT has the highest overall accuracy. In addition to these non-invasive imaging modalities, more invasive options exist, including endoscopic ultrasonography (75–100 % sensitivity), intraoperative pancreatic ultrasonography and intraoperative hepatic ultrasonography. The latter approaches may be necessary in cases where preoperative imaging fails to localize disease [16].

Prognostic Factors

There are several unfavorable prognostic factors in patients with pancreatic gastrinoma. These include: female sex; rapid progression of symptoms; markedly elevated fasting gastrin levels; persistent gastric acid hypersecretion despite optimal medical management; primary tumor size; advanced tumor stage (i.e., lymph node and liver metastases); molecular features including HER2/neu overexpression; and histopathologic features including lymphovascular invasion, perineural invasion, and higher mitotic index (i.e., >2 mitoses per 20 high power fields) [9, 17]. With these factors in mind, there are two main strategies for improving symptom and disease control [e.g., disease-free survival (DFS), progression-free survival (PFS), disease-specific survival (DSS) and overall survival (OS)].

Surgical Management

Treatment options for pancreatic gastrinoma include operative and non-operative approaches. In deciding between these, decision-making is based upon the extent and location of disease, as well as the patient's underlying performance status and medical comorbidities. In determining the optimal approach, treatment outcomes, as well as morbidity and mortality associated with each approach should be considered. However, because of the rarity of pancreatic gastrinoma, the management of this disease is mostly based upon case reports, case series, and expert opinion. As a result, the evidence quality can be considered very low to moderate, but many of the recommendations are moderate to strong.

Reported operative management options include enucleation and resection (e.g., pancreaticoduodenectomy and distal pancreatectomy) [18, 19]. Additionally, it is important to evaluate the liver, because hepatic metastases may be present and therefore warrant treatments such as partial hepatectomy and/or ablation [20–22]. In one of the larger series reported, Norton and colleagues reported that surgical management improved survival in patients with pancreatic and non-pancreatic gastrinomas as compared to non-operative management [20]. More specifically, they compared outcomes in 160 ZES patients who underwent surgical exploration versus 35 ZES patients who did not. Twenty-seven (17 %) of these patients had pancreatic gastrinomas. Overall, the groups were similar in regards to demographics, laboratory values, and imaging findings. At the time of operation, 94 % of patients had a tumor removed, while 51 % had immediate normalization of gastrin levels consistent with biochemical cure. At last follow up (range: 11.8–12 years), 41 % of patients remained disease-free. In this study, the DSS at 15 years was superior in the surgical group (98 %) as compared to the non-surgical group (74 %). Over time, 29 % of the non-operative cohort developed liver metastases as compared to 5 % of the operative cohort. While historically there was controversy regarding the role of surgical management in the treatment of ZES patients, this study suggested that operative treatment increases DSS in patients with ZES while decreasing the development of metastatic disease.

Enucleation

Enucleation of PNET is a well-accepted approach in the management of localized tumors [18]. In one study by Atema and colleagues, 5 of 11 patients (45.5 %) underwent enucleation for pancreatic gastrinomas [8]. One of these five patients (20 %) subsequently underwent completion pylorus-preserving pancreaticoduodenectomy (PPPD) for unresected disease. Another patient had a post-operative course complicated by the development of a chyle leak, which was treated by percutaneous drainage and a medium-chain triglyceride diet. The long-term results in this series were notable for a DFS range from 1 to 13 years with one patient succumbing to metastatic disease, one patient developing a suspected recurrence, and three patients remaining disease-free. While no postoperative pancreatic fistula (POPF) were reported in this small series, it is a well known complication following enucleation of pancreatic tumors. Another study of 60 patients with ≤3.0 cm potentially benign pancreatic tumors were analyzed for POPF rates after enucleation [23]. This study included five pancreatic gastrinoma patients. The authors distinguished deep enucleation [i.e., distance ≤3 mm from the main pancreatic duct (MPD)] from standard enucleation (i.e., distance >3 mm from the MPD). The deep enucleation group (N=30), which included two gastrinomas, had a significantly higher rate (i.e., 70 %) of clinically relevant POPF types B and C versus the standard enucleation (N=30), which included three gastrinomas, and had a lower rate (i.e., 23 %). On multivariate analysis, distance from the MPD independently predicted the incidence of clinically relevant POPF. Beyond the immediate complications of the operation, two patients (40 %) who underwent enucleation of 25-mm and 23-mm sized gastrinomas developed metastatic disease without local recurrence. They succumbed to disease after 10.3 and 16.9 years, respectively. No other patients developed recurrent or metastatic disease. Therefore, based upon the high incidence of POPF, enucleation should be considered with caution, especially in gastrinoma patients.

Resection

In addition to enucleation, surgical resection is a viable option for treating pancreatic gastrinomas. As previously noted, pancreatic gastrinomas may occur anywhere within the pancreas, including the tail (48 %), head (30 %), and body (22 %) [2, 13]. While small, superficial lesions distant (i.e., >3 mm) from the MPD can be considered for enucleation, larger, deeper lesions that are closer to the MPD should be considered for resection. For pancreatic head and uncinate process gastrinomas, pancreaticoduodenectomy (PD) may be performed while for body and tail lesions, distal pancreatectomy (DP) should be utilized. In instances of neck/body tumors, central pancreatectomy is another option. Herein, we discuss pancreatic operations and complications in the setting of gastrinoma.

In a report by Norton and colleagues [24], they studied 81 patients with sporadic and familial gastrinomas. The ZES and MEN-1 patients were divided into four cohorts depending upon the results of preoperative imaging. Group 1 (N=17, tumors <2.5 cm) and group 3 (N=8, diffuse liver metastases) did not undergo operations. All patients in group 2A [N=17; single tumor, 2.5–6 cm (i.e., limited disease)] and group 2B (N=31; ≥2 tumors, ≥2.5 cm, or single tumor >6 cm) underwent laparotomy. Of the patients in these latter two groups, 24 %/58 % had DPs, 0 %/13 % had hepatic resections, 0 %/6 % had PDs, and 53 %/68 % had duodenal resections, respectively. The overall perioperative morbidity rate was 29 %. Complications included pancreatitis (N=2, 2.5 %), POPF (2.5 %), abscess (N=4, 5.0 %), deep venous thrombosis (N=1, 1.2 %), postoperative hemorrhage (1.2 %), and ileus (1.2 %). Long-term complications included small bowel obstructions (N=3, 3.7 %), abscesses (2.5 %) and biliary stricture (1.2 %). During follow-up (mean 6.9±0.8 years), hepatic metastases developed in 6 % of patients in group 2A and 2B. Despite optimal surgical management, no patient was cured at 5 years. In comparison, group 1 patients had a similar 15-year OS rate as group 2A/2B patients (89–100 %). But, the group 3 patients with diffusely metastatic disease that were treated medically had a significantly worse 15-year OS rate (52 %). Taken together, this study demonstrates that: (1) almost 40 % of patients with sporadic and familial gastrinomas have advanced disease without diffuse distant metastases; (2) despite multiple primary gastrinomas and a 70 % incidence of lymph node metastases, tumors can be removed with limited morbidity and mortality; (3) patients with advanced disease who underwent aggressive surgical resection had a 15-year OS rate similar to patients with limited disease who were treated medically. Overall, this suggests that surgical resection plays a role in the management of patients with both ZES and MEN-1 who have advanced disease without diffuse liver metastases.

In a smaller study of 13 patients with ZES and gastrinoma, similar findings were corroborated in patients with pancreatic lesions (N=7). In this series, 6 (46.2 %) patients underwent PD and 3 (23.1 %) underwent DP. The remainder of patients underwent gastrectomy, lymphadenectomy, or duodenal-jejunal resection [25]. In this study, there were no perioperative deaths. However, three (23.1 %) patients had major postoperative complications including anastomotic dehiscence, intra-abdominal abscess and bowel obstruction. Six patients (46.2 %) had developed long-term morbidities, including anemia, bilious emesis, diabetes and failure to thrive. But, irrespective of histology, nodal status or hepatic metastases, 12 of 13 patients (92.3 %) had biochemical cure for an average of 5.2 years (range: 1–6 years). The longest survivor with MEN-1 remained alive and well for 19 years after PD. In this series, the 5-year OS rate was 75 % and the 10-year OS rate was 65 %. Despite the risks, there are clear benefits from surgical management in the treatment of gastrinoma.

Pancreatecoduodenectomy (Whipple Procedure)

Each type of pancreatic resection serves a specific role in the management of patients with multiple or large gastrinomas. In the pancreatic head and uncinate process, lesions, which are not removable by enucleation, should be resected via a PD (Whipple procedure) [26]. This operation can be considered in both sporadic and MEN-1 patients that fulfill the following criteria: (1) large pancreatic head tumor; (2) multiple lymph nodes with findings concerning for lymph node involvement; or (3) following an intra-operative secretin test that fails to show biochemical cure after enucleation of a pancreatic head gastrinoma. Long-term morbidities following PD may include weight loss, diabetes, exocrine pancreatic insufficiency with malabsorption, a difficult reoperative field on upon recurrence (especially in MEN-1 patients with multifocal disease) and increased risk of hepatic abscesses in patients with liver metastases who are treated with chemoembolization [27].

Lymphadenectomy

Pancreatic gastrinomas have a 40 % incidence of lymph node metastases as compared with 70 % for duodenal tumors [28]. A study by Bartash and colleagues evaluated 48 sporadic gastrinoma patients, including 18 patients with pancreatic gastrinomas [9]. After a median postoperative follow-up of 83 months (range: 3–296), 20 patients (41.6 %) had no evidence of disease, 13 patients (27.1 %) were alive with disease, 11 patients (22.9 %) had died from disease, and 4 patients (8.3 %) had died from unrelated causes. In the 41 patients who underwent potentially curative resection, systematic lymphadenectomy with excision of more than ten lymph nodes (N=13) resulted in a higher rate of postoperative biochemical cure (100 %) than no or selective lymphadenectomy (N=28, 62.2 %; P=0.017). Furthermore, there were statistical trends towards prolonged DSS (P=0.062) and DFS (P=0.12). Negative prognostic factors for DSS were pancreatic location (P=0.029), tumor size ≥2.5 cm (P=0.003), preoperative gastrin level ≥3000 pg/mL (P=0.003), and hepatic metastases (P<0.001). Taken together, these data would suggest that systematic lymphadenectomy should be performed, even if no primary tumor is found because it can improve rates of biochemical cure, as well as may improve DSS and DFS in patients with sporadic gastrinoma.

Hepatic Metastases

As previously discussed, Norton and colleagues demonstrated that eight patients with diffuse liver metastases had a significantly worse 15-year OS than patients with limited disease that underwent resection [24]. However, published data would suggest that aggressive cytoreductive surgery with curative intent should still be attempted in patients with liver metastases. In one study of five patients with extensive hepatic metastatic disease who underwent surgical resection, 80 % had all disease removed [29]. In this study, the one patient in whom all gross disease could not be resected continued to have disease progression and died 19 months postoperatively. On the other hand, three patients (60 %) remained disease-free on follow-up at a median of 24-months while two patients (40 %) had biochemical cures at 14 and 32 months. Aggressive surgical management is warranted in patients with liver metastases in order to control disease and achieve symptom relief. However, even when patients undergo curative resection, biochemical cure does not correlate with OS [30, 31].

Thermal ablation techniques have also been applied to the treatment of the hepatic metastases. Although data is limited specifically in gastrinoma patients [32], radiofrequency and microwave ablation have been reported to be effective in the treatment of primary and metastatic PNET lesions in the liver [33]. Thus, ablation is a reasonable option if a lesion is deemed unresectable, but technically ablatable.

Finally, liver transplantation for gastrinoma has been reported in case reports [34] and case series [35]. In the latter series, among 87,280 liver transplantations

(LT) recorded in the United Network for Organ Sharing (UNOS) database from October 1988 through January 2008, 150 LTs (0.17 %) were performed for NETs metastatic to the liver. Eleven (7.3 %) of the 150 patients had gastrinomas. This represents 0.12 % of all LTs during that time period. In this study, 1, 3, and 5-years OS rates were 81 %, 65 %, and 49 %, respectively, in patients undergoing isolated LT for metastatic NETs. Across the United States, the median wait time for patients undergoing LT for metastatic NETs was 67 days. Interestingly, the 5-year OS rate was improved with longer (i.e., >2 months) rather than shorter wait times (63 % vs. 36 %, P = 0.005), suggesting that waiting for confirmed disease stability before considering a patient for LT may be appropriate. In another study of 12 patients who underwent LT for unresectable hepatic NET metastases, 9 of 12 (75 %) patients were alive with a median survival of 55 months [36]. In this series published in 1997, the operative mortality was 8.33 %. The 11 surviving patients had good symptomatic relief following LT. In long-term follow up, two patients died from septic complications or disease recurrences at 6.5 and 68 months, postoperatively. Four of the remaining nine patients (44 %) were alive and without evidence of disease at follow-up of 2.0–103.5 months. Taken together, in highly selected patients at an experienced center, this approach may yield excellent results in patients with stable, but unresectable, liver metastases without evidence of extrahepatic disease.

Vascular Resection and Aggressive Surgical Management

In corroboration with the notion that aggressive hepatic cytoreduction is a critical component of treating gastrinomas, a separate study evaluated 273 patients with PNETs, including 30 patients with gastrinomas (10.9 %) [37]. In this study, 46 patients had major vascular involvement of the portal vein (N = 20), superior mesenteric vein/artery (N = 16), inferior vena cava (N = 4), splenic vein (N = 4), or heart (N = 2). Forty-two of 46 patients had a PNETs removed, including 9 patients (19.5 %) with vascular reconstructions. While there were no deaths, 12 patients (26 %) had complications. However, 18 patients (41 %) were immediately disease-free, while 5 patients (10.8 %) had disease recurrence during follow-up. Therefore, 13 patients (30 %) remained disease-free in long-term follow-up. The 10-year OS was 60 % in this cohort. Taken together, this study would suggest that surgical resection of PNETs with vascular abutment/invasion and nodal or hepatic metastases is indicated.

Laparoscopic Surgery

The role for laparoscopic surgery for gastrinoma resections appears to be limited for several reasons. First, pancreatic gastrinomas are frequently small (<1.0 cm), making localization difficult. Second, and as expected, laparoscopic resection of PNETs is generally more successful when the tumors are localized on preoperative imaging and less successful when they are not. On the other hand, when gastrinomas can be localized in the body and tail, laparoscopic DP is a reasonable option for therapy [38, 39]. Based upon a recent population-based study, application of this approach has tripled in practice in the United States from 1998 to 2009 and has evolved into a safe option in the treatment of both benign and malignant pancreatic lesions [40]. On the other hand, laparoscopic resection of tumors in the pancreatic head has been less widely utilized because of the adjacent major vascular structures, including the superior mesenteric vessels. But, laparoscopic or robotically-assisted laparoscopic PD have evolved into technically feasible and safe procedures in experiences centers [41, 42]. Futures studies are needed to clarify the role of these approaches in the management of ZES patients.

Surgery for Occult Disease

Pancreatic gastrinoma localization is not always straightforward, but the ability to localize a tumor correlates with outcomes. In another study by Norton et al., 58 patients with negative imaging and long histories of ZES were compared with 117 patients with positive imaging results [16]. At the time of exploration by an experienced surgeon, tumors were found in 57 of 58 (98.3 %) patients. In this cohort, 17 % had pancreatic primaries and 10 % had lymph node primaries. Including duodenal primaries (64 %), 50 % had a primary-only, 41 % had primary plus lymph node, and 7 % had liver metastases. Similar to cases of positive imaging, 60 % of patients were cured immediately postoperatively and at a mean follow up of 9.4 years, 46 % remained cured. Only three patients died of disease and all of them had liver metastases, attributed to a long delay to surgical intervention. Taken together, negative imaging studies are not rare in ZES patients. However, surgical intervention is advised in these cases because most lesions can be found at operation and nearly half of patients can be cured.

Surgery in Patients with MEN-1

As has been previously discussed, achieving biochemical cure for patients with MEN-1 associated gastrinomas is difficult due to persistent or recurrent gastric acid hypersecretion from multifocal disease. This fact has been published in several studies. One report from Ellison indicated that in 22 MEN-1 patients treated surgically, only one patient achieved eugastrinemia postoperatively. However, despite a low biochemical cure rate (5 %), resection resulted in an 80 % survival rate at 20 years as compared to 40 % in those who patients that did not undergo resection [31]. In another study of patients with MEN-1 associated pancreatic tumors, patients were classified as asymptomatic (N=8) or symptomatic (N=12) [43]. Following surgical intervention, all patients remained asymptomatic for a mean of 6 years despite the fact that 83 % of the symptomatic patients did not have biochemical cure. This data would suggest surgical intervention is warranted in all MEN-1 patients with ZES, irrespective of symptoms or potential to achieve biochemical cure.

Consistent with these findings, another study evaluated the surgical cure rate reported in 15 series of 242 patients with MEN-1 and ZES treated with local resection without PD from 1990 to 2001 [44]. The surgical cure was very low at 14 %. They then looked at the surgical cure rate reported in 22 series of 17 patients with MEN-1 and ZES treated with PD from 1968 to 2000. The surgical cure was higher at 88 %. This study suggested that the inability to cure patients may be explained by either incomplete resection of multiple small duodenal primary gastrinomas and/or lymph node metastases when only pancreatic lesions are removed. On the other hand, PD removes the entire gastrinoma triangle, including the pancreatic head, duodenum, and draining nodes. Therefore, a more aggressive surgical approach is warranted in MEN-1 patients with ZES in order to achieve biochemical cure, as well as potentially improve survival.

Medical Therapy

Pharmacotherapy can be involved in all aspects of management of patients with ZES. These include: (1) localization of tumors (see section titled "Tumor Localization"), (2) management of gastric acid hypersecretion, and (3) management of malignant disease. As opposed to patients with sporadic, solitary gastrinomas, the gastrinomas in most MEN-1 patients with ZES are multiple, frequently small (<0.5 cm), and associated with lymph node metastases (40–70 % cases) [45]. As a result, MEN-1 patients are rarely cured without aggressive surgical resections, such as PD, as compared to sporadic ZES patients that may be cured with more limited resections. Therefore, life-long medical therapy is necessary for managing gastric acid hypersecretion in almost all MEN-1 patients with ZES, while it is not necessary in patients with sporadic disease who achieve biochemical cure [44, 46–53].

Control of Gastric Acid Hypersecretion Secondary to Gastrinoma

Normal physiologic regulation of the gastric phase of acid secretion includes gastrin, histamine, and cholinergic stimuli. As a result, drugs have been developed in order modulate these targets. Histamine H_2-receptor antagonists (e.g., cimetidine, ranitidine and famotidine) have all been used to control the gastric acid hypersecretion in patients with GERD, PUD and ZES. However, their utility is limited by their lack of adequate control of all three inputs for gastric acid secretion. In addition to their inadequate efficacy in ZES patients, there are multiple drawbacks to these drugs, which include histamine H_1-receptor antagonism, frequent dosing schedules and anti-androgen side effects from cimetidine [45]. In contrast, proton pump inhibitors (PPIs), (e.g., omeprazole, lansoperazole, dexlansoperazole, esomeperazole, pantoprazole, rabeprazole, and llaprazole) control the output of gastric acid secretion irrespective of the degree of gastrin, histamine, and cholinergic stimuli. Furthermore, their advantages include a longer duration of action (i.e., once a day dosing in most patients) and increased potency, making these the drugs of choice for treating gastric acid hypersecretion in ZES patients with or without MEN-1 [45]. Despite the benefits of PPIs, the long-term effects of PPI-induced achlorhydria include possible malabsorption of nutrients requiring gastric acid (e.g., vitamin B_{12}, iron and calcium), as well as induction of hypergastrinemia that may result in increased risk for developing gastric carcinoid tumors derived from mucosal enterochromaffin-like (ECL) cells. Consistent with this fact, more than 90 % of patients with ZES treated with PPIs have ECL cell proliferation, and this especially the case in patients with MEN-1 and ZES [54–58]. Additionally, PPIs are also associated with increased risk of *Clostridium difficile* diarrhea, which contributes to significant increased morbidity, length of stay and mortality in postoperative patients [59].

Another downside to the increased availability of PPIs is its contribution to a delay in diagnosis of ZES [12], because long-term pharmacotherapy can readily control gastric acid hypersecretion. In one prospective study of 72 ZES patients with negative cross-sectional imaging studies, the median duration of symptoms before diagnosis was 9 years [60]. While all patients had control of gastric acid hypersecretion with the PPI, lansoprazole (median dose 60 mg/day, range 15–480 mg/day), 2 of 19 deaths (10.5 %) were due to metastatic gastrinoma and the median survival from the time of diagnosis was 6.6 years. Taken together, this study justifies the use of PPI for symptoms control, but not for cure of disease, even in patients with negative imaging. Finally, in the current era of highly effective gastric acid secretion with PPIs, there is little need for parietal cell (i.e., highly selective) vagotomy or gastrectomy in patients with persistent gastric acid hypersecretion [19, 61].

Primary Control of Gastrinoma

The role of surgery in patients with diffuse, unresectable liver metastases is limited with the exception of highly selected patients undergoing LT. In these patients, pharmacotherapy can be utilized in management of malignant disease.

Somatostatin analogues (e.g., octreotide; Sandostatin, Novartis Pharmaceuticals) have well-known anti-secretory effects in the gastrointestinal tract, as well as in the control of ectopically secreted hormones, including those from PNETs. The most common side-effects include discomfort from drug injections, development of glucose intolerance or hyperglycemia, steatorrhea and cholelithiasis. In a review of 15 studies, including 481 patients, it was clear that the slow-release formulations, including Sandostatin long-acting release (LAR) depot and Somatuline SR/Autogel, achieved symptomatic relief in 74.2 % and 67.5 %, biochemical response in 51.4 % and 39.0 %, and tumor response in 69.8 % and 64.4 % of cases, respectively [62] Newer compounds like the somatostatin analogues SOM230 (pasireotide, Novartis Pharmaceuticals) with pan-somatostatin receptor inhibition needs further investigation to determine its role in the treatment of advanced gastrinoma.

In addition to single agent treatment, combination therapies have been studied. In a small, retrospective report, 11 metastatic gastrinoma patients were treated with both a PPI, as well as 9 of 11 patients received monthly injections of a somatostatin analogue [63]. They then received peptide receptor radioligand therapy [PRRT, (90) Yttrium- or (177) Lutetium-DOTATOC)] for progressive disease. Patients were followed for 6 years by measuring serum gastrin levels and radiological assessment every 3–6 months. There was symptomatic improvement in all patients, as well as a significant improvement in mean serum gastrin levels. The objective response rate was 54 % with disease stabilization in 45 % of patients. The effect of PRRT was maintained after a median of 14 months. With a median time-to-progression of 11 months and means survival time of 14 months, four patients (36 %) died from disease. Mild and transient bone marrow suppression was found in two-thirds of patients from treatment, while one patient (9 %) had transient renal insufficiency. This study suggests that PRRT may be a novel and potentially promising adjunct in the management of inoperable or progressive metastatic gastrinoma.

Sunitinib (Sutent, Pfizer) is FDA-approved for use in patients with unresectable, metastatic, well-differentiated PNETs. It is an orally bioavailable tyrosine kinase inhibitor, which targets PDGFRs, VEGFR-1/2, c-KIT and FLT-3, and has tumor inhibitory effects in patients with advanced PNETs. The most frequent side effects include diarrhea, nausea, vomiting, asthenia, and fatigue [64]. In a study of 171 patients with progressive, advanced PNETs treated with sunitinib (N = 86, 37.5 mg/day) or placebo (N = 85), sunitinib increased the median PFS (11.4 vs. 5.5 months, $P < 0.001$) and objective response rate (ORR, 9.3 % vs. 0 %, $P = 0.007$) [64]. Among the patients enrolled, nine (10 %) in the sunitinib group and ten (12 %) in the placebo group had gastrinomas.

In addition to sunitinib, everolimus (Afinitor, Novartis Pharmaceuticals), an inhibitor of mTOR (mammalian target of rapamycin), has growth inhibitory activity in combination with octreotide in PNET patients [57]. In a phase II study of 160 patients with metastatic PNETs that failed treatment with cytotoxic chemotherapy, everolimus (N = 115, 10 mg/day) or everolimus (10 mg/day) plus octreotide LAR (N = 45) were investigated. The latter combination resulted in a median PFS of 16.7 months versus 9.7 months and ORR of 4.4 % versus 9.6 %, respectively [65]. Among the patients enrolled, nine patients (7.8 %) in the everolimus group and six patients (13.3 %) in the everolimus plus octreotide group had gastrinomas. The most frequent side effects of everolimus included stomatitis, rash, diarrhea, fatigue, and nausea [65, 66]. Taken together, this study suggests that everolimus, with or without concomitant octreotide LAR, demonstrates anti-tumor activity as measured by ORR and PFS, as well as demonstrates that alone or in combination, it is tolerated in patients with advanced PNETs.

In patients with symptomatic, inoperable hepatic metastases and/or progressive liver disease, hepatic artery embolization (HAE) may be utilized because PNETs are hypervascular lesions that derive 70–80 % of their blood supply from the hepatic artery [45]. Radiological interventions have evolved in the treatment of patients with advanced PNETs. These approaches include bland embolization, chemoembolization, radio-embolization, and peptide receptor radioligand therapy using a somatostatin analogue. HAE has been performed with chemotherapeutic agents like doxorubicin, 5-fluorouracil, cisplatin, mitomycin C and streptozotocin. However, HAE can be associated with serious side-effects including: abdominal pain, fever, nausea, vomiting, and liver abscesses [46, 57, 58, 67]. In a review of 15 studies with 896 NET patients with metastatic disease to the liver, patients underwent a total of 979 HAE procedures [68]. Median survival ranged from 10 to 80 months and PFS ranged from 0 to 60 months. The average ORR was 50 % (range: 2–100 %). Overall, the average clinical response rate was 56 % (range: 9–100 %). It is noteworthy that HAE should be avoided in patients with massive tumor burden and severely compromised liver function, poor performance status, sepsis, and other risk factors for treatment-related mortality [68].

A Personal View of the Data

Pancreatic gastrinoma is a rare NET that is responsible for significant morbidity and mortality. The management of this disease depends upon both clinical and pathological factors, as well as the underlying disease etiology (i.e., sporadic or familial). Both medical and surgical therapies are often required in combination or sequentially in order to optimize disease treatment. While surgical resection increases survival in pancreatic gastrinoma patients, those with sporadic disease have a higher chance of biochemical cure than those with familial disease. It is imperative that every patient, including those with metastatic or occult disease, should be evaluated for potentially curative or palliative surgical treatments. In contrast, medical therapy with PPIs can control gastric acid hypersecretion in ZES patients, while anti-tumor therapies play a role in controlling disease progression in the setting of metastatic or unresectable disease.

Recommendations

- For localized, sporadic ZES patients with pancreatic gastrinoma(s), enucleation or resection is the standard management (evidence quality low; strong recommendation).
- For MEN-1 patients with ZES, aggressive surgical management should be utilized, including pancreaticoduodenectomy. (evidence quality low; strong recommendation).

- Systematic lymphadenectomy is associated with increased survival in patients with gastrinoma. (evidence quality low; strong recommendation).
- Patients with metastatic gastrinoma to the liver should undergo surgical resection and/or thermal ablations with curative intent when technically feasible. (evidence quality low; strong recommendation).
- Vascular involvement should not preclude operative approaches involving vascular reconstruction(s) in patients with gastrinoma. (evidence quality low; strong recommendation).
- Symptomatic ZES patients with negative imaging should undergo surgical exploration in order to identify and remove gastrinomas as this affords a high rare of cure. (evidence quality low; moderate recommendation).
- Sporadic ZES patients with hypergastrinemia, despite attempted surgical cure, should be treated with a proton pump inhibitor. (evidence quality low; moderate recommendation).
- MEN-1 patients with ZES should be treated with life-long proton pump inhibition. (evidence quality low; strong recommendation).
- Gastrinoma metastases to the liver can be medically managed with anti-tumor therapies, including somatostatin analogues, sunitinib, and/or everolimus (evidence quality moderate; moderate recommendation).
- Unresectable gastrinoma metastases to the liver may be treated with trans-arterial embolization approaches or liver transplantation in highly selected patients. (evidence quality very low; moderate recommendation).

References

1. Gibril F, Jensen RT. Advances in evaluation and management of gastrinoma in patients with Zollinger-Ellison syndrome. Curr Gastroenterol Rep. 2005;7(2):114–21.
2. Krampitz GW, Norton JA. Pancreatic neuroendocrine tumors. Curr Probl Surg. 2013;50(11):509–45.
3. Epelboym I, Mazeh H. Zollinger-Ellison syndrome: classical considerations and current controversies. Oncologist. 2014;19(1):44–50.
4. Ito T, Igarashi H, Jensen RT. Zollinger-Ellison syndrome: recent advances and controversies. Curr Opin Gastroenterol. 2013;29(6):650–61.
5. Kos-Kudla B, et al. Diagnostic and therapeutic guidelines for gastro-entero-pancreatic neuroendocrine neoplasms (recommended by the Polish Network of Neuroendocrine Tumours). Endokrynol Pol. 2013;64(6):418–43.
6. Tonelli F, et al. Biliary tree gastrinomas in multiple endocrine neoplasia type 1 syndrome. World J Gastroenterol. 2013;19(45):8312–20.
7. Eriksson B, Oberg K, Skogseid B. Neuroendocrine pancreatic tumors. Clinical findings in a prospective study of 84 patients. Acta Oncol. 1989;28(3):373–7.
8. Atema JJ, et al. Surgical treatment of gastrinomas: a single-centre experience. HPB (Oxf). 2012;14(12):833–8.
9. Bartsch DK, et al. Impact of lymphadenectomy on survival after surgery for sporadic gastrinoma. Br J Surg. 2012;99(9):1234–40.
10. Varas M, et al. Pancreatic endocrine tumors or apudomas. Rev Esp Enferm Dig. 2011;103:184–90.

11. Gibril F, Jensen RT. Zollinger-Ellison syndrome revisited: diagnosis, biologic markers, associated inherited disorders, and acid hypersecretion. Curr Gastroenterol Rep. 2004;6(6):454–63.
12. Norton JA, et al. Surgery to cure the Zollinger-Ellison syndrome. N Engl J Med. 1999;341(9):635–44.
13. Cisco RM, Norton JA. Surgery for gastrinoma. Adv Surg. 2007;41:165–76.
14. Fendrich V, et al. Management of sporadic and multiple endocrine neoplasia type 1 gastrinomas. Br J Surg. 2007;94(11):1331–41.
15. Gabriel M, et al. 68Ga-DOTA-Tyr3-octreotide PET in neuroendocrine tumors: comparison with somatostatin receptor scintigraphy and CT. J Nucl Med. 2007;48(4):508–18.
16. Norton JA, et al. Value of surgery in patients with negative imaging and sporadic Zollinger-Ellison syndrome. Ann Surg. 2012;256(3):509–17.
17. Yu F, et al. Prospective study of the clinical course, prognostic factors, causes of death, and survival in patients with long-standing Zollinger-Ellison syndrome. J Clin Oncol. 1999;17(2):615–30.
18. Norton JA, Jensen RT. Current surgical management of Zollinger-Ellison syndrome (ZES) in patients without multiple endocrine neoplasia-type 1 (MEN1). Surg Oncol. 2003;12(2):145–51.
19. Norton JA, Jensen RT. Resolved and unresolved controversies in the surgical management of patients with Zollinger-Ellison syndrome. Ann Surg. 2004;240(5):757–73.
20. Norton JA, et al. Surgery increases survival in patients with gastrinoma. Ann Surg. 2006;244(3):410–9.
21. McArthur KE, et al. Laparotomy and proximal gastric vagotomy in Zollinger-Ellison syndrome: results of a 16-year prospective study. Am J Gastroenterol. 1996;91(6):1104–11.
22. Norton JA, et al. Does the use of routine duodenotomy (DUODX) affect rate of cure, development of liver metastases, or survival in patients with Zollinger-Ellison syndrome? Ann Surg. 2004;239(5):617–25; discussion 626.
23. Heeger K, et al. Increased rate of clinically relevant pancreatic fistula after deep enucleation of small pancreatic tumors. Langenbecks Arch Surg. 2014;399(3):315–21.
24. Norton JA, et al. Comparison of surgical results in patients with advanced and limited disease with multiple endocrine neoplasia type 1 and Zollinger-Ellison syndrome. Ann Surg. 2001;234(4):495–505; discussion 505–6.
25. Thodiyil PA, El-Masry NS, Williamson RC. Achieving eugastrinaemia in Zollinger-Ellison syndrome: resection or enucleation? Dig Surg. 2001;18(2):118–23.
26. Plockinger U, Wiedenmann B. Endocrine tumours of the gastrointestinal tract. Management of metastatic endocrine tumours. Best Pract Res Clin Gastroenterol. 2005;19(4):553–76.
27. Norton JA. Surgical treatment and prognosis of gastrinoma. Best Pract Res Clin Gastroenterol. 2005;19(5):799–805.
28. Sutliff VE, et al. Growth of newly diagnosed, untreated metastatic gastrinomas and predictors of growth patterns. J Clin Oncol. 1997;15(6):2420–31.
29. Norton JA, et al. Aggressive resection of metastatic disease in selected patients with malignant gastrinoma. Ann Surg. 1986;203(4):352–9.
30. Grobmyer SR, et al. Reoperative surgery in sporadic Zollinger-Ellison syndrome: longterm results. J Am Coll Surg. 2009;208(5):718–22.
31. Ellison EC. Zollinger-Ellison syndrome: a personal perspective. Am Surg. 2008;74(7):563–71.
32. Frezza EE, et al. The role of radiofrequency ablation in multiple liver metastases to debulk the tumor: a pilot study before alternative therapies. J Laparoendosc Adv Surg Tech A. 2007;17(3):282–4.
33. Glazer ES, et al. Long-term survival after surgical management of neuroendocrine hepatic metastases. HPB (Oxf). 2010;12(6):427–33.
34. Massaro SA, Emre SH. Metastatic gastrinoma in a pediatric patient with Zollinger-Ellison syndrome. J Pediatr Hematol Oncol. 2014;36(1):e13–5.

35. Gedaly R, et al. Liver transplantation for the treatment of liver metastases from neuroendocrine tumors: an analysis of the UNOS database. Arch Surg. 2011;146(8):953–8.
36. Lang H, et al. Liver transplantation for metastatic neuroendocrine tumors. Ann Surg. 1997;225(4):347–54.
37. Norton JA, et al. Pancreatic endocrine tumors with major vascular abutment, involvement, or encasement and indication for resection. Arch Surg. 2011;146(6):724–32.
38. Gagner M, Pomp A, Herrera MF. Early experience with laparoscopic resections of islet cell tumors. Surgery. 1996;120(6):1051–4.
39. Pierce RA, et al. Outcomes analysis of laparoscopic resection of pancreatic neoplasms. Surg Endosc. 2007;21(4):579–86.
40. Tran Cao HS, et al. Improved perioperative outcomes with minimally invasive distal pancreatectomy: results from a population-based analysis. JAMA Surg. 2014;149:237–43.
41. Winer J, et al. The current state of robotic-assisted pancreatic surgery. Nat Rev Gastroenterol Hepatol. 2012;9(8):468–76.
42. Kendrick ML. Laparoscopic and robotic resection for pancreatic cancer. Cancer J. 2012;18(6):571–6.
43. Skogseid B, et al. Surgery for asymptomatic pancreatic lesion in multiple endocrine neoplasia type I. World J Surg. 1996;20(7):872–6; discussion 877.
44. Norton JA, Fang TD, Jensen RT. Surgery for gastrinoma and insulinoma in multiple endocrine neoplasia type 1. J Natl Compr Canc Netw. 2006;4(2):148–53.
45. Ito T, et al. Pharmacotherapy of Zollinger-Ellison syndrome. Expert Opin Pharmacother. 2013;14(3):307–21.
46. Metz DC, Jensen RT. Gastrointestinal neuroendocrine tumors: pancreatic endocrine tumors. Gastroenterology. 2008;135(5):1469–92.
47. Jensen RT, et al. ENETS Consensus Guidelines for the management of patients with digestive neuroendocrine neoplasms: functional pancreatic endocrine tumor syndromes. Neuroendocrinology. 2012;95(2):98–119.
48. Jensen RT, et al. Gastrinoma (duodenal and pancreatic). Neuroendocrinology. 2006;84(3):173–82.
49. Jensen RT, et al. Inherited pancreatic endocrine tumor syndromes: advances in molecular pathogenesis, diagnosis, management, and controversies. Cancer. 2008;113(7 Suppl):1807–43.
50. Jensen RT. Management of the Zollinger-Ellison syndrome in patients with multiple endocrine neoplasia type 1. J Intern Med. 1998;243(6):477–88.
51. Maton PN, Gardner JD, Jensen RT. Cushing's syndrome in patients with the Zollinger-Ellison syndrome. N Engl J Med. 1986;315(1):1–5.
52. Bonaccorsi-Riani E, et al. Liver transplantation and neuroendocrine tumors: lessons from a single centre experience and from the literature review. Transpl Int. 2010;23(7):668–78.
53. Imamura M, et al. Biochemically curative surgery for gastrinoma in multiple endocrine neoplasia type 1 patients. World J Gastroenterol. 2011;17(10):1343–53.
54. Peghini PL, et al. Effect of chronic hypergastrinemia on human enterochromaffin-like cells: insights from patients with sporadic gastrinomas. Gastroenterology. 2002;123(1):68–85.
55. Maton PN, et al. The effect of Zollinger-Ellison syndrome and omeprazole therapy on gastric oxyntic endocrine cells. Gastroenterology. 1990;99(4):943–50.
56. Berna MJ, et al. A prospective study of gastric carcinoids and enterochromaffin-like cell changes in multiple endocrine neoplasia type 1 and Zollinger-Ellison syndrome: identification of risk factors. J Clin Endocrinol Metab. 2008;93(5):1582–91.
57. Pavel M, et al. ENETS Consensus Guidelines for the management of patients with liver and other distant metastases from neuroendocrine neoplasms of foregut, midgut, hindgut, and unknown primary. Neuroendocrinology. 2012;95(2):157–76.
58. Nazario J, Gupta S. Transarterial liver-directed therapies of neuroendocrine hepatic metastases. Semin Oncol. 2010;37(2):118–26.

59. Biswal S. Proton pump inhibitors and risk for Clostridium difficile associated diarrhea. Biomed J. 2014;37(4):178–83.
60. Wilcox CM, et al. Zollinger–Ellison syndrome: presentation, response to therapy, and outcome. Dig Liver Dis. 2011;43(6):439–43.
61. Metz DC, et al. Use of omeprazole in Zollinger-Ellison syndrome: a prospective nine-year study of efficacy and safety. Aliment Pharmacol Ther. 1993;7(6):597–610.
62. Modlin IM, et al. Review article: somatostatin analogues in the treatment of gastroenteropancreatic neuroendocrine (carcinoid) tumours. Aliment Pharmacol Ther. 2010;31(2):169–88.
63. Grozinsky-Glasberg S, et al. Peptide receptor radioligand therapy is an effective treatment for the long-term stabilization of malignant gastrinomas. Cancer. 2011;117(7):1377–85.
64. Raymond E, et al. Sunitinib malate for the treatment of pancreatic neuroendocrine tumors. N Engl J Med. 2011;364(6):501–13.
65. Yao JC, et al. Daily oral everolimus activity in patients with metastatic pancreatic neuroendocrine tumors after failure of cytotoxic chemotherapy: a phase II trial. J Clin Oncol. 2010;28(1):69–76.
66. Yao JC, et al. Everolimus for advanced pancreatic neuroendocrine tumors. N Engl J Med. 2011;364(6):514–23.
67. Toumpanakis C, Meyer T, Caplin ME. Cytotoxic treatment including embolization/chemoembolization for neuroendocrine tumours. Best Pract Res Clin Endocrinol Metab. 2007;21(1):131–44.
68. Del Prete M, et al. Hepatic arterial embolization in patients with neuroendocrine tumors. J Exp Clin Cancer Res. 2014;33:43.

Chapter 58
Management of Pancreatic Cancer in the Elderly

Francesca M. Dimou and Taylor S. Riall

Abstract As the United States population ages, an increasing number of elderly patients are presenting to primary care physicians, oncologists, and surgeons with pancreatic cancer. Even with aggressive therapy, the prognosis in patients with pancreatic cancer is poor and there many potential complications associated with treatment. In addition, in older patients multiple associated chronic illnesses, decreased functional reserve, and decreased baseline life expectancy make treatment decisions difficult. In population-based studies the majority of older patients with pancreatic cancer do not receive stage-appropriate treatment. The reasons remain unclear but likely include physician nihilism, appropriate patient selection, or patient choice. Older patients need to clearly understand the risks and benefits of treatment in the context of their overall medical condition and cancer characteristics. This will facilitate the shared decision making process and allow for patients to make decisions aligned with their personal preferences. Chronological age alone should not be a contraindication to stage-appropriate aggressive treatment for pancreatic cancer.

Keywords Pancreatic cancer • Elderly • Octogenarian • Pancreatic adenocarcinoma

---

Funding Supported by grants from the UTMB Clinical and Translational Science Award #UL1TR000071, NIH T-32 Grant # 5T32DK007639, AHRQ Grant #1R24HS022134, and Cancer Prevention and Research Institute Grant #RP140020.

F.M. Dimou
Department of Surgery, University of Texas Medical Branch,
301 University Boulevard, Galveston, TX 77555, USA

Department of Surgery, University of South Florida,
1 Tampa General Circle, Tampa, FL 33606 USA

T.S. Riall (✉)
Department of Surgery, University of Arizona, Banner University Medical Center,
1501 N Campbell Ave, Tucson, AZ 85724-513, USA
e-mail: tsriall@utmb.edu

J.M. Millis, J.B. Matthews (eds.), *Difficult Decisions in Hepatobiliary and Pancreatic Surgery*, Difficult Decisions in Surgery: An Evidence-Based Approach, DOI 10.1007/978-3-319-27365-5_58

Introduction

Pancreatic cancer remains a lethal malignancy. In 2014, there will be an estimated 46,420 incident cases and 39,590 deaths from pancreatic cancer [1] with an overall 5-year survival of <7 % [2]. The median age at diagnosis is 71 years and the incidence increases with age. Thirteen percent of newly diagnosed cases and 16 % of deaths from pancreatic cancer occur in people >84 years of age [2]. As the United States population ages, an increasing number of elderly patients are presenting to primary care physicians, oncologists, and surgeons with pancreatic cancer.

The treatment for pancreatic cancer depends on the stage at presentation and pancreatic resection offers the only hope for long-term survival. However, even with aggressive therapy, the prognosis remains poor. In addition, there are significant complications and toxicities associated with the treatment of pancreatic cancer, which can negatively impact the quality of remaining life. In older patients, multiple associated chronic illnesses and decreased functional reserve are associated with higher treatment-'related morbidity and mortality. In addition, decreased baseline life expectancy and varying personal preferences make treatment decisions difficult in this vulnerable population. As such, treatment decisions in older patients with pancreatic cancer are difficult.

Our systematic review was designed to answer the following key questions (Table 58.1): Comparing patients 80 years and older to patients <80 years, what are the short-term outcomes after pancreatic resection (mortality, complications, discharge home)? What is the long-term survival following pancreatic resection for

Table 58.1 PICO table for treatment of pancreatic cancer in elderly patients

P (Patients)	I (Intervention)	C (Comparator)	O (Outcome)
Question 1			
Patients with pancreatic disease requiring pancreatic resection	Pancreatic resection	<80 vs. 80 and older	Morbidity
			Mortality
			Specific complications
			Discharge home
Question 2			
Patients with pancreatic cancer undergoing pancreatic resection	Pancreatic resection	<80 vs. 80 and older	Long-term survival
Question 3			
Patients >70 years old with locoregional pancreatic head cancer (non-metastatic)	Multimodality therapy (surgery with neoadjuvant or adjuvant chemo +/– radiation)	Neoadjuvant vs. adjuvant therapy	% patients completing multimodality therapy
Question 4			
Patients with metastatic pancreatic cancer	Chemotherapy	<70 or 70 and older	Toxicity
			Survival
			Agents

pancreatic cancer in patients? In elderly patients, does a neoadjuvant or adjuvant approach to chemotherapy in resectable disease provide the best opportunity for completion of multimodality therapy? What are the short- and long-term outcomes of chemotherapy for metastatic disease in older vs. younger patients?

Search Strategy

A literature search of English language publications from 2000 to the present was used to identify published data on pancreatic cancer in the elderly population. Ovid MedLine, PubMed, and the Cochrane databases were searched. Terms used in the search were (["pancreatic" and "cancer"] OR ["pancreatic" and "adenocarcinoma"] OR ["pancreatic" and "ductal carcinoma"]) AND ["elderly" or "older" or "octogenarian" or "geriatric"]. For the first two questions, articles were excluded if they did not specifically compare outcomes after pancreatic resection in patients ≥80 years and younger patients (Table 58.1); in key question 2, patients had to have been treated for pancreatic malignancies. For the third and fourth key questions, there were no articles specifically addressing patients 80 and older, so our search was expanded to include studies with varying age cutoffs starting at 65 years and older. The references of all included articles were reviewed and cross-referenced to ensure all articles were identified that addressed this subset of patients. We identified 22 retrospective, observational studies addressing the key questions (Fig. 58.1); ten addressed key question 1, nine addressed key question 2 (not mutually exclusive with key question 1), five addressed key question 3, and seven addressed key question 4. The data was classified using the GRADE system.

Results

Short-Term Outcomes After Pancreatic Resection

Based on national data, fewer than 30 % of patients with locoregional pancreatic cancer undergo surgical resection [3, 4]. In an analysis of the Surveillance, Epidemiology, and End Results (SEER)-Medicare linked data, surgical resection rates in patients with no comorbidities decreased from 39 % in patients 66–70 years old to 5 % in patients 85 and older [5]. However, the reasons for the low observed surgical resection in this population are not clear and may include physician nihilism, appropriate patient selection, or patient choice.

Information regarding surgical outcomes in patients 80 years and older is critical to informing the shared decision making process. Since 2000, seven single-institution retrospective cohort studies and three large, retrospective population-based studies directly compared short-term outcomes after pancreatic resection in patients ≥80 years and <80 years [6–15]. While all studies include patients undergoing

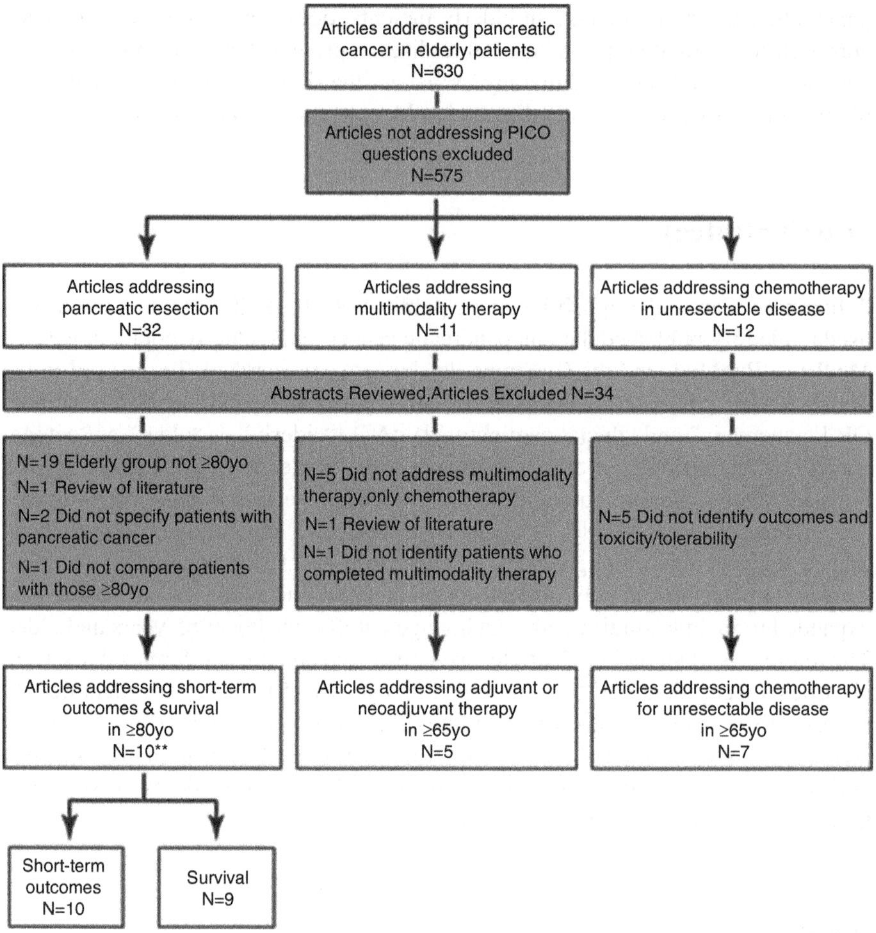

Fig. 58.1 The preferred reporting items for systematic reviews and meta-analyses (PRISMA) flowchart detailing the selection of studies for systematic review. **One study was not obtained from original search strategy and found via cross-reference

pancreatectomy for periampullary cancers, the indications vary across studies with many including pancreatectomy for benign disease.

Mortality Regardless of age, mortality rates varied widely across studies, from 0 to 15.5 % (Table 58.2). Six of the ten of studies reported higher unadjusted mortality rates in older patients [7, 9, 11–14], though many studies were underpowered and this difference did not achieve statistical significance.

The three population-based studies uniformly reported a significant increase in in-hospital or 30-day operative mortality with increasing age (Table 58.2). In an analysis using the Nationwide Inpatient Sample (NIS), Finlayson et al. [7] demonstrated increasing unadjusted mortality rates with increasing age; in-hospital mortality was 6.7 % in patients 65–69 years, 9.3 % in patients 70–79 years, and

Table 58.2 Short-term outcomes following pancreatic resection in patients <80 years and ≥80 years

Author and year	Age group	N	Study type (Quality of evidence)	Mortality	Morbidity	Length of stay (median days)	Discharge home
Chen et al. 2003 [6]	70–79	82	Retrospective cohort (low quality)	12 %	56 %	29	NR
	80–89	16		13 %	51 %	25	NR
Makary et al. 2006 [11]	<80	2,491	Retrospective cohort (low quality)	1.7 %	42 %	10	NR
	80–89	197		4.1%[b]	53 %	11	NR
	≥90	10		0.0 %	50 %	12	NR
Finlayson et al. 2007 [7]	65–69	7,125[a]	Retrospective cohort/population based (moderate quality)	6.7%[c]	NR	17.4 (mean)[c]	89.4%[c]
	70–79	13,478[a]		9.3 %	NR	18.2 (mean)	80.8 %
	≥80	2,915[a]		15.5 %	NR	20.4 (mean)	63.3 %
Riall et al. 2008 [14]	<60	1,780	Retrospective cohort/population based (moderate quality)	2.4%[c]	NR	11[c]	96.5%[c]
	60–69	887		5.8 %	NR	13	93.8 %
	70–79	855		7.4 %	NR	14	79.8 %
	≥80	214		11.4 %	NR	15	61.8 %
Khan et al. 2010 [15]	<80	53	Retrospective cohort (low quality)	1 %	37%[c]	NR	NR
	≥80	564		2 %	51 %	NR	NR
Lee et al. 2010 [10]	<80	703	Retrospective cohort (low quality)	5 %	47 %	10.5	NR
	≥80	74		4 %	51 %	11.0	NR
Hatzaras et al. 2011 [8]	<80	490	Retrospective cohort (low quality)	3.7 %	59 %	11	NR
	≥80	27		3.7 %	52 %	12	NR
Melis et al. 2012 [12]	<80	175	Retrospective cohort (low quality)	0.6 %	44 %	13.7	NR
	≥80	25		4.0 %	68%[a]	20.0	NR
Ogura et al. 2013 [13]	<80	539	Retrospective cohort (low quality)	0.9 %	9.6%[a, e]	26.0	NR
	≥80	22		4.5 %	27.3%[a, e]	31.5	NR
Lee et al. 2014 [9]	<80	4,102	Retrospective cohort/population based (moderate quality)	2 %	OR 1.3 (95 % CI 1.0–1.6)[f, g]	12.0 (mean)	NR
	≥80	475		6 % OR 2.0 (95 % CI 1.3–3.1)[d]		13.9 (mean)	NR

NR not reported

[a]Based on a random sample so numbers are weighted to reflect total population numbers

[b]$p < 0.05$ patients ≥80 years compared to patients <80 years

[c]$p < 0.05$ for chi-square across all groups

[d]Odds of 30-day mortality in patients ≥80 years compared to patients <80 years

[e]Major complications classified as Clavien-Dindo Grade ≥III

[f]Odds of 30-day major morbidity in patients ≥80 years compared to patients <80 years

[g]Major complications defined as organ-space infection, pneumonia, unplanned intubation, pulmonary embolism, ventilator requirement >48 h, progressive renal insufficiency, acute renal failure, cerebrovascular accident, coma, cardiac arrest, myocardial infarction, deep venous thrombosis, sepsis, septic shock, and/or return to the operating room

11.4 % in patients 80 years and older ($p < 0.0001$). Likewise, in a study using Texas state discharge data, unadjusted in-hospital mortality rates increased from 2.4 % to 5.8 % to 7.4 %, to 11.4 % in patients <60, 60–69, 70–79, and ≥80 years ($p < 0.001$), respectively [14]. In the American College of Surgeons National Surgical Quality Improvement Program (ACS-NSQIP) [9], 30-day mortality was 2 % in patients <80 and 6 % in patients ≥80 years ($p < 0.05$). In both the NSQIP (OR 2.0, 95 % CI 1.3–3.1, ≥80 vs. <80 years) [9] and Texas study (OR 4.45, 95 % CI 2.3–8.6, ≥80 vs. <60) [14], the observed increase in mortality in octogenarians remained significant after adjusting for patient characteristics including comorbidity.

The increased mortality in older patients was accentuated at low-volume hospitals (defined as fewer than ten pancreatic resections per year). For patients <60 years, mortality was 2.0 % at high-volume hospitals and 3.0 % at low-volume hospitals. However, for patients ≥80, mortality was 8.7 % at low-volume hospitals and 14.5 % at high-volume hospitals [14].

Complications Overall complication rates following pancreatectomy were high, ranging from 42 to 68 % across studies. Five single-institution studies reported overall morbidity rates and none demonstrated a significant difference between older and younger patients (Table 58.2) [6, 8, 10–12]. Two studies evaluated major complication rates [9, 13]. Oguro et al. defined complications as major if they were classified as Clavien-Dindo III or higher [13]. The 22 patients ≥80 years had a major complication rate of 27.3 % compared to 9.6 % in patients <80 years ($p = 0.008$). From the ACS-NSQIP data, Lee et al. defined major complications as organ-space infection, pneumonia, unplanned intubation, pulmonary embolism, ventilator requirement >48 h, progressive renal insufficiency, acute renal failure, cerebrovascular accident, coma, cardiac arrest, myocardial infarction, deep venous thrombosis, sepsis, septic shock, and/or return to the operating room. The 475 patients ≥80 had a 30 % increased risk of major complications (OR 1.3, 95 % CI 1.0–1.6) after adjusting for potential measurable confounders.

Length of Stay and Discharge Home Length of stay varied significantly across studies. Consistent with the increase in major complications and mortality, length of stay was consistently higher in patients 80 and older (Table 58.2). In addition, octogenarians were less likely to be discharged home. In the Nationwide Inpatient Sample, 89.4 % of patients 65–69, 80.8 % of patients 70–79, and 63.3 % of patients 80 and older were discharged home ($p < 0.0001$) [7]. Likewise, in the Texas discharge data, 96.5 % of patients <60, 93.8 % of patients 60–69, 79.8 % of patients 70–79, and 61.8 % of patients 80 and older were discharged home ($p < 0.0001$) [14]. In patients who were discharged home, increasing age was associated with increased need for home health services. Home health services were required in 13.8 % of patients 66–69 and 31.3 % of patients ≥80 ($p < 0.001$).

Long-Term Survival After Resection for Pancreatic Cancer

Since 2000, seven single-institution studies [6, 8, 10–13, 15] and two population-based studies [5, 7] directly compare survival after pancreatic resection for pancreatic adenocarcinoma in octogenarians compared to younger patients (Table 58.3). The single institution studies have several limitations: (1) small sample sizes, ranging from only 8 to 102 octogenarians, which limits confidence in the estimates and the ability to adjust for variables that differ between the two groups, (2) significant selection bias and confounding by indication, as treatment is not randomly assigned, and (3) significant heterogeneity, with survival rates varying significantly across studies.

Outcomes are mixed across studies with only two studies [5, 11] demonstrating worse unadjusted survival in octogenarians compared to younger patients. In the Makary study, the statistically significant difference in survival was largely due to a decrease in median survival (11 vs. 18 months, $p<0.05$) likely associated with increased operative morbidity and mortality, but 5-year survival was clinically similar between the two groups (37.7 % vs. 33.05, Table 58.3). Finlayson et al. [7] compared survival in a small subset of Medicare patients ≥80 years, 70–79 years, and 65–69 years. Five-year survival was 11.3 % in octogenarians, 15.6 % in patients 70–79, and 16.4 % in patients 65–69 (Table 58.3, $p=0.28$). Of note, this paper further stratified the octogenarians into patients with <2 or ≥2 comorbidities. Patients with <2 comorbidities had similar survival to the 65–69 year old group; 5-year survival was 10 % with >=2 comorbidities compared to 14 % for those with less than two comorbidities (P=NS). One would expect worse in the elderly given their decreased baseline life expectancy, increased comorbidity, decreased functional reserve, and observed higher operative morbidity and mortality with surgery. The similar survival in many single-institution studies suggests significant selection bias, with only the best surgical candidates being selected for resection.

Our group used SEER-Medicare data to evaluate 1,229 patients undergoing pancreatic resection for locoregional pancreatic cancer. This study evaluated the interaction between age and surgical resection comparing resected patients in each age group (<70, 70–79, ≥80 years) to unresected patients 66–70 years old. Unadjusted long-term survival decreased with age (Table 58.3). However, in adjusted models, surgical resection improved survival compared to unresected patients in all age groups despite the increased morbidity and mortality after pancreatic resection in the elderly. Compared to unresected patients 66–70 years of age, resected patients 66–70 years had a hazard ratio (HR) of 0.43 (95 % CI 0.36–0.52); resected patients 70–79 year old group had a HR of 0.47 (95 % CI 0.41–0.53) and resected patients ≥80 and older group had a HR of 0.36 (95 % CI, 0.28–0.45) [5]. Overall the data suggest that carefully selected octogenarians can benefit from surgical resection and enjoy similar long-term survival to their younger counterparts.

Table 58.3 Survival after pancreatic resection for pancreatic or periampullary cancer (<80 vs. ≥80 years)

Author and year	Age Group	N	Study type (quality of evidence)	Median Survival (months)	5-year Survival
Chen et al. 2003 [6]	70–79	82	Retrospective cohort (low quality)	16.0	NR
	80–89	16		17.6	NR
Makary et al. 2006 [11]	<80	1,022	Retrospective cohort (low quality)	18[a]	37.7%[a]
	80–89	102		11	33.0 %
Finlayson et al. 2007 [7]	65–69	49	Retrospective cohort/ population based (moderate quality)	NR	16.4 %
	70–79	91		NR	15.6 %
	≥80	12		NR	11.3 %
Khan et al. 2010 [15]	<80	567	Retrospective cohort (low quality)	18.9	NR
	≥80	53		13.5	NR
Lee at al. 2010 [10]	<80	346	Retrospective cohort (low quality)	18.1[a]	14%[a]
	≥80	45		11.6	<5 %
Riall et al. 2011 [5]	66–69	589	Retrospective cohort/ population based (moderate quality)	16.1[a]	38%[a,b]
	70–74	779		15.8	35 %
	75–79	655		14.9	33 %
	80–84	309		12.5	31 %
	≥85	61		12.3	33 % (2-year survival)
Hatzaras et al. 2011 [8]	<80	490	Retrospective cohort (low quality)	21.9[c]	34.8%[c]
	≥80	27		33.3	33.1 %
Melis et al. 2012 [12]	<80	175	Retrospective cohort (low quality)	13.1	5.8 %
	≥80	25		17.3	4.5 %
Ogura et al. 2013 [13]	<80	316	Retrospective cohort (low quality)	13	NR[d]
	≥80	8		35	38 %

NR not reported
[a]$p < 0.05$ between reported groups
[b]Study reports 2-year survival only
[c]Includes neuroendocrine tumors and pancreatic adenocarcinoma
[d]No patients alive and followed 5 years

Neoadjuvant and Adjuvant Chemotherapy for Older Patients with Resectable Disease

While surgical resection is the only potentially curative treatment option for pancreatic cancer, two thirds to three quarters of patients have positive lymph nodes on final pathology and most patients experience distant, extrapancreatic recurrence even after a margin negative (R0) resection [16–18]. Therefore, in patients with resectable, locoregional disease, a multimodality approach with surgical resection and chemotherapy (with or without radiation) is considered the standard of care.

Studies clearly demonstrate a survival advantage in patients who complete multimodality therapy, but controversy exists regarding delivery of chemotherapy in the adjuvant vs. neoadjuvant setting. In the debate, it has been suggested that patients are more likely to complete multimodality therapy with a neoadjuvant approach, as postoperative complications and failure to thrive following surgery may limit receipt of adjuvant therapy. In addition, a neoadjuvant approach allows for selection of patients with better tumor biology for surgical resection and avoids unnecessary treatment in patients who progress during neoadjuvant treatment.

No studies specifically address the completion of multimodality therapy in octogenarians. We identified five retrospective cohort studies that evaluated completion of multimodality therapy in patients older than 65 years (Table 58.4) [19–23]. These studies were extremely heterogeneous, thereby limiting conclusions. Four single-institution, large retrospective studies addressed receipt of adjuvant chemotherapy after surgical resection; two studies compared patients <75 and ≥75 years

Table 58.4 Completion of multimodality therapy in elderly patients

Author and year	Age group	Timing of chemotherapy	N	% of patients who received multimodality treatment	Survival (months)	Study type (quality of evidence)
Davila et al. 2009 [20]	<75	Adjuvant[a]	811	56.5 %	NR	Retrospective cohort study (low)
	≥75		572	37.7 %		
Horowitz et al. 2010 [21]	<75	Adjuvant	489	54 %	22.7[b]	Prospective cohort study (low)
	≥75		166	29.5 %	22.6[b]	
Nagrial et al. 2014 [22]	<70	Adjuvant	261	51.5 %	22.5[b]	Retrospective cohort study (low)
	≥70		178	29.8 %	21.8[b]	
Cooper et al. 2014 [19]	≥70	Neoadjuvant or adjuvant	179[c]	47.5 % overall	16.1[d]	Retrospective cohort study (low)
			153 neoad juvant/	74/153 (48.3 %) neoadjuvant	15.1[e]	
			26 adjuvant intent	11/26 (42.3 %) adjuvant		
Parmar et al. 2014 [23]	≥65	Neoadjuvant or adjuvant	10,505[f]	11.1%[g]	21[b]	Retrospective cohort study (low)

NR not reported

[a]Adjuvant therapy was either surgery + chemotherapy, surgery + radiation, or surgery + chemoradiation

[b]Survival in patients who received multimodality therapy (surgery and chemotherapy)

[c]Number of patients treated with curative intent (chemotherapy given with neoadjuvant intent or surgery with intent to give adjuvant therapy)

[d]Survival of patients who underwent chemotherapy with neoadjuvant intent (with or without resection, N = 153)

[e]Survival of patients who underwent surgical resection (with or without adjuvant therapy, N = 26)

[f]All patients presenting with locoregional pancreatic cancer without vascular invasion

[g]% of patients with locoregional disease who received multimodality therapy (surgical resection + chemotherapy)

[20, 21] and one compared patients <70 and ≥70 years. Consistently across studies, older patients were less likely to receive adjuvant therapy (29.5–37.7 %) than younger patients (51.5–56.5 %, $p<0.05$ across studies).

Cooper et al. [19] performed the only retrospective study that evaluated receipt of multimodality therapy on an intent-to-treat basis. One hundred seventy-nine patients ≥70 years with pancreatic cancer were treated with curative intent; 153 (85 %) of these patients were treated with neoadjuvant chemoradiation with the intent to resect and 26 (15 %) underwent surgery first with intent to deliver adjuvant therapy. In the neoadjuvant group, 48 % of patients completed multimodality therapy compared to 42 % in the adjuvant group (Table 58.4).

Parmar et al. [23] utilized SEER-Medicare data to identify 10,505 patients aged 66 years and older with locoregional pancreatic adenocarcinoma. Only 5,358 (51 %) underwent treatment with chemotherapy and/or surgical resection. Only 11.1 % of the overall cohort (21.7 % of the 5,385 patients who received treatment) received multimodality therapy, of which 7 % was neoadjuvant and 93 % adjuvant. In patients who received surgical resection as the initial treatment modality, 51.6 % went on to receive adjuvant therapy. In patients who received chemotherapy as the initial treatment modality, only 2.6 % went on to surgical resection. Given the observational, administrative nature of the dataset, the intent of chemotherapy in this group is unclear and it is likely that many did not receive chemotherapy with curative intent. Regardless, the data suggests that in the time period of the study (patients diagnosed from 1992 to 2007) an adjuvant approach to chemotherapy was preferred. It is also striking that so few patients go on to receive resection after chemotherapy, suggesting that outside of specialized centers chemotherapy is not delivered with neoadjuvant, curative intent, or that the rates of completion of multimodality therapy in patients 65 and older are less than those observed at specialized centers.

Across studies, survival was improved with multimodality therapy (Table 58.4). When both surgery and chemotherapy received, survival was similar with neoadjuvant and adjuvant approaches.

Chemotherapy for Advanced and Metastatic Disease

Systemic chemotherapy is standard of care for those with unresectable pancreatic cancer; however, treatment in this setting prolongs survival on the order of weeks to months. There are limited data on outcomes with systemic chemotherapy in the elderly population. We identified seven studies evaluating gemcitabine-based chemotherapy for unresectable pancreatic cancer, including locally advanced and metastatic disease [24–27]. Nakai and colleagues [26] compared patients <75 ($N=114$) and ≥75 ($N=69$) years with locally advanced and metastatic disease. Side effects of gemcitabine-therapy such nausea, anorexia, vomiting, and diarrhea were not significantly different between age groups. Likewise, Yukisawa et al. demonstrated no difference in grade 3 or 4 hematologic (39 % vs. 42 %, $p=0.61$) or non-hematologic (16 % vs. 21 %, $p=0.77$) adverse events in patients <75 and ≥75 years receiving full-dose gemcitabine therapy. These findings were similar to the toxicities reported by Locher et al. in a cohort of 39 patients age 70 and over, where 38 % of patents experienced neutropenia, 28 % experienced thrombocytopenia, and 18 % anemia (grade 3 or 4) [28].

Performance status and not chronological age predicted tolerability of chemotherapy in older patients [24, 25]. Berger et al. [24] evaluated the outcomes of chemotherapy in 53 patients 70 years and older. Patients with an Eastern Cooperative Oncology Group (ECOG) performance status ≥2 tolerated treatment for longer (median duration of therapy 59 days vs. 105 days ECOG <2; $p = 0.009$) and had a greater probability of receiving combination therapy. Across studies, older patients experienced similar benefits with chemotherapy. In a group of 66 patients with unresectable pancreatic cancer receiving gemcitabine, 23 % patients ≥70 and 16 % patients <70 obtained partial responses. Median survival times were 311 days in patients ≥70, 292 days in patients <70, and 127 days in patients who did not receive gemcitabine [29]. Likewise, tumor growth control (66.6 % vs. 59.6 %), time to progression (119 vs. 104 days), and overall survival (240 vs. 220 days) were comparable for patients <70 (N=57) and ≥70 years (N=42) receiving gemcitabine-based chemotherapy, respectively [30].

Recommendations

Despite increased operative morbidity and mortality in older patients, with aggressive therapy, carefully selected octogenarians can enjoy similar long-term survival when compared to their younger counterparts across various disease stages. Chronological age alone should not be a contraindication to surgical resection. Older patients considering pancreatic resection for pancreatic cancer should be informed of their operative risk in the context of their overall medical condition. In addition, they need to understand the long-term prognosis with and without aggressive therapy, allowing patients to make decisions aligned with their personal preferences. When performed in this age group, surgical resection should be done at high-volume centers.

When aggressive therapy is chosen for locoregional disease, a multimodality approach with both surgical resection and chemotherapy (with or without radiation) is recommended. The data demonstrate that outcomes are better in carefully selected older patients (>65) who receive multimodality therapy compared to surgery alone. However, data are insufficient to recommend a neoadjuvant or adjuvant approach. When both modalities are received, survival is similar in the neoadjuvant or adjuvant groups. The only study addressing receipt of multimodality therapy on an intent-to-treat basis with both approaches shows a slight increase in receipt of multimodality therapy with a neoadjuvant approach.

In older patients with unresectable disease (>70), gemcitabine-based chemotherapy in carefully selected patients is well tolerated and survival benefits are similar to those observed in younger patients, and such treatment should be offered to older patients. There are not data regarding toxicity or survival of newer chemotherapeutic regimens (i.e. FULFIRINOX – 5-flourouracil, leucovorin, irinotecan, and oxaliplatin, and others) in older patients with advanced disease.

A Personal View of the Data

Even with aggressive therapy, the prognosis for patients with pancreatic cancer remains poor. After potentially curative resection, only 70–80 % of patients survive 5 years [3, 31–33]. When metastatic disease is present, patients rarely survive more than 6 months [34] and chemotherapy in this setting improves survival on the order of weeks. In addition, there are significant complications and toxicities associated with the treatment of pancreatic cancer, which can negatively impact the quality of remaining life. Even at high-volume, specialized centers, pancreatic resection has a 30–40 % incidence of surgical complications [35], prolonged hospital stay [14, 36, 37], a 2–5 % operative mortality [35, 38, 39], and readmission rates in excess of 30 % [36]. Many patients require skilled nursing care after surgery and are unable to be at home with their families [7, 14]. Chemotherapy can cause nausea, vomiting, diarrhea, dehydration, neutropenia, thrombocytopenia, anemia, liver damage, and other adverse symptoms. Abdominal radiation can lead to diarrhea, radiation enteritis, and bowel obstruction.

Given the poor prognosis of pancreatic cancer and the significant toxicity associated with treatment, patients face complex treatment decisions that are extremely preference sensitive. These decisions are even more difficult in older patients, whose associated chronic illness and decreased functional reserve increase their probability postoperative complications which has a potential negative impact on the quality of their remaining life. In the age of personalized medicine, clinicians should not take a one-size-fits-all approach. It may be the observed "underutilization" of pancreatic resection in part reflects good patient selection and patient preference.

Older patients must evaluate the trade offs between quantity and quality of life in the context of their cancer characteristics, overall medical condition, and their treatment goals. Given all the information, two patients with the same cancer and personal characteristics may have markedly different treatment goals and choose different treatment options. Chronological age alone should not be a contraindication to stage-appropriate aggressive treatment for pancreatic cancer.

Recommendations

- Age alone should not be a contraindication to surgical resection. The decision regarding surgical resection in octogenarians should be made context of their cancer characteristics, overall medical condition, and their treatment goals (evidence quality moderate; strong recommendation).

- When aggressive therapy for locoregional disease is chosen, a multimodality approach with chemotherapy and surgery (+/− radiation) is recommended (evidence quality moderate; strong recommendation).
- Surgical resection in older patients is best performed at high-volume centers (evidence quality moderate; strong recommendation).
- A neoadjuvant approach should be considered in older patients with borderline resectable and resectable pancreatic cancer as it may increase rates of completion of multimodality therapy and avoid resection in patients who will not benefit (evidence quality low; weak recommendation).
- In older patients with unresectable disease who desire aggressive treatment, gemcitabine-based chemotherapy should be offered. Further studies are necessary to assess the toxicity and survival of newer regimens in older patients (evidence quality moderate; strong recommendation).

References

1. Siegel R, Ma J, Zou Z, Jemal A. Cancer statistics, 2014. CA Cancer J Clin. 2014;64(1):9–29.
2. http://seer.cancer.gov/statfacts/html/pancreas.html (http://seer.cancer.gov/statfacts/html/pancreas.html) on 7 Sep 2014.
3. Bilimoria KY, Bentrem DJ, Ko CY, Stewart AK, Winchester DP, Talamonti MS. National failure to operate on early stage pancreatic cancer. Ann Surg. 2007;246(2):173–80.
4. Riall TS, Townsend Jr CM, Kuo YF, Freeman JL, Goodwin JS. Dissecting racial disparities in the treatment of patients with locoregional pancreatic cancer: a 2-step process. Cancer. 2010;116(4):930–9.
5. Riall TS, Sheffield KM, Kuo YF, Townsend Jr CM, Goodwin JS. Resection benefits older adults with locoregional pancreatic cancer despite greater short-term morbidity and mortality. J Am Geriatr Soc. 2011;59(4):647–54.
6. Chen JW, Shyr YM, Su CH, Wu CW, Lui WY. Is pancreaticoduodenectomy justified for septuagenarians and octogenarians? Hepatogastroenterology. 2003;50(53):1661–4.
7. Finlayson E, Fan Z, Birkmeyer JD. Outcomes in octogenarians undergoing high-risk cancer operation: a national study. J Am Coll Surg. 2007;205(6):729–34.
8. Hatzaras I, Schmidt C, Klemanski D, Muscarella P, Melvin WS, Ellison EC, et al. Pancreatic resection in the octogenarian: a safe option for pancreatic malignancy. J Am Coll Surg. 2011;212(3):373–7.
9. Lee DY, Schwartz JA, Wexelman B, Kirchoff D, Yang KC, Attiyeh F. Outcomes of pancreaticoduodenectomy for pancreatic malignancy in octogenarians: an American College of Surgeons National Surgical Quality Improvement Program analysis. Am J Surg. 2014;207(4):540–8.
10. Lee MK, Dinorcia J, Reavey PL, Holden MM, Genkinger JM, Lee JA, et al. Pancreaticoduodenectomy can be performed safely in patients aged 80 years and older. J Gastrointest Surg. 2010;14(11):1838–46.
11. Makary MA, Winter JM, Cameron JL, Campbell KA, Chang D, Cunningham SC, et al. Pancreaticoduodenectomy in the very elderly. J Gastrointest Surg. 2006;10(3):347–56.
12. Melis M, Marcon F, Masi A, Pinna A, Sarpel U, Miller G, et al. The safety of a pancreaticoduodenectomy in patients older than 80 years: risk vs. benefits. HPB (Oxf). 2012;14(9):583–8.
13. Oguro S, Shimada K, Kishi Y, Nara S, Esaki M, Kosuge T. Perioperative and long-term outcomes after pancreaticoduodenectomy in elderly patients 80 years of age and older. Langenbecks Arch Surg. 2013;398(4):531–8.

14. Riall TS, Reddy DM, Nealon WH, Goodwin JS. The effect of age on short-term outcomes after pancreatic resection: a population-based study. Ann Surg. 2008;248(3):459–67.
15. Khan S, Sclabas G, Lombardo KR, Sarr MG, Nagorney D, Kendrick ML, et al. Pancreatoduodenectomy for ductal adenocarcinoma in the very elderly; is it safe and justified? J Gastrointest Surg. 2010;14(11):1826–31.
16. Griffin JF, Smalley SR, Jewell W, Paradelo JC, Reymond RD, Hassanein RE, et al. Patterns of failure after curative resection of pancreatic carcinoma. Cancer. 1990;66(1):56–61.
17. Katz MH, Wang H, Fleming JB, Sun CC, Hwang RF, Wolff RA, et al. Long-term survival after multidisciplinary management of resected pancreatic adenocarcinoma. Ann Surg Oncol. 2009;16(4):836–47.
18. Smeenk HG, Tran TC, Erdmann J, van Eijck CH, Jeekel J. Survival after surgical management of pancreatic adenocarcinoma: does curative and radical surgery truly exist? Langenbecks Arch Surg. 2005;390(2):94–103.
19. Cooper AB, Holmes HM, des Bordes JK, Fogelman D, Parker NH, Lee JE, et al. Role of neoadjuvant therapy in the multimodality treatment of older patients with pancreatic cancer. J Am Coll Surg. 2014;219(1):111–20.
20. Davila JA, Chiao EY, Hasche JC, Petersen NJ, McGlynn KA, Shaib YH. Utilization and determinants of adjuvant therapy among older patients who receive curative surgery for pancreatic cancer. Pancreas. 2009;38(1):e18–25.
21. Horowitz DP, Hsu CC, Wang J, Makary MA, Winter JM, Robinson R, et al. Adjuvant chemoradiation therapy after pancreaticoduodenectomy in elderly patients with pancreatic adenocarcinoma. Int J Radiat Oncol Biol Phys. 2011;80(5):1391–7.
22. Nagrial AM, Chang DK, Nguyen NQ, Johns AL, Chantrill LA, Humphris JL, et al. Adjuvant chemotherapy in elderly patients with pancreatic cancer. Br J Cancer. 2014;110(2):313–9.
23. Parmar AD, Vargas GM, Tamirisa NP, Sheffield KM, Riall TS. Trajectory of care and use of multimodality therapy in older patients with pancreatic adenocarcinoma. Surgery. 2014;156(2):280–9.
24. Berger AK, Abel U, Komander C, Harig S, Jager D, Springfeld C. Chemotherapy for advanced pancreatic adenocarcinoma in elderly patients (>/=70 years of age): a retrospective cohort study at the National Center for Tumor Diseases Heidelberg. Pancreatology. 2014;14(3):211–5.
25. Hentic O, Dreyer C, Rebours V, Zappa M, Levy P, Raymond E, et al. Gemcitabine in elderly patients with advanced pancreatic cancer. World J Gastroenterol. 2011;17(30):3497–502.
26. Nakai Y, Isayama H, Sasaki T, Sasahira N, Tsujino T, Kogure H, et al. Comorbidity, not age, is prognostic in patients with advanced pancreatic cancer receiving gemcitabine-based chemotherapy. Crit Rev Oncol Hematol. 2011;78(3):252–9.
27. Yukisawa S, Ishii H, Matsuyama M, Kuraoka K, Takano K, Kamei A, et al. Outcomes and tolerability of systemic chemotherapy for pancreatic or biliary cancer patients aged 75 years or older. Jpn J Clin Oncol. 2011;41(1):76–80.
28. Locher C, Fabre-Guillevin E, Brunetti F, Auroux J, Delchier JC, Piedbois P, et al. Fixed-dose rate gemcitabine in elderly patients with advanced pancreatic cancer: an observational study. Crit Rev Oncol Hematol. 2008;68(2):178–82.
29. Yamagishi Y, Higuchi H, Izumiya M, Sakai G, Iizuka H, Nakamura S, et al. Gemcitabine as first-line chemotherapy in elderly patients with unresectable pancreatic carcinoma. J Gastroenterol. 2010;45(11):1146–54.
30. Marechal R, Demols A, Gay F, de Maertelaer V, Arvanitaki M, Hendlisz A, et al. Tolerance and efficacy of gemcitabine and gemcitabine-based regimens in elderly patients with advanced pancreatic cancer. Pancreas. 2008;36(3):e16–21.
31. Cress RD, Yin D, Clarke L, Bold R, Holly EA. Survival among patients with adenocarcinoma of the pancreas: a population-based study (United States). Cancer Causes Control. 2006;17(4):403–9.
32. Riall TS, Nealon WH, Goodwin JS, Zhang D, Kuo YF, Townsend Jr CM, et al. Pancreatic cancer in the general population: improvements in survival over the last decade. J Gastrointest Surg. 2006;10(9):1212–23; discussion 23–4.

33. Simons JP, Ng SC, McDade TP, Zhou Z, Earle CC, Tseng JF. Progress for resectable pancreatic [corrected] cancer?: a population-based assessment of US practices. Cancer. 2010;116(7):1681–90.
34. Thota R, Pauff JM, Berlin JD. Treatment of metastatic pancreatic adenocarcinoma: a review. Oncology (Williston Park). 2014;28(1):70–4.
35. Winter JM, Cameron JL, Campbell KA, Arnold MA, Chang DC, Coleman J, et al. 1423 pancreaticoduodenectomies for pancreatic cancer: a single-institution experience. J Gastrointest Surg. 2006;10(9):1199–210; discussion 210–1.
36. Reddy DM, Townsend Jr CM, Kuo YF, Freeman JL, Goodwin JS, Riall TS. Readmission after pancreatectomy for pancreatic cancer in medicare patients. J Gastrointest Surg. 2009;13(11):1963–74; discussion 74–5.
37. Riall TS, Eschbach KA, Townsend Jr CM, Nealon WH, Freeman JL, Goodwin JS. Trends and disparities in regionalization of pancreatic resection. J Gastrointest Surg. 2007;11(10):1242–51; discussion 51–2.
38. Balcom JH, Rattner DW, Warshaw AL, Chang Y, Fernandez-del Castillo C. Ten-year experience with 733 pancreatic resections: changing indications, older patients, and decreasing length of hospitalization. Arch Surg. 2001;136(4):391–8.
39. Trede M, Schwall G, Saeger HD. Survival after pancreatoduodenectomy. 118 consecutive resections without an operative mortality. Ann Surg. 1990;211(4):447–58.

Index

J.M. Millis, J.B. Matthews (eds.), *Difficult Decisions in Hepatobiliary and Pancreatic Surgery*, Difficult Decisions in Surgery: An Evidence-Based Approach, DOI 10.1007/978-3-319-27365-5

D

E

J

L

M

Q

R

CPI Antony Rowe
Chippenham, UK
2017-01-11 22:36